P9-DKE-308

# History of Pharmacy

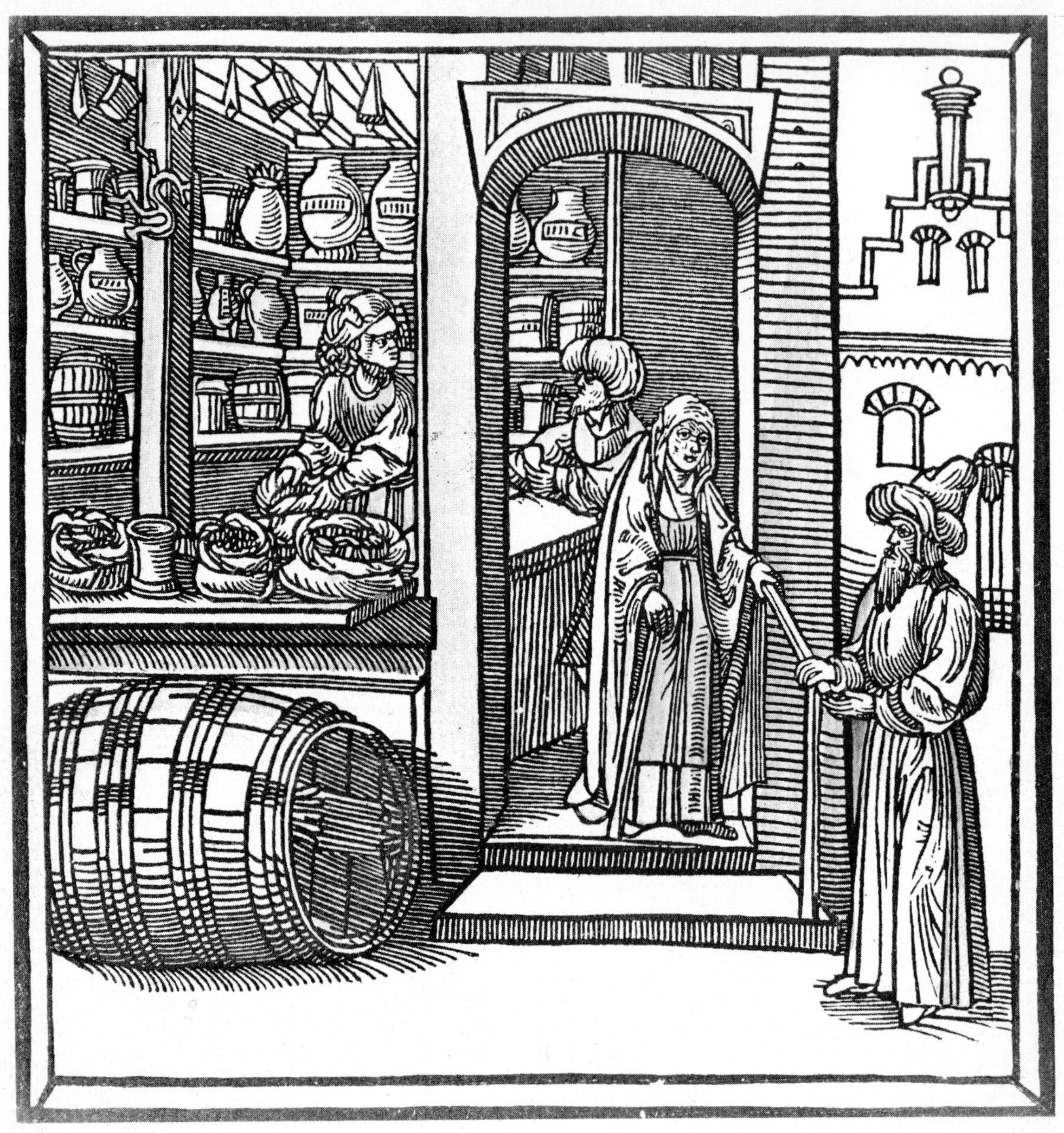

*Frontispiece.* Over the centuries the pharmacy has changed its appearance superficially, but its basic elements remain ever the same. The pharmacist, too, has retained his basic role in society as drug expert—while drugs and his relationship to them and to the patient are reshaped by historical events. These two illustrations underscore this unity in diversity during pharmacy's long history by juxtaposing an allegorical woodcut of 1515 and a photograph of an American pharmacy of the 1960's (woodcut from Quiricus de Augustis' The Light of the Pharmacist, Brussels edition of 1515; photograph of pharmacy in Oklahoma City, U.S.A., courtesy of C. J. "Connie" Masterson family).

Kremers and Urdang's

# History of Pharmacy

Fourth Edition

*Revised by*



GLENN SONNEDECKER, Ph.D.
*Professor of History of Pharmacy, University of Wisconsin*

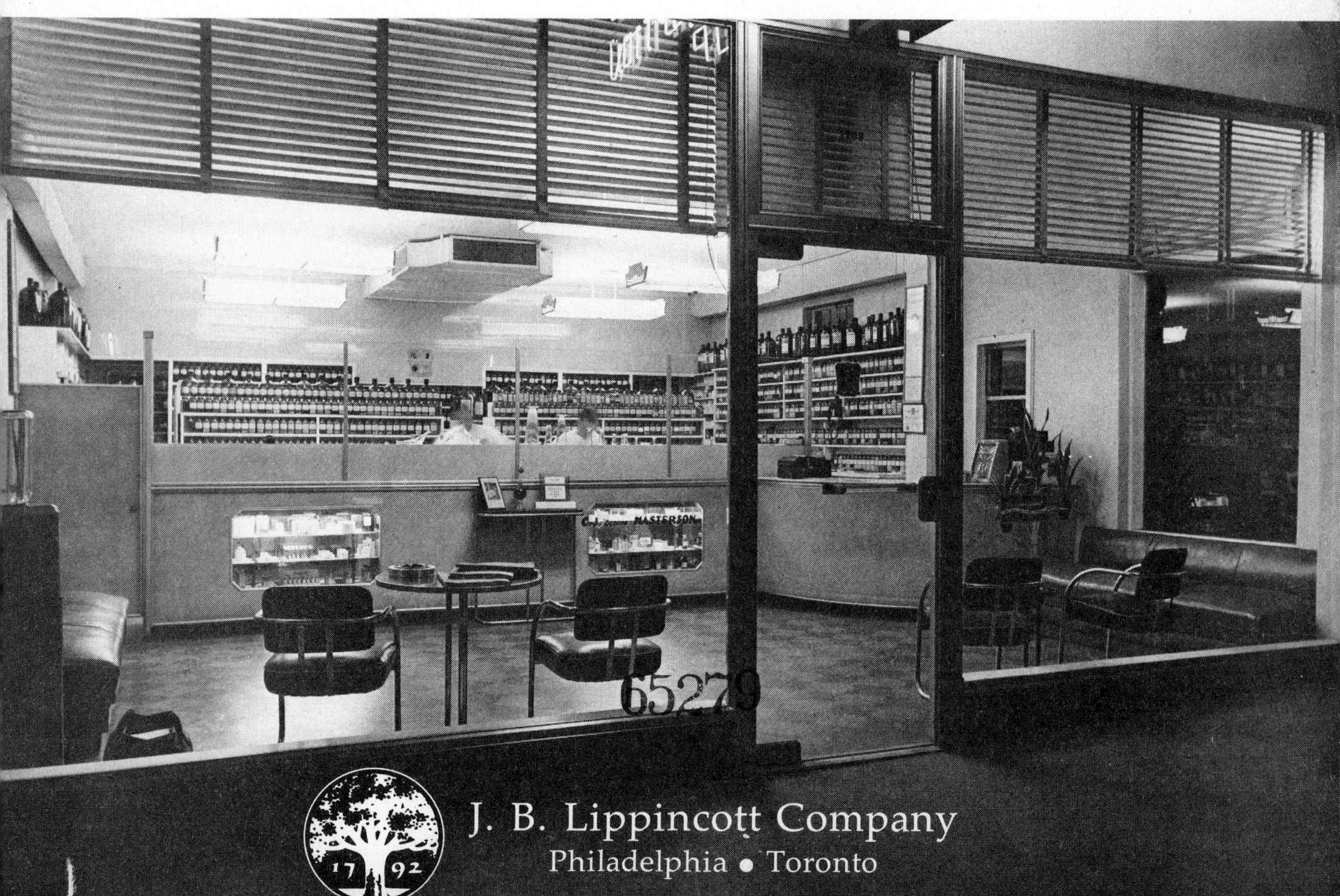



J. B. Lippincott Company
Philadelphia • Toronto

ISBN 0-397-52074-3

Library of Congress Catalog Card Number 75-40104

Printed in the United States of America

6 5 4 3 2 1

**Library of Congress Cataloging in Publication Data**

Kremers, Edward, 1865–1941.
Kremers and Urdang's History of pharmacy.

Bibliography: p.
Includes index.
1. Pharmacy—History. I. Urdang, George, 1882–1960 joint author. II. Sonnedecker, Glenn Allen. III. Title. IV. Title: History of pharmacy.
[DNLM: 1. Pharmacy—History. QV711.1 K92h]
RS61.K73 1976 615'.4'09 75-40104
ISBN 0-397-52074-3

# Preface

The evolving fusion of knowledge and responsibility designed to provide safe, effective drugs and health supplies comprises a significant component of one of man's most basic concerns and thus also of his history. An account of this development merits the attention of the general reader, but more particularly this book is intended to give the pharmacy student some additional perspective to guide his reshaping of traditions and improving of the services and the satisfactions which he expects in the profession.

The history of pharmaceutical science and technology has the cumulative, progressive quality that characterizes the history of science at large; the history of the pharmaceutical profession shows the character of social history, with its unforeseen regressive turns of events, its conflicts of interests, and their resolution by trends and forces that would elude comprehension solely in terms of science or any other type of endeavor or opinion circumscribed by a given time or group.

This sociohistorical view of pharmacy evolving as a profession in the Western world is what we have tried to portray. The materia medica—and the science and technic that transform it—cannot be ignored here, but the serious study of pharmacy's history from that viewpoint must be left to another occasion and framework. Likewise, there are large areas of the world—both primitive and highly civilized, in remote and more recent time—whose interesting pharmaceutical endeavors had to be ignored in the task of producing a manageable volume focused on the sources of historical growth that seemed most relevant to American pharmacy.

Despite this limitation of scope, the Kremers-Urdang *History of Pharmacy* has remained since the first edition (1940) the most ambitious work of its kind in English, showing us the truly international character of pharmacy and its development—clarifying without oversimplifying the context of that development.

In the Preface to the first edition, Edward Kremers observed, "The organization and plan of this *History of Pharmacy* go beyond the merely chronological order which is so common in books of this kind. Facts and events have been grouped in accordance with their organic relationships, thus presenting an integrated picture. . . ." The original concept and arrangement have been proved sound by time, and therefore have been retained through four editions.

The main initial difficulties encountered by Edward Kremers and George Urdang likewise have persisted. They found that "material available for the book, while extensive, tends to be scattered and partial. . . . The authors have been faced with the persistent problem of selecting, rejecting, subordinating, and coordinating this mass of material with particular reference to the needs of American students." This means, in terms of the present revision, that important segments of pharmaceutical history still are mentioned only in passing, if not ignored altogether—such as the history of medications, specific problems and contributions of minority groups, and cultural areas outside the Western European tradition—either because specialized historical research has been too sparse or because the narrative would bulk too large for a textbook. It was, as Kremers originally noted, "necessary constantly to keep in mind the varying pedagogic demands to be made on the book"; as a result, the organization permits it to be "used for courses of different lengths by omitting certain chapters or portions of chapters."

This challenge of selecting and presenting a systematic account that would serve a pharmacy student's needs—to help satisfy the urge we all share to know something about where we came from—has dominated the work through three revisions. At the same time, trying to fill a broad gap in the American literature of pharmacy, the authors could not ignore the mature practitioner, or the reference needs of libraries, or the layman or historian seeking a lead to information on some pharmaceutical development. The original authors therefore tried to give the book dual service as a reference volume by including (beyond textbook requirements) precise detail in the narrative, careful documentation, and an encyclopedic supplement. In the second edition, they took the first step in a plan for broadening geographic coverage.

These reference features were welcomed by those whose interests required more than a textbook. Yet, teaching experience and reports from elsewhere convinced me that the scholarly weight of the book was not being too happily sustained by the average student. Nor could the scope be readily encompassed in the normal course. So, to make the book more palatable to the student, and yet retain as much of the reference value as possible, a great deal of textual detail has been moved out of the way, to the Notes and References and Appendices, where it can still be consulted; but some material has been reluctantly omitted for textbook purposes. For elusive reference data, the reader may sometimes find it useful to check the earlier editions (1940, 1951, 1963).

An attempt has been made in the present revision to bring the entire text into accord with historical findings since the third edition appeared, to take into account events and their consequences on the pharmaceutical scene during the intervening years, to correct whatever errors came to my attention, and to edit the text with the aim of communicating effectively the development of the pharmacist's role through the sweep of history.

Anyone who has examined this historical structure, brick by brick, must be respectful of the design and the effort of the pharmacist-historians Edward Kremers and George Urdang, which gave a solidity and successful expression to pharmacy's heritage unprecedented in English. How did it come about?

In his Preface of 1940, Edward Kremers explained that for years he "had the desire and intention of writing a history of pharmacy. Well meaning friends have prodded him on to the task. . . . The manifold and insistent duties of the author's teaching work left little leisure for the sustained effort necessary. Moreover, much detailed study and collecting of material has been essential in preparing such a history of pharmacy." This collection has continued to grow under Kremers' inspiration, maintaining its place as a resource unique in the United States and seldom equaled in Europe. It may therefore be permissible to consider Madison, Wisconsin, the birthplace of the history of American pharmacy.

One of the great American pharmacists, Kremers had the intellectual grasp of history to create the volume before us, but—not himself a professional historian—he could not meet the insatiable demand for time and concentration to give his dream reality. At the end of his career, however, Kremers had the satisfaction of bringing to Madison a pharmacist and pharmaceutical journalist who had become the first in Germany to earn a doctorate on the basis of historical studies centered about his own profession. At the University of Wisconsin, George Urdang, without official position at first, dedicated himself to giving fulfillment to Kremers' long-standing plans for a *History of Pharmacy*.

"The effective stimulus leading to the actual writing of the book was the presence and help of a colleague, Dr. George Urdang, whose entire time could be devoted to the work. The general plan and organization of the book are the senior author's," Kremers noted, "while the actual composition, documentation, etc. have been done by Dr. Urdang, to whom full credit should be given for the manner in which this difficult and arduous task has been performed."

In his preface to the second edition Urdang commented, "Shortly after the publication of the first edition, in 1941, Edward Kremers, the man who gave the initiative to the writing, died, and the responsibility of making the present revision was assigned to his coauthor. The author of this revision is glad that there was no need for a change of the arrangement, with its attempt at a sociologic integration instead of a mere chronologic narration. . . . This new book has been changed in its content but not in its spirit and its goal. It has remained 'a guide and a survey,' to be used for teaching as well as for reading, as a book of reference so far as data and dates are concerned, and a book presenting and evaluating concepts."

As had Urdang in Germany, the pharmacist-writer responsible for the two more recent versions of the book had been a pharmaceutical journalist who became the first in this country to earn a doctorate on the basis of historical studies centered about his own profession. Those studies were nearing completion when Urdang penned the above lines and added some kind words about his "friend and assistant, Glenn Sonnedecker."

In 1960 the second of the book's original authors died. To try to carry forward the working center for pharmacy's history that these two had established at Madison, including the preparation of this fourth edition, has been my privilege.

There has been much talk of the need for ensuring that a man professionally educated be a man generally educated also—in pharmacy, a practitioner equipped for a high level of citizenship within the profession and within his community. One natural bridge between the humanistic and the technical is formed by the profession's own history, which seems essential to an adequate understanding and philosophy of the pharmacist's role in society. For such reasons, many of the schools devote a course or a substantial part of a course to the historical development of pharmacy, and it appears as a required subject in all course patterns shown in the influential study, *The Pharmaceutical Curriculum* by Lloyd E. Blauch and George L. Webster, on the ground that "no subject so readily lends itself to developing in the pharmacist the orientation he should have as a professional person, to producing in him a sense of appreciation for, and pride in, his profession."

To provide an introduction to the knowledge and the values furthering that purpose, and as a basis for discussion and more specialized reading, the *History of Pharmacy* was written.

GLENN SONNEDECKER

# Acknowledgments

Many colleagues generously provided assistance and suggestions to help improve this fourth edition. Two historians of pharmacy who have been helpful above all others kindly agreed to formal collaboration for systematic updating of certain chapters. David L. Cowen, Professor Emeritus at Rutgers, The State University of New Jersey, has assisted with Chapters 9 to 11 on the American colonies, the Revolutionary period, and the young republic. John L. Parascandola, Associate Professor at the University of Wisconsin at Madison has assisted with Chapters 3 and 18 on the changing medicaments in relation to the modern pharmacist and on the contributions by pharmacists to modern science and industry. While responsibility for the final form of these and other chapters remains my own, the contribution by Professors Parascandola and Cowen is one I value highly.

Of equal importance, if in a different way, have been the remarkable resources for the history of pharmacy offered by the University of Wisconsin Library and its librarians, particularly Librarian Dolores Nemec of the F. B. Power Pharmaceutical Library and its associated Kremers Reference Files.

Among European colleagues, concrete suggestions and valuable guidance concerning the chapters on pharmacy in their own countries have been generously given by Rossana Ventura (Italy), Pierre Julien and Georges Viala (France), Erika Hickel (Germany), and Melvin P. Earles (Britain). Concerning Britain, comments valuable to the revision were received from Ernst W. Stieb of Toronto and T. Douglas Whittet of London.

As noted in Appendix 5, George B. Griffenhagen of Washington, D.C. kindly undertook the updating of the unique international guide to museum collections, just as he was responsible for the original compilation. Chapter 13 on American pharmaceutical legislation benefitted greatly from the advice of my knowledgeable colleague, Robert W. Hammel of Madison, Wisconsin. I am also grateful for various suggestions kindly contributed by Alex Berman of Cincinnati and Robert G. Mrtek of Chicago. Not least of all, I appreciate the tolerance (as well as typing assistance) of Cleo Sonnedecker during my long preoccupation with this work.

Any book that goes through repeated revisions becomes increasingly an amalgam of the thought and work of various individuals, not only those whose publications have been drawn upon and cited in footnotes, but others who generously responded to requests for advice during work on previous editions. It is hard to identify them all, much less adequately recognize their contributions, but mention may be made at least of Howard Bayles, Alex Berman, Henri Bonnemain, Maurice Bouvet, Louis Irissou, David L. Cowen, George B. Griffenhagen, Robert W. Hammel, Rafael Folch Andreu, Guillermo Folch Jou, George E. Osborne, Wolfgang Schneider, Ernst W. Stieb, and T. Douglas Whittet.

Publishers and organizations who have permitted quotations, answered queries, or provided illustrations have been thanked privately, but their collective contribution deserves recognition here also.

As George Urdang dedicated the second edition to "the memory of his friend Edward Kremers," so I dedicate this edition in the same spirit to both of them, with the high respect and grateful memory shared by so many pharmacists everywhere.

GLENN SONNEDECKER

# Contents

## Part One
## Pharmacy's Early Antecedents



## Part Two
## The Rise of Professional Pharmacy in Representative Countries of Europe

## Part Three
## Pharmacy in the United States

*Section One* **The Period of Unorganized Development**



*Section Two* **The Period of Organized Development**

## Part Four
## Discoveries and Other Contributions to Society by Pharmacists



## Appendices

PART ONE

# Pharmacy's Early Antecedents

# 1

# Ancient Prelude

Wherever civilization arises we find "pharmacy," because it fulfills one of man's basic needs. This effort to grasp from nature whatever might shield us from affliction became old as a service before it was new as a "profession." Its origins have disappeared into the veiled millennia—perhaps as much as a million years—that hide the origin of man himself.

Various opinions about pharmacy's origin continue to be put forward, because speculation is tempered only by logic and analogy when there is not much real evidence. More is known about prehistoric man's diseases, for many traces of damage to his body were recorded indelibly in bones that awaited the archaeologist's shovel. But the earliest random and desperate efforts to use natural resources as "drugs" to fend off such damage left scarcely an enduring trace.

For prehistoric man, we suppose that therapy would not be first of all drug therapy. Disease came upon him with such mysterious ways and frightening forces that, as an imaginative and rational being, he must have concluded that "supernatural" countermeasures were called for—measures that for *him* were a part of the ordinary natural world. The "magic" thus invoked ultimately was reinforced by a custom of using plants and other objects in ways that brought their friendly spirits to bear on the evil powers manifested by disease. Even if only a blind empiric groping over many tens of thousands of years should be postulated, it would be understandable that by the time of the earliest written records, about four thousand years ago, the accumulated materia medica had come to include quite a number of substances that we call pharmacologically active, as well as substances having only the higher spirit-powers (which we call inert). This trend of speculation about the origin of pharmaceutical endeavor seems reasonable in the light of the pharmaco-magic beliefs of millions of our contemporaries.

Clearly, magic and empiricism each played an important role in finding and employing remedies. Yet, it can be said that "neither empiricism nor magic stands at the beginning of the internal employment of remedies by men but the animal function, the instinct."[1] Instinct was affirmed or denied by an increasingly selfconscious empiricism. This empiricism became the foundation of medical and pharmaceutical "science" as observations were systematized and constantly purified by inductive and deductive reasoning. In the whole field of medicine so much remained beyond ordinary observation, explanation or control that for thousands of years magical-religious practices tended to pervade medical practices. Only in our own millennium have they been placed gradually in a separate category.

This is not the place to argue whether the great civilizations of the ancient Far East or of the Middle East were the earliest and the most original, pharmaceutically speaking. The linguistic problems of comparative study are so challenging and the dating of ancient evidence is so often speculative that we remain uncertain about the locus of many medical and technologic innovations of antiquity, and the directions in which their influence ran.

The Far Eastern civilizations hold great historical interest for their early achievements and their imperfectly understood influence on Western culture, especially as mediated by the ancient Greeks and the medieval Arabs. Interesting accounts of premodern pharmacy in the Far East, and its rich materia medica, now may be read in Western languages to a certain extent.[2]

However, pharmacy in the West sees its early antecedents most clearly in the river valleys of the Nile, the Tigris and the Euphrates. Today's ruins once throbbed with magnificent civilizations as remarkable in their own time as the later westerly cultures that they helped to shape.

## BABYLONIA-ASSYRIA

In a southern Babylonian kingdom of city states, in the region of today's Iraq, the Sumerians developed a system of cuneiform writing by about 3000 B.C., thereby entering the historical period. They and the heirs of Sumerian civilization—Babylonia and, later, Assyria—left thousands of clay tablets in the ruins of their remarkable civilizations. Their history remained locked in the clay until about a century ago, when a few men recaptured enough of the "lost language" to make serious attempts at translation. Today we have a fairly clear picture of the general development of this part of the ancient world, although research adds continuously to our knowledge. However, knowledge of medicine and pharmacy in Babylonia-Assyria remains fragmentary.

### General Therapeutic Concepts

The ideologic fundamentals of Babylonian-Assyrian medicine have been described as follows:

> . . . as a consequence of the persistent hold maintained by the belief in signs of all kinds, disease became primarily an omen, the interpretation of which on the part of the priest as diviner supplemented the efforts of the priest as exorciser; while the priest as healer availed himself of both these aids to supplement his efforts in the direct treatment of the disease. These three aspects of Babylonian-Assyrian medicine—exorcism, divination and medical treatment—blend together to form a composite picture in which it is not always possible to distinguish the different strains.[3]

Illness was a divine punishment, and healing a purification. Medicine thus attained a fixed place in the religious ideology, in the immemorial purification from sin through penance, called "catharsis." This concept of catharsis, which entered into various religions, found its most famous expression in the sacrifice of Jesus Christ, who gave his life to purify sinful mankind. The fact that medicine in antiquity (i.e., in Babylonia-Assyria, Egypt and, partly, in Greece) stood within the ideology of "catharsis" categorizes it as "archaic" medicine.[4]

This interests the pharmacist specifically because it explains the original meaning of the Greek word *pharmakon* (see Appendix 7), from which we have made the term "pharmacy" and its derivatives. From the religious ideology of catharsis there emerged the word and the concept *pharmakon,* in the sense of a means of purification through purging. This idea—first spiritual, then pharmacologic—finds a still more direct expression in the term "cathartics" for especially effective purgatives.

Ancient cultures always must be considered from the standpoint of their outlook on life afforded by their own spiritual, geographic and economic conditions. Thus it would be unfair to accept as proof of an "unscientific" spirit the fact that Babylonian-Assyrian, ancient Egyptian, and the early part of Greek medicine contained a great deal of "magic." For these peoples, magic was a part of systematized "science." It went hand in hand with empiric discoveries,[5] and no doubt was harmonized with them.

## Drugs

We find a comprehensive materia medica in these times of "archaic" medicine. When R. Campbell Thompson examined many hundreds of the clay tablets (excavated from the library of King Assurbanipal of Assyria), he was able to identify 250 vegetable drugs and 120 mineral drugs. He also found that alcoholic beverages, fats and oils, parts of animals, honey, wax and various milks were then being used medicinally.[6]

The Assyrians already were using many, if not all, of the minerals mentioned by the Greek Dioscorides in his famous book on materia medica (1st century after Christ). Excrements also played a part in the Babylonian-Assyrian therapy, because filth was expected to disgust the evil spirit that had invaded the body of the patient and cause it to leave forthwith.[7]

Botanical drugs included, for example, pine turpentine, styrax, galbanum, hellebore, myrrh, asafoetida, calamus, ricinus, mentha, opium, glycyrrhiza, mandragora, cannabis, crocus, thymus.

The forms in which the Assyrians prepared drugs for administration included medicated wines, draughts, mixtures, ointments, embrocations, cataplasms, enemas, poultices, plasters, lotions, infusions, decoctions and fumigations.

The oldest pharmaceutical document now known tells how the Sumerians prepared some of these drugs, perhaps about 4,000 years ago. It contains a series of drug formulas such as the following:

"Pulverize the seed of the 'carpenter' plant [perhaps *Gymnosporia serrata* Loes], the gum resin of the markasi plant, [and] thyme; dissolve it in beer; let the man drink."[8]

Mesopotamian drug formulas such as this one typically were not quantitative (although their Egyptian counterparts were). This is curious, since the system of weights and measures invented by the Babylonians has been considered to be one of their contributions to civilization.

Their materia medica "includes substances which presuppose a broad acquaintance with many chemical operations, and elaborate procedures are implied in the text in order that the substances listed may have been obtained."[9]

Incantations and magic were so much a part of Mesopotamian culture that it may be sheer accident that they form no part of the earliest drug formulary known. After all, it is a single clay tablet, only partly legible, which probably was one "page" of a longer document. Later records illustrate how incantations gave drugs their healing power or enhanced it. Probably some substances eventually were recognized to have inherent healing power that made them useful without priestly intervention.[10] But many centuries passed before a new interpretation of the causes of disease (abandoning the supernatural) removed the magico-religious core of pharmaceutical and medical practices as exemplified in both ancient Mesopotamia and Egypt.

A class of preparers of remedies and cosmetics is said to have arisen, called "pasisu," but we find no details about when it appeared or about its position in relation to medicine. In Sippar at the time of the great Babylonian king Hammurabi (about 2111 B.C.), retailers of drugs seem to have plied their trade in a particular street.[11]

## Mythology and the Healing Arts

The Babylonian-Assyrian gods Ea and Gula are mentioned most frequently in the incantations often interspersed among drug formulas. Of special interest is the fact that a serpent cult and the use of the serpent as a venerated symbol appear already in

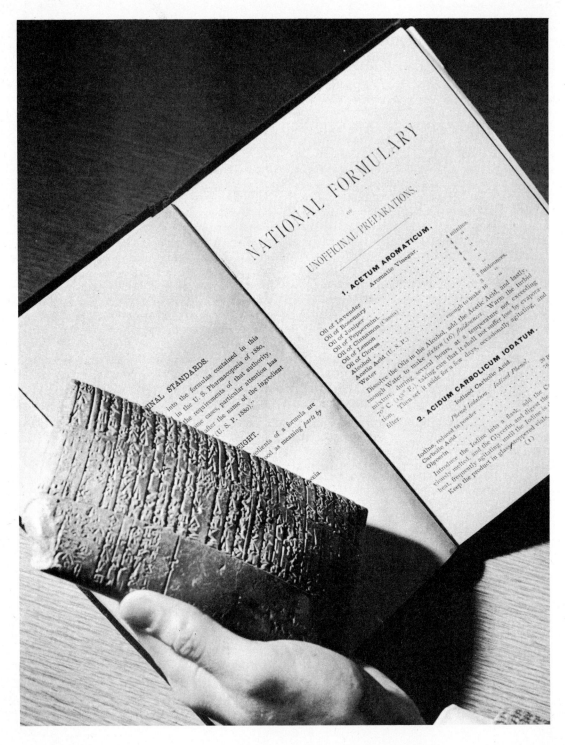
NATIONAL FORMULARY
OF
UNOFFICIAL PREPARATIONS.
1. ACETUM AROMATICUM.
Aromatic Vinegar.
Oil of Lavender
Oil of Rosemary
Oil of Juniper
Oil of Peppermint
Oil of Cinnamon (Cassia)
Oil of Lemon
Oil of Cloves
Alcohol
Acetic Acid (U. S. P.)
Water
2. ACIDUM CARBOLICUM IODATUM.
Iodized Carbolic Acid.
Phenol Iodatum. Iodized Phenol.
Iodine, reduced to powder
Carbolic Acid
Glycerin
STANDARDS.

Babylonian-Assyrian mythology. A medical god, Ninazu was "the lord of physicians," and his son, Ningischzida, functioned as messenger of the gods.[12] Their symbol was a rod and serpent, reminding us of the modern symbol of medicine, although that comes to us from the later Greek culture.

In Babylonia observation of the planets and the stars laid the groundwork not only for the science of astronomy, but simultaneously for the pseudoscience of astrology. Since the course and constellation of the stars had a supposed relationship to life on earth, it is understandable that this belief found specific applications in early medicine and pharmacy.

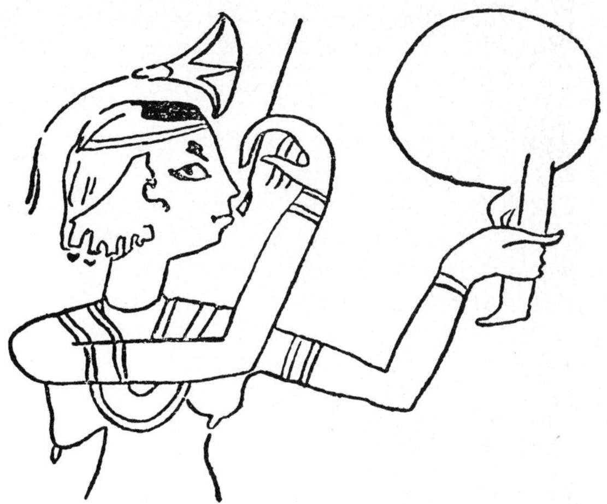

An ancient Egyptian artist caricatures a girl who holds a mirror in one hand and, with the other, applies red-ochre rouge to her lips (about 1200 B.C.). She knew other cosmetic devices such as eye and face pigments, perfumes, hair dye, wigs, cleansing unguents and elaborate make-up kits. The Papyrus Ebers includes cosmetic as well as therapeutic formulas, and artifacts testify that even before the earliest written history human vanity had established the importance of cosmetics. (From the Oriental Institute, Univ. of Chicago *in* Hughes, G. R.: J. Soc. Cosm. Chem. *10*:159–176, 1959)

## EGYPT

The Babylonian-Assyrian and the ancient Egyptian cultures were closely related. Both had a theocratic foundation, and theurgic medicine prevailed in both of them. Egyptian medicine appears to have been less dominated by metaphysical concepts, but there is an obvious similarity between the Assyrian and the Egyptian medical texts;[13] and there were epochs during which the magic elements in Egyptian medicine gained in prominence.

The ancient Egyptian hieroglyphics baffled modern man, who wished to read what Egyptian life had been like. Then, in 1799 the famous "Rosetta stone" was found near the Rosetta mouth of the Nile. It bore a trilingual inscription in hieroglyphics, in demotic characters (the simplified hieroglyphics in use since about 700 B.C.) and in Greek. This gave the Frenchman J. F. Champollion the first clue toward deciphering hieroglyphics. Since then, much progress has been made in translating and interpreting the records of ancient Egypt that survive. Yet, many problems challenge even the best Egyptologists—not least of all the puzzle of identifying drugs referred to in medical papyri.

← This clay tablet is believed to be the oldest pharmaceutical document whose contents are known. It was probably toward the end of the third millennium B.C. when a Sumerian took a reed stylus, wrote drug formulas in the slab of soft clay, then baked the tablet. In the background can be seen a modern American successor to this earliest formulary, the first edition of the *National Formulary* (1888).

(The cuneiform tablet shown is a replica cast from the original in the University of Pennsylvania Museum, Philadelphia.)

### Medical Papyri

Eight medical papyri thus far are translated and commented on. All of them were written between about 1900 and 1100 B.C.[14], but much of the knowledge in them probably is far older.

The Ebers papyrus (bearing the name of a German Egyptologist, Georg Ebers) contains the greatest number of drugs and formulas, but the medical papyri as a group testify to the extensive attention accorded the preparation and the use of drugs.[15]

*Ebers Papyrus.* Containing remnants of various earlier treatises, but complete as written and more than 20 meters long, the Ebers papyrus has attracted scholars again and again. The work is so difficult that it has been said of even the most recent translation[16]:

> The identification of many names of diseases, symptoms and drugs by Ebbell is the result of long labor . . . yet even on superficial reading of the translation, one becomes doubtful as to the reliability of these identifications. In most cases they are mere conjectures . . .[17]

The text is dominated by drug formulas and, when taken with other evidence, suggests that the pharmaceutical side of medical care received more attention than it did in ancient Greece later on, when medical concepts left a relatively large place for dietetics. In crude form, the Egyptians knew most of our modes of administering drugs by 1500 B.C., such as gargles, snuffs, inhalations,

Small excerpt from the Ebers papyrus, about 1500 B.C., which mentions about 700 medicinal substances used by the ancient Egyptians. The complete document, almost 22 yards long, is in the cursive (hieratic) script. (From J. Berendes: *Geschichte der Pharmazie,* Leipzig, 1898)

suppositories, fumigations, enemas, poultices, decoctions, infusions, pills, troches, lotions, ointments and plasters. In the Ebers papyrus alone, these various forms have been found to embrace more than 700 drugs, in more than 800 formulas.

The drugs were drawn from the plant, the animal and the mineral kingdoms, but botanic drugs predominate for internal use—such as acacia, castor bean, wormwood, date, fennel, fig, garlic and poppy seeds. There appear to be references to such mineral substances as alum, iron oxide, limestone, sodium carbonate, salt and sulfur. Excrements of various animals were used occasionally, as we noted in Babylonia-Assyria. Beer, milk, wine and honey were popular vehicles for drugs. Honey and wax were often used as binding agents in the formulas.[18]

A representative formula reads:

Another to clear out purulency:

| | |
|---|---|
| Hyoscyamus | 2 ro |
| Dates | 4 ro |
| Wine | 5 ro |
| Ass's milk | 20 ro |

are boiled, strained and taken for four days.[19]

Such quantitative formulas—favored by the ancient Egyptian practitioners and usually lacking in Babylonian formulas—customarily specify measures rather than weights, even for dry substances. A "ro" (as in the above formula) is about 15 ml. The 4 days specified as the course of treatment occurs commonly in Egyptian pharmacotherapy and may originate in magic formula rather than in clinical observation.

Mortars, hand mills, sieves and balances were commonly used in technologic operations such as pharmaceutical compounding.

Copies of the drug formulas were handed from one practitioner to another and from one generation to the next. Sometimes a scribe ignorant of medicine would simply combine in his copy several simple ingredients listed originally as separate prescriptions, which may have contributed to the rise of polypharmacy.[20]

Straightforward formulas occupy so much space in the Ebers papyrus that the incantations of the introduction, intended for general application, tend to be subordinated. Although the Egyptologist Ebbell prefers to look on them merely as "evidence of the piety of the Egyptians,"[21] it appears that they were for use whenever a remedy was applied or a bandage loosened, and that they were intended to reinforce the drugs with divine power against "afflictions [caused] by a god or goddess, by a dead man or woman, etc."

*Edwin Smith Papyrus.* A treatise that revealed the surgical side of Egyptian medicine is perhaps as important as the Ebers papyrus and is impressive because of its organization, wealth of information and freedom from magical elements. Since its publication, including the translation and the commentary by the pioneer American Egyptologist James Henry Breasted (an erstwhile pharmacist), respect for the medicine achieved by so ancient a people has increased considerably. The distinguished medical historian Henry Sigerist called the work of Breasted "one of the most accomplished editions that has ever been made of an ancient text."[22]

## Egyptian Medicinal Plants

The opinion has been expressed that there were not many medicinal plants native to ancient Egypt due to topographic peculiarity. Bounded on the east by the Arabian desert and on the west by the Libyan desert, Egypt's populace was restricted to the valley inundated by the Nile. On the other hand, Theophrastus (4th century B.C.), quoting the verses of Homer, praises the many and efficacious medicinal plants of ancient Egypt; Dioscorides (1st century A.D.) mentions the Egyptian origin of 80 vegetable drugs that he described. We may suppose that the ancient Egyptians cultivated other plants originally not native to their country and used them medicinally.[23] For example, pomegranate was not indigenous to Egypt but must have been cultivated extensively there about 1100 B.C.[24]

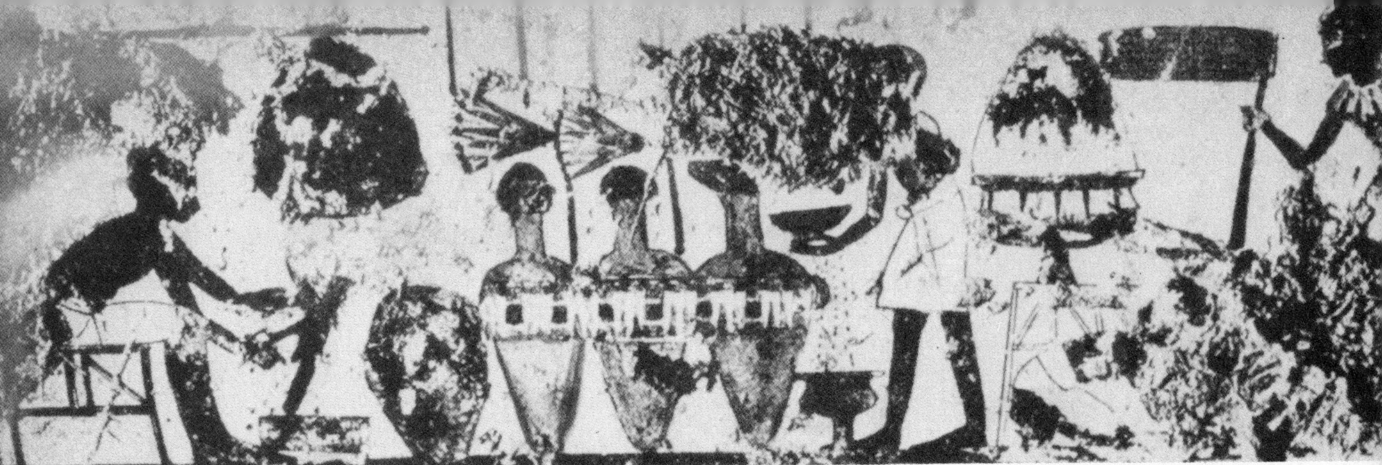

Ointment workroom portrayed prior to 1400 B.C. in an Egyptian tomb painting. The following interpretation seems probable (although not entirely certain), based on comparison with classical representations of ointment rooms (left to right across the double page):

The man at the extreme left appears to be hewing a plug for a container, or perhaps wood for the fire. In front of him are a basket and three vase-shaped containers, probably containing the crude ingredients used by these ancient preparers of medicines. To the right a workman holds a sieve over a container on the floor. Next to him, a pedestal-table presumably bears a large mound of finished ointment. The next two workmen are comminuting crude ingredients, the one at the start of the right half of the panel using a mortar. The kneeling man appears to be shaping some of the cooled finished ointment into balls for transport. To his right an ointment cook stirs, in a kettle on the hearth, the melting animal fat with other ingredients until it has the proper consistency. (After W. Wreszinski, *Atlas zur altaegyptischen Kulturgeschichte,* Plate 356.)

## Mythology

As in other ancient countries governed or influenced by theocratic rule, medicine was supposed to have originated with some mythologic deities, in Egypt notably Thoth, Osiris, Isis, Horus and Imhotep. Gradually, Imhotep became more and more the divine representative of medicine in Egypt. He was originally a real personage, one of the earliest of known physicians. He lived about 3000 B.C. and was deified 2,500 years after his death. The Greeks reportedly saw in Imhotep (whom they called Imouthes) a representation of their own god of the healing arts, Asklepios.[25]

The specialization of pharmaceutical activities also found expression in Egyptian mythology. The secret of pharmacy had been revealed, according to Egyptian mythology, to the divine Horus by his mother, Isis. The tasks of the divine house of medicine and of the chamber of embalmment were assigned to a special god, Anepu (called Anubis by the Greeks), who thus might be regarded in one respect as the pharmacist of the gods.[26]

## The Practice of Medicine and Pharmacy

We noted in ancient Babylonia-Assyria a group of preparers of medicine, of whom we have no detailed knowledge. However, they did not play an important part in the development of medicine and pharmacy. The variety of preparations of drugs used in Egyptian medicine that required professional skill implies a more definitely distinguished group of preparers of medicine.

Such a group did exist, although the exact character and refinement of "pharmacy" at such a remote time eludes us. To present any systematic account of pharmaceutical practice requires scholarly conjectures and assumptions based on single passages or even a half-understood phrase in the ancient hieroglyphics.

With this in mind, attention can be given to conclusions put forward (here in free translation) by the medical Egyptologist, Frans Jonckheere:

The personnel of pharmacy included two echelons, in Egypt: a group of specialist-functionaries

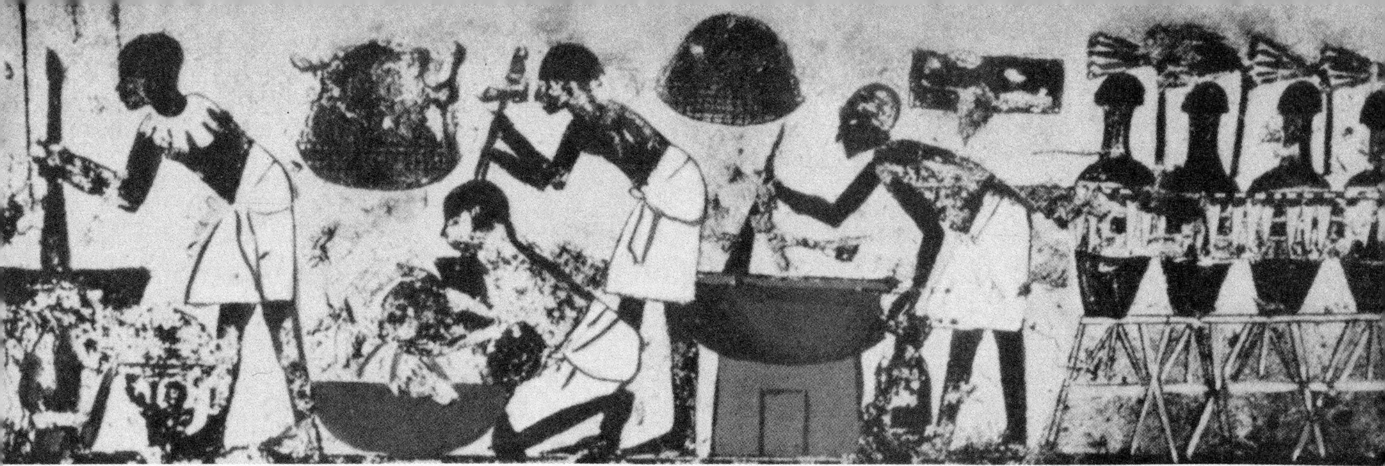

and a complex of technical services, the first being hierarchically above the latter.

In the category of well-informed pharmaceutical workers we should place especially the "chief of the preparers of drugs" and the "conservator of drugs," perhaps associating with them a "priest-herbalist."

In the group of technicians, one perhaps distinguishes "collectors of drugs" and "laboratory aides."

Here, then, carrying or not a particular name, are those who form a class of "pharmacists," so to speak.

The evidence duly attesting to this medical auxiliary—not physician and not layman—reduces to nothing the notion that medical prescriptions were executed in a laboratory annexed to the temple, by "priest-physicians."

On the other hand, it forces the partisans of the idea of pharmaceutical work being in the hands of physicians alone to correct their point of view, and it invites them to accept, at the side of the man of healing art, the presence of an assistant charged with the preparation of remedies, a task that he at times fulfilled in the home of the patients.

In conclusion, the classic opinion ought to be erased that the place is in Rome—and in part of the 4th century solely—for the first appearance of a specialist, the *pigmentarius,* for preparing and delivering the prescribed products, in view of our "preparer of remedies," a lower echelon of a veritable pharmaceutical organization of which we have been able to catch only a glimpse in the complex administrative cadre.[27]

To what extent do these views clash with what Henry Sigerist had written earlier?:

There was no pharmacist in ancient Egypt. The physician himself compounded his remedies or his servants did it under his supervision, just as he and his assistants probably gathered the necessary ingredients and stored them in the house. . . . Drugs imported from abroad were probably stored in royal warehouses, whence the physicians could obtain them.[28]

The two views are not as incompatible as they may seem to be at first. What meaning should we expect of the term "pharmacist" as applied to conditions in Egypt 3,500 years ago (or for that matter, America 100 years ago)? In any event, both scholars see a probable assistant or associate of the physician with special responsibility for pharmaceutical work. The pharmaceutical associate may well have depended on stocks held in what Sigerist termed the "royal warehouses" as the source for drugs imported or gathered from the countryside by the "collectors of drugs." A counterpart in Jonckheere's evidence is the "House of Life" where apparently drugs were both collected into storage (under the "conservator of drugs") and prepared, at least in certain instances, by "those who fabricate the medicaments." There was a designation for the "chief of those who fabricate the medicaments," quite distinct from his medical functions, but it must be noted that at least in the House of Life this "chief" was also chief of the royal physicians among various other titles.

In reading recent studies of individual papyri it is also hard to escape the feeling that the person who practiced medicine often practiced pharmacy as well, even though pharmaceutical work may have been more distinct and distinctive—at least at the more centralized level—than we once believed.

In positing pharmaceutical activities in medical care distinct from priestly ministrations and temple "laboratories" (yet not denying a theurgic foundation), Jonckheere and Sigerist stand together against past views. If tomorrow the Egyptian sands yield additional documents, the picture may unify or, more probably, it may diversify into several different and clearer pictures, by supplying evidence of how different the medical practices were in different periods of Egypt's long history.

For example, Hermann Grapow believes that ancient Egyptian medicine, revealing a "scientific character," reached its full development before 1600 B.C. but, in the time of the New Kingdom, degenerated into sorcery.[29] This statement suggests an explanation for the differences of opinion as to the "magical" or "rational" character of medicine in ancient Egypt. In the more than 3,000 years of the empire's changing destiny, there were periods of cultural blossom in which rationalism reached a high degree, and others in which the dogmatic fetters were drawn tighter. However, there was never a time in which the theocratic regime and the theurgic ideology lost their grip. Hence, even in periods of comparatively rational medical practice, there still remained the "archaic" superstructure.

The high standard of the ancient Egyptians' medicine and therapy under a theocratic system earns our respect, but for further developments we look to the astonishing culture achieved by the Greeks about a thousand years after the Egyptians reached their zenith.

## GREECE AND ROME

There are few pharmaceutical differences between ancient Greece and Rome since the Romans adopted most of their customs from the Greeks and from them largely drew their ideas regarding medication.[30]

The Greeks, living on both sides of the Aegean Sea and on its islands, received many outside stimuli from both Mesopotamia and the Nile valley. So if we compare the drugs and the forms of medication used by the ancient Egyptians with those used later on by the Greeks, we find that the differences are neither very great nor very important. The rise of the oldest and best known medical schools, Cos and Cnidos, on the main sealanes to the Orient facilitated a fruitful connection between ancient Egyptian and Greek medicine.

It is pertinent to recall the special character of ancient Greek civilization, which impressed itself so indelibly on the Western world and created what we call European culture. In contrast with the ancient Oriental peoples with their disregard of the individual, the Greeks (Attic and Ionian especially) based their culture on individuality. With the appearance of famous physicians different opinions were presented on behalf of the different schools of thought; and these varying viewpoints were defended in public. As a result, secrecy and mystery were replaced gradually by communication and critical discussion.

### Mythology and Temple Medicine

A penchant for natural explanation and critical examination of old dogmas did not make the Greeks intolerant of religion or its place in healing. Rather, we find our own "modern" view that lay medicine must pursue diagnosis and treatment of disease within the framework of natural science, yet must not deny that the supernatural may have a separate place in the patient's resources.

At this stage medicine still had a severely limited scope of effectiveness, and it was a scientific merit of the best Greek physicians that they did not claim overmuch. Such modesty could not have been very satisfying to a desperately ill patient. Hence, we are not surprised at the popularity of the unlimited possibilities offered by several deities and demideities to whom healing qualities were attributed—for example, Apollo, among others. Prometheus was especially referred to as a preparer of remedies.

Beginning in the 7th century B.C., Asklepios gradually superseded Apollo as the greatest of healing gods. In his legend we find that the centaur Chiron taught Asklepios his pharmaceutical knowledge about drug plants growing in the Thessalian plains. Sanctuaries devoted to healing the sick were erected all over Greece, wherein dwelt the kindly but powerful spirit of Asklepios, aided by his two daughters, Hygeia and Panacea. What happened there finds an analogy in places of religious pilgrimage today. The image of Asklepios embodied so many of the finest qualities of medicine that he became a divine ideal for lay physicians, and the "staff of Asklepios" still remains the official symbol of medicine all over the world.[31] The bowl and sacred serpent carried by the god's daughter Hygeia, as she aided him in the visions of supplicants, became symbolic of health and then, in modern centuries, an internationally recognized symbol of pharmacy.

Beside this Greek version of temple medicine, there flourished a secular system of medical practice, the finest exponent of

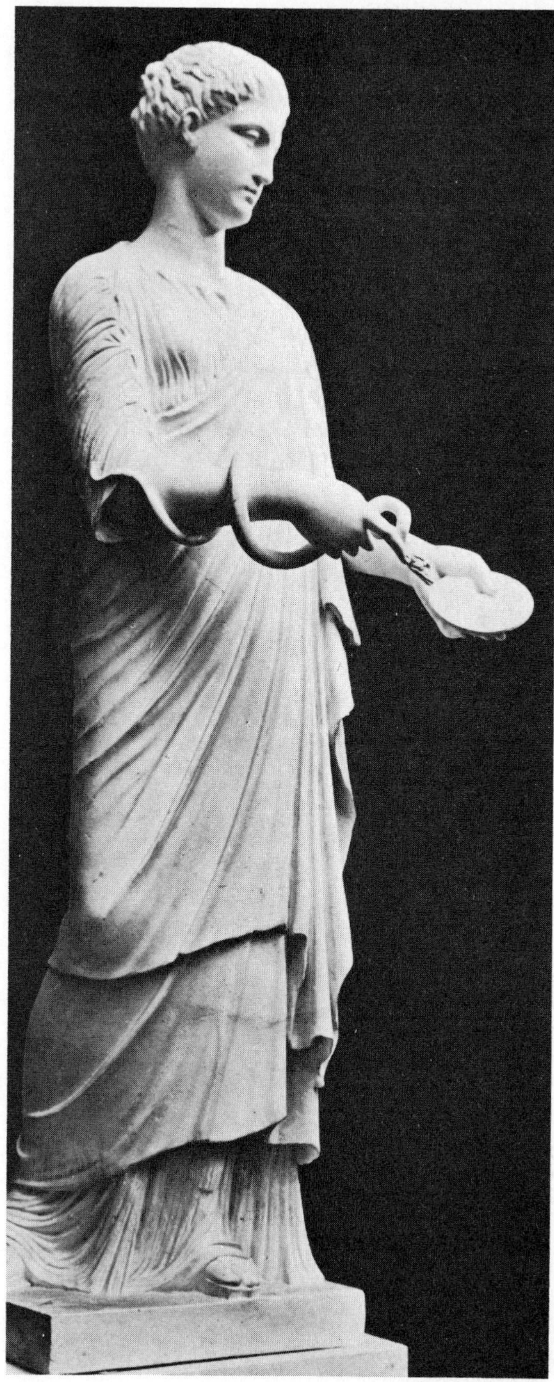

Classical statue of Hygeia, goddess of health in ancient Greece, who served beside her father, the great healing god Asklepios. Hygeia holds her traditional adjuncts—a sacred serpent of miraculous powers and a bowl (containing a healing potion?). As the staff and entwined serpent of Asklepios became the world-wide symbol of medicine, so the bowl and serpent of Hygeia have become in modern times an internationally recognized symbol of pharmacy. (From the Wellcome Historical Medical Museum, London; cast from an original in the Louvre, Paris)

which was the Hippocratic school. It rejected a theurgic conceptual basis for dealing with disease. Though by that time concepts and therapeutics usually found their explanation in the natural world, they eventually were shaped considerably by speculative philosophy, from which "science" could not yet be extricated.

## Philosophy and Its Influence on Medical Concepts

Greece originated the systematized reasoning about phenomena of the universe and the place of the human being in it that we call philosophy. The very term "philosopher" has been derived from the Greek words *philos* (friend) and *sophia* (wisdom). Through the Greeks, wisdom has become available to everyone who seeks to be its friend.

Most of the philosophers were eager to explain nature and its phenomena in a rational way. They dealt likewise with the healing arts and even sometimes practiced them. The most important problem facing these early philosophers was this: What rational explanation can be found both for the origin of the kind of world that human beings are living in and for the diseases that are their lot? Above all, it was the nature of matter that asked for an investigation. The most alluring idea was that of one essential and fundamental substance from which everything in nature developed. Four Greek philosophers in turn conceived one fundamental principle after another. The fourth of these, Empedocles (b. 504 B.C.) believed that four states of matter—combining ideas of his predecessors—were the "roots of all things." In his theory of the so-called four elements, it was proposed that the components of all matter, including the animal (hence human) body, were water, air, fire and earth.

According to Empedocles and his followers, health was the result of equilibrium of these four elements in the body, and disease was the result of a disequilibrium.

The question naturally arises, why were the four elements eventually called "Aristotelian" elements in preference to "Empedoclean"? The answer is that Aristotle, a strong proponent of the four-element theory, was so famous as a philosopher and a natural scientist that he overshadowed by far all the other Greek philosophers working in the same field. For thousands of years—up to our time—he has been regarded (to quote the Italian Renaissance poet Dante) as "the Master of those who know."[32]

Another Greek philosopher who influenced medicine and pharmacy was Pythagoras (580–489 B.C.). The father of the so-called Pythagorean proposition and the founder of a special philosophical-religious sect, he also, in all probability, discovered that the relation between musical pitch and the length of vibrating cords can be expressed in definite numbers. This discovery was regarded by the Pythagorean sect as a confirmation of the Babylonian-Assyrian mystical evaluation of numbers. The number seven was considered especially significant, as expressing the idea of a relationship between the seven then–known planets (each of them assigned to and symbolizing one of the gods) and the seven metals that had been identified. This relationship can be exemplified as follows:

| *Planets* | Jupiter | Mars | Mercury | Moon | Saturn | Sun | Venus |
|---|---|---|---|---|---|---|---|
| *Greek Gods* | Zeus | Ares | Hermes | Selene | Cronos | Helios | Aphrodite |
| *Roman Gods* | Jupiter | Mars | Mercurius | Luna | Saturn | Apollo | Venus |
| *Metals* | Tin | Iron | Mercury | Silver | Lead | Gold | Copper |
| *Symbols* | ♃ | ♂ | ☿ | ☾ | ♄ | ☉ | ♀ |

It was assumed that through the planets the gods influenced happenings on earth. This influence gradually became attributed to the planets themselves; hence, the factors revealing these influences at work were sought in the position of the stars at a particular time. On this basis the pseudoscience of astrology developed, although other forms of this system of belief appeared already in early Mesopotamia. For pharmacy, astrology implied that the time when plants were to be collected, and even when some preparations were to be compounded, had to be chosen according to astrologic considerations.

Another Greek idea that survived more than two thousand years, in modified form, has had greater scientific respectability and consequence for pharmaceutical research: atomic theory. It was conceived in a speculative way by Leucippos and Democritus (about 440 B.C.). According to these philosophers, the world consists of indivisible small corpuscles that differ in shape and position but not in substance. The antique theory of atomism gave a boldly mechanistic explanation to motion and qualitative change.

## Hippocratic Medical Writings

It was after the development of the theory of the four elements that Hippocrates entered the scene. This man posterity has termed "father of medicine." He was born about 460 B.C. on the island of Cos and died about 370 B.C. in Thessaly. However, "scholars have given up the use of the word Hippocrates as denoting an historical person who was the author of at least some of the books that are contained in the Hippocratean Corpus,"[33] because probably not a single book in this corpus (collected at Alexandria during the 4th and 3rd centuries B.C.), can be associated definitely with Hippocrates himself.[34]

While the scientific and ethical level evidenced in these writings was not achieved by one great man only, it was representative of some of the best Hippocratic practitioners during the 5th through the 3rd centuries B.C.

*Hippocratic "Humors."* In the Hippocratic corpus the concept of the harmony of the four elements (of which the body was supposed to consist, according to Empedocles and others) was replaced by the concept of the harmony or disharmony of the "four humors" as the cause of health or sickness. These four humors paralleled the four elements. This concept remained an explanatory theory and did not become a binding doctrine. The authors of the Hippocratic corpus were empiricists, believing in the healing power of nature and believing that the task of the physician is to help nature to help herself. "The great Hippocratic group imply the doctrine of humors in their phraseology and outlook on symptoms, but it is in the background, and nowhere are the humors described."[35]

*Drugs and Therapeutics.* Although the regulation of diet occupies the most important place in the Hippocratic Corpus, we also find many drugs, mainly of vegetable origin—the total ranging between 200 and 400 drugs, depending upon the definitions employed in studies of these bulky writings. Often the dividing line between dietary regimen and pharmaceutical regimen was thinly drawn by Hippocratic physicians, in their overall strategem to strengthen the healing power of nature and bring the patient back to a healthful equilibrium.[36]

Pharmaceutical processes mentioned in the Hippocratic corpus are manifold and include the preparation of fomentations, poultices, gargles, pessaries, pills, ointments, oils, cerates, collyria, lohochs, troches and inhalations. Narcotics were known and used (juice of the poppy, henbane seeds and mandragora). The frequent references to purgatives, sudorifics, emetics and enemas are due to the Hippocratic theory that the first requirement of medical treatment has to be the

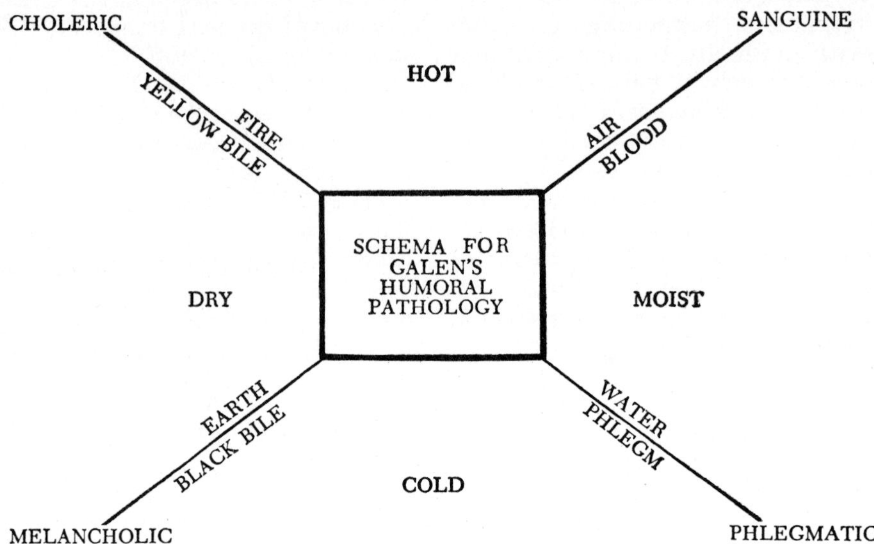


A diagram clarifies and simplifies relationships in the theoretic framework of humoral pathology. The *four humors,* whose balance and distribution were fundamental to the living organism, are given below the diagonal lines. Each of the *four elements* comprising all matter is adjacent *(above the line)* to its analogous humor. In the space above and beneath each diagonal are the two *qualitative characteristics* associated with each elemental substance.

*Temperament,* as well as one's health, reflected the humoral state, hence the designations at the *end* of each diagonal line. The etymology of each term of temperament reminds us of its ancient association with one of the humors.

purification of the body from illness-producing excess of humors.

This purification represented a bodily catharsis and led to a change in the concept of the word *pharmakon* from the original meaning of a charm (whether healing or poisonous) to the Hippocratic meaning of a purifying remedy. Later, it became the general designation for remedy.

Simplicity, freedom from irrationalism and, especially, the idea that each individual represents a unit that has to be treated as such, are important features of the Hippocratic theory and therapy. For this reason, throughout the ages, whenever medicine had lost itself too much in complexities and disregard for the individual patient, the battle cry could and can be heard: "Back to Hippocrates!"

*Hippocratic Oath.* The Hippocratic contribution of the rudiments of scientific method had far-reaching consequences in medical care through the centuries. Yet, Hippocrates is more widely remembered in recent times through association of his name with the first-known manifestation of medical ethics. Still today a host of medical graduates annually commit themselves to the "Hippocratic Oath" (and a paraphrase of the oath in pharmaceutical terms is taken by some pharmacy graduates). Was this ancient Greek expression of medical ideals in fact penned by the famous Hippocrates? Probably not, as we must say about so many other writings linked to his name.

Apparently the oath was composed shortly after the death of Hippocrates, not later than the fourth century B.C. However, it expresses ideas not then dominant, but those of the Pythagorean philosophical-religious sect. Therefore, adherents of this sect must have composed the oath. Since it mirrored the ideas of a Greek minority, it did not become popular until the end of antiquity, when "a new religion [Christianity] arose that changed the very foundation of ancient civilization." The similarity of the Pythagorean concepts to those of Christianity, together with the desire of Greek physicians in Rome to maintain their exclusive rights, gradually made the Hippocratic Oath generally recognized.[37]

### The School of Alexandria

The victorious sweep of Alexander the Great through the Eastern world brought in its wake the spread of the Greek way of thought over this enormous area. The founding of Alexandria in 331 produced a new cultural center that soon overshadowed in importance the old seat of Greek wisdom, Athens.

Under the Greek dynasty of the Ptolemies there developed the famous library where, for instance, the Hippocratic Corpus was preserved. A medical school there not only replaced but outshone its predecessors at Cos and Cnidos. At Alexandria different medical sects developed. The most important sects became known as "empiricists" or "experimentalists" and as "methodists."

"Empiricists" followed the Hippocratic idea of therapy based primarily on experience, allowing its adherents conclusions but not speculations. Its main representative was Herophilus (about 300 B.C.) who was a more ardent advocate of the use of drugs than the Hippocratic physicians were.

The "methodists" followed a special "method" (propagated by Themison about 300 B.C. and elaborated by Soranos about A.D. 100), which was based on a theory that disease resulted from too weak or too strong tension of the walls of the ducts in the body or, as they called it, the *status laxus* or the *status strictus*. The former condition called for strengthening by physical exercise and irritating drugs; the other called for relaxation and soothing drugs. Since this theory was based on the "solids" rather than the "humors" of the body, it is termed one kind of solidar pathology.

### Pharmaceutical Botanists

Before, during and after the time of Hippocrates there was a group of experts in medicinal plants. Their group name, *rhizotomoi* (from the Greek word *rizoma*, the mass of roots of trees), reflects frequent use of roots in Greek therapy.

> The *rhizotomoi* were erudite pharmacobotanists whose writings, if they had come to us, would probably fill the niche between Homer and Hippocrates and would show where the representatives of the Hippocratic period got their knowledge of medicinal plants. The fragments, which we know, are not less valuable than the writings of Dioscorides and contain the very earliest descriptions of medicinal plants.[38]

The rhizotomoi collected the indigenous vegetable roots and sold them. In addition they themselves often practiced medicine. Probably the most important representative of these rhizotomoi was Diocles of Carystos (4th century B.C.). He is considered to be the source for all Greek pharmacotherapeutic treatises between the time of Theophrastus and Dioscorides. Another famous rhizotomist, Crateuas (1st century B.C.), left the earliest known illustrated herbal.[39] Later, his depictions of medicinal plants illustrated the classic treatise on materia medica by Dioscorides (fl. A.D. 60), the ancient pharmaco-botanist most respected and influential down to early modern times. Deservedly so, for he dealt with his subject so much in the spirit of an applied science that probably he merits the appellation as the first real pharmacognosist.

Whether Dioscorides actually practiced medicine remains uncertain. It is probable that he accompanied the Roman armies through Asia Minor and also traveled in Italy, Greece, Gaul and Spain, collecting in-

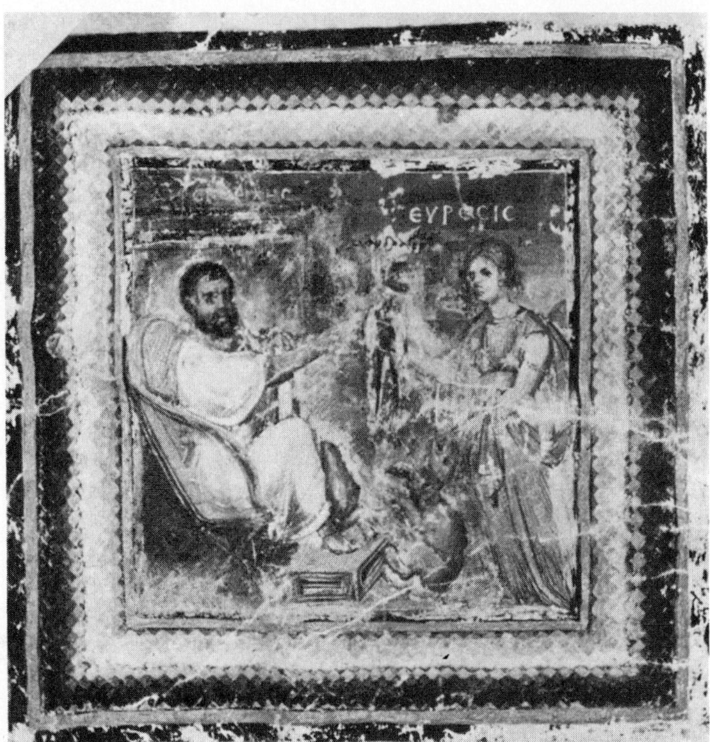


Early in the 6th century this illustration was painted into a manuscript copy of Dioscorides' work on pharmacy and applied botany, an antique cornerstone of pharmaceutical science. Probably it is the oldest illustrated work of its kind that has survived. The artist depicted a sage (intended to be Dioscorides, *seated)* receiving a forked mandrake root *(center)* from a female figure (Eurasis, *right*). The magical power of the mandrake has forced the dog *(bottom, center)* back on its haunches in a paroxysm of agony, which reflects one of the superstitions about this solanaceous drug that commanded awesome respect up to modern times. (Codex Vindobonensis, Med. Gr. 1, f. 4r., Austrian National Library, Vienna; from MacKinney-Smith Fund Collection of Medical Miniatures, University of North Carolina)

formation about plants of possible use in medicine. He not only described the drugs of his time and explained their effect but also arranged his description systematically.

Dioscorides' *De materia medica libri quinque* was translated into English (1665) and today is still kept in print as a classic representing an intellectual milestone in the development of pharmacy and botany.[40] The contents of the five books are arranged as follows: Book I: aromatics, oils, ointments, trees; Book II: living creatures, milk and dairy products, cereals and sharp herbs; Book III: roots, juices, herbs; Book IV: herbs and roots; Book V: vines and wines, metallic ores.

Dioscorides knew the preparation of leadplaster from fats and lead oxide. He mentions the processes of purifying woolfat, of making extracts by maceration followed by evaporation (e.g. extracts of glycyrrhiza) and of expressing the fresh juice of plants and concentrating it by exposure to the sun. He knew the differences among medicinally-used gums, such as acacia, tragacanth and the gums of cherry, plum and almond. He explained the usual adulterations and suggested means of discovering them. His remarks on the collection of drugs are excellent. His directions for storage, since they are the first known and the basis for many later writers, may be quoted:

> Flowers and sweet-scented things should be laid up in drug boxes of lime wood; but there are some herbs which do well enough if wrapped up in papers or leaves for the preservation of their seeds. For moist [liquid] medicines some thicker [impermeable] material such as silver, or glass, or horn will agree best. Yes, and earthenware if it be not thin [permeable] is fitting enough, and so is wood, particularly if it be box-wood. Vessels of brass will be suitable for eye-medicines and for

liquids and for all that are compounded of vinegar or of liquid pitch or of Cedria, but fats and marrows ought to be put up in vessels of tin. (Translation by John Goodyer.)

## Galen

As personified by Hippocrates, Greek medicine of the 5th and 4th centuries B.C. gave the world healing arts in a new spirit; to Dioscorides it is indebted for fundamentals of materia medica and to Pliny for a summary of ancient knowledge. What entitles Galen to be added to this illustrious group?

Galen was born in Pergamon (ca. A.D. 131), practiced and taught in Rome as a great physician and natural scientist, and about A.D. 201 died in his native town. What carried his name through the ages was the fact that he created a system of pathology and therapy that ruled western medicine for 1,500 years. This was possible because of the logic of his system, the reverence for his authority and the lack of experimental methods that would readily reveal fallacies embedded in his brilliant writings.

Galen drew from all available sources whatever he thought worthwhile (mostly without giving any references), typically mentioning "not those he copied but those he attacked!"[41] There was at least one exception: Hippocrates. For Galen saw it as his mission to complete and systematize the work ascribed to "the father of medicine." It was indeed, essentially in the form of "Galenism" that Greek medicine was transmitted to later ages.[42] What Galenism means could, and has, occupied volumes, since the medical philosophy in Galen's works or ascribed to him provided a wide-ranging guide to scientific medicine and to thought about "man's body in health and disease."

Here it is possible to give only a few indications and examples of how and why Galen's name has remained one of the best remembered also in pharmacy—in a practical sense at least through the 17th century and in the profession's collective memory up to our own time.

A fundamental principle in Galenism as applied to pharmacy was the transformation of humoral pathology, hence of therapeutics, into a rigid dogma—attributable more to Galenic practitioners than to Galen himself.

The school of Hippocrates had formulated the theory of the four humors (paralleling the four elements), the correct balance of which meant health, while every disturbance of this balance spelled disease. There were the four humors: blood, phlegm (supposed to come from the brain), yellow bile ( supposed to be secreted from the liver) and black bile (supposed to come from the spleen and the stomach). Each one of these humors had definite qualities. Blood was moist and warm; phlegm, moist and cold; yellow bile, warm and dry; black bile, cold and dry. Furthermore, there was a definite connection between predominance of any one humor in the metabolic system and an individual's temperament. The diagram (p. 16) gives an idea of these relationships.

Of general importance were Galen's efforts to test the action of drugs, both qualitatively and quantitatively, according to these characteristics. Having attributed observed diseases to specific imbalances of the humors, one could classify drugs (on a scale of four degrees) according to the presumed strength of their counteraction against particular diseases.

To illustrate, Temkin says, "Supposing that the patient suffered from a disease where the affected part was ten units warmer than normal and seven units drier, the remedy had to be ten units colder than normal and seven units moister, provided that the diseased part was located superficially. If it was situated more deeply, an adjustment had to be made, lest the remedy lose its power before reaching the diseased part."[43]

Drugs that were supposed to have only one quality were classified as "simples," while those with more qualities were considered "composites." There were also so-called "entities," drugs with specific effects that did not fit one of the regular systematic categories. Examples of these are emetics and purgatives, poisons and antidotes, which were said to be effective through their "whole substance."

Thus a rational and systematic guide for selecting medicinal treatment became available (even though eventually seen to be "wrong" in modern times). Not its least appeal was the order it brought to drug therapy; as implied by "the therapeutic anarchy that followed its destruction [which] made itself felt beyond the middle of the nineteenth century."[44]

Galen prepared his medicaments himself and had a very high opinion of the efficacy of well chosen and prepared remedies. He had not only an *iatreion,* the usual room of the Greco-Roman physicians for the preparation of remedies, but also an *apotheca* or storeroom.

Galen described 473 drugs of vegetable, animal and mineral origin. In addition, a profusion of drug formulas is found in his medical treatises. Three famous remedies that gained a worldwide reputation for a millennium and a half because of his recommendation, although in use before his time, were *hiera picra* (holy bitter), *terra sigillata* (sealed earth) and *theriaca* (treacle).

Pharmacy continued to be dominated by Galenic concepts until in the Renaissance the whole medical system, now tradition-bound, finally came under serious attack by Paracelsus, whose weaponry included a new approach to selecting and preparing remedies. What had begun in ancient Rome as the exciting contribution of a single intellect had become a confining authority that came to dominate the course of history in medicine and pharmacy.

### Retail Trade in Drugs

In Greece as well as in Rome the necessity of well organized medical care was gradually recognized. There developed a system of providing community-paid physicians who, however, were allowed to charge wealthy people. Since these practitioners took care of the pharmaceutical part of treatment likewise, there was no similar official recognition and regulation of pharmaceutical activities, although there were groups of drug preparers and sellers in existence.

Indeed, it had become common comparatively early for Greco-Roman physicians to have these specialists compound medications for them. Pliny complained about this tendency,[45] and Galen admonished his colleagues to do their drug compounding themselves and not delegate this function to the pigmentarii. In any case, the physician remained the one who applied or gave the medicaments to the patients under his care, and it was his responsibility to see that the drugs had been prepared properly. The division of labor and responsibility between the physician as the prescriber and the pharmacist as the legitimate agent for preparing prescription medication and dispensing it to the patient still had not become a recognized concept, still less an accepted reality.

The preparers and sellers of drugs and cosmetics were known in Greece as *rhizotomoi, migmatopoloi, pharmakopoeoi, pharmakopoloi, myropoeoi* and *myripsoi;* in Rome as *pharmacopoli, circumforanei, sellularii, seplasiarii, unguentarii, aromatarii, pharmacopoei, medicamentarii, pharmacotritae, pharmacotribae* and *pigmentarii.* (For explanations, see the Glossary: Appendix 7.)

Limited by meager evidence, it has been hard to assess whatever changes in the structure and the administrative arrangement of pharmaceutical services had arisen in the "golden age" of Greek culture as compared with the Egyptian zenith reached 1,500 years before in a quite different intellectual climate. Perhaps more important for the future of pharmacy was the potential created by striking advances in the knowledge of drugs and the refinement of technics and by the embryonic scientific methods that now characterized the best medical thought and practice.

While theurgic concepts had long since been thrust aside, the rational technics were not yet sufficiently complex nor was medical care sufficiently mature to split pharmacy and medicine into two distinct specialties. Some practitioners served as both physician and pharmacist, others had a pharmaceutical assistant, and still others were relying more and more on special dealers to prepare certain compounds as well as gather, as of old, the crude drugs needed.

Certain groups may have been little more than collectors or dealers in herbs (such as the *rhizotomoi*); others were merely street-corner quacks (the *pharmakopolos* had that reputation). Some (the *seplasiarii*) settled down in permanent shops to vend remedies. If at first they specialized in cosmetics, they later branched out into medicinal salves and plasters. In any event, the fact that these different groups existed suggests that during Greek and Roman antiquity there was no distinct profession or class comparable with the pharmacist of later periods.[46]

## FOUR ROMAN MEDICAL AUTHORS

Medicine in Rome was almost monopolized by Greek physicians. For example, the great Galen and Dioscorides both came from Greek colonies in Asia Minor. Among other medical writers working in Rome the four cited here represent highly influential works dating from the 1st century B.C. to the 7th century A.D.: Celsus, Scribonius Largus, Pliny and Paulus.

### An Influential Medical Encyclopedia

Aulus Cornelius Celsus, like his great contemporary Pliny, was in all probability not a physician but a learned and medically experienced encyclopedist. As part of a large encyclopedic work, he wrote *De Medicina*, one of the best practical treatises on medicine written in Greco-Roman antiquity. Its great influence after the late 15th century came about partly by accident. Pope Nicholas V discovered Celsus' forgotten manuscript and had it published in 1478 when no other classical book on medicine or medicaments was in print. But there were less accidental virtues to recommend the author: his wide scope, evaluative attitude, and excellent Latin style. Roman medicaments and other pharmaceutical matters discussed by Celsus may be consulted in a modern English translation.[47]

### The First Dispensatory?

The *Compositiones* of the Roman physician Scribonius Largus, written about A.D. 43,[48] might be categorized as an early dispensatory. It defends, in the preface, a thorough and plentiful use of medicaments, opposing the medicinal nihilism that existed even in those early days. Scribonius Largus says:

> We have to condemn all those who intend to deprive medicine of the use of remedies, the name "medicine" being derived not from healing *(a medendo)* but from the power and efficiency of the medicament *(medicamentum)*. All those should be praised who try whatever is possible to save the sick patient.

The work by Scribonius Largus contains only a few simples *(simplicia)* and most of his formulas for compounded medicaments *(composita)* contain many ingredients. Scribonius describes the preparation and gives the first definition of opium, insisting on the use of immature poppy capsules as the source of opium (reserving the designation *meconium* for the inspissated juice of poppy leaves). He perceptively warns against substituting the juice of the leaves for the juice of the unripe capsules, "as the *pigmentarii* prepare it in order to make a profit."[49]

### All Science His Province

Pliny was a Roman general, admiral and diplomat with a passion for collecting and compiling the entire scientific knowledge of his time. He was a contemporary of Dioscorides, in the first century A.D., writing in part on the same subjects and often using the same sources. While Singer gives Dioscorides full credit, he characterizes Pliny as

> the compiler par excellence, the learned collector who will put down anything he is told or can read without verification. Scientifically the work is, therefore, worthless. . . [yet] read throughout the ages, alike in the darkest as in more enlightened periods, copied and recopied, translated, commented on, extracted. . . .[50]

Pliny's work continues to be of special interest, particularly because most of the books that Pliny used have been lost (he himself spoke of more than 2,000!). The reflection of a vast lost library that can be found in Pliny's encyclopedic *Natural History* has attracted study by a number of historians.[51]

**End of an Epoch**

This group of Greco-Roman medical authors is completed chronologically with Paulos Aegineta (7th century), whose *Seven Books on Medicine* represent essentially a critically selected compendium, with commentary. It was composed from the writings of earlier authors, principally Dioscorides, Galen and Oribasios of Pergamon.[52] Paulos Aegineta gives a complete picture of Greco-Roman medications.

Paulos lived at Alexandria when the Arabs took possession of this old stronghold of Greek science and remained there under the Arabian government. He therefore represents, in his person as well as in his activity, the transmission of Greco-Roman medical wisdom to the Arabs.

In Babylonia and Egypt, in Greece and Rome, we have glimpsed some of the foundation stones on which the Arabs and, later, medieval Europe were to build a more distinctive "pharmacy." In this ancestral sense, as an "ancient prelude," these early civilizations capture our interest. However, we value them properly only if we think of them as rather an astonishing climax after eons of brutalized life and of primitive reaction to the profound mystery of disease.

# 2

# The Arabs and the European Middle Ages

## THE ARABS

With the conquest of a great part of the ancient civilized world in the 7th and 8th centuries by a group of Semitic tribes called Arabs, suddenly this primitive people became the heir and administrator of the surviving remnants of Greco-Roman culture. The literature found in Egypt, Syria and Byzantium provided a basis for Arabic civilization, especially translations of Greek manuscripts into Syriac and Arabic (mainly by the Nestorians).

Nestorius, patriarch of Constantinople, had been condemned for heresy by the Council of Ephesus in 431. Banned by the official church, the "Nestorians" who held his beliefs established themselves in Persia, Syria, India and other oriental countries. Among this sect were many scientists, who took into exile their books and their wisdom and became teachers of the world into which they immigrated. Their schools became famous (Nisibis, Edessa and Gondêschâpûr). When the Arabs entered the politico-cultural scene, this special kind of Greco-Oriental synthesis offered itself. Thus it could be said that

> The Arabic civilization was at bottom the Hellenized Aramaic and Iranian civilizations as developed under the aegis of the caliphate and expressed through the medium of the Arabic tongue.[1,2]

From the 9th to the 13th centuries a flood of book manuscripts written in Arabic testified to this flourishing of culture on the basis of a marriage between the Greek and the oriental spirit. However, in medicine as in other sciences and philosophy, this culture was the product of many nations under the aegis of the caliph in a predominantly Muslim society.

> The term Arabian does not necessarily imply an Arab, for the Persians and Nestorians in the East, and the Spaniards and Jews in the West, took the principal part in the development of medicine which was expressed in the Arabic language . . . the language of the learned in the Empire of Islam just as Latin was the linguistic medium of the educated in Western Europe.[3]

### New Literature Created

This poetic language conveyed an outpouring of literature in every field of intellectual endeavor, not least of all in the health field. Translations of the most respected writings on medicine and pharmacy from earlier civilizations stimulated writers in Arabic to contribute new material of their own. Among the earliest known writers on pharmaceutical subjects were Theodoq (d. ca. 709 A.D.), court physician to the governor of Iraq, who wrote on drugs, drug products and their nomenclature, and the more famous physician Ibn Masawaih (called Mesue, Sr., d. 857), the son of a pharmacist, whose treatise on aromatic medicinal plants survives.[4] Among these substances, wrote

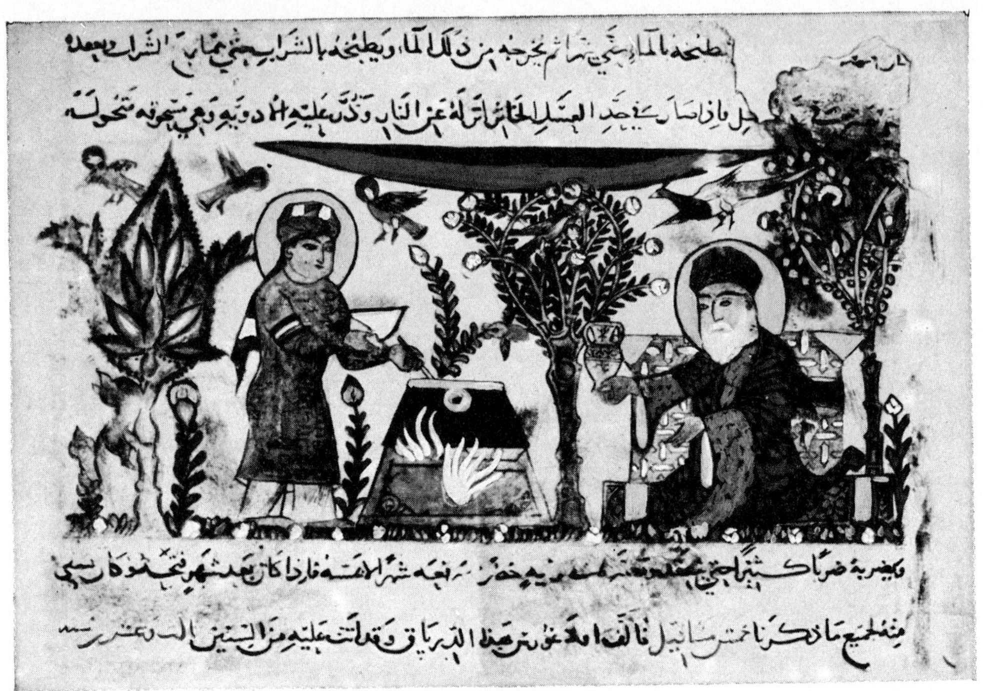

This miniature in an Arabic manuscript of the early 13th century depicts the preparation of drugs. A liquid remedy is being mixed over a fire in the open air, where flora and fauna symbolize the pharmaceutical bounty of nature. The bearded figure (*right*) holds out an ornate ceramic drug container. This manuscript was based on Galen's treatise concerning electuaries.

Masawaih, are five principal ones: musk, ambergris, aloe, camphor and saffron.

Subsequent writers in Arabic produced scores of such specialized treatises. Although they are remarkably varied, four main types of drug-oriented contributions have been characterized by the pharmacist-historian Sami K. Hamarneh. These are, briefly:

1. *Formularies and compendiums,* which offer a collection of formulas or recipes for medications, systematically arranged (e.g., A–Z by drug names), including instructions for formulating the drug products and, sometimes, for their therapeutic use. One Arabic prototype is the compilation by Sābūr b. Sahl in the 850's (titled al-Agrabadhin al-Kabīr). This product of the Eastern caliphate was followed in the next century by the earliest known formulary to be written on the Iberian peninsula, in the Western Caliphate. Its author, the physician Ibn 'Abd Rabbih, gave his formulary a title *(al-Dukkān)* meaning "The Apothecary Shop." In it 'Abd Rabbih said he wished to discuss "all useful medications that could be manufactured [in the pharmacy]: syrups, robs and conserves, electuaries, confections, sternutatories, eye salves, oily extracts, and all types of medicated powders, spiced perfumes, and cosmetics. . . the methods and techniques employed in the preparation of these remedies and their modes of action on diseases, as best as I can, and as recommended by the ancient sages."

The next several centuries brought a suc-

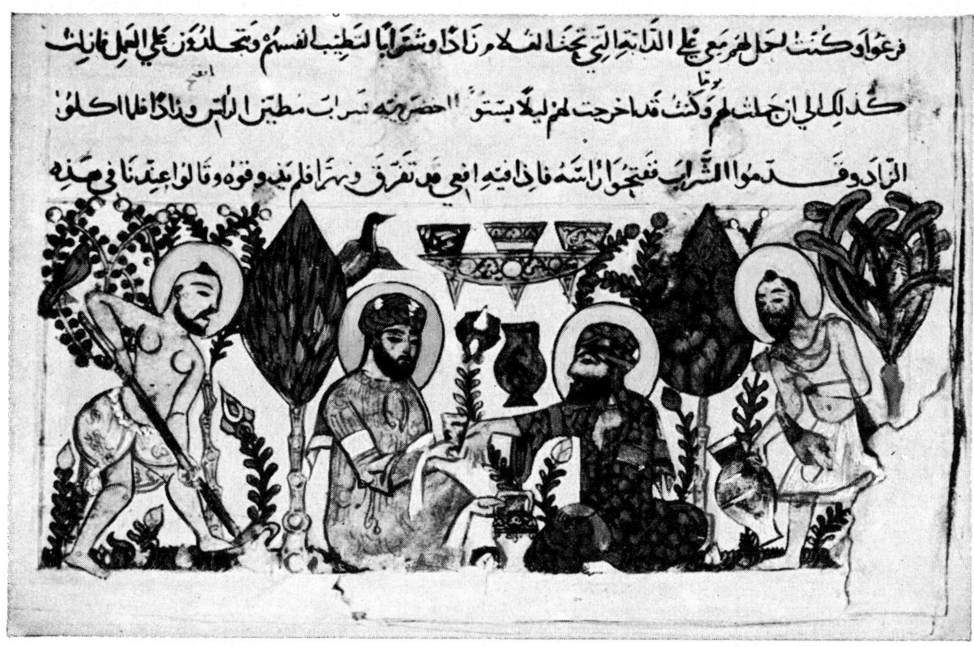

This companion to the illustration on the facing page shows the preparation of theriac, a complex antidote that Galen's recommendation helped to raise to the level of an internationally renowned panacea. Between and above the two central figures are various drug containers from which they are measuring the ingredients. Two assistants (*extreme left and right*) obtain supplies of crude drugs for the compounders. (Miniature from ms. in Austrian National Library, Vienna; reproduced from Zekert, O.: Chem. and Druggist *120*:728, 1934)

cession of Arabic manuscripts in the same category, either compilations of drug formulas as free-standing treatises or as a section in broader encyclopedic works on medicine. Some were prepared specifically for use in Islamic hospitals, for example, one by Ibn al-Tilmīdh in the 12th century. At their best, these formularies were practical and precise, essentially free of superstition, and gave attention not only to adjustment of dosage for different purposes, but to possible side effects and to additive effects when several drugs are administered together.

2. *Herbals and books on the materia medica,* which were strongly influenced by the Greco-Roman authority, Dioscorides. But gradually, Islamic workers made significant additions to natural medicinal products from their own soil or from their venturesome trading expeditions. Medicinal plants were especially interesting in an economy so dependent upon agricultural products. By the 10th century various forms of Arabic treatises in this category were readily available to practitioners of medicine and pharmacy and their students.

One culmination of this type of literature was al-Biruni's work in the 11th century, which described more than a thousand simples (i.e., the crude uncompounded drugs), recognized pharmacy as a separate branch of the healing art and provided a masterful summation of pharmaceutical knowledge.[5] Still more comprehensive, however, was the materia medica of Ibn al-Bayṭār, the most renowned Islamic medical botanist of the thirteenth century. He mentions about 1800 botanical drugs, 145 mineral drugs and 130 drugs from animal sources—in a sophisticated work that reportedly cites about 150 other authors. It instructed pharmacist-readers for several centuries throughout the Middle East and to some extent in the West.[6]

3. *Toxicology treatises,* which responded to the risks of being poisoned accidentally or intentionally—since poisoning was then popular as both a personal and political weapon. These special manuals described the toxic substances and their action, the toxic symptoms, and the often complex and wondrous antidotes. Some of this lore had come out of India; and indeed the whole realm of Islamic drugs and pharmacy owed a debt to the older Indian civilization, with which there were close commercial and cultural ties. A separate chapter or even separate treatises were written about various forms of "theriac," a universal antidote of complex composition from Greco-Roman antiquity. Indeed, by this time the therapeutic repute of theriac had inflated to the status of a panacea. Hamarneh concludes that Arabic "literary contributions on toxicology, antidotes, and theriac, from Hunayn in the ninth century to Ibn al-Ṣūrī in the thirteenth, were tremendous."

4. *Diet and drug therapy in relation to human ecology,* was accorded even more attention than that given to the subject by the ancient Greeks, Hamarneh concludes. A central concept was that the sick person requires a different mode of living and different food and drink than does a healthy person, and the importance of unpolluted air for good health was clearly recognized. As early as the 9th century, the renowned translator Ḥunayn b. Ishāq gave impetus to this line of development through his translation of relevant Hippocratic and Galenic treatises, then through his own writings on the subject.

This Islamic literature, as Hamarneh demonstrated in various investigations, has been an impressive force in shaping the distinctive occupation that we call pharmacy.[7] Even more than the Roman encyclopedists noted earlier, Islamic writers responded to the practical need to try to systematize and elaborate all medical knowledge into great encyclopedic works. Just four Islamic encyclopedists will be mentioned as examples—men whose influence extended across the Mediterranean where their works helped to develop medicine and pharmacy in Europe.

One of the most capable was al-Rāzī (Latinized Rhazes; d. ca. 925), a physician who took a pioneering interest in scientific chemistry. His comprehensive review of ancient Greek and early Arabic medical knowledge was reinforced by his own experiences. He gave much attention to "the most effective as well as most palatable methods of administering medicaments—in which preference is given to the pill form—and gives recipes, many of them very complicated, against specified diseases."[8]

A medical encyclopedia more systematic and concise than that by al-Rāzī was the *Royal Book* by 'Ali Ibn 'Abbās (Latinized Haly Abbas, d. 994). His work showed concern for the ethics of medical care and the part on drugs was held in highest esteem.

Later, Ibn Sīnā (Latinized Avicenna, d. 1037) wrote a five-part "Canon" of medicine that considers about 760 drugs in the pharmaceutical part. His Canon was an immense work with great influence, although its originality has been disputed. Probably the most renowned of all Islamic scientists, Ibn Sīnā was especially respected for his theoretic expositions. Separately, he wrote a specialized tract on cardiac drugs.[9]

His contemporary in the western caliphate of the Islamic empire, Abu-l-Qasim al-Zahrawi (Latinized Abulcasis; d. ca. 1013), wrote a medical encyclopedia still more pervaded by pharmaceutical concerns. It was especially his 28th chapter (the *Liber servitoris*) that became so highly regarded throughout Europe, particularly as a manual of medicinal chemistry.[10]

The presentation of two books, apparently written by Europeans around the 13th century, as the work of two famous medieval Arabs, Mesuë Senior and Jābir Ibn Hajjaj, illustrates the esteem which Arabic pharmaceutical and medical science commanded eventually on European soil. The authority of this pseudoauthorship coupled with impressive content made both volumes influential on generations of European pharmacists—the pseudo-Mesuë's *Grabadin* as a masterful exposition on the composition of medicaments, and pseudo-Jābir's (or Geber's) *Summa perfectionis* as a summation of chemical knowledge.[11]

## The Practice of Pharmacy

The great attention paid to the science and the art of pharmacy by the medical authors of the Arabic world influenced, and strengthened the basis for, the development of pharmacy.[12] The drug armamentarium became enlarged considerably. Persian and Indian drugs unknown to the Greco-Roman world—camphor, cassia, cloves, cubebs, musk, nutmeg, rhubarb, sandalwood, senna and tamarind, to name only a few—were described. Of equal importance were new modes of drug therapy that required considerable skill on the part of the preparer—for example, confections, conserves, juleps and lohochs.

These advances in pharmaceutical knowledge and technic on the one side and medical knowledge on the other, in connection with a growing recognition of governmental responsibility for the health of the people in the Arabic world, fostered a division of labor between pharmacy and medicine and, finally, the creation of a public health system in which the profession of pharmacy was given a definite place of its own.

Before the 8th century, medical care had remained largely the "Medicine of the Prophet," especially hygienic rules and pre-Islamic folk medicine. Then, beginning about four decades after Muhammad's pilgrimage to Mecca, a growing emphasis on the health field and a professionalized medicine can be discerned.

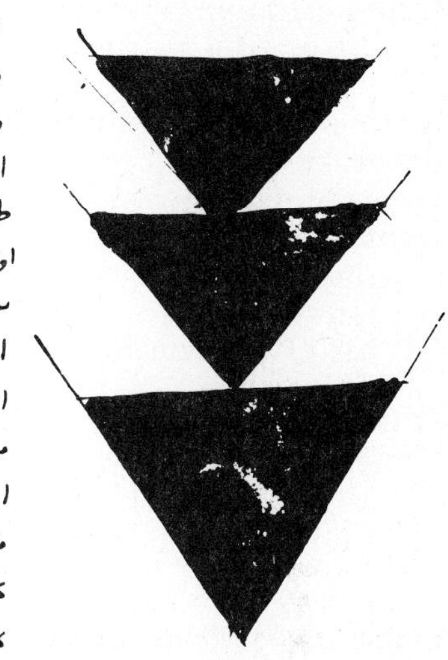

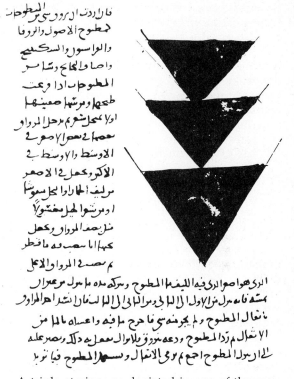

A triple strainer as depicted in one of the earliest known drawings of pharmaceutical equipment for instructional purposes. It is found in a late medieval Arabic manuscript of the famous 28th treatise of Abū-l-Qāsim al-Zahrāwī of Cordova (10th century). A decoction poured into the top strainer filtered through successively finer strainers arranged underneath. Such strainers often were woven of horsehair. (Veliyuddin ms. 2491, copied 1265 A.D., f. 39 v. and 40 v.; from Süleymaniye 'Umūmī Kütüphanesi, Istanbul; see Hamarneh, Sami K.: J.A.Ph.A. (Pract.) *21*:91, 1960)

Probably in the early 8th century a "state hospital," much as we understand the term, was founded in Damascus—perhaps the first hospital in Islam.[13]

Under the caliph al-Mansur, Baghdad became a dazzling capital city (in the years following 762), a center of learning as well as of administration.

The vigorous development of intellectual life and health facilities makes it understandable that drug shops which we dare call pharmacies had appeared by the early 9th century. Pharmacy emerged as a calling distinct from medicine. Shops specializing in medicines and spices appeared, especially around Baghdad, although often in the hands of uneducated dispensers. In higher esteem among the citizenry were a minority of better educated practitioners called "sayādilah," a term even today associated with a qualified pharmacist in Arabic lands. From the old Arabic manuscripts, Hamarneh concluded:

> From the first half of the ninth century on, pharmacists were examined and licensed by the Muḥtasib and their shops were routinely inspected. . . . Aside from the privately owned apothecary shops, there were also dispensaries attached to hospitals. These were often directed and operated by professional, educated pharmacists and their aides. They collected and preserved materia medica simples and compounded remedies and dispensed or sold medications to the sick in the hospitals or to others who came to the out-patient clinics. There are also records of botanical gardens adjacent to hospitals where medicinal herbs were cultivated. Laboratories for the manufacture of electuaries, syrups, and other frequently needed medications often were connected with hospital pharmacies.[14]

Thus, pharmacy had become, said the contemporary al-Biruni (973–1051), "the art of knowing the materia medica simples in their various species, types and shapes. From these, the pharmacist prepares compounded medications as prescribed and ordered by the prescribing physician." Within this concept, society found a specialist of great utility, one readily distinguishable from the alchemists on one side and the physicians on the other. "al-Attar" remained as a competitor, a personage who also dealt in drugs but traditionally specialized in aromatics. These "attārīn" remind us of the "seplasiarii" of ancient Rome, who settled down in shops and expanded in scope from fragrant cosmetics to a wider range of pharmaceutical products.

However, in the elaboration of pharmaceutical technic and knowledge and in the acceptance of responsibility by a pharmaceutical class within an ordered health system, the Arabs made a distinctive place for pharmacy going well beyond pharmaceutical function either as a sideline of a medical practitioner's offices or as technical commerce of ordinary marketplace vendors.

This Arabic development helped to establish and shape Western pharmacy as we know it.

## TRANSIT WAYS OF KNOWLEDGE

Sicily and Spain especially served to channel Greco-Arabic medicine into the Latin West (the 7th to the 12th centuries). Sicily was a center of Arabic culture from the time Syracuse fell to the Arabs (878) until the Normans conquered the island (completed 1091). In Spain, Cordova became a cultural capital as well as the political capital of Islam's Western caliphate by the 10th century. Of the Spanish centers where scholars were busily translating out of the Arabic, Toledo especially yielded an exciting outpouring of Arabic learning that was soon widely absorbed and discussed among Western scholars. Much of this knowledge, of course, had its roots in classical Greece.[15]

Greek science returned to Western Europe by three routes: through the continuous tradition of Southern Italy, through the Eastern (Byzantine) Empire and through the Arabians. Until the period of the Renaissance, the most important of these was the Arabic route. It was the main current even in Salerno, where the three streams met.

With Salerno, we reach European soil to see what was happening to European medicine and pharmacy meanwhile, between the rise of Islam and the time of the Renaissance—that is, during the Middle Ages.

## MEDIEVAL EUROPEAN PHARMACY

The conquest of the ancient Roman Empire of the West, especially of Italy, by German tribes (the Vandals, the Longobards, the Visigoths and the Ostrogoths) found only a shadow of Rome's old glory and culture. Italy had been haunted for centuries by civil war, hostile invasions and epidemic diseases that depopulated and demoralized the country. In such a situation, the disparagement of earthly life and wisdom—a significant trend of early Christendom—not only found broad acknowledgment and success but often led to the destruction of works of pagan art and science.

The German invaders now continued the work of cultural destruction. They were all the more prone to do so because their increasing belief in the healing power of faith and of relics of saints could not be harmonized easily with some of the scientific wisdom that survived from antiquity.

Thus, the first tutelary saints for medicine and pharmacy, which in a measure replaced the old pagan deities of medicine, began to appear about the 5th century. Cosmas and Damian, Arabian Christians, were twins martyred in the persecutions under Emperor Diocletian during the 4th century. They became the most celebrated patron saints of medicine and pharmacy in all the countries of Christendom. Later, they were supplemented by other saints; but until today, especially in Catholic areas, Damian best represents divine guardianship over the services of the pharmacist.[16]

### Monastic Medicine and Pharmacy

During the early Middle Ages, individuals with some knowledge of the old intellectual treasures tried to rescue at least those parts that had practical value. Most important was Marcus Aurelius Cassiodorus (490–585), a learned Roman and chancellor of the great Ostrogothic king Theodoric, in Ravenna (Northern Italy). He induced the king to create a magistrate especially empowered to safeguard relics of classical antiquity.[17] Cassiodorus himself founded a kind of classical academy in which the cultivation of medicine and pharmacy played an important part. In his "fundamental book of medieval science," Cassiodorus established the rule that the monks who acted as physicians were required to consult Dioscorides' writings, read Latin translations of the works of Hippocrates and Galen, and study the work of Caelius Aurelianus, a Roman medical compiler of the 1st century. Thus, the activity of Cassiodorus was basic to monastic medicine as well as to the survival of such independent scientific medical life as could exist during the period from the 5th to the 10th century.

What results did Cassiodorus get?

> Conditions developed in Ravenna and other centers that were very similar to those in Alexandria. And granted that there, too, the medical men may have been chiefly members of the church, their medicine was anything but monastic. The medical literature of the period is entirely Latin. . . . By the end of the 6th century a fairly large number of classical books had been translated into Latin.[18]

This "fairly large number of classical books" represented only a small part of ancient medical wisdom. Moreover, it was used almost exclusively by a small group of persons.

Then the empire of Theodoric the Great disappeared, and new swarms of barbarian invaders put an end to that modest attempt toward a cultural renaissance. In those times of perpetual bloodshed and destruction, study was "almost exclusively restricted to the clergy, because only the church was a safe asylum provided for the studious. . . Thus was born monastic medicine."

> Medicine, after having played a most important part in Roman civilization, withdrew into the shadow of the church and became, under the influence of Christian dominance, a dogmatic medicine in which the first and most important point was faith. Faith alone could cure the body and the soul of the sufferer and was the essential point in the help of the sick.[19]

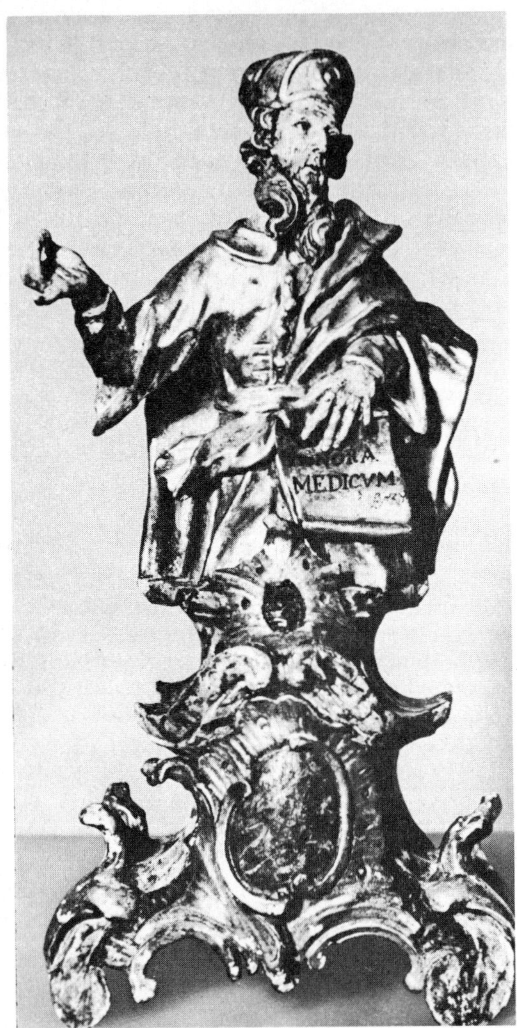


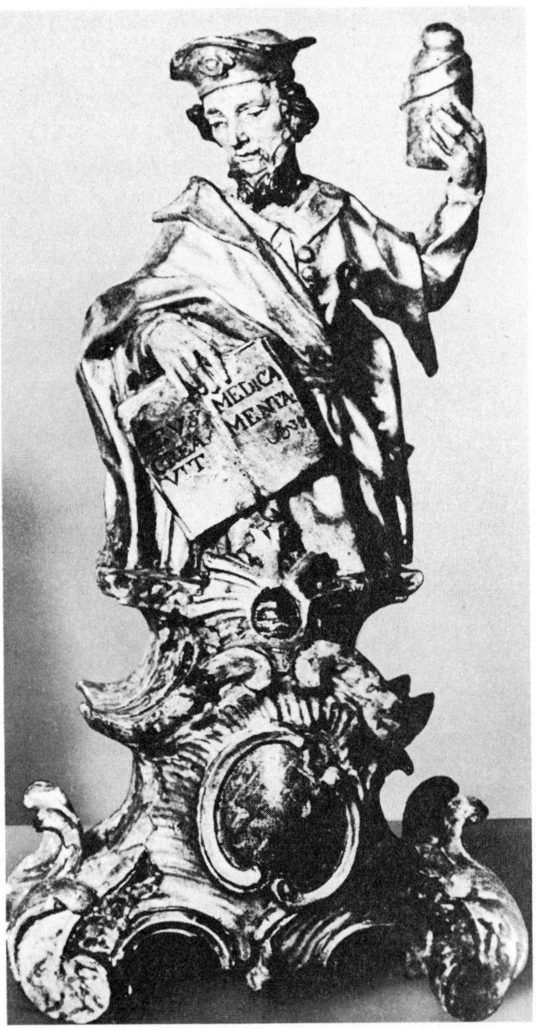


Pharmaceutical work has been conducted under the protecting hands of diverse religious figures; in Christendom, it has been associated above all with the saints Cosmas and Damian. Their martyrdom and legendary feats of healing inspired works of art from at least as early as the 11th century. These small wooden figures were carved by Ferdinand A. Hiernle of Lower Bavaria in the 18th century. Saint Damian (*right*) is shown holding a book open to the aphorism, *God has created drugs,* while, in his other hand, he holds aloft a drug container. The twin brothers from ancient Aegea seem to symbolize the twinship of medicine and pharmacy; Saint Damian particularly has been considered to be guardian of both pharmacy and surgery. (From Verbandstoff-Fabriken Paul Hartmann AG: Kostbarkeiten aus der Apotheke, Heidenheim/Brenz, 1952; photographs by Maximilian Doerr)

Therefore, little opportunity was provided for the development of science or for the enlightenment of men by science. In many monasteries monks heeded the advice of Cassiodorus that they collect and use the old manuscripts. But only the few Latin treatises that the monks had rescued could be studied, principally "those of Celsus, Scribonius Largus, Pliny the Elder (to a slight degree only), and Caelius Aurelianus."[20] The Greek manuscripts that they had collected and preserved for posterity they could not use, "being unable to read Greek." These manuscripts did become important several centuries later in the time of the Renaissance, when scholars eagerly searched the cloisters of Italy and elsewhere for original Greek medical manuscripts and found copies in a number of institutions.

Meanwhile, a more modest literature arose to fill the gap, generated in that small sector where there was a possibility of the cultivation and the practice of scientific medicine.

> What was mostly needed was short treatises, abstracts, epitomes, giving brief instructions for practice. A new literature arose, consisting of short treatises on urine, pulse, fever, dietetics, prognostic, bloodletting and, above all, endless prescriptions were written. These treatises sometimes were given the form of epistles or of dialogues, or of catechisms. They were anonymous, many of them falsely bearing the great names of Hippocrates, Galen, Democritos, Apuleius to give them more authority. . . . This literature lasted, unchanged in character, until the 11th century. The turning point in the literary development was made by the translations of Constantine of Africa. They started a new movement, inaugurated a new literature, which from now on invariably had traces of Arabian influence.[21]

Before the invaluable translations of Constantine of Africa, the European scientific world had available the work of Dioscorides; parts of the treatises of Hippocrates, Galen, Celsus, Scribonius Largus, Pliny the Elder, Caelius Aurelianus, Oribasios and Alexander Trallianus; and some anonymous and pseudonymous abstracts. Two such abstracts, "undoubtedly the most popular treatises for many centuries, [were]. . . . the Passionarius Galeni and the herbal of Pseudo-Apuleius."[22] Thus, knowledge of the materia medica to be used against sickness in the Middle Ages—before Greco-Arabic medical literature filtered into Europe—depended largely on secondhand compilations based on extant remnants from antiquity.[23] Descriptions of indigenous botanical drugs and directions for their medicinal use were available in a few fragments of ancient medical literature in Latin and, here and there, in books or lists written in Old English, Irish, French and German (including the famous Old English "leech books").

The medicopharmaceutical literature of the monasteries reached its climax in the Latin poem about herbs (entitled *De viribus herbarum,* or *Macer floridus)* probably produced toward the end of the 11th century by Odo of Meune, abbot of Beauprai, and in treatises (*Physica* and *Causae et curae*) by the abbess Hildegard of Bingen (1098–1179). The *Macer floridus* was a popular book and perhaps the first independent herbal to be produced in the medieval West, but its author used older Latin sources, and perhaps also drew on Arabic authors through the writings of Constantine the African. Certainly Hildegard did.[24]

The light of science had burned only gloomily in the Middle Ages. It was oxygen of Arabian origin that would make it bright again.

## The School of Salerno

By their nature, monastic medicine and pharmacy were dogmatic, their most important element being faith. A growing tendency developed among the clergy to discover presumed traces of Christian ideas in some Greco-Roman philosophers and physicians and, later on, even in Arabian masters; and thus they rationalized the use of pagan wisdom in a dogmatic Christian world. This tendency opened the way for the systematic reconquest and acceptance of lost antique knowledge from Arabian sources and later on from the Greek originals that became available.

The 7th to the 12th centuries saw Islam and Christianity in intimate contact in Spain and Sicily. So mainly it was from these two areas that the Latin West drew Greco-Arabian knowledge (see page 28). A little seaside town, Salerno near Naples, was destined to play an important part in this development.

The famous school of Salerno dates from about the 8th century. Probably not of ecclesiastic origin, "the whole character of the school was that of an isolated laical institution, a *civitas Hippocratis,* in the midst of purely clerical foundations, and there is significant silence about Salerno in the ecclesiastic chronicles."[25] Gradually Salerno became the seat of a guild of physicians, attracting not only patients but also students.

Arabic influence there continued to increase. An "antidotarium" by a Jewish physician called Donnolo (913–970) was based on Arabic sources.[26] After Constantine the African had come to Salerno (middle of the 11th century) these infiltrations became fundamental. In him the West had the first of the Latin translators of Arabian manuscripts, who "translated everything that came into his hands. . . ."[27] Constantine thus influenced the European medical world enormously. Instead of mere fragments of ancient wisdom, there were suddenly available systematic and complete works that opened entirely new vistas. The effect became obvious within and outside Salerno.

Even the famous book of materia medica called *Circa instans* (the opening words of the book) may be basically a treatise by Constantine, as revised and enlarged by Mathaeus Platearius (mid-12th century).[28]

Another drug book renowned in the late Middle Ages, the *Antidotarium magnum,* apparently drew heavily on the Arabic drug formulas that Constantine had translated, as well as on late classical and early Byzantine drug formulas. A copy of this "Large Formulary," written in a Swiss monastery about 1190, contains about 1,100 such formulas, some quite complicated, and marginal annotations about them by Mathaeus Platearius.

This rich store of pharmaceutical lore was overshadowed later by what seems largely a modified extract of the *Antidotarium magnum* just mentioned. This small formulary contained only 140 formulas in the mid-13th century. It became identified with the name Nicholas, and since several editors had that same name, the genealogy of the treatise eventually became a puzzle. The *Antidotarium Nicolai,* translated into various languages, by the late 13th century had become the official textbook on materia medica at the University of Paris, and it continued to influence pharmaceutical literature strongly until the 18th century.[29]

Of the knowledge emanating from Salerno, however, the work most influential on health practices of Europeans was of quite different character. A health manual, the so-called *Regimen sanitatis,* consisted of dietetic and pharmaceutical rules in verse form. The original collection of 364 verses presumably was edited and annotated about the year 1300, by one of the most progressive and chemically oriented physicians of the late Middle Ages, Arnald of Villanova. Although perhaps not intended originally for laymen, the treatise soon became popular, and after the invention of printing it appeared in all European languages in upward of 300 editions, accumulating additional verses and commentaries through the decades. The relatively simple and inexpensive pharmaceutical measures advocated in its pages probably was not the least appealing feature of this popular health guide for a continent.[30]

At Salerno the writing and translating, the education of practitioners, the special studies available there, all interacted to earn its repute as the leading European medical center of pre-modern times, which became a model for developments elsewhere.

## UNIVERSITIES EMERGE

The late medieval development of the health sciences in Europe depended ultimately, not upon any single center, but fundamentally upon the key to accumulated knowledge held by the translators. They conveyed Greco-Roman learning and its Arabic transformations into Latin as the common language of learned Europeans. During the 12th and 13th centuries many of the key medical works that we have had occasion to mention became available in manuscript translations. The invention of printing greatly extended Arabian influence on European medicine, and even before the end of the 15th century some key pharmaco-medical works originated or dominated by Arabic thought were off the press—for example, the pseudo-Mesue's *Grabadin,* the *Antidotarium Nicolai,* Abulcasis' *Liber servitoris,* Serapion's *De simplici medicina,* Rhazes' *Liber ad almansorem,* and others.

In other sectors, Europe was undergoing a similar expansion of knowledge and a cultural stimulus. For the most part, it was the teachers at clerical schools (*scholae*) who renewed the study of philosophy and science, despite the heathen origin of the exciting new translations. It seemed a responsibility, however, to prove or to disprove such knowledge from the viewpoint of dogmatic Christianity. Scholarship of a high order thus became dedicated to religious hair-splitting in lieu of more dispassionate research. What has been called medieval Western "scholasticism" was mainly the grandiose attempt of the Christian Church to arrive at a dogmatic system in which science and philosophy—as inherited from antiquity and more recently developed—were harmonized with religious thought. "The doctrines of medical science were a finished book—just as the authorities of the Church were final—they might be commentated, expounded, interpreted . . . but not contradicted nor seriously questioned."[31]

Though under such conditions real scientific progress could not be expected, yet there was an urge for knowledge that expressed itself in the development of places of higher learning. These "universities," although up to the 15th century and sometimes even later under the influence of the Church, were open to the layman for education in the arts and sciences. True, these universities were the main seats of scholasticism, but they were simultaneously the places where new ideas originated and were nurtured when the time was ripe.

By the early 13th century, European institutions of higher learning had been founded at Salerno (medical school, 848; university, 1180), Parma (1025), Paris (university, 1110–1113; with medical school from 1205), Bologna (1110–1113), Oxford (1167) and Cambridge (1209). During the 13th century, 13 more universities were founded (7 in Italy, 2 each in France, Spain and Portugal). The 14th century brought the first Germanic universities (Prague, 1347; Vienna, 1365; Heidelberg, 1385).

Before the Renaissance, pharmacy had not become sufficiently independent as a profession to find a special academic place, except as expressed in materia medica courses of early medical schools. In the 11th century and perhaps even earlier, however, public pharmacies began to appear in Southern Italy and Southern France, and probably in other places. With the transmission of Arabian medicine and polypharmacy to Europe, conditions that caused the creation of public pharmacies in urban centers of the Middle East thus produced similar institutions in European states.

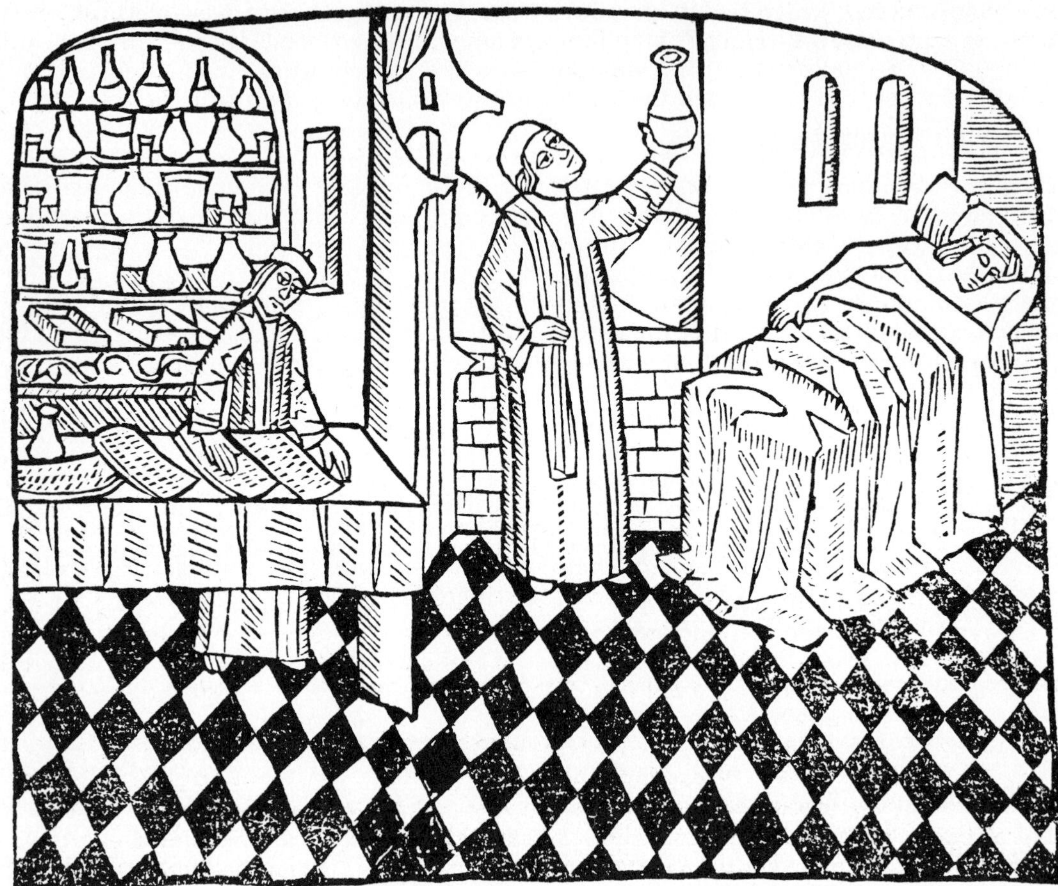

A late-medieval artist carved on a block of wood this scene showing a pharmacist at work (*left*), while a physician examines a urine sample (*center*) from the patient in bed (*right*). Is it the earliest depiction of the concept of the "triad of medical care" to appear in an English book? The illustration introduces Book 7 (medical counsel largely derived from Constantine the African) of the encyclopedia *On the Properties of Things,* by Bartholomew the Englishman, which came off the press at Westminster about 1495. Bartholomew probably wrote his great work between 1230 and 1240. (From the University of Wisconsin Library)

Pharmacy, with its beginnings in the instinctive defense against disease by primitive peoples, had developed under several diverse influences. It was part of the work of priests at first; later it fell among the duties of lay practitioners of medicine and pharmacy combined. It found its own form and expression in the culture of Greece and Rome. However, only under the influence of the Arabic wisdom and pattern did pharmacy take firm root in European soil as a distinctive institution of public welfare, to be respected, regulated and further developed.

## THE BIRTH OF EUROPEAN PROFESSIONAL PHARMACY

Sometime between 1231 and 1240 the German Emperor Frederick II issued an edict that was to be the Magna Charta of the profession of pharmacy.[32] Although promulgated by an emperor of the Holy Roman Empire of the German nation, the edict applied only to that part of his realm called the kingdom of the Two Sicilies.

Three regulations of the edict created pharmacy as an independent branch of a governmentally supervised health service. They won nearly universal application in the centuries that followed. Two additional regulations were highly consequential in the development of pharmacy in most of the countries coming under German politico-cultural influence.

The three essential regulations were:

1. *Separation of the pharmaceutical profession from the medical profession.* This rule, transgressed now and again by both parties, nevertheless constituted the charter of pharmacy as an independent profession. This separation acknowledged the fact that the practice of pharmacy required special knowledge, skill, initiative and responsibility if adequate care of the medicinal needs of the people was to be guaranteed. Forbidding any business relation between physician and pharmacist, the law tried to establish the ethical principles that the only function of the healing professions should be professional service, and that the sick should not be exploited.

2. *Official supervision of pharmaceutical practice.* Thus was acknowledged the importance of pharmacy as a public health service for the protection of the public.

3. *Obligation by oath to prepare drugs reliably, according to skilled art, and in a uniform, suitable quality.* This requirement acknowledges the necessity, not only of reliable remedies, but also of their uniform preparation. Thus it might be considered the first European legal reference to a pharmaceutical standard, a harbinger of later pharmacopeias.

The two sections of the law that did not find general application (especially not in the Anglo-Saxon countries) were:

1. *The limitation of the number of pharmacies*

2. *Governmentally fixed prices for remedies*

The provisions and the context of this legal milestone in the history of pharmacists suggest that a fairly well developed system of public pharmacies must have emerged already in the 13th century. Whether these pharmacies developed from the monastic dispensaries, or from general stores in which the trade with drugs became more and more specialized, has been debated. In the history of the period both trends can be discerned. However, the clerical dispensaries, open to the general public and therefore competitors of the private pharmacies, were transferred to private owners at a relatively late period. In the case of the Swiss city of Basel, "monastic and private pharmacies existed for a long time side by side. . . . Only the discontinuance of the monasteries after the reformation about 1528 caused the monastic dispensaries to disappear." In countries that retained or restored the Catholic faith, as in Bavaria and Austria, such public monastic pharmacies existed until the early 19th century.[33]

The first European nonmonastic pharmacists, like the nonmonastic physicians in the Middle Ages, undoubtedly owed most of their scientific knowledge and practical skill to their clerical predecessors.

> Monasticism has eternally to its credit that it afforded to culture a sanctuary in the midst of barbarism and with far reaching result sowed the seeds of civilization simultaneously with those of the healing art where the Roman legions had never penetrated.[34]

The seeds of pharmacy, growing out of the field of medicine, had found fertile soil in the late Middle ages. The citizen's need for a publicly responsible specialist in drugs lay partly in avoiding exploitation in a field so vulnerable to quacks, and partly in providing expertness in a field so demanding in the range of knowledge and skills required to make and dispense medicaments. A central function of the pharmacist, for 600 years or more, would be particularly to prepare medicaments and to try to assure that each conformed to specifications authorized. The character of the pharmacist's work, and his place in society therefore would be shaped by successive important changes in the character of medicaments themselves, beginning already during the Renaissance.

PART TWO

# The Rise of Professional Pharmacy in Representative Countries of Europe

# 3

# Changing Medicaments and the Modern Pharmacist

### THE IDEA OF THE "RENAISSANCE"

The Renaissance meant a return not only to the original writings of the Greeks but also to Greek spirit, to the esteem of Attic Greeks for individualism and, with this, to their liberty of thought.[1] It meant that fetters imposed on European intellect by the Arabian and clerical scholasticism were removed. It meant the rebirth of independent thought, with the promise and the challenge to the imagination that it offered. It opened new worlds of thought, discovered new horizons, created unexpected possibilities. After Columbus reached America in 1492 this spirit was given opportunity for physical expansion and expression. Those who followed Columbus did so with the creative vigor demanded of them by the richness and the promise of the new world. Vasco de Gama found an all-water route to the East Indies 6 years later in 1498, and the treasures of the Far East were brought closer to eager hands by the discoverers. The introduction of printing with movable type, which came at about this time, brought the knowledge of the new discoveries, inventions and ideas within quick and easy reach.

Now began that admirable intellectual competition of European individuals and peoples that made Europe, small though it was, the dominant continent in the world. As in all fields of science, so in medicine and therapy the new developments fathered a

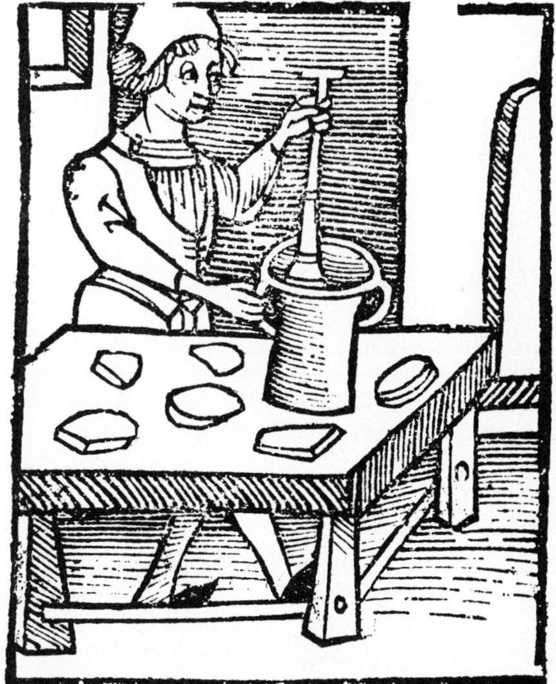

Medicinal chemicals came into wider use internally with the Renaissance. This woodcut from a famous drug book of that time shows a contusion mortar being used to grind up "Armenus," a variety of cupric carbonate, which was then obtained particularly from Armenia. (*Hortus Sanitatis*, Chap. 13, Strasbourg, about 1507; from the University of Wisconsin Library)

number of varying ideas or systems that followed one upon the other. Many of these systems gained international acceptance, influencing the materia medica and, through it, pharmacy.

## PARACELSUS AND CHEMICAL DRUGS

The spirit of the Renaissance permeated European science as well as other intellectual disciplines and led in time to the "scientific revolution" of the 16th and 17th centuries, associated with the names of Copernicus, Vesalius, Galileo, Descartes, Newton, Harvey and others. Gradually and at first cautiously some of the long-established scientific theories came to be challenged. The year 1543 is a particularly important landmark in the history of science, when Nicolaus Copernicus stated (in *De revolutionibus orbium coelestium*), contrary to then current belief, that the earth moves around the sun, and Andraeus Vesalius (in *De humani corporis fabrica*) questioned certain of the anatomical views of Galen.

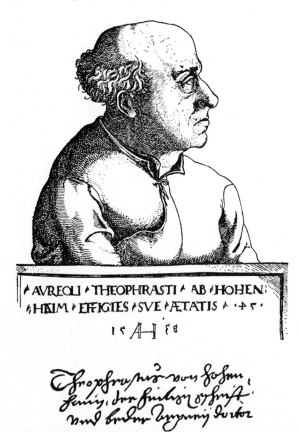

The 16th century produced another important figure who performed an analogous revolutionary deed in medicine and pharmacy by attacking old theories and opening the door to new findings. He was the Swiss physician Theophrastus Bombastus von Hohenheim, called Paracelsus (1493–1541).[2] Before Paracelsus, various modifications of two main hypotheses concerning pathologies played their part again and again: the humoral and the solidar pathologies (see pp. 17 & 19). Paracelsus introduced instead the concept of the body as a chemical laboratory. As a result of advocacy by Paracelsus and his followers, the internal use of chemical remedies (mineral salts and acids, and substances prepared by chemical processes such as distillation and extraction), which had occurred sporadically before him, was made a matter of principle and study. He coined the famous phrase that "it is not the task of alchemy to make gold, to make silver, but to prepare medicines."

Paracelsus opposed the concept of humoral pathology and, especially, the systematization into which it had been pressed by Galen and Avicenna. In every way possible he tried to deprive these two main representatives of

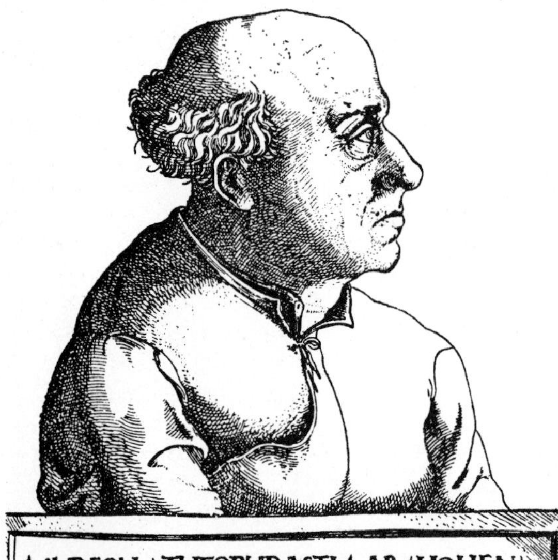
AVREOLI THEOPHRASTI AB HOHEN:
HEIM EFFIGIES SVE ÆTATIS

This portrait of Paracelsus conveys the rugged, bold quality of his thought and action. It is a copper engraving made (1538) toward the end of Paracelsus' life, probably based on sketches of Paracelsus himself by A. Hirschvogel. Below the portrait is his autograph, reproduced from a letter, which may be translated, "Theophrastus von Hohenheim, Doctor of Theology and of both Medicine and Surgery." (From Stillman, J. M.: Theophrastus Bombastus von Hohenheim called Paracelsus, p. 162, Chicago, Open Court)

Greco-Roman and Arabic medicine and pharmacy of the esteem in which they were held. In 1527 he started his lectures at Basel with a startling attack against the medical tenets of his time.

"Only a few," he said, "practiced medicine successfully. Too closely did we cling to the words of Hippocrates, Galen and Avicenna, as if they were oracles. It is not the adornment by titles, eloquence, linguistics and book wisdom that makes the physician, but the knowledge of the secrets of nature." Paracelsus promised to read about practical and theoretic medicine according to his own notes, which he assured his students he did not "beggarly collect out of Hippocrates and Galenos," but had taken "from the best possible teacher, to wit, from my own experience and experimentation." He declared that "there will be no reference to complexions and humors which, while thought to be the cause of all diseases, have widely prohibited the understanding of them, their origin and their critical course."[3]

In his own speculation on the basic nature of matter he did not drop the idea of the four "Aristotelian" elements as such. However, Paracelsus considered them as "also consisting of the . . . tria prima."[4] These three primary principles, "sulphur, mercury and salt" were by no means simply identical with the substances generally understood by these names. Sulfur represented the principle of combustibility; mercury that of liquidity and volatility; salt, being permanent and resisting the action of fire, represented that of stability. In Paracelsus' own words, "all that fumes and disappears in vapors is Mercury; all that burns and is consumed is Sulphur; all that is ashes is also Salt."

Disease was caused, according to Paracelsus, by a local separation of one of these three principles from the other two. While this view may not seem very different from the old concept of imbalance of the humors, it did have the advantage of emphasizing the localized nature of disease. Disease was not viewed, as in the Galenic system, as being a disequilibrium of the entire body, but was believed to be localized in a given organ. Paracelsus also stressed the need for a treatment that would be specific for that particular disease. The action of a remedy, he felt, did not depend upon qualities such as moistness, but on its *specific* healing virtue, which was determined by its chemical properties.

Pharmacy was enriched by Paracelsus, not only by the introduction into internal therapy of quite a number of chemicals, but also by his endeavor to extract the "healing virtue" from the more or less inert substances in which he thought it to be hidden. This idea led Paracelsus to prepare alcoholic tinctures and extracts, essences and—supposedly the most essential products—the so-called "quintessences." According to the Paracelsian concept, tinctures as well as extracts originally were considered to be "chemicals" or, to use a more descriptive early synonym, as "spagyric" products—from the Greek words *spao* (to separate) and *ageiro* (to assemble).

By emphasizing those aspects of Paracelsus' theories that led to advances in medicine and pharmacy, we risk making him seem too "modern" and "scientific." It should be emphasized that his system of medicine was embedded within a larger religious, mystical philosophy (which is too complex to be considered here). For example, his conviction that there was a unity in the universe, which tied all things together, led him to believe that the heavenly bodies influence the organs of the body and the remedies used against disease.

Paracelsus' search for effective remedies was thus not carried out on strictly empirical and scientific grounds.

In this light, his often ridiculed revival of the old theory of "signatures" becomes understandable. Paracelsus was a faithful believer, to whom a benevolent Providence was an indisputable dogma. He was not surprised to find Nature hinting at the therapeutic bounty of her store of raw materials, sig-

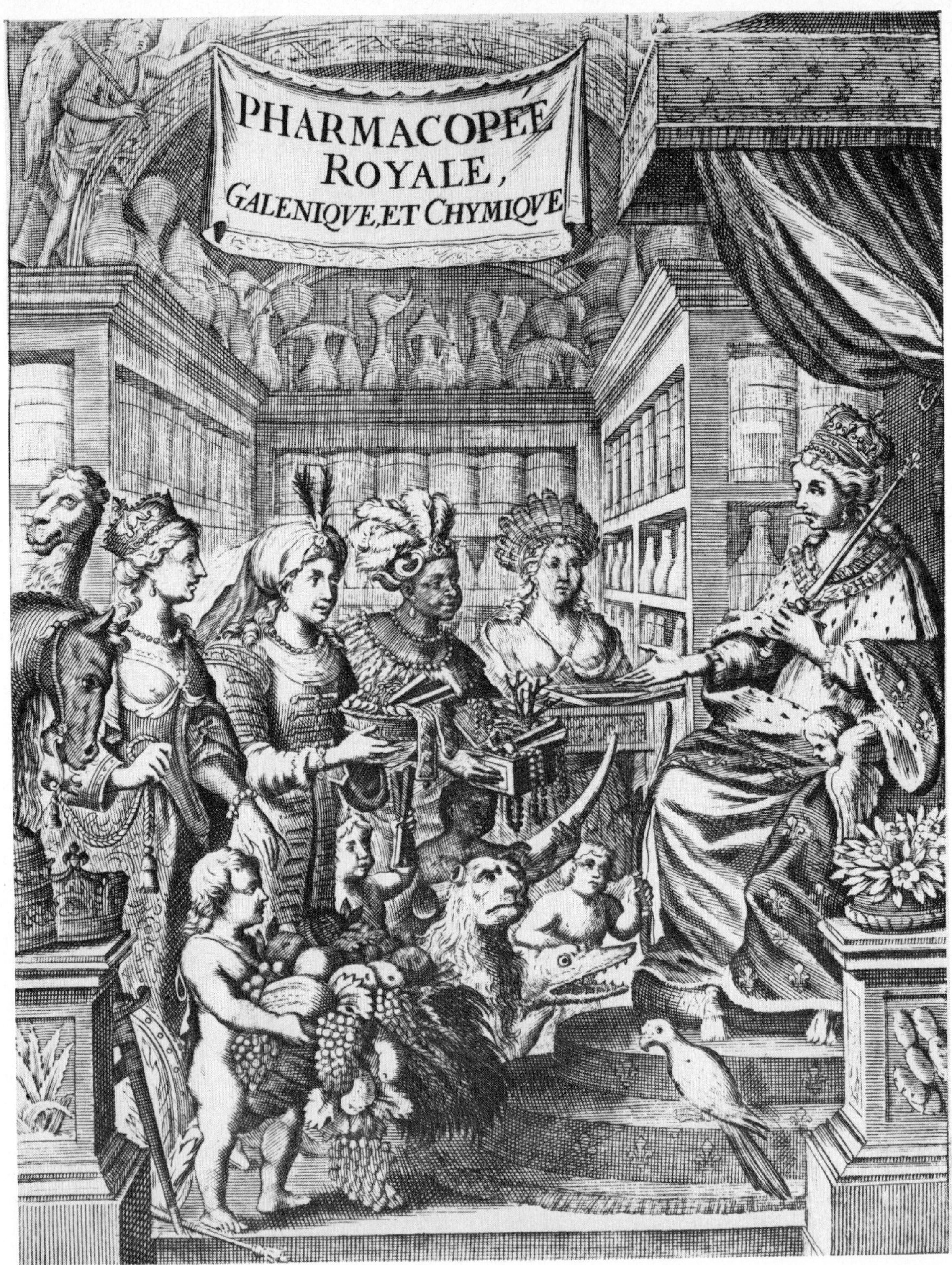
PHARMACOPÉE
ROYALE,
GALENIQUE, ET CHYMIQUE

nified by characteristics of their outer appearance (e.g., turmeric, or yellow root, to be used against jaundice). What else were these but specifics "signed" by the Lord himself, with direct designations as to their specific usefulness? Far from being strange to the Paracelsian way of thought, the theory of "signatures" offered him a welcome divine confirmation of his thinking.

While Paracelsus' relation to the rise of pharmaceutical chemistry is complex and easily oversimplified, it can be said that he did influence tremendously the transformation of pharmacy from a profession based primarily on botanic science to one based on chemical science. If Paracelsus himself was not the most important innovator, it was he who inspired the "Paracelsians" of the subsequent century to bring to therapy a whole new outlook by the chemical procedures that they developed and by the definition of chemical drugs that thus were created.[5] Under the influence of the followers of Paracelsus, many chemical remedies were introduced into the pharmacopeias of Western Europe in the 17th century.[6]

## IATROCHEMISTRY AFFECTS PHARMACY

Paracelsus was a mystic as well as a revolutionary empiricist. He not only believed in the doctrine of the signatures, but assumed the presence of a mysterious vital force. He called it *archaeus,* endowed with the power of dominating all processes of life. This idea of a vital force and the concept that sickness reflects chemical changes in the body produced by a morbid mood of the *archaeus* are expressed still more definitely in the medical system of the great Flemish physician Jean Baptist van Helmont (1577–1644). He is famous as the discoverer of carbonic acid, which he called *gas sylvestre,* thus originating the concept and the term "gas." However, the real founder of the doctrine of "iatrochemistry" was François de le Boë Sylvius (1614–1672). His theory was a kind of compromise between humoral pathology and the ideas of Paracelsus.

The vantage point of de le Boë Sylvius' theories is what he called "fermentation." He believed that food is transformed through saliva and a ferment secreted from the pancreas, and that blood becomes the life-maintaining substance he thought it to be through certain ferments carried into the bloodstream from the gall bladder and the lymph glands. These continuous transformations, influenced by the body temperature (*calor innatus*) and the spirits of life (*spiritus*), result in either alkaline or acid end products. If both are in the right proportion qualitatively as well as quantitatively, the person concerned is healthy.

Disease, on the contrary, is caused by an "acrimony" or excess of either the acid or the alkaline substances, or their being at a wrong place. According to iatrochemical theory, this acrimony leads to a change in the blood, the bile or the lymph. Hence all diseases were subdivided into those based on alkaline or an acid acrimony. The drugs used in treating them had to be of a contrasting nature, either acid or alkaline.

This medico-chemical theory became naturally the basis for preparing new chemical drugs. It was welcomed still more as a convenient guide for selecting from among a myriad of drugs already known, and as an explanation of their empirically observed effects.

←

The medicinal bounty of nature has always impressed pharmacists and laymen alike. On this allegorical title page, angels (*top*) hang out a banner proclaiming that it ornaments the Royal Pharmacopeia (1672) prepared by the French pharmacist Moise Charas. Below, the royal profession of pharmacy on her throne receives the products of the animal, the vegetable and the mineral kingdoms from representatives of the continents (*l. to r.*) Europe, Asia, Africa and the Americas. (A humanized camel, *far left,* is more interested in looking critically at the reader!)

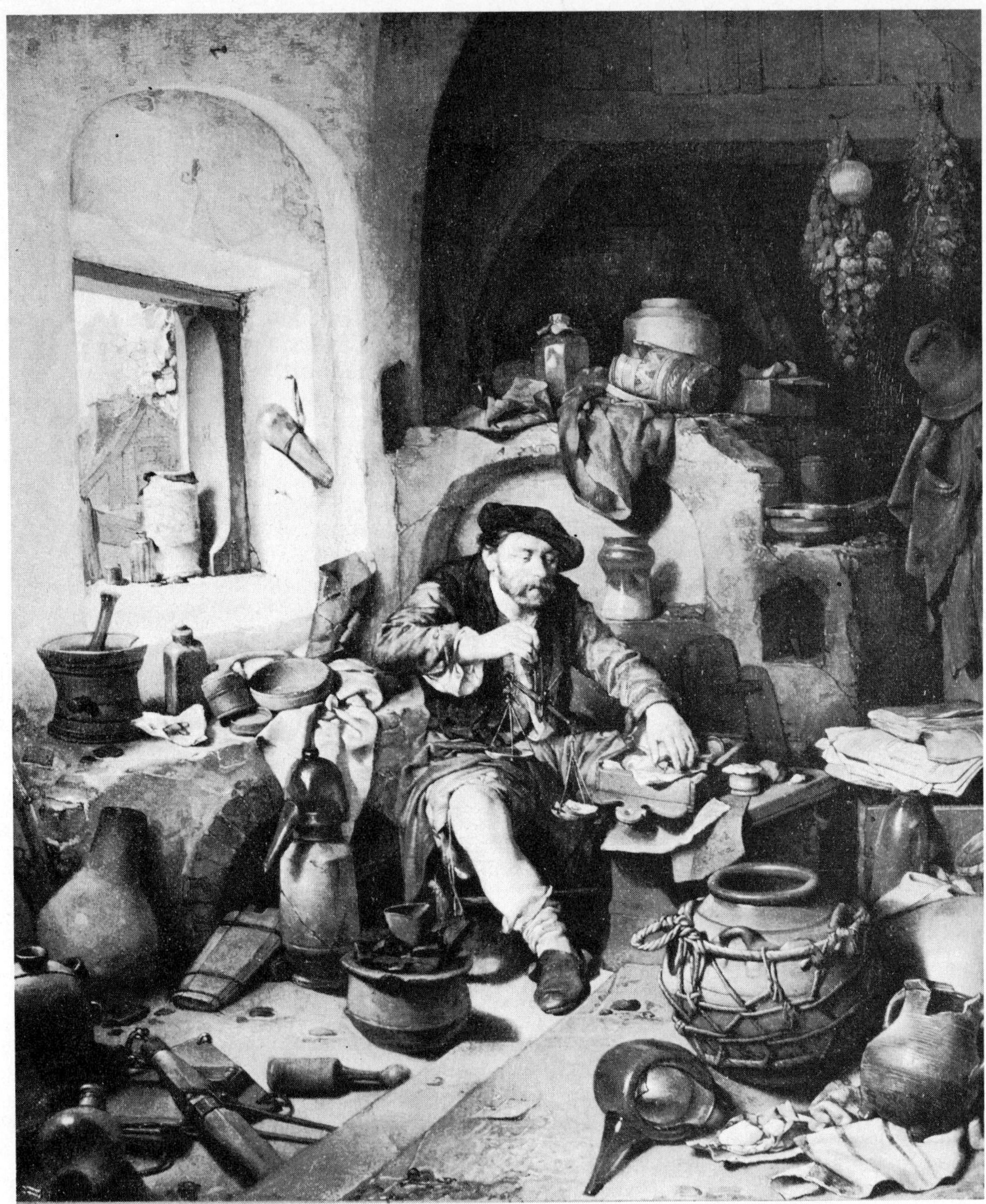

A needy European alchemist sits among a litter of equipment, weighing out a chemical for one of his experiments in making gold. A traditionally secret and nonscientific art, alchemy remained foreign to both the spirit and the methods of modern pharmacy or chemistry. Although no forerunner of the pharmacist, the alchemist transmitted or invented equipment and technics of value to pharmaceutical development. (17th-century painting by Cornelis P. Bega of The Netherlands, in the Fisher Collection, Fisher Scientific Company, Pittsburgh)

This felt need for an adequate explanation of known effects attracted a number of physicians of the 17th and the early 18th centuries to another hypothesis, the iatrophysical or mechanical theory, developed some decades before de le Boë Sylvius' hypothesis by the Italian physician Santorio Santorio (1561–1636). It was based on the concept of the body as a kind of engine, following mainly physical laws.[7] This outlook led Santorio to invent the first instrument intended to measure body temperature, a predecessor to our clinical thermometer, and to make the first systematic attempt to explain, by as exact means as possible, what we call metabolism.

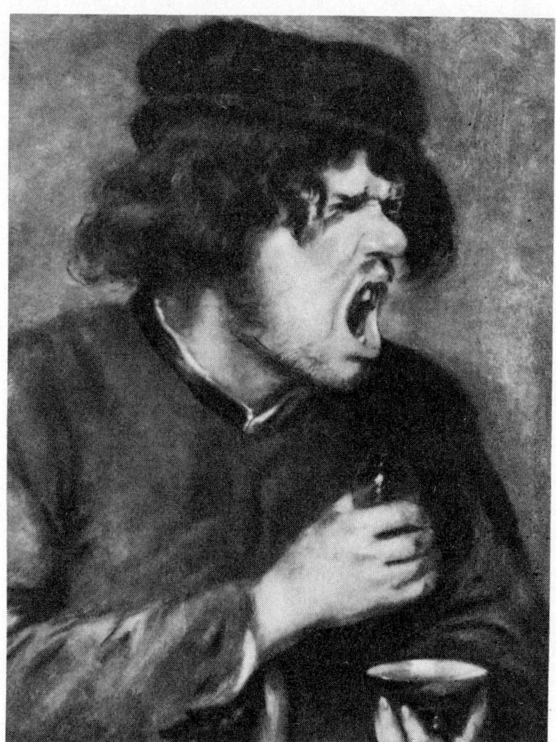

This 17th-century painting conveys vividly the reaction of a rustic patient to the copious, unpleasant draught that one could expect to receive from a pharmacist before investigations had yielded the active constituents of drugs in more concentrated, palatable and reliable forms. (From 1941 calendar of the Nederlandsche Maatschappij ter Bevordering der Pharmacie; original canvas by Adriaen Brouer located at Frankfurt am Main)

## DRUGS FROM THE NEW WORLD

Another important factor influencing European therapeutics in the 16th and 17th centuries was the introduction of many new drugs from foreign lands, particularly the Americas. The most important of these drugs were cinchona and ipecac, but many other plant drugs of the New World—such as curare, tobacco, cascara sagrada, and coca—also found their way into European medicine. Ackerknecht has commented that these exotic drugs "undermined ancient tradition in no less an effective way than the cures of Paracelsus."[8] It became obvious that the book of Dioscorides and other Graeco-Roman and Arabic works did not contain all of the drug lore of the world, and the "specific" action of drugs such as cinchona (which apparently cured only the so-called intermittent fevers) was difficult to fit into the traditional Galenic categories.

## A CENTURY OF SPECULATIVE THEORIES

The attacks upon the Galenic tradition in the 16th and 17th centuries had destroyed its monopoly upon therapeutic thought, although Galen still retained a significant influence upon medicine. The humoral theory had not been replaced, however, by any systematic theory of pathology and therapeutics having universal acceptance. The 18th century saw various attempts to create comprehensive medical systems, however, producing theories that were certain to be speculative and debatable, since the health professions still lacked experimental technics for establishing the site and the mechanism of drug action.

A new kind of solidar pathology was announced in Halle by Friedrich Hoffmann, the

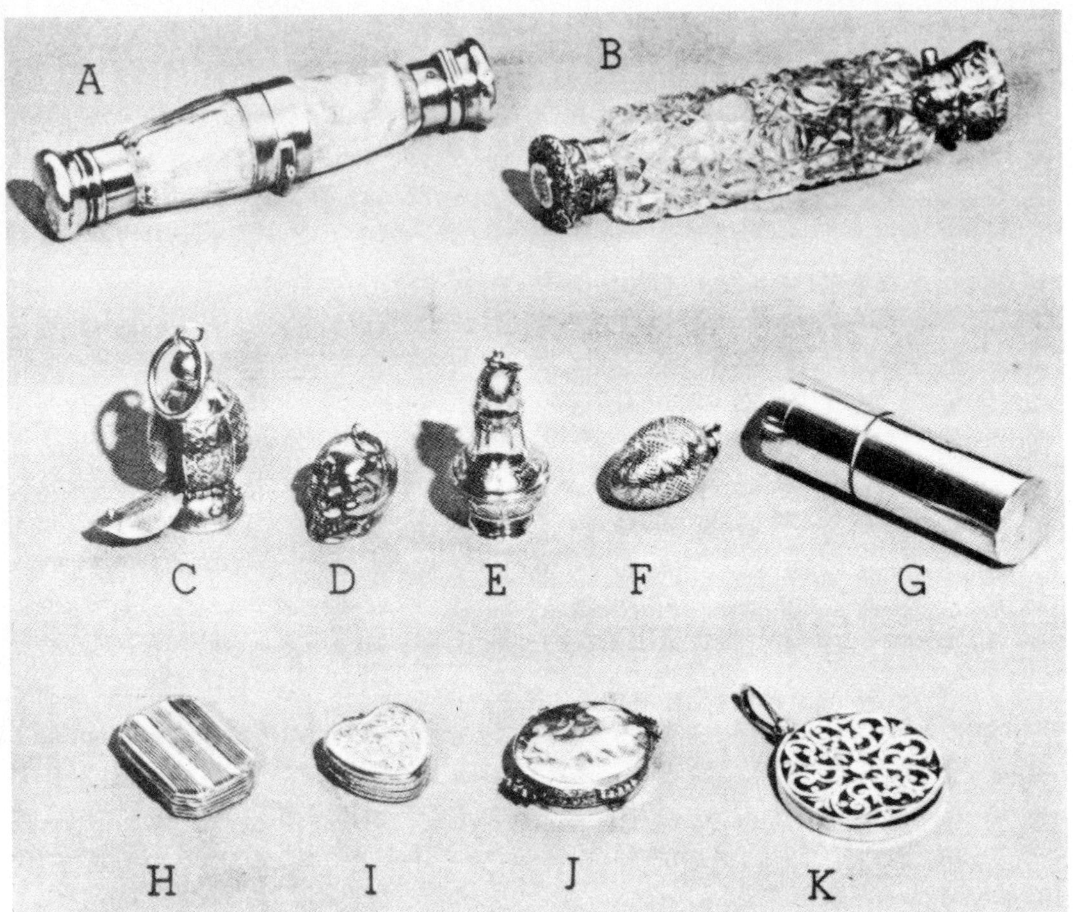


Elegant containers made more impressive the old drugs whose actual effects were usually doubtful or nonspecific. Supposedly anti-infective aromatics intended to neutralize the "ill air" were carried in containers such as the multicompartment pomander (*C*), which held ambergris (16th century), and other pomanders (*D, E, F*) of later vintage. The vinaigrettes (*H, I, J*) were small silver boxes that held a bit of sponge charged with aromatic vinegar (early 19th century). The locket (*K*) contained camphor. The silver pill box (*G*) is a rare example (ca. 1800), but pocket "pill boxes" have never gone completely out of style. Bottles (*A, B*) for smelling salts (ammonium carbonate with lavender-scented ammonia water) were popular when swooning was fashionable. (Artifacts from the Drake Collection, Academy of Medicine, Toronto, Ont.; *see* Drake, T. G. H.: J. Hist. Med. *15*:31–44, 1960; photograph from University of Wisconsin.)

famous inventor of many remedies (1660–1742). According to him life depends—as the ancient Soranos assumed—on a normal tension of the solid parts of the body. However, unlike Soranos, Hoffmann taught that these solid parts are not the ducts but the fibers. He assumed a hypothetical ether-like fluid acting through the nervous system upon the fibers and keeping them in a state of partial tonic contraction, and also keeping the humors of the body in the motion necessary for life.[9]

This materialistic theory had its antipode

in the ideology of Ernst Stahl (1660–1734), at Halle. His concept of illness and therapy was named *animismus,* because Stahl considered the soul (Latin: *anima*) the highest principle of life, balancing all bodily functions by a distinct rhythmic movement. This movement produced a certain tension called tonus. The individual was ill if this tonus was not normal. The task of remedies was to help the anima to restore normal tonus.

Similar to the animism of Stahl was the "vitalism" of the Frenchman P. J. Barthez, in which the soul was replaced by the so-called vital principle (1778).

In England two theories in particular gained wide acknowledgment. (1) William Cullen (1710–1790) postulated that all bodily functions are regulated by a so-called nervous principle, which in cases of illness tries to restore normal conditions by convulsion or by atony. Therefore, the remedies had to be either irritating or emollient. (2) The hypothesis of the Scottish physician John Brown (1735–1788), a pupil of Cullen, was that not the nervous principle itself but the stimuli that set it in motion are decisive for health or sickness. Normal life is a harmony between excitability and the incessant external and internal stimuli acting on the body; all diseases thus have their final cause in a disproportion between the excitability of the organism and the stimuli (too strong or too feeble) that affect it.

## HOMEOPATHY AS AN EXAMPLE OF MEDICAL SECTARIANISM

Speculative medical systems did not completely disappear, of course, with the end of the 18th century. While attempts to generate a comprehensive system of medicine, based upon a monistic pathology, were perhaps less common in the 19th century, a number of medical sects, based upon unorthodox and highly speculative theories, grew up to challenge the prevailing therapeutic practices of orthodox practitioners. One of the most interesting of these sects, particularly from a pharmaceutical point of view, was homeopathy, which has been described as "an offshoot of 18th century theorizing."[10] This peculiar pharmacologic system was proposed around the turn of the 19th century by the German physician Samuel Hahnemann (1755–1843). Somewhat later this system found wide acknowledgment and sectarian cultivation, particularly in the United States (see Chap. 11).[11]

*The "Simile" Principle.* The general idea of homeopathy is to incite the defense mechanisms of the body by adequate irritation, rather than to attack the disease as such. This leads to the *simile* principle, which states that disease is cured by remedies that produce symptoms resembling the disease in question. Drugs are tested on healthy individuals to determine the type of symptoms they produce, and thus their therapeutic indications. Hahnemann called his theory "homeopathy" (from the Greek *homoion*-similar) as contrasted to traditional therapy, based upon the ancient principle of using remedies with properties opposite to the symptoms of the disease, which he called "allopathy" (from the Greek *alloin* - different).[12]

*Minute Doses.* This irritation concept also provides a rationale for the use of astonishingly minute doses in homeopathic practice. In the late 19th century this application of very small doses for the purpose of irritation found support in the so-called "biologic fundamental law" promulgated by the German physicians Rudolf Arndt and Hugo Schulz. This "law" states that "minute stimuli initiate the activity of living organisms and those of medium strength promote it, while strong stimuli slow it down and very strong ones stop it."

Naturally, the question concerns the degree of "minuteness" that still allows for an inciting effect, and it is understood that dilutions transgressing the limits drawn by modern chemistry and physics are beyond scientific evaluation and hence beyond consideration.

In his prescriptions Hahnemann himself insisted on the use of only a single active drug at a time. His followers often have been less rigorous in regard to the prescribing of mixtures and compounded drugs. Another pharmaceutical principle required that the homeopathic tinctures be made from fresh crude drugs (not dried). Because of such special requirements,[13] homeopathic drugs in the United States often have been dispensed by homeopathic physicians themselves or, in metropolitan areas, through special pharmacies.

Writing of Hahnemann's homeopathy, the medical historian Erwin Ackerknecht concludes: "The dogmatism of his system separated it from the main stream of scientific development, and now it lives on as a cult with a relatively small following."[14]

Other medical sects, such as "Thomsonianism" and "eclecticism" (discussed in Chap. 11), also waned as the 19th century progressed and medical science advanced, but unorthodox medical sects still have not completely disappeared from the health-care scene even today (witness chiropractic).

## BACKGROUND TO MODERN PHARMACY

An important advance of medical science during the first half of the 19th century, in pathologic anatomy, focused medical thought on the localized changes revealed by careful observations and the advancing technics of microscopy. A brilliant line of investigators begins with Morgagni (1682–1771) of Bologna, continues with Corvisart (1755–1821) and Laennec (1781–1826) of Paris and is brought to its culmination by Rokitansky (1804–1878) and Skoda (1805–1881) of Vienna.[15]

According to this school of thought, maladies were localized in the ill parts of the body and made obvious by anatomic changes. There were generalized diseases too, their habitat being the blood. Nevertheless, even these general diseases were supposed to have a tendency to localize themselves. Thus there were no sick individuals but only distinct, anatomically demonstrable pathologies. The consequence of this theory was to relegate therapeutic efforts more and more to the knife of the surgeon and to condemn or at least to deprecate internal medication that was of necessity more general in its effects. By mid-century this spirit of skepticism became an actual therapeutic nihilism.[16]

The man whose work crowned the development of solidar pathology, Rudolf Virchow (1821–1902), founded cellular pathology, which has continued to dominate medical biology to the present day. His theory, briefly stated, is as follows: The cell is the bearer of life. Disease is the reaction of the cell to abnormal stimulation. According to Virchow's own statement, "the organism is not a unified but a social arrangement." The influence of the work of Virchow

> . . . enabled doctors to realize that the point of onslaught of remedies in the organism are not the organs in general but the cells. We now know that there are peculiar affinities between particular cells and particular chemical substances.[17]

On this ground pharmacy and drug therapy took on renewed meaning and purposefulness, although it has been pointed out that cellular theory did not truly make its impact felt on therapeutics until the chemotherapeutic work of Paul Ehrlich.[18] Once all but annihilated by Viennese nihilism, internal therapy again commanded respect. As cellular pathology was joined with the new chemistry and bacteriology, experimental pharmacology began to chart the world of drug therapy during the second half of the 19th century in terms that we understand today.

### Immunology and Medical Bacteriology

The scientific basis for massive conquests of disease during the past century had a remarkable empiric beginning in the field of immunology.

The first disease against which an artificial immunity was produced was smallpox. For many hundreds of years people in Eastern countries, such as China, had practiced inoculation with smallpox. This practice involves the artificial communication of the disease from one individual to another, for example by scratching a person's arm with a needle that has been dipped in infectious material from a smallpox pustule on the body of a victim of the disease. The hope was that the inoculated person would thus contract only a mild case of smallpox and thereafter would be immune to the disease. The technique of inoculation with smallpox, which was introduced into Western Europe in the 18th century, is, of course, a risky procedure. In some cases it led to a severe, even fatal, case of the disease.

A far safer method was developed by the English physician Edward Jenner (1749–1823). Leaning on earlier empirical observations by European farmers and on his own experiments, he reported in 1798 on his success in inducing in humans the harmless cowpox, which he found produced an immunity against smallpox. Jenner's technique of "vaccination" (from the Latin *vacca*, cow) was at first criticized on such grounds as the belief that the transference of diseased animal material into humans had a debasing influence, but eventually the procedure was widely adopted.

Immunology could only be placed on a scientific basis after the development of the germ theory of disease. While certain individuals had suggested since the 17th century that microorganisms might be the cause of disease, this theory did not receive widespread acceptance until the French chemist Louis Pasteur (1822–1897) and the German physician Robert Koch (1843–1910) had provided convincing evidence to support it. Pasteur's demonstration that microorganisms could spoil wine and beer, and could cause diseases in silkworms, led the British surgeon Joseph Lister in the 1860's to introduce antisepsis (through the use of disinfectants in the treatment of wounds). Later this was followed by asepsis. Pasteur also developed methods of producing weakened or attenuated cultures of pathogenic microorganisms (vaccines) for immunization purposes. Robert Koch, who developed the basic techniques of modern bacteriology, isolated the anthrax bacillus in 1876 and the tubercle bacillus in 1882; and he clearly established that diseases in higher organisms, including man, could be caused by microorganisms.

Another important facet of immunology is serum therapy. We are indebted to the German physician Emil von Behring (1854–1917) for the knowledge of how to produce antitoxins in the blood serum of animals by immunizing them with specific toxins. In the early 1890's, von Behring and his colleagues developed an antitoxin against diphtheria, thus greatly reducing the mortality rate from this dreaded childhood disease.

Immunization procedures have since been developed against many other diseases, such as cholera, plague, poliomyelitis and measles.[19] What this development means to pharmacy becomes evident from the fact that the so-called biological products—serums, vaccines, toxins, antitoxins, etc.—have become one of the important parts of the responsibility and the service of the pharmacist. Moreover, it is now difficult to imagine the practice of pharmacy or medicine without the variety of medicated and sterilized gauzes, cottons and other surgical materials, and of sterile parenteral medications, the manufacture and use of which are based on the principles of antisepsis and asepsis.

## Chemotherapy Ascendant

During our own century drug therapy has been unfolding largely under the banner of "chemotherapy," which rests on the theory of relationships between chemical constitution and pharmacologic action. Paul Ehrlich (1854–1915) was the founder of this new concept and line of development (although his work was, of course, based upon the many scientific advances during the century pre-

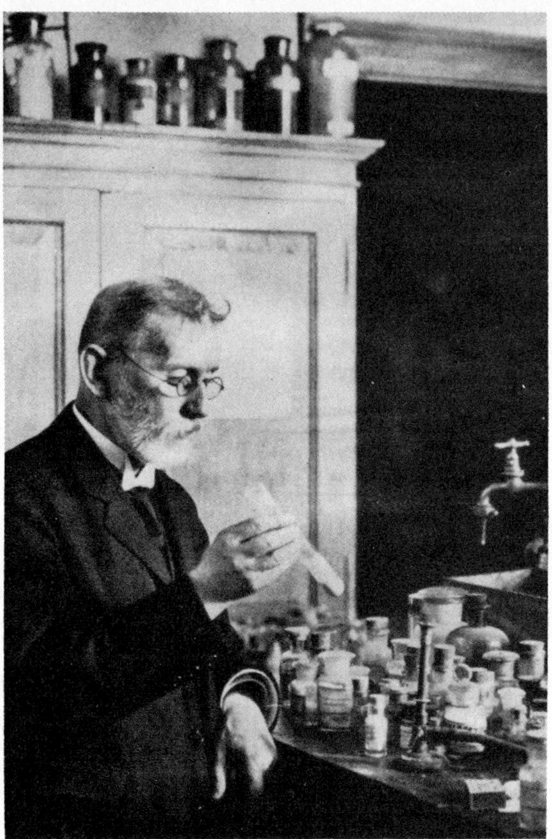

The principal founder of chemotherapy, Paul Ehrlich (1854–1915), at work in his laboratory in Germany. (From National Library of Medicine)

ceding him).[20] Although a number of useful drugs had been synthesized in the late 19th century, these agents had provided symptomatic rather than curative treatment (e.g., analgesics). In modern chemotherapy we see in a sense the realization of the dream of the Paracelsians (the preparation of chemical remedies specific for particular diseases).

Ehrlich's approach was based on the belief that it should be possible to treat an infectious disease by administering a toxic chemical that had great affinity for a pathogenic microorganism but little affinity for human tissues. After it had been shown in 1905 that atoxyl (an organic arsenic compound) could destroy the trypanosomes that caused sleeping sickness, Ehrlich and his coworkers synthesized and tested hundreds of related arsenic compounds. Their aim was to find a substance that had the trypanocidal activity of atoxyl but was devoid of its damaging action on the optic nerve of higher animals. Clinical trials in 1910 showed that the 606th compound to be prepared and tested, arsphenamine (tradenamed "Salvarsan") was effective in treating sleeping sickness and also syphilis. The success of Salvarsan, in spite of its serious side effects, led to a great deal of optimism about the prospects for chemotherapy.

This direct attack on morbific agents in the body by means of chemicals, without doing unbearable harm to the cells containing the microbes or to the body at large, was called "chemotherapy" by Ehrlich. There is a tendency to extend use of the term, originally meant only for internal treatment, to include external attack on microbes as well. The discoverer of penicillin, Alexander Fleming, favored (1946) the use of the term chemotherapy "to cover any treatment in which a chemical is administered in a manner directly injurious to the microbes infecting the body. In this latter sense antiseptic treatment comes under chemotherapy—call it local chemotherapy if you like."[21]

After a frustrating quarter century, during which the concept and the methods of Ehrlich could not be made to yield another major breakthrough, the announcement came from Gerhard Domagk in 1935 of the curative action of Prontosil (4-sulfonamid-2′,4′-diaminoazobenzol) against streptococcal infection in man—a success foreshadowed 3 years earlier by tests in mice.[22] Like arsphenamine, this compound was a chemotherapeutic specific. It was soon shown that Prontosil was broken down in the body to produce sulfanilamide, which was the active disease-fighting agent. A series of related compounds (sulfonamides or "sulfa drugs"), effective against various bacterial infections, were synthesized by modification of the parent compound, sulfanilamide. The sulfonamides opened up the area of antibacterial therapy; previous chemotherapeutic agents (such as Salvarsan) were effective only against protozoa-like microorganisms such as trypanosomes. In America by 1955 the official compendia of drug standards recognized no less than 13 sulfonamides, not counting simple variations of the basic drugs.[23]

Repeated success in the "sulfa era" is important not only for the specific diseases brought under control but for the tremendous stimulus and the hints it gave to research workers and the resultant industrial optimism that led to heavier investment in pharmaceutical research.

Despite optimism and progress concerning theories of relationship between chemical structures and pharmacologic actions, the role of empiricism and quasi-accidental discovery have been displaced only slowly from pharmaceutical research since the time of Paul Ehrlich. Evidence in point may be seen in the massive random screening programs which were set up following the sulfanilamide discoveries. This effort, especially directed toward finding effective antimalarial and anticarcinogenic compounds, has yielded valuable new drugs.

The fruitfulness of chemotherapy as originally conceived pointed the way toward additional discoveries and understanding of drug action since the 1930's (even though many of these are used beyond the area of infectious diseases), such as the new diuretic, antihypertensive and psychotropic drugs.

Meanwhile, newer theoretic concepts have illuminated probable relationships between chemical structure and biologic activity, but their predictive value has been rather limited. In fact, it was stated by one prominent drug researcher in 1959 that recent major discoveries in medicinal chemistry owe little to such concepts.[24] One dramatic illustration of this disconcerting circumstance can be found in the antibiotic drugs.

The story of the exciting accident and the perceptive observation through which Alexander Fleming discovered penicillin (1928) is one well known. Equally remarkable was the wait until other Britons (Chain, Florey and Heatley in 1939) sensed the import of the discovery clearly enough to take up a vigorous investigation, which brought the drug into therapy—with an important assist from American pharmaceutical industry, universities and government—in time to meet urgent military demands of the early 1940's.[25]

Less well known is the fact that the term (and the vague notion) of "antibiosis" occurred to the Frenchman Paul Vuillemin as early as 1889. Twelve years earlier still, Louis Pasteur himself mentioned the phenomenon of antagonism between living organisms. A whole series of half-forgotten observations of antibiotic action among micro-organisms had come out of European laboratories before the turn of the century; even the effect of a *Penicillium* mold was recorded in the 19th century.[26] However, it was the observation by Fleming that proved to be consequential, in that it gave the Oxford group headed by Florey and Chain the direct lead they needed to isolate the little penicillin that was given to a London policeman on February 12, 1941.

Penicillin represented the most startling advance in medicine and pharmacy since the initial success of Ehrlich, and opened up the "era of antibiotics." Discoveries in the antibiotic field have been based almost exclusively upon an empirical search for naturally-occurring products, rather than upon synthetic work involving structure-activity relationships. This fact is underscored by the frantic testing of thousands of antimicrobial substances in the ensuing decade, of which less than ten found noteworthy use in therapy.[27] However, the practical value of these few antibiotics has improved the life chance of the human race, first notably extended by the American discovery of streptomycin by Selman Waksman and associates in 1944 and then within a decade by the wider resource of broad-spectrum antibiotics, which is still being explored.

It has been said that "chemotherapy" is a revival of the "iatrochemistry" of old—based upon the doctrines of the Paracelsians and systematized by François de le Boë Sylvius, but this certainly is not the case. De le Boë Sylvius' system was another attempt at a scheme of comprehending and explaining the whole of medicine. Above all, it was a medical speculation, although using the contemporary chemical concepts as its basis. Ehrlich's chemotherapy (unlike iatrochemistry) was restricted to a special area of chemico-biological attack, in which chemical considerations play the dominant part. The term "chemotherapy" itself points to the distinction, giving chemistry precedence over therapy, just as the term "iatrochemistry" gives preference to *iatros* (the physician), i.e., to the medical side of the concept thus designated.

The cellular pathology of Virchow, which provided the ground on which chemotherapy developed, may be regarded as a European attempt to formulate a general explanation of the fundamental nature of health and sickness and, by implication, to give a guidepost for therapy. However, recent years have brought several more specific medical, medico-chemical and biologic theories and discoveries that, like the aforementioned immunology and medical bacteriology, have a great influence on therapy and, hence, on pharmacy.

### Vitamins and Hormones

Among modern discoveries prominent places are held by the avitaminoses—diseases caused by a lack of some of the substances found in food (substances now known under the name of vitamins)—and, furthermore, by the regulative effect of the hormones.

The word "vitamin" derives from the Latin vita (life) and amine, the chemical class to which the inventor of the term (1912) erroneously considered the vitamins to belong. The many-branched research on the vitamins came largely only in our own century, because the earlier blinding revelation of medical bacteriology had made it difficult to grasp, in all its far-reaching consequences, the concept of disease as caused by the *absence* of something rather than by the presence of infectious organisms.[28] Since 1913, the United States and England have contributed the most to newer knowledge of the vitamins. Chemists associated with the agricultural experiment stations in Wisconsin and Connecticut played instrumental roles in the identification of the first vitamins, "fat-soluble A" and "water-soluble B." The vitamins have been found in foodstuffs of both vegetable and animal origin and have been synthesized in growing number.[29]

The word "hormone" is taken from the Greek, meaning "to excite." The hormones, products of the glands of internal secretion, became of practical importance in therapeutics only after experiments of a Franco-American in the 1880's, the physiologist C. E. Brown-Séquard. With the unfolding of endocrinology, a few endocrine extracts (e.g., suprarenin and thyroiodin) were made already in the 19th century, but, like vitamin therapy, effective hormonal therapy is mainly a research child of our own century. The first hormone to be isolated in pure form was adrenaline (epinephrine) in 1901. A cornerstone in the development of hormonal therapy was the discovery of insulin by the Canadian physician F. G. Banting, in collaboration with McLeod, Best and Collip in 1922.[30] Its manufacture on a large scale was made possible by the far-sighted assistance given to these scientists by an American pharmaceutical firm, Eli Lilly and Company. This firm developed the processes for mass production and put the experience thus obtained at the disposal of other manufacturers who agreed to meet established standards and to submit the products to controlling tests. Thyroxin was isolated from the thyroid gland in 1915 (E. C. Kendall of the Mayo Foundation). More recently, the so-called "sex hormones" have gained therapeutic importance. The first naturally-occurring androgenic hormone to be obtained in crystalline form was isolated from male urine in 1931 (Butenandt and Tscherning). The hormones from animal sources have been, like the vitamins, synthesized in increasing number.

Another important outgrowth of hormone research was the development of hormonal oral contraceptives, which are synthetic modifications of naturally-occurring steroid hormones. The first clinical trials of oral contraceptives were begun in 1956 by Gregory Pincus and his colleagues. Since the first oral contraceptive product was approved by the Food and Drug Administration of the United States in 1960 their use has expanded rapidly to the point where millions of oral contraceptives are consumed daily in various parts of the world, in spite of concern about certain undesirable side effects. Their impact upon society, in terms of their effect upon sexual mores and population control, will affect human history but cannot yet be fully assessed.[31]

### Psychopharmacology

Psychoactive drugs, such as stramonium and opium, have been used in the treatment of mental illness for centuries. In the 19th century, cannabis, chloral hydrate and other drugs were introduced into psychiatry.

The first striking therapeutic success in this area, however, did not occur until 1952, when chlorpromazine was shown to be effective in the treatment of psychotic patients, in clinical trials carried out in France. Its use in psychiatry was suggested by the French surgeon Henri Laborit, who had first used the drug (synthesized by the Paris pharmaceutical firm Specia in 1950) to help prevent postoperative shock, because of its ability to abolish anxiety. Chlorpromazine had two distinct advantages over hypnotics and other drugs previously used in psychiatry: (1) in doses large enough to be effective it leaves consciousness unclouded, thus allowing the patient to remain responsive to psychotherapy, and (2) it induces lack of interest in the environment, thus minimizing anxiety and excitement.

The success of chlorpromazine opened up the field of psychopharmacology. Other psychoactive drugs, such as reserpine and meprobamate, were soon introduced to treat mental disease and psychoneurotic symptoms (such as anxiety and depression).[32] Moreover, this is another pharmaceutical development that has an impact on society at large, as a majority of the mentally ill under medication, who might otherwise be institutionalized, soon resume activity in their home communities. While this class of drugs has proved to be extremely valuable in the treatment of mental disorders, concern has been expressed in some quarters that our society may be "over-using" psychoactive drugs to alleviate common emotional distress (such as anxiety).[33]

## INTERACTIONS WITH PHARMACY

Every change in medical concepts that influenced therapy made itself felt in the practice of pharmacy. The question is how far did these influences extend?

Therapy (hence pharmacy) is based mainly on empiric or experimental observations. But even without new observations, changing medical theories could still alter the combinations of remedies. They could influence physicians in their choice of drugs. Finally, through the medical profession, theories could deny the usefulness of drugs altogether. However, new drugs could hardly be found in the wake of new theoretical concepts not based on or followed by experimental work.

The consequences derived from this fact are obvious: There was no basic change of types of medication until the modern development of the underlying basic sciences. Chemistry first, and bacteriology later, furnished broad substantial and experimental possibilities for the creation of new kinds of drugs, and experimental physiology and pharmacology finally offered a new way of testing, checking and verifying the assumed effects. Until the late 18th century, there were continuous, more or less haphazard additions to the official materia medica, but hardly any deletions.

It has often been overlooked that the masses of the medical practitioners were more indifferent toward the changes in theories than the heated discussions published by the medical elite seem to indicate. Only some of the physicians followed new speculative theories for which there could not yet be experimental tests. Furthermore, many of these—and even the creators of the theories—were by no means fanatical adherents. Thus we know that François de le Boë Sylvius, for example, made liberal use of the old and tried remedies that had no justification according to his own chemical theory.[34] This conflict between theory and practice we meet again and again, and it always ends with the victory of practice.

A case in point is offered by the conservative medical teachers who were bound to Galenic theory at the University of Paris in the 17th century. Leaders in the fight against iatrochemistry, with its presumed specifics against certain diseases, they likewise were antagonized and confounded by the arrival of new drugs coming from America.

> These were herb preparations which like the chemical preparations exerted violent, in fact specific, effects without the addition of other materials. Foremost of them was quinine [at that period not the alkaloid but the cinchona bark]. "An impertinent innovation," it was called by Guy Patin, but its effect in malaria was too apparent to allow any of its opponents to hold out against its use for long. Even the Paris faculty had to admit it shamefacedly.[35]

Even if the "Galenists" had to admit drugs of the new school in formularies appearing under their authority, they retained those of old.

It has been pointed out above that in the pharmacopeias the authorities had for a long time merely added the new drugs to the old ones. Thus the first edition of the *Pharmacopoeia Augustana* (1564) contained about 1,100 medicaments.[36] Yet that "number is relatively small when compared with that of the official and unofficial pharmacopeias of the 17th century resulting from the union of Galenical and chymiatric remedies."[37] One of the best-reputed pharmacopeias of the 18th century (*Pharmacopoeia Wurtembergica*, 1741) contains 1,952 different drugs and formulas.

When in 1746 the Royal College of Physicians of London published a "purified" revision of the *Pharmacopoeia Londinensis*, purged of a number of outmoded drugs, it considered itself "to be the first medical society in Europe which shall have duly undertaken this reformation."[38] After acceptance of the chemical theories of Lavoisier, such "purifications" of pharmacopeias (i.e., the omission of many old formulas containing dozens of ingredients) became more general. When the first *Pharmacopoeia Borussica* appeared (1799), decisively influenced by the great pharmacist-chemist M. H. Klaproth, medical as well as pharmaceutical practitioners complained so vehemently about its radically simplified materia medica that some of the omitted drugs were again included in the 1827 edition of the Prussian standard.

In addition to the official standards, there has always been an unofficial literature dealing with drugs not admitted to the official books. That literature grew with the increasing trend toward pruning and simplifying the pharmacopeias. Many of the complicated preparations, sanctioned more by tradition and fading belief than by effect, disappeared altogether. However, a greater number remained, altered or unaltered, and formed the contents of unofficial books. Thus the "extra" pharmacopeias (England), the *officines* (France), the *Ergänzungsbücher* (Germany), the "dispensatories," the "national formularies" and the "recipe books" (America) came into being.

Still another factor helped prevent the disappearance of useful drugs merely because they did not fit into a medical system. Even during periods dominated by certain medical theories there always were influential and esteemed eclectic physicians who went "back to Hippocrates," i.e., who aided the healing power of nature with all reasonable and available means regardless of theory. Among such famous physicians were the English practitioner Thomas Sydenham[39] (1624–1689), whom his grateful contemporaries called the English Hippocrates; the Dutch physician and teacher Hermann Boerhaave (1668–1738),[40] and the German C. W. Hufeland (1762–1836).[41] These men greatly influenced the practice of medicine.

The common people, conservators of folk medicine, also held fast to traditionally proven remedies and continued to use them. Sometimes drugs that had lost official acknowledgment because they were not in harmony with the dominant medical theory were preserved by popular use and, later on, with the rise of a new and more satisfactory theory, were again officially approved. A good example is cod-liver oil.[42]

From the early 19th century on, the development of scientific chemistry progressively replaced botanic drugs by better chemical drugs, and even threatened to eliminate the former entirely by a modern materialization of the Paracelsian idea of the "essential." The vegetable drugs, insofar as their usefulness was too obvious to be denied, were investigated chemically, in order to isolate and identify their active constituents and, finally, to synthesize them. Alkaloids, glucosides, vitamins and hormones are among the important results of this development.

As pointed out above, iatrochemistry and, still more, chemotherapy were "medical" theories mainly with regard to their application to medicine. However, they were based on chemical concepts. Sylvius was not only a physician but, within the limits of his time, an excellent chemist as well. It was his knowledge of chemistry that made him conceive a medical system in which chemical concepts played an important part. Ehrlich, the founder of chemotherapy, passed the medical examinations but, throughout his life, practiced chemistry, not medicine. He did not take his ideas from medicine and support them by chemical knowledge; he took them from chemistry and transferred them to medicine. From the effect in vitro, both men assumed a like or similar effect in vivo.

The empirico-experimental root of medical chemistry, growing up from the soil of pure chemistry and sending its branches into the air and the area of medicine, made possible the fruits that we are enjoying today. Furthermore, the origin of medical chemistry explains why, in this epoch of therapy, pharmacists then played such an important role in the finding of new remedies—for example, such men as the discoverer of morphine, the German Sertuerner, and the discoverers of quinine, the Frenchmen Caventou and Pelletier.

As the requirements in methods and facilities grew, much of this investigative basis of modern therapy has been elaborated elegantly and fruitfully in the laboratories of pharmaceutical industry.

The development of therapeutic thought and practice, as explained above in its relation to pharmacy, has been common to Western civilization in general. Was that the case likewise in regard to the particular development of professional pharmacy in the important cultural centers of Europe, in Italy, France, Germany and England? As a matter of fact, it was not.

# 4

# The Development in Italy

Pharmacy's development received early stimulus from the heavy Mediterranean trade in drugs that funneled through Italian ports and from frequent contacts with Islamic concepts of ordering society, including pharmaceutical services.

Italy is the classic soil of European pharmacy as it is that of most of the European professions and arts. The law of the German ruler of the Two Sicilies, Frederick II (see pages 35 and 467), although promulgated in Italy and for Italian territory, was born more out of the German spirit. The first real Italian legal regulation of the duties of both physicians and apothecaries known are the Venetian *statuta* promulgated in 1258.[1] Although they resemble the edict of Frederick II, the *statuta* mention neither a limiting of the number of pharmacies nor governmentally fixed prices for remedies. The statutes forbade the practice of medicine by the pharmacist, and specifically stated that he was not allowed to examine the urine of patients, which up to the 17th century was one of the most important means of medical diagnosis. Official supervision of the drug trade, wholesalers as well as retailers (the latter called *speziarii* and *aromatarii*), had existed in Venice as early as the 12th century.[2]

## ORGANIZATION INTO GUILDS

Italian pharmacies were not created by governmental edict but existed long before legislation dealt with them. Consequently, they had found their natural place within the framework of the guild system—an organization that had a special dignity and task, particularly in Italy.

We know of guildlike associations already in ancient Rome, where somewhat shadowy predecessors of the pharmacists, the *seplasiarii* (see page 21 and 485), are said to have been united in such a guild.[3] They were founded mainly for social and welfare purposes, and the regulating of conditions of trade.[4] In wartime they could be mobilized for military purposes.

The organization of merchants and craftsmen into guilds, according to the kind of goods sold or manufactured, is one of the most significant features of the Middle Ages. During the period of feudalism the guild system created a bourgeoisie regulating both production and distribution.[5] However, there were great differences in the manner in which the guilds in the several countries fulfilled their task. In France, England and Germany the guilds were restricted largely to the internal organization, regulation or administration of their special occupation. In Italy, much more than elsewhere, they were also political, important cogs in the governmental machinery of the city republics up to the 17th century.

In Florence, physicians and pharmacists combined in the same guild, together with some others, toward the close of the 12th cen-

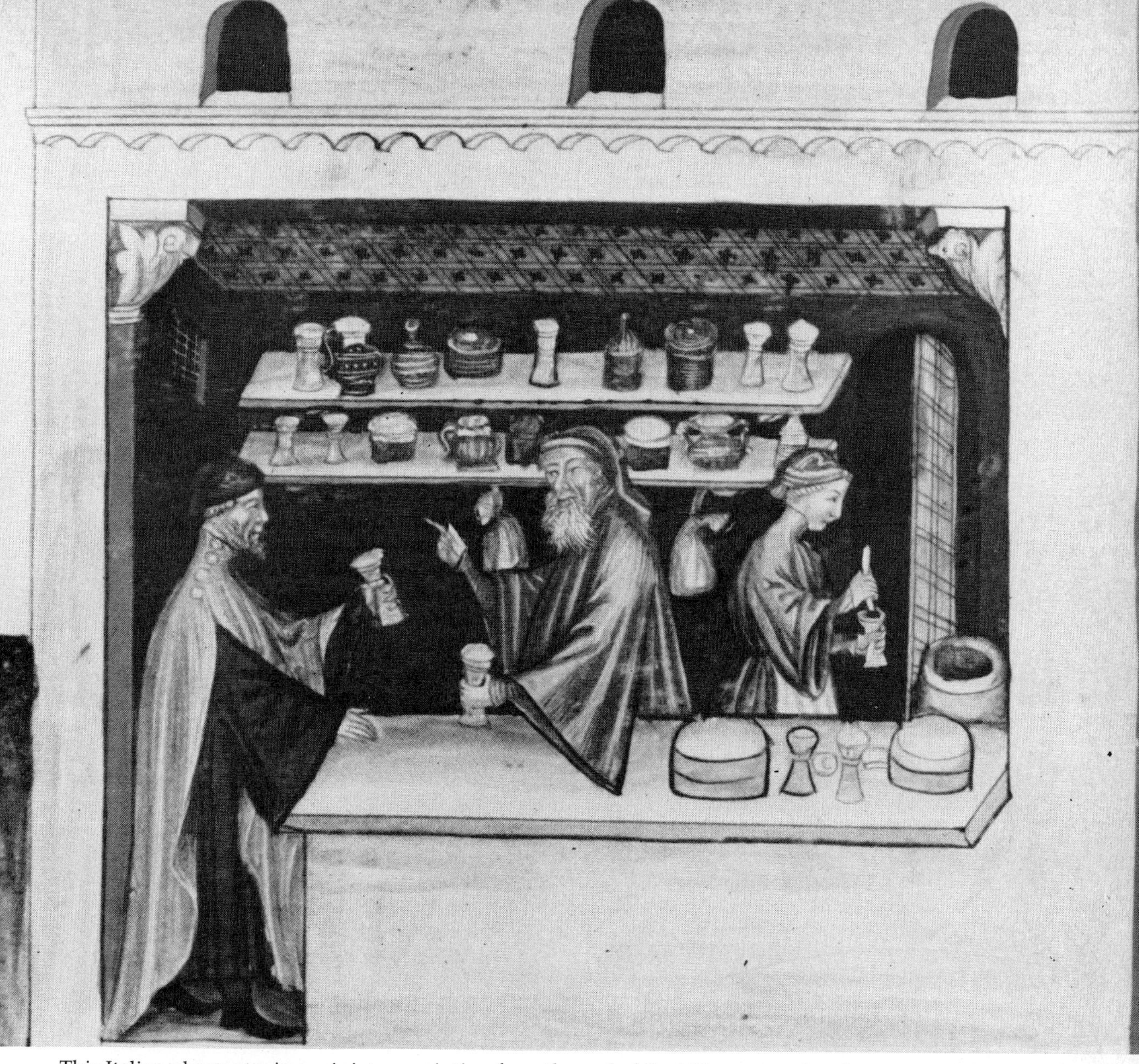

This Italian pharmacy, in a miniature painting from the end of the 14th century, has features reminiscent of its Arabic antecedents. It is typically small and open to the street, with a counter that folds up at night to close off the pharmacy from both the elements and intruders. Its shelves hold drug containers made of glazed ceramic, for which both the process of manufacture and the geometric ornamentation came out of the Middle East. The manuscript *(Tacuinum Sanitatis)* in which this scene appears probably originated near Venice, at that time a principal center for the trade in drugs and other spicery from the Arabic world. (Austrian National Library, ms. n. s. 2644; from Art and Pharmacy, II, Deventer, Netherlands, De Ysel Press, 1958)

tury.[6] When, in 1236, the principal trade corporations of Florence were divided into two divisions, i.e., the seven major arts and the fourteen minor arts, the distinction was one both of technic and of class.[7] As group six, the guild of physicians and pharmacists belonged to the major arts, the arts of higher esteem.

In the membership lists of the various guilds (1297–1444) about 70 different callings were represented. Among these the pharmacists and the wholesalers of drugs outnumbered all the others. That is understood readily if we recall that at this time Italy (more particularly Florence, Genoa and Venice) governed the entire European trade in oriental drugs and spices.[8] Guild statutes (1349) mention no less than 206 different articles as belonging to the monopoly of the pharmacists or spicers. Their trade extended to many products that at this time were rare and costly, such as book manuscripts and wax candles. Even funerals, especially those of the wealthier citizens, were conducted by the pharmacists.[9] Supervision was rigid. Once a year the pharmacies were inspected by a commission of the guild. Drugs not meeting the requirements were confiscated and the culprits excluded from professional practice for variable periods.

The part played by the guild of physicians and pharmacists in Florence was characterized by Staley: "a great guild it truly was . . . it yielded to none in the loftiness of its aim and in the splendor of its achievements."[10]

In various other Italian cities, guilds of pharmacists—either separate or together with physicians—first appear in records of the 13th and subsequent centuries.[11]

The oldest Italian pharmaceutical guild still existing is the Nobile collegio chimico farmaceutico founded in time immemorial and solemnly renewed in 1429 by a special edict of Pope Martin V.[12] The tasks of the guild were (1) the care of poor and sick members, (2) the "immatriculation and location" of all pharmacists who have passed the examinations, (3) the regulation of the distance between pharmacies, (4) the regulation of the prices for remedies, (5) the collection of taxes, to be delivered to the government and (6) the supervision of the producers and the retailers of food, liquors, pastries and medicinal herbs. These tasks can be regarded as traditional for the Italian pharmaceutical guilds.

Of course, pharmaceutical conditions were not uniform in the different states established on Italian soil between the 13th and 19th centuries. Thus, there were variations in the important provision for separating the medical and the pharmaceutical professions. While all commercial association between the professions was forbidden (although not always rigidly enforced) in Southern Italy, Rome, Pisa and many other Italian states,[13] the Florentine statute (1313) allowed the pharmacist to employ a physician in his shop and the physician to employ a pharmacist. A similar regulation appears in the Mantuan statute of 1303. In Pistoia, and later in Florence, similar arrangements permitted physicians and pharmacists to share in the ownership and income of a pharmacy. The pharmacist was forbidden to reimburse the physician for individual prescriptions, however.

In most Italian towns it was customary for the physician to see his patient in a pharmacy, or at least to be available through the pharmacy.

Until the close of the 16th century the cultural influence of the powerful city-states made their institutions a model for other parts of Italy. From the 12th to the 16th centuries Italy was once more the cultural center of the world. Pharmacists of Northern Europe, as well as physicians who desired a better education than they could acquire at home, came to the renowned Italian universities (especially Padua, Bologna, Pisa and Ferrara). This cultural development rested on the wealth acquired by the city-states. Their merchant princes, such as the Medici of Florence, not only controlled the oriental spice trade but were international bankers as well. The Italian trade, including drugs,[14] extended from Constantinople, Damascus, Alexandria and Tunis to southern Germany, France, London, Lisbon, Antwerp and Bruegge in the north.[15]

## EARLY LARGE-SCALE MANUFACTURING

The Italian drug trade was supplemented very early by the development of a chemical industry, the first on European soil. In 1294 Venice was producing corrosive sublimate and cinnabar and, somewhat later, sugar of lead, borax, soap, sal ammoniac, Venetian talc and Venetian turpentine.[16] A very important pharmaceutical export was Venetian treacle (from Latin, *theriaca,* an antidote, q.v. p. 489). Another was the famous Venetian troches of vipers, legally required in some European states for the local preparation of treacle.[17]

In Italy we also observe for the first time industrial pharmaceutical activity by the monasteries. Thus the monastery of the church of Santa Maria Novella in Florence was famous for distilled waters and cosmetics that the monks prepared and sold.

## STATUS IN SOCIETY

The important role played by Italian pharmacy and pharmacists in the political and social life of the country found one expression in public esteem as well as in the equipment of the pharmacies. The Italian pharmacist was always considered a patrician. In Venice the profession was officially recognized as an *arte nobile;* and pharmacists were granted the right to marry Venetian ladies of noble rank. During the middle of the 14th century, the Florentine pharmacist Matteo Palmieri was ambassador of his country to the court of the King of Naples.[18] Up to the present there has always been a number of pharmacists active in Italian politics and represented in the literature of their country. Even in the military service the social and professional recognition of the calling found early expression, putting the pharmacist on an equal level with the physician. This has been true from the establishment of the modern Italian kingdom up to our time.

The Italian pharmacies of the Renaissance expressed status by rooms of architectural beauty, with equipment that today is highly valued by connoisseurs of Italian art[19] and is the pride of many museums and private collections.[20] The development of pottery from a simple handicraft to an art was especially stimulated by Italian pharmacy. Private pharmacists, hospitals and the high nobility competed with each other in adorning their shops or pharmaceutical workrooms and storerooms with precious faience jars and jugs to hold precious medicaments.

## FROM GUILD TO GOVERNMENT RULE

Italian trade and wealth declined after the discovery of America and, particularly, of the all-water route to the East Indies. As early as 1501, King Manuel of Portugal wrote to the Venetian government that there was no longer a reason for Venetian merchants to send ships to Egypt (and the Levant), suggesting that they should rather buy their oriental goods in Portugal.[21] The time of the Italian intermediate trade was a thing of the past. The drugs of the Orient were brought directly to Europe by the Portuguese and, later, by the Dutch; the drugs of the New World were made available first by the Spaniards and then by the English. In the unhappy Italian situation of the 17th century, "Venice and Genoa were on the road to decadence, Lombardy was pillaged by the Spanish, French and Germans, the small Italian states were tormented by the fights of princes."[22]

The political importance of the guilds declined with the declining wealth and political power of the Italian municipalities. However, under government authority they retained a certain internal authority within their own occupational fields.

Conditions changed in the 18th century, which was characterized politically by interference on the part of Austria, the rise of Savoy in the North, and the re-establishment of the southern Italian kingdom as the King-

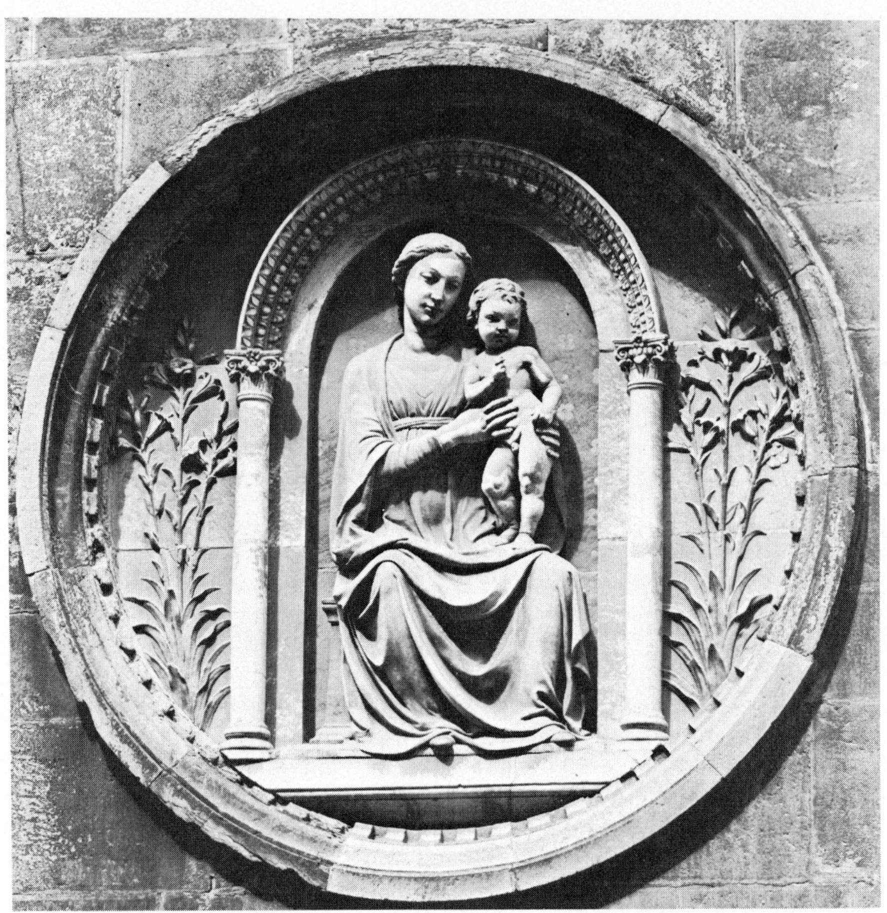

The lustrous guild of physicians and pharmacists in Florence, Italy, commissioned the sculptors della Robbia to execute their emblem (*above*) as a polychrome medallion, one of a series dedicated by various professions and practical arts (15th century). Its superb composition, serenity and grace may still be admired today high on the south gable of the church Or San Michele. Other churches, too, bear mute evidences of the patronage of the rising class of early modern pharmacists. (Photograph from Ed. Alinari, Florence.)

dom of Naples. It was Austrian regulations for Lombardy (1778) that gave the impulse for progressive pharmaceutical legislation in Italy as a whole. One of the most important innovations was the limitation of the number of pharmacies, allowing one pharmacy to 5,000 inhabitants in the Northern Italian territory then under Austrian rule. However, the organization of pharmacy in the various Italian states existing before 1870 differed greatly. In some of them the number of pharmacies was not limited; in others one pharmacy was allowed to 3,000 inhabitants, as in Rome, or a certain distance was required between the pharmacies, as in Naples.[23]

The new Italian Kingdom established in 1870 gradually reduced these variations to a uniform system. From 1888 registered pharmacists were authorized to practice their profession anywhere in Italy, and were allowed the unrestricted opening of pharmacies. Unfortunately, the new pharmacies opened under this law were for the most part in the large cities. Severe competition destructive of standards developed in the metropolitan districts; while in the country the need for well distributed pharmacies was not met. The unrestricted and uncontrolled establishment of new pharmacies thus proved of no advantage either to pharmacy itself or to the public.[24] Therefore in 1913, a new set of restrictions replaced the freedom of the law of 1888, after long controversy.

With the new enactment, regional differences in pharmaceutical requirements—vestiges of the varied states and principalities of earlier centuries—finally disappeared. Everywhere, the opening of a pharmacy henceforth was considered a privilege

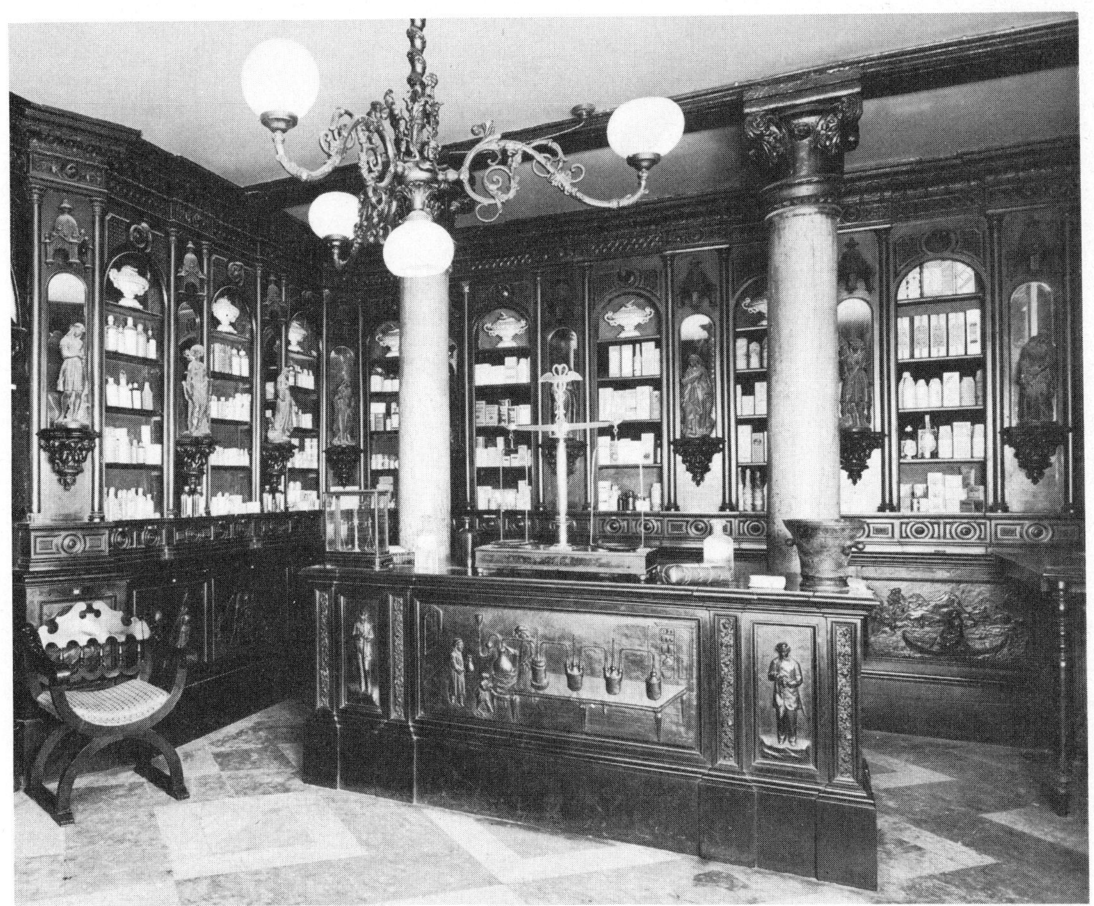

The beautiful old Farmacia Daniele Manin still serves the populace of Venice at Campo San Fantin. The terra-cotta sculptures that watch over the work of Pharmacist Guiseppe Zaini and his associates are thought to be the work of the brothers Zandomeneghi, of the 19th-century school of Cannova. (Photograph copyrighted by Foto Giacomelli, Venice.)

to be earned through a government-administered competition. The number and distribution of pharmacies became government-controlled: 1 pharmacy per 5000 citizens, and, in the cities, at least 550 yards apart. If one eventually became a pharmacy owner it was a lifetime privilege.

The old permanent privileges, granted by rulers or by municipalities, were supposed to be closed out within a 30-year grace period. If not sold by then, a government competition would be held to pass the pharmacy into new hands (although exceptions later proved to be a political necessity). In rural areas where the practice of pharmacy was less attractive and less prosperous, subsidies were provided to induce better geographic distribution of pharmacists—a method traditional in Sweden and some other countries. The dispensing of all medication packaged as separate doses was reserved to pharmacists. For prescription medications on an official list, prices were government-controlled. A system of inspection and control of pharmaceutical services in Italy was funded by license fees.[25]

Social change beginning in the 1950's, especially an upsurge in the number of young pharmacy graduates flooding from the universities, compelled the government to consider relaxing the restriction on the number of pharmacies authorized and other reforms. The question was complicated by the reluctance of old pharmacists to give up their pharmacies and retire, especially with the continuing devaluation of Italian currency. This movement culminated in a revised pharmacy law adopted by the Italian parliament in 1968, which brought notable changes.

Pharmacies in Italy henceforth could be bought and sold freely among pharmacists, but subject to certain limitations (e.g., minimum five-year interval, to minimize speculation). *New* pharmacies, however, still could be opened by private pharmacists only by government permit awarded through competitive examination. The closing of municipally-owned pharmacies, foreseen already in the 1913 law, has not materialized. Indeed, under current law municipalities and civil hospitals could preempt up to half the permits.

While control of the number of pharmacies has been continued, the 1968 law dropped the ratio from 5000 to 4000 persons per pharmacy (in cities over 25,000), and the minimum distance between them dropped (from 550) to about 211 yards. The traditional social rationale for assuring that a pharmacy will have a reasonable number of clients is that it compensates for the government ceiling placed upon the pharmacist's fees, as well as helping to maintain the professional viability of a pharmacist's establishment. To try to deal with the problem of equitable distribution of medical care, pharmacists who practice in a rural community of less than 5000 population are given preference when permits are granted for opening new pharmacies in larger towns. It remains to be seen whether this provision will entice enough young pharmacists to practice for a time in areas needing more accessible pharmaceutical service.[26] As in various other countries, ownership of private pharmacies is limited to pharmacists (or, in the case of a corporation, pharmacists must own control). Pharmacists are aided by a technician-class of assistants.[27]

A pharmaceutical organization, the Federazione Ordini dei Farmacisti Italiani, with headquarters in Rome, works in close contact with the governmental authorities. There is an Ordini dei Farmacisti in every province, as a branch of the government and under the authority of the provincial governmental administration. Membership is compulsory for pharmacists, since authority has been delegated to the Ordini to register pharmacists and to discipline those who overstep legal or ethical bounds (similar, for example, to the Pharmaceutical Society of Great Britain).

## DEVELOPMENT OF EDUCATION

How one prepared for the practice of pharmacy during the earlier period of organized pharmacy in Italy may be exemplified by the Venetian statutes (1565). A student had to serve 5 years as an apprentice and another 3 years as a clerk; finally, he was required to pass a rather rigid examination, after which he became a pharmacist fully qualified to operate a pharmacy of his own.[28] Such requirements were more or less general for a long period.

The Austrian legislation of 1778, abovementioned, regulating pharmacy in Northern Italy (Lombardy), made academic study and examination a requirement for pharmacists in this area. This requirement was extended in 1805 to the Napoleonic Kingdom of Italy during its short life. Pharmaceutical education thus, gradually, was transferred from the craft-like schooling by the guilds to the Italian universities. Here as elsewhere, the trend toward science-based higher education was never reversed by later political events.

Traditionally, admission to a university course in pharmacy was limited to those holding a secondary-school diploma from a *lyceum,* a selective program preparatory to university-based careers. Under democratizing pressures common to higher education in various parts of Europe, Italian universities threw open their doors in 1970 to all students with diplomas from any type of higher secondary school (whether lyceum, technical school, or commercial institute). The entering student is ordinarily 19 or 20 years old, since Italian secondary schools require somewhat longer and higher education than those in the United States.

The 4-year professional course, standard for some decades, continues as preparation for practice in a pharmacy. Since 1967, however, most pharmacy faculties of Italy have introduced a second pharmacy curriculum of 5 years, as preparation for students intending to enter a manufacturing laboratory, toxicologic work, or a pharmacy. The basic structure of both curricula is a foundation of general scientific studies followed by specialized pharmaceutical education.

Another change during this period cut the practical-experience requirement in half. Instead of a 1-year probationary period in a pharmacy after university studies, the neophyte now receives 6 months of controlled experience before becoming fully qualified as a pharmacist (permissible *during* the 4-year curriculum, but in the 5-year curriculum permissible only *after* the academic studies).

Unlike in some European countries, in Italy the university diploma alone does not entitle one to the practice of pharmacy. Qualification is by a postgraduate board examination, somewhat analogous to American custom, but with noteworthy differences. The examining board, consisting of university professors as well as practitioners of pharmacy, sets both oral and practical examinations. A successful candidate may practice as an employed pharmacist. To have the full responsibility of owning and operating a pharmacy, a pharmacist—after at least five years of practice—may take a further competitive examination (as previously mentioned).[29]

After the close of the 17th century the Italian pharmacists as a class no longer contributed importantly to the advancement of the pharmaceutical sciences. This was in spite of the high standards for the practice of pharmacy and the social rank of the pharmaceutical practitioner. Whereas in France and Germany a constellation of pharmacists went on to attain high standing as scientists and, therefore, recognition for their profession, the attainments of Italian pharmacists rarely went beyond the compilation of treatises for the practice of their calling. A possible explanation may be that, throughout the triumphant development of chemistry from the latter part of the 18th through the 19th century, progress came largely from researches conducted in France, Germany, England and Sweden. The great scientific achievements of the Italians lay rather in the spheres of physics and medicine.

**Early Medicinal Botany**

Italian pharmacists and their apprentices utilized botanic gardens or maintained their own, for their learning in botanic science was one hallmark of their calling and its ascendant repute.

By the 14th century, plots of medicinal herbs, theretofore notable as an adjunct of monasteries, had appeared as part of private gardens. One of the earliest known belonged to the famous author Matthaeus Sylvaticus at Salerno, who wrote a dictionary of simple drugs and their uses (*Pandectae . . .*, ca. 1317). Similar gardens flourished about this time at Castelnuova and Naples. In 1545 the famous botanic garden at Padua was established, which might be called the first in a modern sense.

The first chair at a European university for pharmacognosy *(lettura dei semplici)* was established in Padua (1533), and others soon followed.[30] The well known botanist Ghini taught there. One of his students published (1544) a famous commentary on Dioscorides that continued in use through numerous editions and translations as the encyclopedia of herbal materia medica of the Renaissance.[31]

## DEVELOPMENT OF A LITERATURE

The early pharmaco-botanical gardens and cabinets of materia-medica specimens were supportive of early pharmaceutical education, whether through guild or university. Equally important—certainly more significant for the development of European pharmacy at large—was the pharmaceutical literature generated in Italy during the Middle Ages and the Renaissance.

At first, the authors of pharmaceutical interest came from the ranks of medicine, as was the case in other countries of the Western world. One of the earliest guides to the practice of pharmacy printed in Europe was written in the middle of the 15th century by the physician Saladin di Ascoli.[32] This book tells the neophyte pharmacist how to collect, prepare and preserve drugs properly. It explains the terms then used in pharmacy and materia medica. It even describes the behavior appropriate to a proper pharmacist, in the author's view. Perhaps it does not go too far to say that Saladin's book was "the first real treatise on pharmacy in a modern sense . . . which became the model for all later textbooks of pharmacy and for centuries was the indispensable vade mecum [i.e., reference manual] of the apothecary."[33]

It was a harbinger of the growing independence and stature of a separate occupation of pharmacy when Italian pharmacists began to generate their own pharmaceutical treatises. Especially noteworthy is The Greater Luminary *(Luminare majus),* written by the pharmacist Joannes J. Manlius de Bosco toward the end of the 15th century (published 1494), which became an authoritative guide for pharmacists in several countries and cities.[34] Another practicing pharmacist, Paulus Suardus, followed with a widely used text called The Treasure Chest of the Pharmacists (*Thesaurus aromatariorum*, 1512).

→

Title page of an Italian book by Pharmacist de Sgobbis of Venice (1682). Pharmaceutical books before the 18th century often had artistic title pages, sometimes including riotous symbolism. In the central panel a pharmacist (*right*) envisions the colloquy that his pharmaceutical studies give him with sages of the past. Ships bear exotic drugs to him, through waters infested with sea serpents. The hill (*left*), with miners underground and flora and fauna above ground, represents the medicinal resources of the three natural kingdoms. These the pharmacist can put in the service of mankind if he possesses the virtues and the knowledge represented by allegoric figures around the edge of the design.

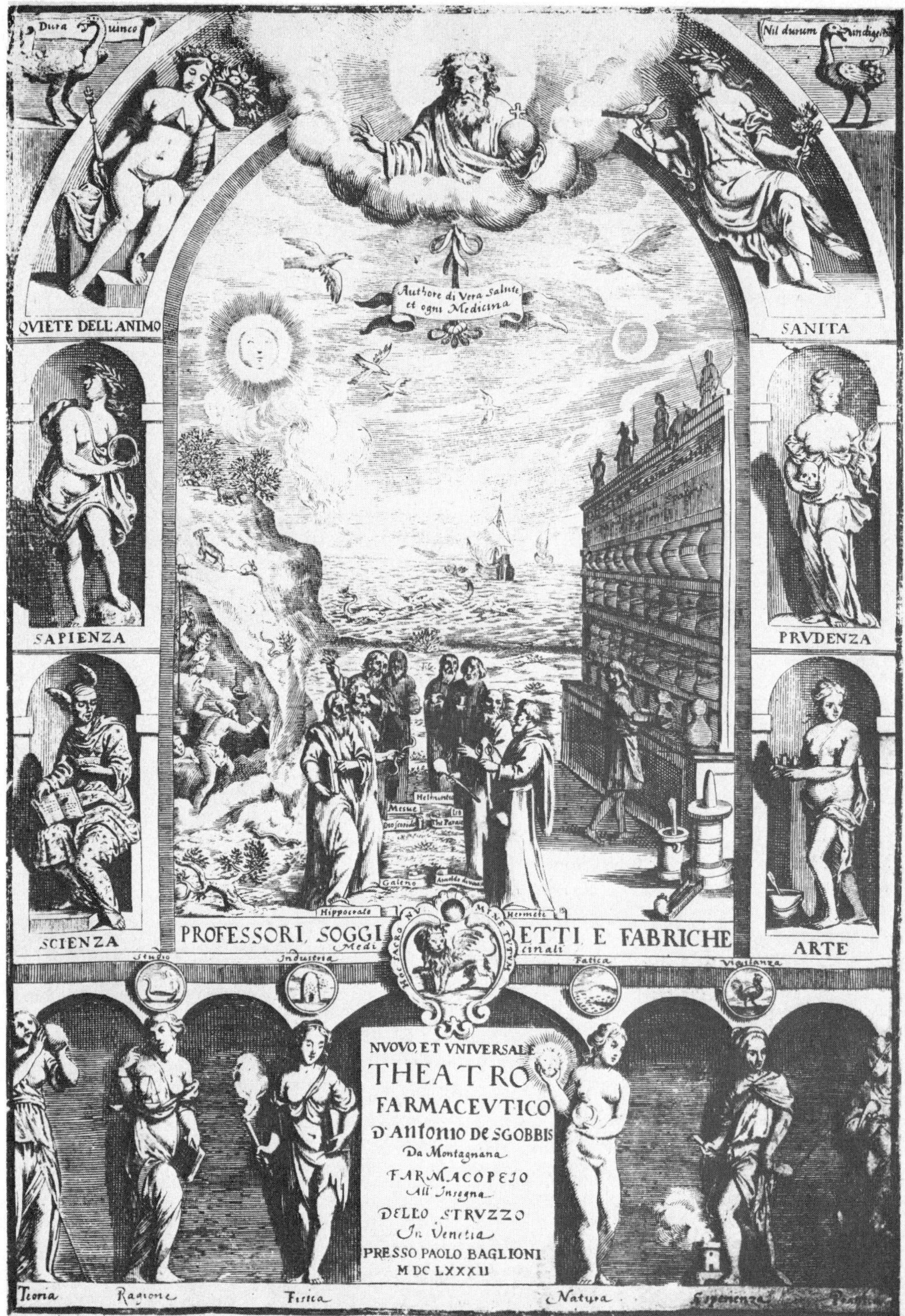
Authore di Vera Salute et ogni Medicina
QVIETE DELL'ANIMO
SANITA
SAPIENZA
PRVDENZA
SCIENZA
ARTE
PROFESSORI, SOGGIETTI E FABRICHE Medicinali
Hippocrate
Galeno
Mesue
Hermete
Studio
Industria
Fatica
Vigilanza
NVOVO, ET VNIVERSALE
THEATRO
FARMACEVTICO
D'Antonio De SGOBBIS
Da Montagnana
FARMACOPEJO
All' Insegna
DELLO STRVZZO
In Venetia
PRESSO PAOLO BAGLIONI
M DC LXXXII
Teoria
Ragione
Fisica
Natura
Esperienza
Pratica

The tradition of such professional manuals reached one culmination in the 17th century with a real pharmaceutical encyclopedia, which in some ways foreshadows the later "universal pharmacopeias." Written by the owner of the esteemed Ostrich Pharmacy in Venice, pharmacist Antonio de Sgobbis da Montagnana, it contains comprehensive directions for the management of a pharmacy and describes and illustrates all the pharmaceutical processes and apparatus (*Nuovo et universale theatro farmaceutico,* 1662; frontispiece reproduced on p. 65).[35] After the end of this century, the Italian pharmaceutical treatises no longer attained much renown beyond the borders of Italy.

The genesis of a special class of literature to unify the specifications for drugs lies partly in Italy. A renowned early attempt was made by the Florentine guild of physicians and pharmacists, when it issued a pharmaceutical formulary in 1499 (titled *Nuovo receptario).* In the preface, the physicians observed that,

> the ill in our city are exposed to many dangers; for our pharmacists, whether in the city or environs, have committed many errors because of the various ways of preparation, choice, care, and manufacture of the simple and compound drugs necessary. . . .[So] apothecaries should follow this [*New Formulary*] not only in the stated city but also in the surrounding area, and in your jurisdiction, with regard to preparation, choice, compounding, and protection of drugs. In so far as all these matters are regulated with honesty, love, diligence, and care, then not only will the apothecaries carry out their work without error but the physicians also may be able to perfect their practice without any fear and for that achieve, with the help of God, praise and great reward.[36]

Since the guild intended this book to be obligatory for pharmacists, it often has been considered the first European "pharmacopeia." The lack of evidence of a legal enforcement of these standards (which the modern usage of the term pharmacopeia implies) leaves the status of the *Nuovo Receptario* in doubt. Other Italian city-states, after a few decades, followed the lead of Florence by issuing their own drug standards (beginning with Mantua in 1559). In the pages of these early local pharmacopeias one sees reflected the nationalistic tendencies and the character of pharmacy as it had developed in the various political units.[37] The long struggle to unify the Italian peninsula as a single country came to fruition in 1870; but the standards for drugs were not unified for the entire country until 1892 when the first edition appeared of the *Farmacopoea ufficiale del regno d'Italia.*

A periodical literature of pharmacy began at the end of the 18th century with reports in Italian journals of physics and of chemistry, and then was given primary attention for the first time in Italy with the founding (1824) of the *Giornale di farmacia, chimica e scienze affini.* The 20th century has brought many specialized pharmaceutical journals, but one particularly representative of the practicing pharmacist is the official organ of the Italian Pharmacists' Association, *Il Farmacista* (f. 1947). (For references to some additional pharmaceutical journals and books of Italian pharmacy, see Appendix 6, p. 422.)

# 5

# The Development in France

Italy cradled European professional pharmacy, but almost simultaneously a similar development took place in France. Pharmacy had emerged in a form we can recognize by about 1300 and, during the preceding century or so of maturing, legal regulations separating pharmacy and medicine and setting other requirements reminiscent of the edict of Frederick II had become effective in Montpellier, Arles and Marseille. Indeed, requirements at Montpellier antedate the others in Southern France and Italy. Perhaps as early as 1180, the preparer of drugs (the especiador) obligated himself in many ways when taking the professional oath after a qualifying examination.[1] It is suggestive that these three French centers of early professional structuring all lay on the Mediterranean, geographically exposed to interaction with Italian and Arabic influences.

There has always been a close connection between Italy and France. During the last centuries of the Roman Empire, Ancient Gaul was more a Roman province than a colony. Thus France felt itself to be a legitimate heir to Roman civilization, almost to the same extent as was Italy. One fundamental difference influenced the political and cultural development of both peoples, the difference in the elements composing the populations of the two countries.

The original Italians did not amalgamate appreciably with the northern peoples who overran them for longer or shorter periods. In all their dominant features, they remained a Mediterranean people. In France, on the contrary, the pre-Roman inhabitants (Aquitani, Celtae and Belgae), then the Romans, then the several Germanic tribes who overran the country (Visigoths, Burgundians and Franks) and, finally, the Normans, blended into a new and almost homogeneous people. The French are one of the most striking examples of amalgamation of different peoples into a single nation, united by the same customs and language, the same aims and thoughts. In 486 Clovis, a chief of the Franks, definitely put an end to Roman rule in the north of France, and settled a German tribe on French soil. For a time, France and Germany constituted a united empire. However, this unity was political only. The division of France from Germany in 987 was but the recognition of their different racial and cultural developments.

## ORGANIZATION INTO GUILDS

The intermediate cultural position of France between Germany to the north and Italy to the south finds expression in the evolution of French pharmacy. In France, as in Italy during the Middle Ages, pharmacy found its place in the guilds. However, unlike the great Italian guilds, these French associations were nonpolitical. They were professional or commercial organizations, based on decree of royal, parliamentary or local authorities.[2]

The fact that until the reign of the House of Bourbon (1589) many feudal lords governed their territories like sovereigns and that, later on, until the great revolution (1792), the individual municipalities enjoyed wide administrative independence, did not prevent a rather uniform development of pharmacy throughout France. The guilds were given far-reaching self-determination in all matters concerning admission to the profession, education of apprentices and their examination, the limitation of the number of pharmacies, and the care of poor colleagues and their widows and orphans.[3] In general, wise use was made of the right of self-government.

There were three kinds of regulation of pharmaceutical life: by the central government, by local authorities and by the pharmacists themselves (that is, by their associations). The last type of regulation was the most common.[4]

By the 13th century the field of pharmacy had developed sufficiently, here and there, to generate a group consciousness and identity. A century or two earlier we find only traces of individual practitioners, the pharmacist's forerunner sometimes being called "pigmentarius" (e.g., Angers in 1093; Poitou in 1123).[5] An early guildlike association in French pharmacy arose in Avignon (1262), where sellers of drugs joined with an association of spicers. At Dijon, also in the late 13th century, we know that pharmacists owned a kind of association-headquarters building *(domus apothecariorum)*.[6] In Paris, at least as early as the middle of the 13th century, pharmacists had an association together with spicers and others in more or less related callings.

To this association King Philip IV entrusted (1312) the control of weights and balances used by all retailers, thus making the pharmacists and spicers the appointed custodians of the standard weight.[7] Outside of Paris similar regulations were issued, most of them making the pharmacists the appointed inspectors of the balances and the weights used by all retail merchants.

If the number of physicians in a community was not large enough to form a special medical group, they united with the pharmacists. At times, surgeons, pharmacists and barbers were in the same association. However, the special pharmacy guilds were predominant. Of 199 guilds in which pharmacists are known to have participated, 103 were exclusively pharmacy associations.[8]

By means of these guilds, the pharmaceutical profession in France gained and maintained a high standard. As measured by the values of that time, the requirements for entrance into the profession were high and strictly enforced.

The applicant had to be of legitimate birth and of the Roman Catholic faith; he had to know sufficient Latin to read intelligently the formularies and the prescriptions; in addition, the guildmasters often asked whether the applicant's family was wealthy enough to enable him to buy a pharmacy later on.

> Most of the apprentices were recruited from the rich bourgeoisie of the towns, very often from the apothecaries' families. The son succeeded the father, the nephew the uncle. That explains the numerous dynasties of apothecaries. In Rouen, for instance, a widow Chandelier practiced [the profession] in 1214 and eleven members of the family practiced pharmacy in that town from 1600 to 1786.[9]

The statutes of many guilds restricted the number of apprentices. Generally, only one apprentice was allowed for each pharmacy.[10] Even the number of pharmacies was often limited, sometimes by statute as in Nancy and Nice,[11] sometimes by other means—for instance, by the requirement that each pharmacist coming from another district pass a local examination.

In a number of cases the limitations—restricting membership in French guilds to certain cliques—apparently went too far. An edict of 1539 improved the situation by the drastic remedy of banning the guilds of

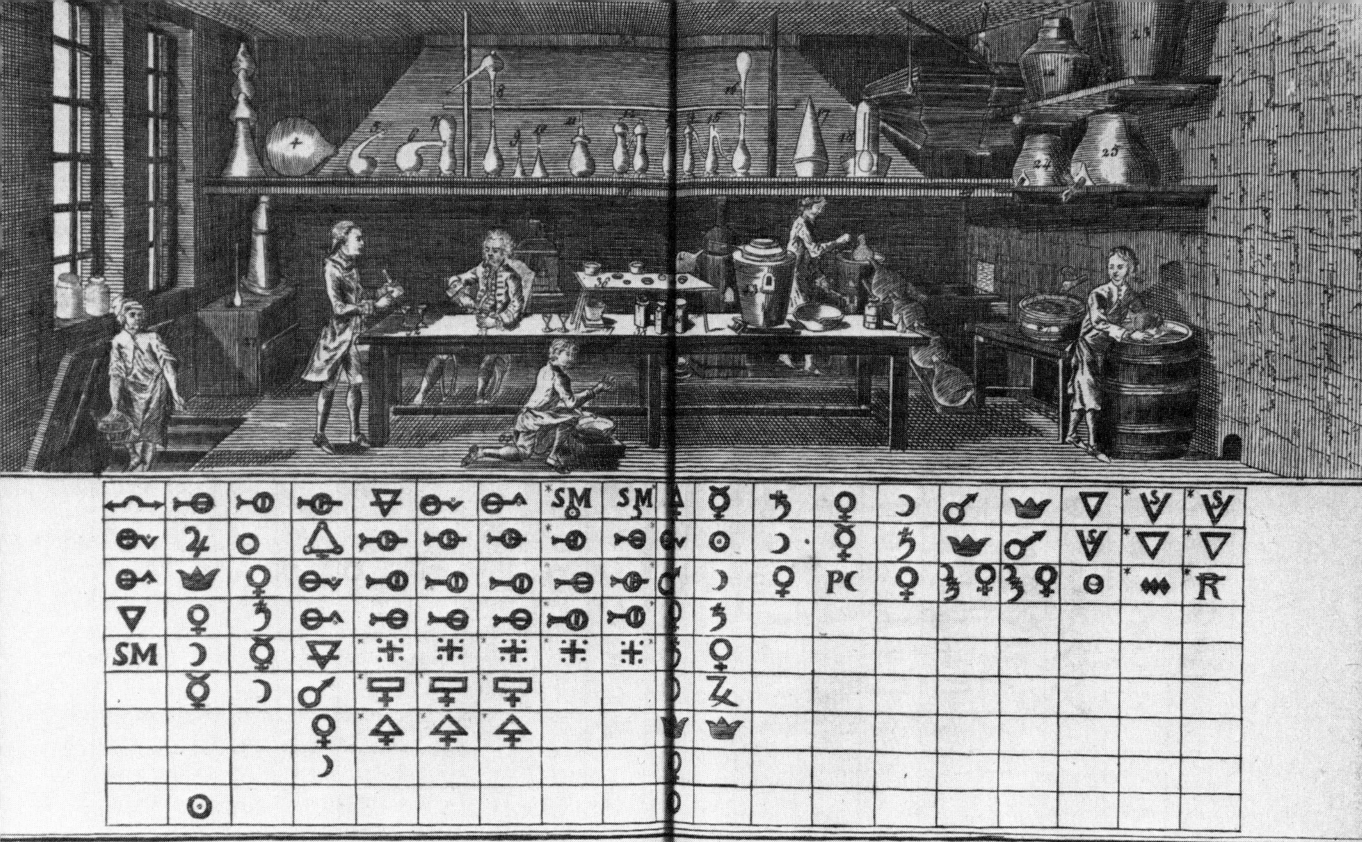

The French pharmacist Etienne François Geoffroy stated the existence of chemical affinities for the first time (Memoirs of the Parisian Academy of Science, 1718), and published the above table (using the chemical symbols of the time) to illustrate the presumed relationships. The engraving showing in detail a contemporary laboratory appeared with the table in Diderot's *Encyclopedie; . . .*, Lausanne, 1780–82, Vol. 2. (From National Library of Medicine)

trades and professions as they then existed.[12] Subsequently, many new guild statutes based on a model statute approved by the king were issued in the late 16th and early 17th centuries.

## PHARMACISTS AND SPICERS

In a Parisian book on the trades and professions of 1270 (*Livre des métiers* by Etienne Boileau), the term *apothicaire* appears, as it does in other French documents about this time. However, members of the profession of pharmacy were at that time more commonly called *épicier* (spicer).[13] The fact that the designation *apothicaire* did not become general until about 1400 proves that until that time neither the public nor the governmental authorities had seen much difference between the apothecary and the spicer.

Due to the lack of sharp distinctions of rights and privileges, there had never been much love lost between the two groups. Each accused the other of trespassing; each required and had enacted legislation for its benefit, dealing particularly with the situation in the capital, Paris.

An edict in 1484 forbade the practice of pharmacy by spicers.[14] Another ordinance (1514) separated the small spicer from the apothecary-spicer. The small spicer was forbidden to practice pharmacy, which, according to the ordinance, "requires much art, science, experience and knowledge of drugs as well as of the compounding of prescriptions which enter into the human body." However, the apothecary (pharmacist) was permitted to practice both occupations simultaneously.

Contending ambitions and fluid boundaries of function—which would continue to haunt pharmacists in other centuries and circumstances—made pharmacy's privilege unstable. Within a generation pharmacists too had to choose between the two callings (1553). Then the king reunited the hostile groups within the same guild (1560). Repeated amendment of the ordinances governing the competing groups into the 18th century reflects the conflict of interest and the friction between them.[15]

The attention paid to the spicers by the French authorities until the early 18th century finds explanation in the economic importance of these tradesmen, especially the importers and wholesalers (and often retailers) of spices and drugs from the Orient and later from America. Their influence in certain French cities along the changing routes of import (until the end of the 16th century mainly Marseilles and Lyons, and later Bordeaux, La Rochelle, Nantes and Rouen) was so great that at times professional pharmacy was overshadowed by the spicers.[16]

The definite separation of the pharmacists and the spicers of Paris was brought about by a royal declaration in 1777 that replaced the old guild with the quite different Collège de Pharmacie. This declaration allowed to the spicers the wholesale trade in drugs, the retailing of a few specifically enumerated drugs and trade in all herbs and roots in their natural state, requiring no preparation or compounding.

The disagreements between the pharmacists and the spicers were not peculiar to France, but occurred in all countries and still occur today among pharmacists, herbalists and merchants. The French quarrel with the herbalists culminated in a law (Germinal, 1803) that stabilized the situation. After having proved their knowledge by examination, the herbalists were given a certificate entitling them to sell indigenous crude drugs. Licenses are no longer granted to herbalists, and, when the owner of an old herb shop dies, the doors are closed.[17]

## FROM "APOTHICAIRE" TO "PHARMACIEN"

The social status of the French *apothicaire* from the 14th to the 18th century was doubtless that of a patrician. His social position was maintained in spite of the fact that his duties included not only the preparation but the administration of medicated clysters (enemas), which were a therapeutic fad from the 15th to the 18th century. Louis XIII received no less than 312 clysters within a year! Only when the apothecaries became the target of ridicule by poets, especially Molière (a development which fortunately coincided with the passing of the fad), did the administration of clysters come to seem degrading.

It is sometimes overlooked that Molière, in his famous play *Le malade imaginaire,* scoffs at physicians and apothecaries in quite the same manner and that, for him, the *apothicaire's* involvement with clysters was only a welcome occasion for added ridicule. At any rate, in French public opinion the designation *apothicaire* gradually became associated with the ridiculous picture drawn by the caricaturists, which may have had something to do with the profession preferring the new name *pharmacien.* The term made its appearance in the 17th century and became official with the establishment of the Collège de Pharmacie in 1777.

The giant syringe used for the application of clysters was too good a motif not to be taken advantage of by caricaturists, such as the great master of French politico-satirical graphics, Honoré Daumier, long after clysters, and especially their application by *apothicaires,* had ceased to be a fashion.

The attacks of Molière and his literary contemporaries were to a large extent directed against the high prices charged for remedies. In France prices fixed by the government

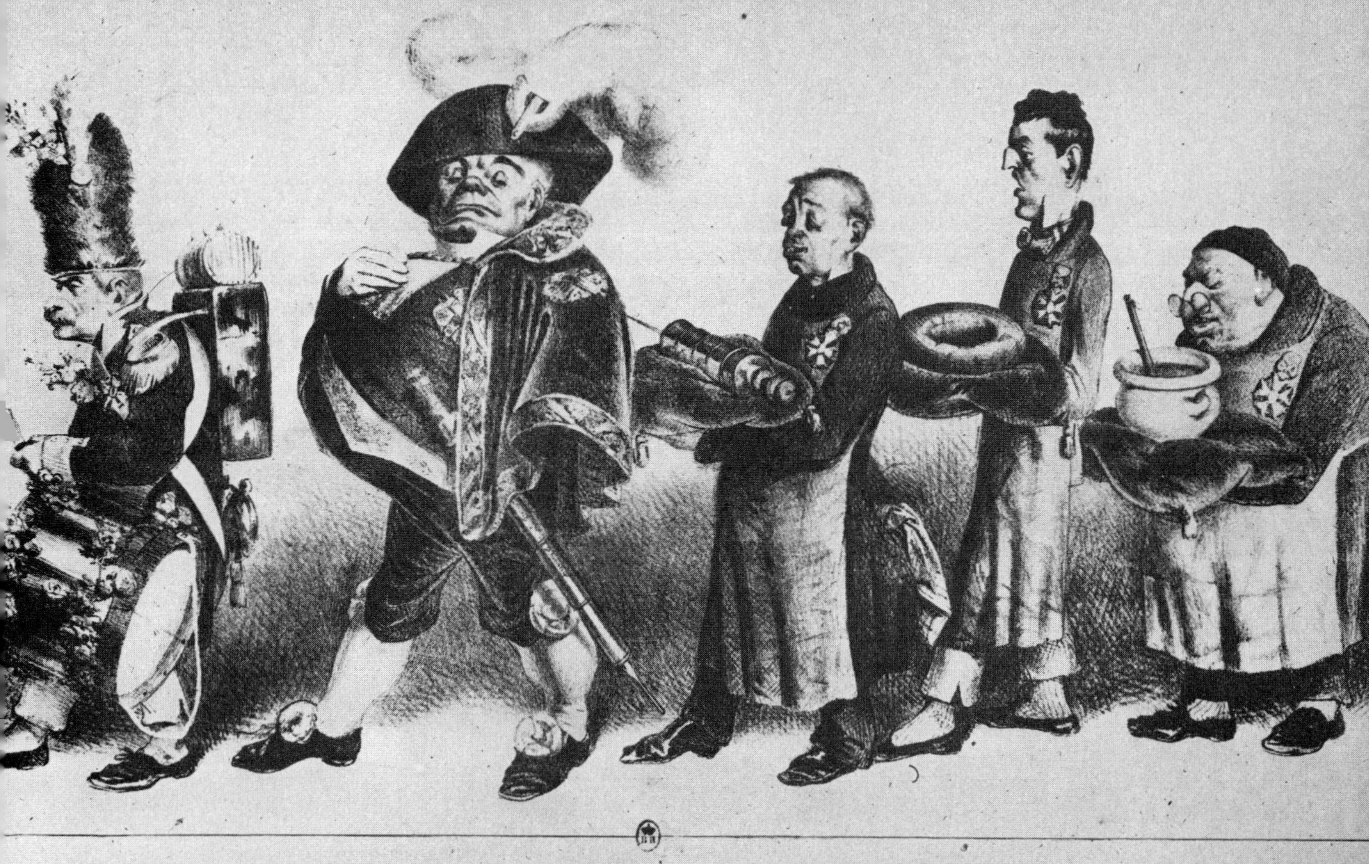


The French pharmacist's erstwhile duty of administering medicated enemas stirred the polemical imagination of the great caricaturist, Honoré Daumier. On the surface, his "Cortège" (*above*) purports to show "the commanding General of the Pharmacists, prince Lancelot Tricanule, upon his entry into the chamber of Peers." Who, in reality, is this officious and vacuous general with a huge enema-syringe instead of a sword, followed by aides bearing auxiliary equipment? Actually, the barb was thrown at General Mouton (Count Lobau), who had offended by ordering fire-hoses turned on public demonstrators (1831) and, immediately afterward, had received his field-marshal's baton and a peerage. (From *La Pharmacie & la Médecine dans l'Oeuvre de H. Daumier,* Les Pharmaciens Bibliophiles, Paris, 1932.)

were never a general institution, and we know of pharmaceutical invoices which, indeed, seem to be very high.[18]

## PHARMACISTS AND PHYSICIANS

Pharmacists and physicians, who are so closely associated in their professional life and are the common target of sarcasm, nevertheless often have had conflicts, possibly because of their close relationship. However, nowhere did these quarrels reach such a degree of malice as in France. As early as 1271, the medical faculty of Paris were admonishing the apothecaries not to trespass on the field of medicine; on the other hand, some French physicians in their turn sold medicines (as late as about 1470).[19] The scarcity of learned physicians sometimes drew pharmacists into the practice of medicine. For example, in 1724, a royal ordinance permitted the pharmacist to visit the sick if no physician was available.[20]

The quarreling between the professions,

launched by the physician Symphorien Champier in the early 16th century, had gained notoriety the world over. Vitriolic treatises were met by countertreatises. In Germany and in England, echoes of these French publications[21] were heard later, a classic source of barbs to be hurled at pharmacists on the one hand, or against physicians on the other.

Another quarrel arose about 70 years later, in which medical authors used the old arguments but tried new means as well, with the clearly expressed intention of ruining the pharmaceutical profession. Guy Patin, the famous head of the faculty of medicine at the University of Paris and a conservative clinician, was campaigning against the use in medicine of what he considered to be dangerous chemicals. He and his associates wanted pharmacists to refuse to dispense prescriptions containing chemicals. The pharmacists' answer that they felt obliged to dispense all prescriptions ordered was considered a declaration of war.

Nevertheless, common sense triumphed over hatred, prejudice and presumption. In 1666, the Faculty of Medicine at Paris legitimatized the therapeutic use of the controversial antimony (in the form of wine of antimony) "as a purgative," and the Parlement de Paris even gave governmental blessing to this decision.

These early conflicts may be viewed as more than a curious episode in history; they illustrate a recurrent handicap to orderly, well developed services wherever the pharmacist's role lacks clear and well regulated boundaries. In countries where merchants on one side or physicians on the other have collided with the pharmacist's presumed responsibilities (e.g., in America) controversies have arisen again and again. France, having experienced fruitless overlap and friction, came, in the 18th century, to a firmer designation of the role reserved to the pharmacist and to a higher level of development.

## ORGANIZATION OF FRENCH PHARMACY SINCE 1777

The Royal Declaration of April 25, 1777 ushered in modern French pharmacy. By establishing the Collège de Pharmacie as an administrative as well as an educational institution, the declaration replaced the old guild, and strictly stated the tasks and the rights of professional pharmacy. Thus a definite borderline was drawn between activities considered to be pharmaceutical, and hence reserved to pharmacy, and those open to everyone, including the herbalists. The declaration forbade the selling of drugs by religious hospitals and societies (a practice which had been rampant before),[22] and it authorized pharmacists to educate their rising generation without medical interference.

The French Revolution changed little more than the name of the tested institutions—after a short, painful trial of "free" pharmacy, which meant pharmacy thrown open to anyone, without educational requirements. A decree (March 2, 1791) had declared everyone entitled to practice any profession or trade! One immediate result was that uneducated owners established numerous stores called pharmacies everywhere in France, especially in Paris. This put an end to revolutionary enthusiasm for liberty in the field of pharmacy. A month later, a new decree (April 14, 1791) announced the return to the customary regulation of the practice of pharmacy.

In 1796 former members of the Collège de Pharmacie set up a new association, called the Société libre de Pharmacie de Paris. A Société de Pharmacie de Paris, founded (1803) to provide scientific interchange and stimulus, gained an illustrious reputation. Analogous local societies were founded in other scientific centers of French pharmacy.[23]

The defense of the commercial interest of pharmacy was left to other and younger associations,[24] (especially L'Association [now Fédération] générale des syndicats Pharmaceutiques, founded in 1876).

Meanwhile, the organization of French pharmacy has been changed entirely.[25] Since 1945 there has been an all-inclusive pharmaceutical association called L'Ordre des pharmaciens. Membership is compulsory for (a) community pharmacists, (b) pharmacists responsible for the manufacture of pharmaceutical proprietary products, (c) pharmacists responsible for pharmaceutical wholesale distribution, (d) pharmacists not belonging to groups a, b or c—for instance, hospital pharmacists, bio-clinical analysts (whether or not their laboratories are attached to a general practice of pharmacy), pharmacists responsible for shops belonging to prepaid-benefit societies, and also the assistant pharmacists. It has to be kept in mind that in France large-scale manufacture of pharmaceuticals, as well as pharmaceutical wholesale activities are regarded as "pharmaceutical practice" and are by law under the control of registered pharmacists. In May 1974 there were 29,453 pharmacists registered, to serve a population of some 52 millions. Anyone not listed as a member of the Ordre and active in one of the capacities enumerated is practicing pharmacy illegally and is subject to punishment.

The aims of the Ordre (enactment of May 1945) are "to assure respect for the professional duties, [and] to assure the defense of the honor and the independence of the profession." The organization is given a certain professional jurisdiction. Its councils (one for each of the four groups named and regional councils for the community pharmacists) are supposed "to ferret out violations of a professional nature, which only too often escape the jurisdiction of the common courts and are sanctioned by the latter."[26]

The Société de pharmacie de Paris has become (1946) the Académie de Pharmacie, thus underlining still more the purely scientific character of this institution and putting it on the same level with the time-honored Académie de Médecine.

While French law has not restricted the number of pharmacies severely, compared with some other countries, it does try to ensure fairly even distribution of pharmaceutical service and sets some limit to their number. In the country as a whole, a little more than 3,000 persons are served by each pharmacy. Besides other conditions to be met, a new pharmacy may open only where the development of inhabitants per pharmacy would be at least the ratios shown below (for localities in three population categories):

3,000 to 1, for populations of more than 30,000

2,500 to 1, for populations of 5,000 to 30,000

2,000 to 1, for populations of less than 5,000[27]

In case the needs of the populace demand, the prefect may authorize the establishment of pharmacies beyond the number stipulated above.

This pattern has been attempted to make pharmaceutical service reasonably available to the patient while, at the same time, giving reasonable opportunity for a full-time, dignified practice of pharmacy. It is a delicate balance, threatened since the 1950's by a mounting number of university students in pharmacy and affecting the professionally nurtured character of the pharmacist's establishment.

## DEVELOPMENT OF THE PHARMACIST'S ESTABLISHMENT

Up to the late 16th century, the French pharmacies were mostly open-fronted, with the pharmacist working in the public gaze, not unlike the early pharmacies of Islam and Southern Italy. The equipment gradually became more elegant; but, with few exceptions, only the pharmacies of hospitals or religious societies equalled the luxury of Italian pharmacies of the Renaissance. In the 17th cen-

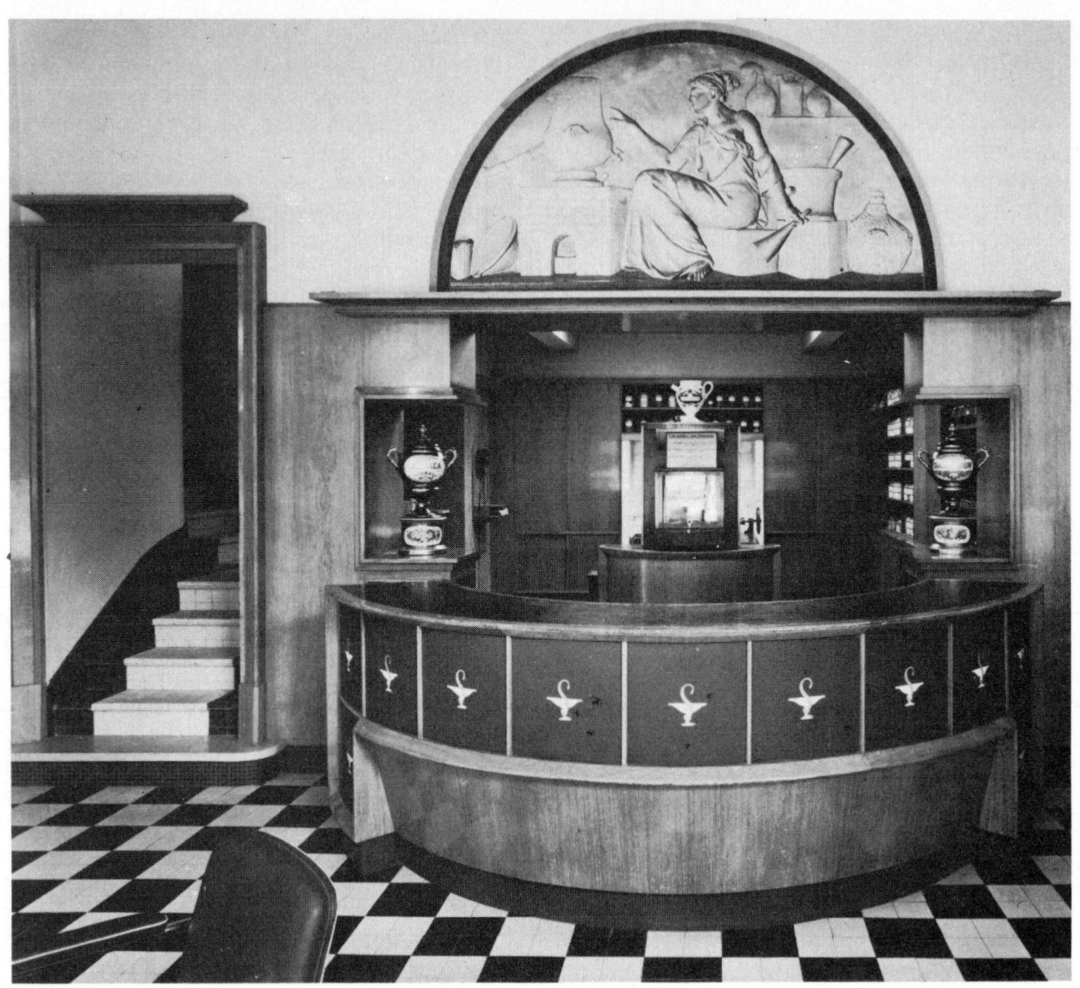

Old and new elements combine to preserve French elegance in the Claude Pharmacy at L'Aigle (Orne). The graceful curve of the main dispensing counter is ornamented by rhythmic repetition of pharmacy's symbol, the Bowl of Hygeia; the bas-relief overhead probably represents the goddess Hygeia herself, sitting among antique pharmaceutical equipment. (Photograph from A. I. H. P.)

tury, faience drug jars from French potteries (Nevers, Rouen, Moustiers) greatly improved the appearance of the pharmacies. After the close of the 18th century, matched sets of elegant drug containers from French porcelain manufacturers also went onto the shelves. Indeed, it was the discovery of the kaolin of St. Yrieix by a pharmacist, M.-H. Vilaris of Bordeaux, that made the French porcelain industry possible.

Products of French pottery even became distinguishing symbols of pharmacy. The so-called *chevrettes*—specially shaped jugs for medicinal syrups, honeys and oils could be legally displayed only by pharmacists.[28] A Parisian ordinance forbidding the spicers to use the so-called *pots à canon* (containers of cannonlike shape for ointments, electuaries, etc.) gave this type of container likewise a pharmaceutical distinction.[29]

As these embellishments suggest, a French pharmacy is often well appointed, and is always devoted primarily to professional activities. Legally limited to 21 categories of stock, a French pharmacy has as sidelines only such products as perfumes, insecticides, special dietary aids and the like.[30]

Since each pharmacy serves about the same population, on the average, as a pharmacy in the United States, the much more uniform professional appearance and specialization of French pharmacies seems striking to American pharmacists. While factors accounting for this are complex, it is important to recall that physicians do not preempt any significant part of the pharmacist's practice and, secondly, that well-trained pharmacists have biologic (clinical) analysis as a second professional function. About 70 per cent of all such laboratories were directed by pharmacists in 1950. Pharmacies that do not conduct the actual testing may obtain commissions for forwarding specimens to such a laboratory and handle the test reports. While physicians are divided in their attitude toward this function of French pharmacy as a public service, pharmacists tend to see clinical laboratory work as a means of utilizing their scientific education more fully in a second professional sense, despite a countercurrent of industrial and economic change within the practice of pharmacy itself.[31]

### Pharmaceutical Inspection

During the first centuries of professional French pharmacy, the supervision either was entirely the responsibility of the physicians or was dominated by them. In 1336, for example, the faculty of medicine in Paris was charged with the inspection of the pharmacies. Then an ordinance (1353) created a commission consisting of the head of the pharmacists' guild, two master pharmacists appointed by the municipal authorities and two members of the medical faculty. Mixed commissions of this type appeared everywhere, although medical dominance over pharmacy was maintained. Supervision by pharmacists exclusively was rare.[32]

The previously mentioned law of 1803 made the supervision of the pharmacies the function of commissions elected from the staffs of the schools of medicine and pharmacy in Paris and of the departmental councils of hygiene in the provinces. After another century, a new law (1908) established the supervision by pharmaceutical inspectors, not only of the pharmacies but of the entire drug trade. "Pharmacy was thus freed from a servitude which has lasted too long and which could only injure its reputation by illusory control and repression."[33] Present legislation provides for full-time and part-time inspectors appointed by the Ministry of Health.

## LARGE-SCALE MANUFACTURING

In the development of the French pharmaceutical industry pharmacists played a large and important part. One of the first in France to manufacture chemicals and galenics on a large scale was the pharmacist Antoine Baumé, the inventor of a number of technical improvements, which he proved in his own manufacturing laboratory and generously made known to his colleagues. His price list (1775) shows about 2,400 preparations, among them about 400 which can be considered chemical.

Some of the early French discoverers of alkaloids, for instance Joseph Pelletier (quinine) and P. J. Robiquet (codeine), made their discoveries the basis of large-scale manufacturing. Furthermore, in the 17th and the 18th centuries, community pharmacies contributed most of the proprietary remedies on the market, and continued to do so. For it has been characteristic of the French proprietary industry that, beyond a few very large drug manufacturers, there stand "countless small manufacturers, each of whom specializes in one or two remedies," and that in the 1920's still "fully 50 per cent of the licensed pharmacists in France are engaged in this business, most of them in a small way."[34] From this group of practicing pharmacists emerged Stanislas Limousin, the inventor of the apparatus for administration of oxygen, of wafer-capsules and, above all, of parenteral ampuls.[35]

Around the middle of the 19th century, French pharmacists created the first cooperative of national scope covering pharmaceutical industry and commerce. The similar venture undertaken by London apothecaries in the early 17th century (see page 102) was only local in scope and restricted to the members of the Society of Apothecaries of London. This cooperative, the Pharmacie centrale de France, whose shareholders are exclusively French pharmacists, developed into one of the world's large pharmaceutical manufacturing and wholesale enterprises. It affects practically all aspects of the life of French pharmacists.

The abilities growing out of French pharmacy thus nourished in important ways the growth and contribution of modern pharmaceutical manufacturing. Yet, it was that very development which seriously undermined the scientific foundation for the eminence of at least a practitioner elite. For the rise of industrial production inevitably "curtailed the individual pharmacist's chemical and pharmaceutical manipulation, and stifled the scientific life of the *officine* [i.e., the community pharmacy] in a torrent of prefabricated specialties."[36]

## DEVELOPMENT OF EDUCATION

During the time of the guilds the applicant for apprenticeship had to meet high social, financial and educational requirements. To become a master he had to pass difficult examinations. In Marseilles such examinations were required as early as the 13th century. A Parisian ordinance in 1484 stated that the candidate had to prove his knowledge of drugs and of the compounding of medicaments by undergoing a protracted and difficult examination and, lastly, had to perform his "masterpiece," by preparing a number of galenics requiring special technical skill and scientific knowledge. This masterpiece became a general requirement throughout France up to the 18th century.[37] (It was in this tradition that state boards of pharmacy in the USA during the late 19th and early 20th century asked candidates to compound complex prescriptions.) The prospective pharmacist also usually had to serve a certain time as a clerk *(compagnon)* before he could become a candidate for mastership. The entire time thus spent varied from 2 to 8 years as apprentice, to a total time of 4 to 10 years as apprentice and clerk.[38]

Academic studies were introduced comparatively early, and gradually became general. Already in 1536 a Parisian ordinance required apprentices of pharmacy to attend two lectures each week relating to the art of the apothecary, given by a member of the faculty of medicine. In Poitiers (1588) only those candidates who had attended lectures on the art and the science of pharmacy for 1 year could become masters of pharmacy.

In the famous University of Montpellier the doors were always open to the students of pharmacy of the entire world. In 1588, the pharmacists at Montpellier established, at their own expense, an instructional collection of drug specimens, and the practicing pharmacist Bernardhin Duranc was appointed curator, obligated to exhibit and explicate the materia medica to the assembled students three times a year. It was a significant, if limited, beginning, opening the doors of the university for the first time to instruction by a master apothecary. Indeed, Duranc appears to be the first practicing pharmacist to become officially a member of the teaching staff of a European university.

During the 17th century pharmacy matured academically at Montpellier in successive steps: Henry IV created a chair for surgery and pharmacy (1601); the famous master pharmacist Laurent Catelan lectured on medicinal herbs and demonstrated the art of pharmacy (1605); and Louis XIV created a chair of pharmaceutical chemistry (1675).[39]

In Paris the Garden of the Apothecaries (founded by the pharmacist Nicolas Houel on the basis of a special ordinance of Henry III, October 1576, and preserved and enlarged during several centuries by the pharmacists' guild) provided general scientific instruction for the apprentices of pharmacy. Other courses were given primarily at the Garden of the King (founded 1635).[40] These courses were supplemented by private courses on pharmaceutical chemistry given by some of the famous pharmacist-chemists, such as Lefebvre and Lémery in the 17th century and Rouelle and Baumé in the 18th century.

These courses had to be a private undertaking, because the several attempts of the Parisian guild to organize official academic instruction met with the same lack of fair professional sentiment on the part of physicians that has been noted earlier. Official courses twice launched (1705–1723, and 1753–1765) had to be abandoned because of opposition by the Paris faculty of medicine. They were resumed after replacement of the guild by the society called the Collége de Pharmacie (1777) and were continued during the lifetime of this institution. The successor organization established its own "free school" after the Revolution, which evolved into the present-day faculties of pharmacy of the University of Paris.

The legislation of 1803 provided six higher schools of pharmacy for the education of pharmacists of the first class, who were permitted to practice pharmacy throughout the nation. It also provided for the examination of pharmacists of the second class, who were allowed to practice only in the district where they passed their examination.

Having pharmacists at two different levels of qualification was not without problems (as other countries have found likewise); and in 1909 the second-class category of pharmacist was abolished. Although other provisions of the educational structure have also been altered periodically, the basic requirement until the 1960's consisted of a secondary schooling at the university-preparatory level, a pre-university year of apprenticeship with an officially-authorized pharmacist (until 1962) and a four-year university curriculum, offered by several types of university faculties.

Pharmaceutical education, meanwhile, has been considerably affected by the intense reexamination of French higher education in general during the late 1960's. The old faculties were replaced in 1969 by a new structure of "universities of studies and of researches." Twenty-three universities of pharmaceutical studies were designated.[41] At Paris the famous old "Faculté de pharmacie" has been divided in two. One half became part of the University of Paris-South (Paris XI), housed in impressive new facilities in the suburb Châtenay-Malabry. The other half became part of the University René-Descartes (Paris V), retaining the building in the old university quarter, so long known and honored internationally.

Each part consists of three of the new academic structures ("U. E. R."):[42] one devoted mainly to the professional curriculum leading to the diploma qualifying as a pharmacist; and two others where research predominates. Each of the two parts of the Paris faculty has been given a somewhat different focus: At the University René-Descartes, the three structures comprise pharmaceutical and biologic sciences; mechanisms of action of medicaments and poison; and human and experimental biology. At the University of Paris-South, the three comprise pharmaceutical and biologic sciences; therapeutic chemistry; and hygiene, including the protection of man and his environment.

The admission standard to study phar-

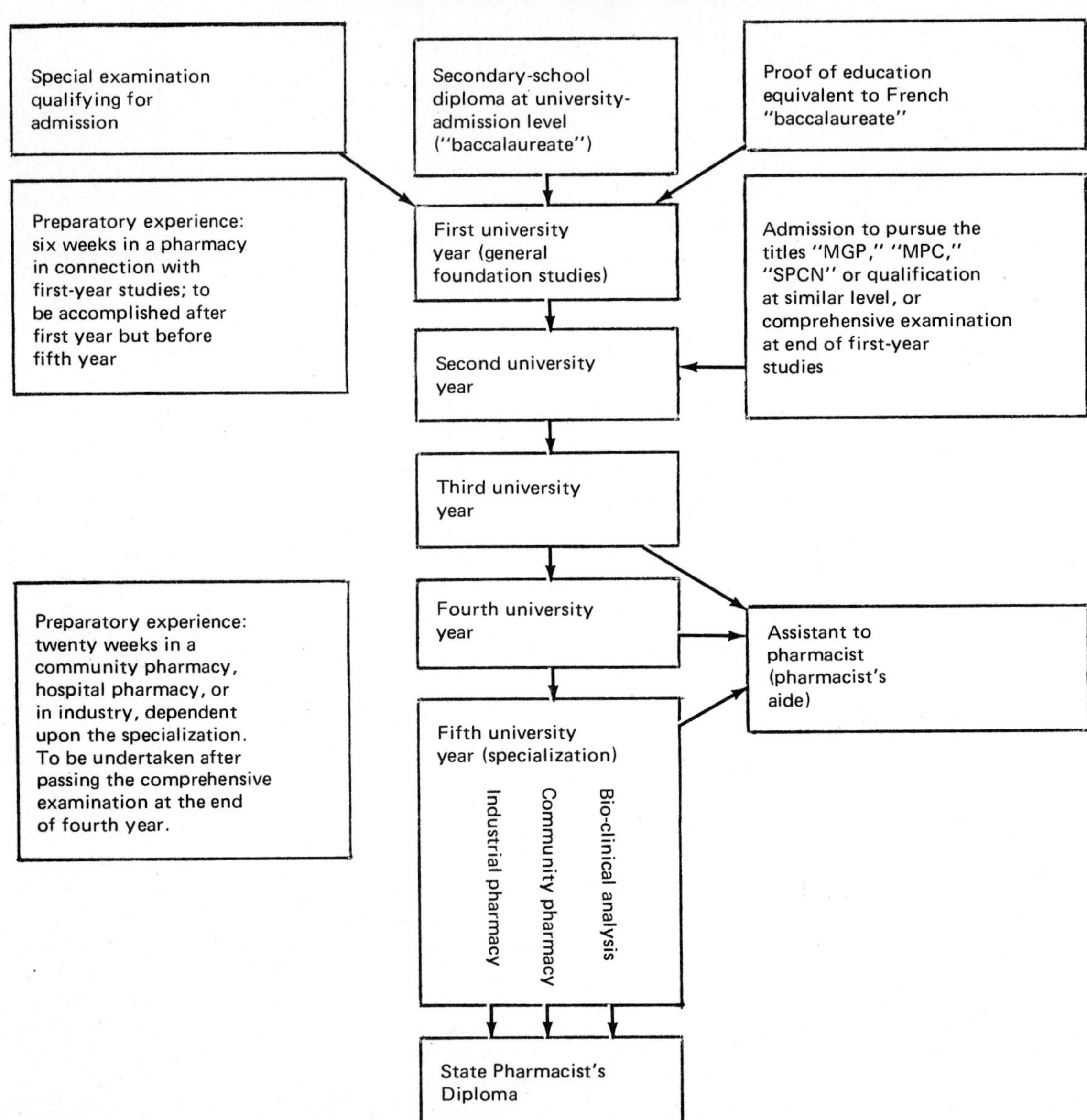


macy continues to be the "baccalaureate" diploma from a secondary school, at a higher level than an American high-school diploma (sometimes said to be equivalent to perhaps two pre-professional college years in the USA).

The formal curriculum in pharmacy at French universities requires at least 4½ years. The main subjects studied are: (a) mathematics and statistics; (b) the physicochemical sciences of inorganic and organic chemistry, mineralogy, analytical chemistry and physics; (c) the natural sciences of botany, cryptogamy, zoology, and parasitology; (d) the biological sciences of biochemistry, hygiene, toxicology, microbiology, and pathology; and (e) the professional subject areas of chemical pharmacy, galenical pharmacy, materia medica, pharmacodynamics, and pharmaceutical legislation.

Part of the reform introduced a terminal specialization in the fifth year. The student chooses one of three options or specialized tracks: community pharmacy, industrial pharmacy, or clinical laboratory analyses (termed "biology")—the latter having a long tradition among French pharmacists as one of their health-care services. One dilemma was resolved in favor of maintaining the "unity of the diploma;" that is, any of the three specializations would lead to a diploma giving the legal right to practice as a pharmacist.

The in-service portion of the requirements (controlled experience) was reduced in 1962 to two unequal parts: a six-week stint after the first university year, then an additional twenty weeks interposed during the last years of the five-year program. Part of the qualifying experience may be obtained in a manufacturing laboratory or a clinical-analytical laboratory, if a student has chosen one of those options in which to specialize, and the remainder is served in a community pharmacy. Postgraduate programs are of course available for those who elect to carry specialization to a more advanced level. Those students who leave the university without completing the full curriculum may elect to qualify as "assistant pharmacists," a technician category initiated in 1969–70. (The chart on the opposite page shows in simplified form the relationship of the educational requirements after 1968.)[43]

Before the changes in pharmaceutical education could be effectuated, some rather difficult issues had to be resolved during the 1960's: interchangeability of diplomas with other members of the European Economic Community; how to reconcile the push for specialization with the traditionally encyclopedic character of pharmaceutical education; and whether adequate specialization could be achieved and still legally accord the right to practice pharmacy to all graduates.

## DEVELOPMENT OF A LITERATURE

The professional spirit that has animated the development of French pharmacy through many decades likewise found expression in a professional literature. The early treatises that guided pharmaceutical work derived largely from Islamic sources, as was true throughout Southern Europe. By the 16th century, when we saw the academic interests of pharmacists becoming more visible, the best French practitioners had reached the stage of generating original literature of their own. Probably the earliest was Michel Dusseau's manual of pharmaceutical technique published in 1561. After the mid-17th century the number of books by French pharmacists increased, the authorship of some so illustrious that their names survive in the history of science, beyond the parochial circle of pharmacists themselves—men such as Charas, Lefebvre, Lémery, and Geoffroy.

It was also in the 17th century that the first local pharmacopeia of France appeared (Lyons, 1628), which was soon emulated by other cities. This local approach to unifying drug standards was not superseded entirely until 1818, when the first edition of the *Codex medicamentarius. . .* became an obligatory pharmacopeia for the whole of France.

A rich literature began with the Journal of the Society of Pharmacists of Paris in 1797—just 4 years after the launching of its German prototype—then periodicals branched out diversely during the 19th century. Many contributions to their pages influenced phar-

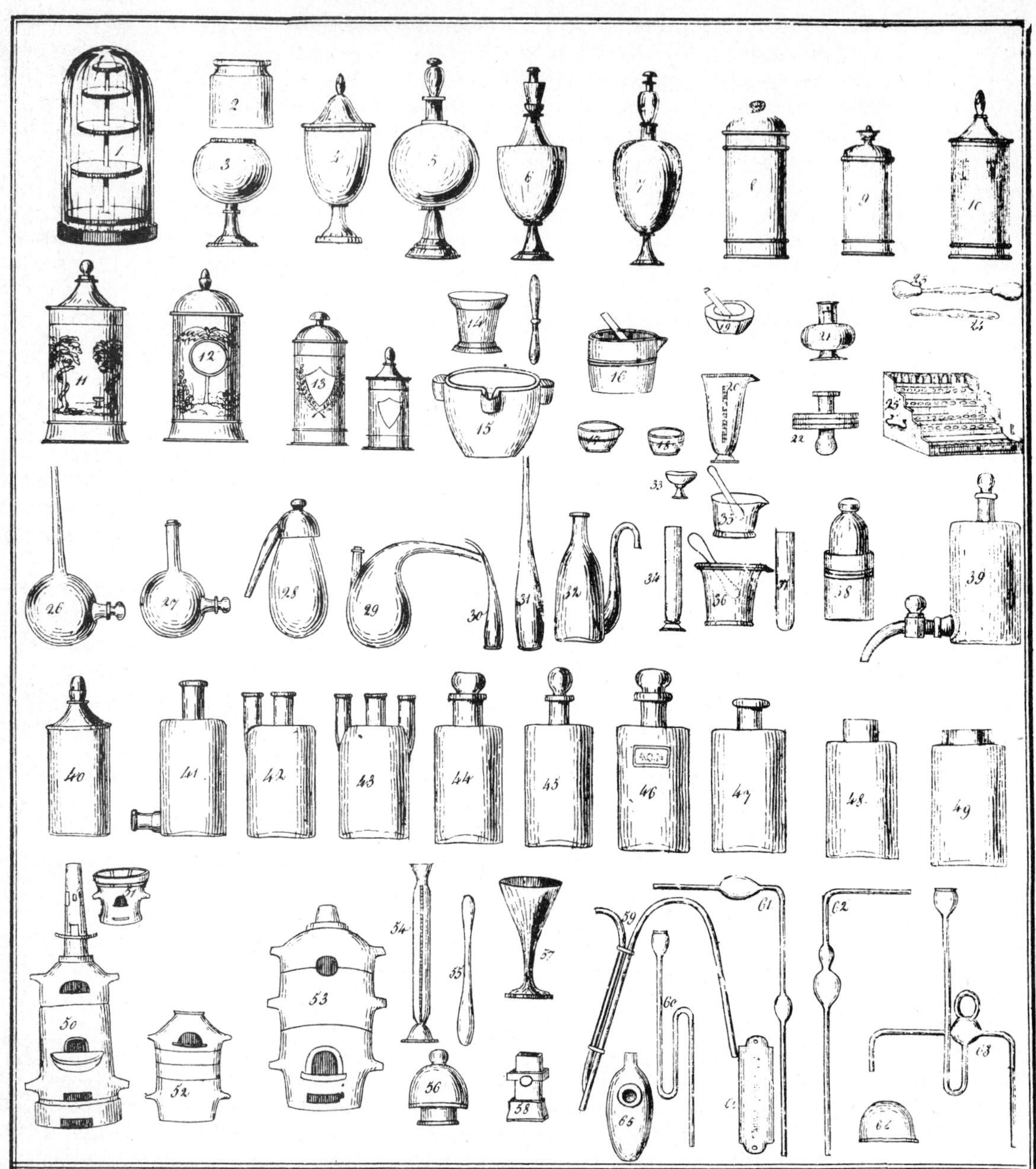

The character of French pharmacies and their small laboratories, about the middle of the 19th century, is almost tangibly conjured up by this parade of equipment. Reproduced from a price list of a Paris dealer, the numbered items (*left* to *right*) are:

*1.* Mahogany display rack with cylindrical glass cover

*2, 3.* Leech jars

*4.* Jar for medicaments

*5, 6, 7.* Show-window bottles (globe-shaped, urn-shaped and egg-shaped) macy and health care far beyond the borders of France, including America.

The authors often drew stimulus from the scientific and clinical milieu of Paris, where pharmacy interacted with science and medicine in a way seldom surpassed.[44] (*Appendix 6* includes additional literature references, p. 424, for those who wish to consult French historical sources at first hand.)

## PROMINENT PHARMACISTS AND SCIENCE

The prominence of the names of pharmacists in the French development of science was no minor or transitory phenomenon. Already at the end of the 18th century, the famous chemist J. A. Chaptal observed that, "The relations between chemistry and pharmacy are so intimate that they have been considered for a long time as one and the same science . . . ."[45] By the nature of the pharmacists' central task of drug making, they carried over into general chemical work an "emphasis on factual, empirical data at the expense of theory," which in this period may have been more advantage than handicap, as one leading pharmacist after another made his mark as a superb analyst or top-notch experimentalist.

During the 19th century, moreover, pharmacist-chemists continued to apply their chemistry-based resources with great versatility in such diverse fields as biology,

←

*8, 9, 10.* Conserve jars with convex, Paris-market and Chinese cover styles, respectively
*11, 12, 13.* Ceramic pharmacy jars, with Chinese, acorn and convex cover styles, respectively
*14.* Cast iron mortar, with pestle
*15.* Marble mortar
*16.* Serpentine mortar
*17, 18.* Small serpentine mortars, with and without lip
*19.* Agate mortar with pestle
*20.* Graduated measure
*21.* Lamp for spirit of wine (i.e., ethyl alcohol)
*22.* Bulb of barometer
*23, 24.* Pestles of guaiac and of boxwood
*25.* Reagent box
*26.* Long-necked, round-bottom flask with ground-glass stopper
*27.* Same without tube
*28.* Cucurbit (i.e., boiler) with distillation head
*29.* Tubulated retort with ground-glass stopper
*30.* Curved adapter or coupler
*31.* Straight adapter or coupler
*32.* Florentine receiver
*33.* Eye cup
*34.* Footed cylinder
*35.* Mortar of twice-baked porcelain
*36.* Glass mortar with pestle
*37.* Test tube
*38.* Disinfecting bottle
*39.* Bottle with stopcock, for syrup of ether
*40.* Undecorated conserve jar with Chinese-style lid
*41.* Woulf flask with one tube below
*42, 43.* Woulf flasks with two and three tubes above
*44, 45, 46.* Glass-stoppered bottles, one with glass-label
*47.* Necked bottle for distilled water
*48.* Salt-mouth, short-necked bottle
*49.* Wide-mouthed bottle for herbs
*50.* Furnace with cupeler
*51.* Furnace with basin
*52.* Tube furnace
*53.* Reverberatory furnace
*54.* Alkalimeter
*55.* Spatula
*56.* Cupping glass
*57.* Glass for experiment
*58.* Ingot mold
*59.* Siphon
*60.* S-tube
*61.* Pipette
*62.* Blowpipe
*63.* Burrette
*64.* Oval cupping glass, English
*65.* Infant feeding-bottle
*66.* Drawer label.
(Photograph, University of Wisconsin, from a brochure of Ancienne Maison Acloque, Vimeux Vieillard & Cie, successors)

hygiene, therapeutics and toxicology. "In this sense," Alex Berman concluded, "science was cultivated by many 19th-century French pharmacists, for its own sake, where-ever its applications might lead . . . . The cumulative results were impressive: new therapeutic agents were uncovered, new elements brought to light and characterized, and various significant techniques and apparatus were introduced."[46]

Thirty-two pages of the history of French pharmacy written by André-Pontier and 48 pages of Bouvet's history[47] are devoted to a brief enumeration of famous French pharmacists from the 17th to the present century. These men intensively and often decisively promoted scientific progress in the different branches of the natural sciences. While so doing, some of them served their country in prominent positions with remarkable success. Some names have already been mentioned. A few further examples (for whom biographic notes may be found in Appendix 7) are Balard (1802–1876), Bayen (1725–1798), Caventou (1795–1877), Parmentier (1737–1813), Pelletier (1788–1842), Proust (1754–1826), Robiquet (1780–1840), G. F. Rouelle (1703–1770) and his brother H. M. Rouelle (1718–1778), Sérullas (1774–1832), Soubeiran (1797–1858) and Vauquelin (1763–1829).

Thirteen pharmacists were members of the French Academy of Science before 1803; six pharmacists were members of this Academy in 1936 and eleven pharmacists were members of the French Academy of Medicine.[48]

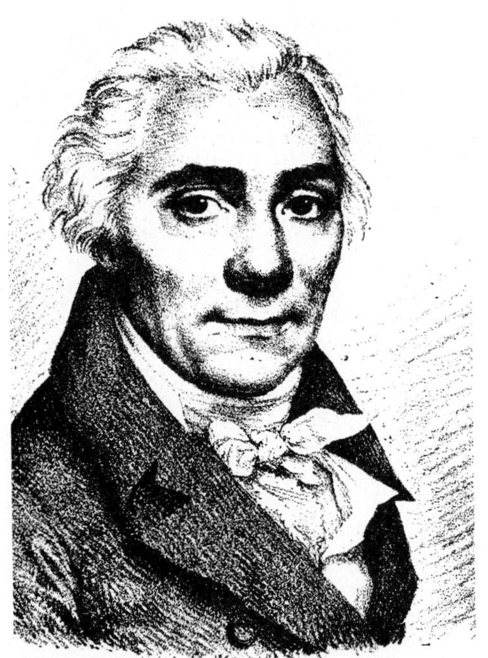

Born on a humble Normandy farm, L.-N. Vauquelin became a pharmacy owner in Paris, eventually reaching a scientific distinction that earned him the title of Chevalier of the Legion of Honor and his appointment by Napoleon as director of the school of pharmacy at Paris, and later as professor of chemistry in the Jardin des Plantes. (Drawing by J. Boilly, 1820; Collection L. Sergent; reproduced from Bull. Soc. Hist. Pharm. No. 65, 1929)

## HOSPITAL AND MILITARY PHARMACY

Modern hospital pharmacy was born in Paris in the early 19th century. As a specialty, it constituted one of the unique features in the development of pharmacy in France and was without precedent in other countries, even in Germany where French pharmacists encountered their most formidable scientific and professional rivalry.[49]

The role of the hospital pharmacist in this period has been characterized and distinguished from both monastic and lay predecessors as follows:

For one thing, he was a lay practitioner and not a member of a religious order. Unlike the English hospital apothecary of the 18th and early 19th century, he did not assume the dual role of pharmacist and minor medical practitioner. The Parisian hospital pharmacist was a municipal employee, selected on the basis of a competitive examination *(concours)* and, after 1814, recruited from those having completed an internship in hospital pharmacy. The internship became more and more important during the course of the century, not only for staffing hospital pharmacies but also in stimulating young pharmacists to become scientists. This new hospital pharmacist was generally oriented toward research and was often an excellent analytical chemist working in the fields of biochemistry, toxicology, and hygiene. Thus, with the passing of the years, a tradition of scientific eminence was established, and we see the hospital pharmacists of Paris acquiring advanced degrees, becoming members of learned societies and professors in the various Faculties, making original discoveries, and publishing in learned journals.[50]

As in the community pharmacies, clinical laboratory work has been an important function of hospital pharmacists, but recently its volume and complexity make it difficult for the hospital pharmacist to fulfill his traditional role of joint director of the pharmacy and the medical biochemical services.

Hospital pharmacy holds a special place in military service, where we find the French pharmacist first mentioned in 1630.[51] From the beginning he was placed on the same footing with the surgeon. The permanent office of "apothecary-major of the battlefields and the armies of the king" was created in 1766 (a title usually abridged to "apothecary-major general").[52] To accord with the title of *médecin inspecteur général* held by the leading military physician, this title was replaced (1824) by the designation *pharmacien inspecteur général.* The French military pharmacists, called *pharmaciens-chimistes,* have enjoyed (since 1928) ranks equal with those of the army physicians.

In the pharmacists' effort to avoid subordination to military medicine, "the most significant factor was the impressive display of their scientific accomplishments—a display without precedent in pharmacy of the English-speaking world, and unmatched by military pharmacy in other European countries at that time."[53]

Many of the best-known French pharmacists have seen service in the army, such as J. A. A. Parmentier (1737–1813). Although famous for research in food chemistry, which earned his election to the French Academy of Sciences, Parmentier remained for most of his career in military pharmacy. He was Chief Pharmacist at Invalides, and eventually became Inspector General of the Health Department of the Armies of France.

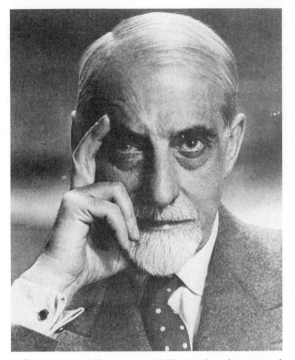

Ernest F. A. Fourneau (1872-1949), who owned a pharmacy for many years, rose to international fame as a brilliant investigator in pharmaceutical chemistry. For 30 years he directed the chemotherapeutic laboratory of the Pasteur Institute, whose research paved the way for sulfonamide products, produced pioneer antihistaminic agents and yielded other significant discoveries. When Fourneau sent the above picture to George Urdang (1947), he inscribed it on the back, "With cordial homage from a pharmacist."

The pharmacist-general Ch. Laubert, of the so-called *Grande armée* of Napoleon I, enjoyed the special confidence of the Emperor.

After the siege of Moscow in 1812, Napoleon planned a mint to stamp coins out of the gold and the silver that the French had found in the conquered city. When asked whether he knew someone who could set up and operate a mint, the Emperor answered, "Don't we have our pharmacist-general? I commission him with everything!"

It was this remarkable versatility—if in a different context—that led Alex Berman to say after long study of French pharmaco-scientific developments: ". . . The historian becomes aware of dominant characteristics not present in the development of pharmacy in the English-speaking world, namely a rich diversity and versatility and an impressive scientific orientation which resulted in contributions to the fields of chemistry, hygiene and public health, toxicology and therapeutics."[54]

# 6

# The Development in Germany

## THE BEGINNINGS

Pharmacies may have appeared in Germany during the 13th century, but questions of definition leave uncertainty. During the Middle Ages, the number of pharmacists in German communities remained too small to make pharmaceutical guilds or guildlike associations possible. Pharmacists were forced at times to join a guild of another calling, since some cities in Germany (and the German-speaking part of Switzerland) did not allow tradesmen not belonging to a guild to operate businesses.

For example, in esteemed guilds in Kassel and in Basel, comprised of leading commercial groups and members of the intellectual professions, pharmacists not only were guild members but often were elected to office.[1] German pharmacists often objected to becoming members of the guilds of ordinary retailers, and in such a "marriage of convenience" only the commercial side of the pharmacist's activity was subjected to guild regulation.[2]

## SYSTEMS OF PHARMACY OWNERSHIP

### Feudal Grants of "Privilege"

Controls guaranteed to merchants and craftsmen by their guilds—for example, the "closed shop" and the monopoly of sale and of manufacture of specified products—were accorded by the ruling authority through a *privilegium*, that is, special privileges granted on the basis of duties carefully stipulated in a signed and sealed document carrying full legal power.

Such a contract—typical of the feudal system, especially in Germany—was bestowed on a pharmacist, for example, by an individual ruler or by an aristocratic governing body of a principality of the Holy Roman Empire. This *privilegium* could be of various types. It might concern the pharmacists' establishment, in which case the recipient of the "privilege" would have to buy the building. Another type of "privilege" might contain a proviso that it would end with the grantee's death or, conversely, that it would be hereditary. It might be a type granted by a ruler without restriction, in which case the pharmacist at any time could sell this exclusive right to operate a pharmacy in the area specified.[3] An "exclusive" right—by no means rare up to the 17th century—excluded the establishment of another pharmacy in the community or the area concerned, no matter how large the population might grow.

Either with or without the "exclusive" right, privileges remained the usual legal basis of pharmacies in the Germanic states until the early 19th century. From then on, no new "privileges" were granted, generally speaking, although the old ones were not invalidated.

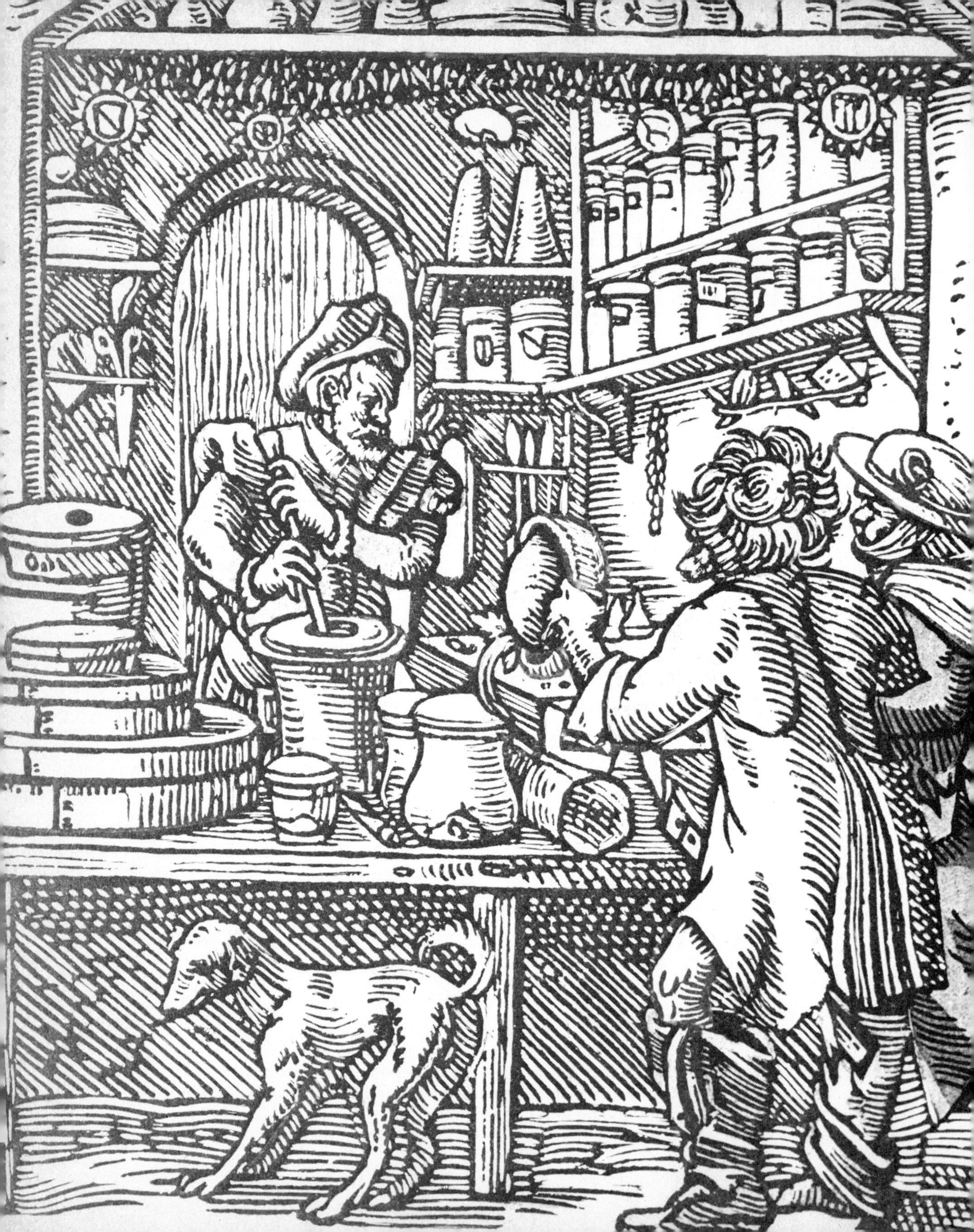

## Concession System

The arbitrariness and the unlimited authority reflected in the old feudal mechanism were replaced by a competitive system of granting a government "concession" to operate each pharmacy serving a specified segment of the population. The concession system recognized a new time, without abandoning the German values of regulated order, dignity and quality in pharmaceutical development.

If we ignore minor differences in provisions among the various German states, the procedure may be summarized as follows: The town, or area in a town, where a pharmacy was deemed to be needed, issued a public announcement. Interested pharmacists were invited to apply. A commission compared the qualifications of the applicants, but, in general, the right to operate the pharmacy (the "concession") tended to be awarded to the employed pharmacist who had been longest in practice.

These valuable rights could be neither sold nor inherited in some German states. However, in the largest state (Prussia), a concession holder could nominate his successor—which, in practice, was almost equivalent to the right of sale or of hereditary transmission. The government could say "no" to a nomination, but seldom did so. The "concession" for a pharmacy practically assured a large and prosperous professional practice, so it was a sought-after property of high value, (and hence called a *Real-Konzession*). Such concessions carrying the "right of presentation" were discontinued even in Prussia beginning in 1894.

The pattern of awarding a permit for a new pharmacy, or a vacated old pharmacy, was by competitive selection among applicants (termed a "*Personal-Konzession*) under which the selected pharmacist had the right to operate the pharmacy only during his lifetime.[4] Unlike the speculative value of a "real" concession, the "personal" concession changed hands on payment of only the value of the stock and equipment, and possibly a certain amount for any capital improvememts made.

Until after World War II German pharmacists operated under any one of three types of permit; for, when one of the German states modified its permit system, the action was not retroactive. Hence in some pharmacies rights that had been granted in a remote time persisted:

1. *Privilegia* could be disposed of quite as the owners might desire.
2. *Real-Konzession* could be transmitted by sale or inheritance, but government confirmation of each transfer was required.
3. *Personal-Konzession* gave the right to the operation and the income of a particular pharmacy for a person's lifetime on the basis of professional merit and, especially, of length of service as an employed pharmacist. Being a personal concession to a particular pharmacist, it could not be sold or inherited.

Exceptions to these categories were usually pharmacies owned by communities, by organizations or by the old aristocracy.

## Municipal and Princely Pharmacies

A few pharmacies in certain German states were owned by the government or by former

←

Country folk visiting their village pharmacist in the 16th century. This woodcut from a booklet about various German crafts and professions had in rhyme, beneath it, the pharmacist saying (in German):

In my pharmacy I have placed
Much material of pleasant taste.
Sugar with spices I prepare.
Of cathartics and clysters I likewise take care.
Also to strengthen the sick and the weak
Many a self prepared tonic I seek.
For all this, on a doctor's advice I lean
Who has the patient's urine seen.

(Woodcut by Jost Amman; rhymes by Hans Sachs, in Eygentliche Beschreibung . . ., Frankfurt a/M, 1568; through Illustrierter Apotheker-Kalender, Stuttgart, 1925.)

SANVS ET HVC ÆGER
NVLLO DISCRIMINE CVRRANT
INDIGET ET DIVES
PAVPER ET ARTE MEA
GALENICA
CHYMICA
PRECIOSA
PRECIOSA
SALVS INFIRMORVM
ACIDVL
ACIDVL
ACI DVLÆ
ACI DV LÆ
Caspar am Ort Invent.
Wolfgang Kilian
PHARMACIA

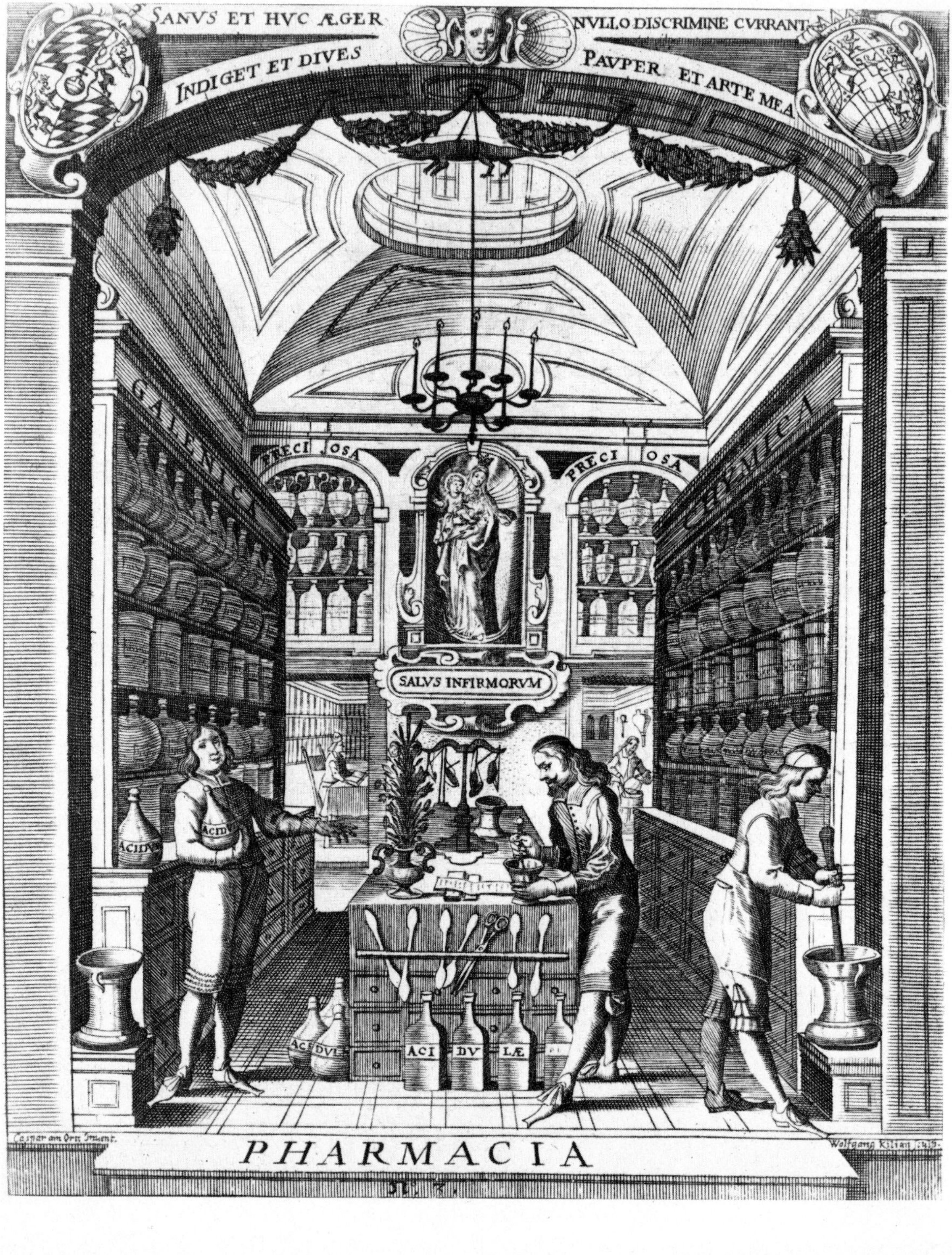

sovereigns, after World War II. Most of these had been established in the 16th and 17th centuries as the court pharmacies of German princes.[5] Then pharmacies often had also been operated by the larger municipalities, especially in the imperial cities, which possessed the same governmental sovereignty as the German princes of the time.[6] The municipalities did not derive the advantage from their pharmacies that they had expected, so they leased or sold them. Still, in modern times, communities in some of the German states (Anhalt, Baden, Hessia and Thuringia) had governmental permission to establish pharmacies in places where the government considered them to be needed. These pharmacies were leased to pharmacists who were selected in the usual way, by public contest in which the length of service as an employee in pharmacies played a decisive part. (In 1934, Hessia still had 23 such communal pharmacies among a total of 128.)

As with the early municipal pharmacies, the first German attempt at socialized pharmacy—that is, pharmacy as an institution of the state, conducted by pharmaceutical officials—failed financially. The Duke of Brunswick tried this experiment as early as the second half of the 18th century, when he bought the pharmacies in his country, created a central pharmaceutical administration and laboratory, and a central department for the purchase of all drugs and supplies. After 20 years, during which neither the expected profit was achieved nor better service rendered to the public, the pharmacies were sold to private individuals.[7]

All of these different systems of regulation found in the history of German pharmacy agree in one decisive principle: the limitation of the number of pharmacies. This principle was abandoned in Prussia for only one year (1810), with the introduction of general liberty to practice any calling *(Gewerbefreiheit)*. Another exception, for almost a century, was Hamburg—a city influenced by England as a result of its location and trade—where anyone who could prove his pharmaceutical knowledge was permitted to open a pharmacy. However, the difficulties of maintaining professional standards and order brought back, in 1818, a limitation on the number of pharmacies in relation to the population served.

The general tradition of controlling the number and the distribution of pharmacies—at a certain price in freedom of opportunity and decision—did achieve a high and unusually uniform level of professional practice, appearance and pride in the German pharmacies, all of which have been devoted exclusively to health-related and technical services.

**Limitation Overthrown**

A fundamental turn away from the traditional limitation on the number of pharmacies came at the close of World War II, when the four military occupation zones of Germany became regulated under different concepts and circumstances. The American zone introduced the freedom of establishing pharmacies; the British and French zones remained in principle with the "concession" system; while in the Soviet Eastern zone the pharmacies gradually came under socialized government operation. This process continued until a new regulation was issued after the founding of the West German republic.

Then came court proceedings culminating in the "Karlsruher Urteil," a decision under the postwar constitution that made freedom of location of pharmacies general after 1959 throughout the West German republic. To be sure, the special pharmaceutical rights and privileges were not rescinded, but they were made worthless by a wholly new situation that permitted new pharmacies to mushroom

←

Hospital Pharmacy at Munich, as represented in a mid-17th-century engraving by W. Kilian. (From M. Geiger Microcosmus Hypochondriacus, facing p. 240, Munich, 1652; through The National Library of Medicine)

from the German land. Whereas in 1951 there were about 5,000 community pharmacies operating in West Germany, two decades later the number had more than doubled. The average number of citizens served by each pharmacy had fallen from 9587 in 1950 to 5122 in 1970. The universities, in the early 1970's, could accommodate only a fraction of the qualified students who wished to study pharmacy.

While many young pharmacists tended to see the breakdown of the old ownership restrictions in terms of opportunity, there were calls from older pharmacists for "vigilance, lest the high professional standing of German pharmacy is lost." The President of the Hamburg Chamber of Pharmacists in 1960 said, "The past experiences in Germany and in other countries abroad clearly indicate that this road [freedom of location] should not be attempted again."[8]

What makes the freer system more problematic for German pharmacists in recent years has been the introduction of a new class of supportive personnel into the pharmacies, which seems almost to create a new

Characteristic German pharmacy of the 17th century. A pharmacist is handing medication to a patient at the walk-up dispensing window (*left*), while other pharmacists busy themselves at the prescription counter (which has a vertical rack for hand-held balances for weighing drugs). On the small furnace (*right foreground*) is an air-cooled alembic for distillation. The crocodile overhead was symbolic of the natural science to which pharmacy has been devoted. (Engraving from early 17th century, studio of A.-C. Fleischmann, Nuremberg, in William Helfand Collection; photo from The Smithsonian Institution)

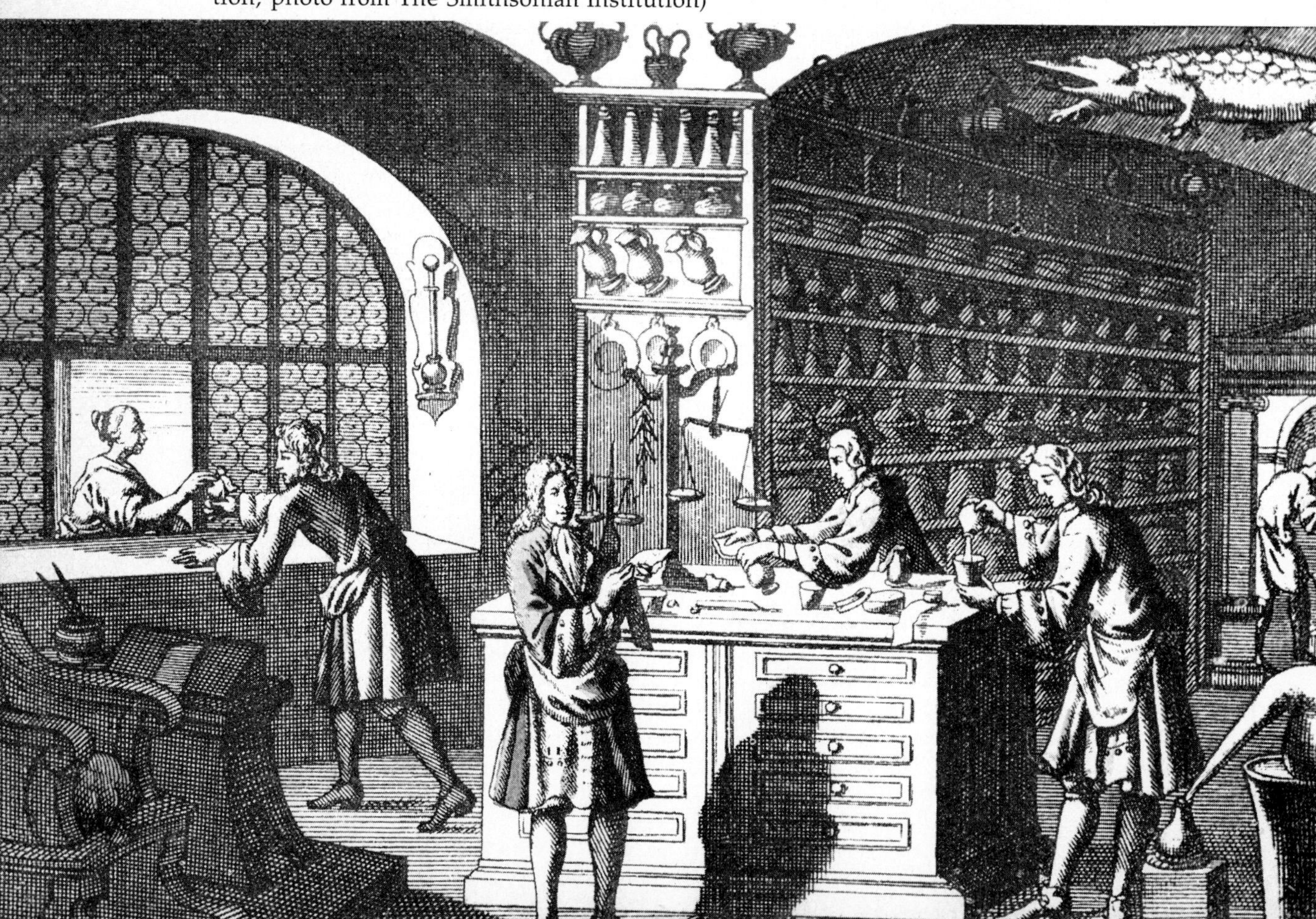

pharmaceutical calling and has proved attractive among German youth who do not undertake work toward some type of university degree. Under conditions set by a law effective since 1968, the educational requirement for a technical assistant to a pharmacist is two years of study (having considerable pharmaceutical content) in a special school, followed by a half year of on-site training in a pharmacy before examination.[8a]

## MONOPOLY; PRICES; "DROGERIEN"

Most of the *privilegia* issued between the 14th and the 18th centuries contained instructions about the management of the pharmacy and enumerations of monopolies granted the pharmacist, often including even such products as sugar, spices, liquors, wine, tobacco, coffee and chocolate. Some of these were used in medicine and were costly substances. However, the main reason for reserving them for sale by pharmacists was a presumed need to assure a livelihood to an essential group whose professional function was too limited quantitatively. For example, a privilege granted a pharmacist in Landsberg a.W., in 1585, explicitly stated that he must be given a monopoly of the trade in spices, wine and liquors, because it would be impossible for him to earn his livelihood from the sale of medicaments only.[9] The same idea was expressed in many laws, ordinances and edicts. The Count of Schleiz in the 17th century, for example, admonished the town authorities to protect the pharmacy from illegal competition by ordinary retailers lest "this precious jewel so very useful for town and country becomes damaged or even perishes!"[10] Later on, the monopoly rights of the pharmacists became restricted more and more to medicaments. Nevertheless, the fundamental concept of governmental obligation to protect the pharmacies in behalf of the public welfare has not been changed.

A consequence of the German principle of maintaining a just balance between the rights and the duties of the people by legal regulation was that governmental limitation of competition had to be supplemented by governmental protection of the people from abuse of this restriction. This implied early introduction of regulated prices (e.g., the legal system of Frederick II of Hohenstaufen) for remedies sold by pharmacists who held monopolistic privileges.[11] It gave rise to elaborate lists of governmentally fixed prices, which in modern form still regulate commercial relations between the pharmacists and the public, with intended mutual benefit.

The price lists of all the smaller German states and the individual towns,[12] which with a few exceptions had gradually disappeared in the 19th century, were replaced in 1905 by the first governmentally fixed drug prices obligatory for the entire German Empire. New editions have been issued periodically in accord with changes in wholesale prices.

This *Arzneitaxe* not only fixes prices for drugs, but also sets fees for the pharmaceutical work done in filling prescriptions, in accordance with the amount of time required and the technical skill involved.[13]

Even after the monopoly rights of pharmacists gradually came to be limited to remedies, there was sporadic quarreling between the pharmacists and would-be competitors. Many of the edicts and laws concerning pharmacy through the centuries tried to deal with this subject.[14] Again and again, the governments of the various German states stated the kinds of products reserved to pharmacies and those that might be sold elsewhere.

The original tendency to reserve all dispensing of remedies to pharmacists underwent a gradual change. Concessions had been made to the *Materialisten,* a combination of retail grocer and hardware dealer. Further concessions opened the retail trade in spices and cosmetics to everyone. In 1872 the first of a series of Imperial edicts took out of the pharmaceutical monopoly all unprepared and unmixed drugs—with the exception of a number of very potent ones—and all preparations sold avowedly for use as cosmetics, foodstuff, dietetic aids and preventives (even if these had some properties that seemed healing or palliative). One result was a new art of advertising, developed to remove from the pharmaceutical monopoly as many remedies as possible by labeling them cosmetics or dietetic aids or, above all, as preventives (even though the primary use of some such products was medicinal).

As the edicts did not enumerate what was allowed for free trade but only stated the kinds of preparations reserved to the pharmacies, many possibilities for interpretation were left open. Out of these possibilities gradually developed a distinct class of shops called *Drogerien,* specializing in the sale of technical chemicals, cosmetics, dietetic aids, spices, candy, dyes, toiletries, varnishes and all those drugs and remedies that were not restricted to pharmacies, or that could be so interpreted.

These shops (in superficial appearance like below-average American drugstores, but without any potent drugs or prescription service) are operated by *Drogisten* (literally "druggists," but in no respect being or considered to be pharmacists). The owners of the *Drogerien* have had since 1872 a quite separate and very active organization. While the number of such shops has tended to decline in recent decades, there are still more *Drogerien* than there are *Apotheken* (pharmacies).

Having achieved their position on the basis of a contention that no special pharmaceutical knowledge is needed to sell "harmless" drugs, the *Drogisten* later changed their tune. Since the early 20th century they have clamored periodically for official recognition as a kind of second-class pharmacist (with certain privileges not permitted general storekeepers), and as part of this move they organized special schools for their apprentices.

After World War II the *Drogisten* sought permission to deal in all drugs not requiring a prescription, without success. The group of non-prescription drugs restricted to pharmacies remains the same as before (in the USA sought, but not authorized, for pharmacies as a so-called "third class" of drugs). The shops of the German "druggists" *(Drogisten)* retain their special character, but still in selling drugs have no special privileges different from a supermarket or other types of retail shops. Neither the law on the practice of pharmacy of 1960 nor the drug law of 1961 shrank the area over which the German pharmacist has responsibility. The drug law sharpened stipulations concerning the claims made for drugs, their manufacture, the special registration of proprietary specialties, the distribution of drugs and the safeguarding and the control of their use. During the early 1970's the appropriateness of further elaboration of controls over medicinal products again was being debated in the "Bundestag" and in the press. A proposed second drug law contained a number of controversial features affecting drug manufacturers, and indirectly the pharmacist and the patient.[15]

## DEVELOPMENT OF EDUCATION

During the early period, the professional education of the German pharmacists was not so well regulated as it was in France. Lack of cooperative self-determination left the regulation of pharmaceutical education to circles outside of pharmacy. Thus until the end of the 17th century the numerous decrees concerning pharmacy contain only vague remarks concerning professional education, although examination of competency was required (e.g., in Bavaria after 1595 physicians administered oral, written, and practical examinations to pharmacy candidates).[16]

An apprenticeship of 6 years was customary as a learning period. A satisfactory knowledge of Latin was a general requirement needed to read pharmaceutical books of the time as well as prescriptions. Since no fixed course of study was specified, however, German pharmacy on the whole could scarcely rise above the level of technical skill until after the 17th century.[17]

This situation changed in the course of the 18th century. Obligatory examinations based on definite requirements, first introduced in Prussia in 1725, gave German pharmacists a place among the representatives of the scientific professions. Thereafter, in Prussia, two classes of pharmacists existed.

Those of the second class, who were permitted to practice in small towns only, were not required to study academically. They had to serve their apprenticeship (usually 5 years) and a clerkship (usually 6 years) and then pass an examination before their provincial medical board (*Collegium medicum*).

The pharmacists of the first class were required to serve longer (at least 7 years) as clerks after their apprenticeship and had to attend a course at the higher *Collegium medicum* in Berlin, an institution mainly for the scientific education of military physicians and surgeons. This course consisted of lectures in chemistry and botany, discourses on the chemicals used in remedies, their preparation and "the chemicophysical reasons" for the several kinds of preparations and, lastly, practical pharmaceutico-chemical instruction. This division of the Prussian pharmacists into two classes disappeared in 1854.

During the last third of the 18th century the German pharmacists themselves had begun to increase their educational opportunities. A series of private institutes, devoted to the education of pharmacists, was established. Some of these became famous far beyond the German frontiers. For example, the institute of the pharmacist Johannes Bartholomaeus Trommsdorff in Erfurt (1770-1847) had many students from foreign countries. The Prussian government acknowledged the education acquired in this institute as equivalent to the study "at Berlin or at universities."[18]

This trend continued in the 19th century when Bavaria, in 1808, made university study obligatory for pharmacists; and the other German states soon followed Bavaria's lead.[18a]

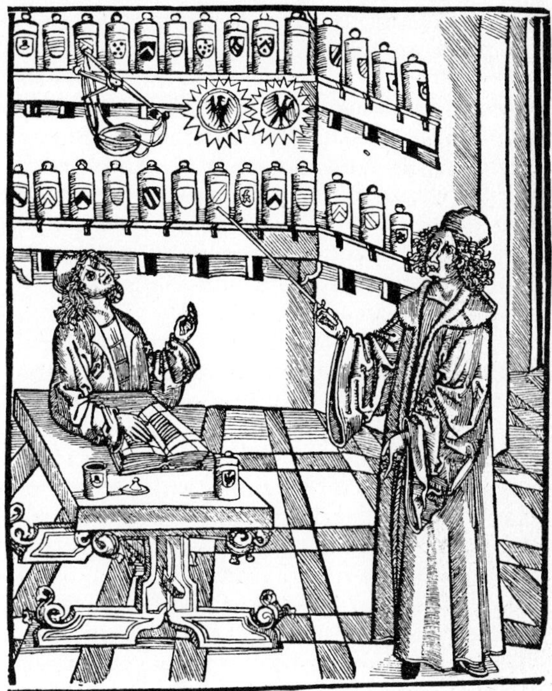

Interior of a pharmacy as depicted in a woodcut published in 1505. Probably it shows a pharmacist seated at a work-table before an open drug book, discussing a formulation with a physician, who is pointing to a medicinal ingredient. (On the edge of the top shelf can be seen a folded hand-balance for weighing and, apparently, the coat of arms of the nobleman under whose jurisdiction the pharmacy is operating.) (From A. Neuburger: Erforschung . . ., p. 257; original in H. Brunschwig, Kunst zu destillieren . . .)

The present educational requirements to practice pharmacy in Germany became effective in 1971, superseding a previous pattern that had persisted in its fundamentals since 1935.

*Preliminary education:* Under both the old and new law, an entering pharmacy student must have had 13 years of preliminary education, including the type of secondary school that prepares for university studies (a *Gymnasium*). This reaches a level sometimes estimated as equivalent to 2 to 3 years of preprofessional college studies in the United States.

*Professional studies* occupy 7 semesters of successful work, one semester less than under the previous law. The university subjects and the extent of laboratory instruction are legally defined in far more detail than in the United States.

*Examinations:* After the first 2 years of university education, written and oral examinations (*Vorexamen*) test the level of general scientific knowledge, thus qualifying an applicant to proceed to the final stage. Upon completion of the specified university program, written and oral examinations that cover the entire range of the university curriculum are taken.

*Pharmacy internship* consists of one year of practical training (*praktische Ausbildung*) in a pharmacy authorized for teaching purposes, which follows the university studies and the second-stage examination. Under the previous (1934) law, there was a 2-year apprenticeship *before* university study; then after graduation, an additional year of "probationary practice" was required before full responsibility for owning or managing a pharmacy could be assumed. Before World War II the probationary year served a secondary purpose in alleviating the scanty pharmaceutical service in rural districts. The expectation was that half the probationary time of young graduates would be served in a village having a single low-income pharmacy, in return for little more than room and board.

The lengthy, demanding apprenticeship, for centuries characteristic of the pharmacy tradition in Germany thus has given ground before the stepwise advance of academic studies, as in other countries. Yet, substantial formal learning continues in certain directions during the internship period still today—certainly more than occurs in most internships of the USA.

*A final examination,* following the internship, completes the qualification for the practice of pharmacy. This third-stage examination (*Dritter Prüfungsabschnitt*) is administered by the student's university in collaboration with the administrative/regulatory body (*Apothekerkammer;* see pp. 97f.) acting on behalf of the state.[19]

## SUPERVISION OF PHARMACY

For a long period the inspection of German pharmacies was generally the duty of physicians. By 1642 an edict issued for the town of Brandenburg officially admitted the cooperation of a pharmacist. Only after another 80 years did this local regulation become general for the entire Prussian kingdom. In some other German states the supervision of pharmacies was placed entirely in the hands of pharmacists (as in Hessia, Saxony and Thuringia). However, the Prussian system of cooperative inspection by a medical official and a pharmaceutical practitioner persisted and, since 1935, has been obligatory for the entire German Reich. The pharmacist participating in the inspection is coordinate with, not subordinate to, the physician. He has a 5-year term as an honorary official (with the title *Pharmazierat* or in special cases even *Oberpharmazierat*). The inspection of the retail trade in drugs outside pharmacies, hence the inspection of the *Drogerien,* is the responsibility of pharmaceutical practitioners.

## SOCIAL STANDING

The position of the German pharmacist socially has been similar to that of his French colleague, a typical representative of the middle class. Throughout the centuries, representatives of pharmacy have been awarded all the honors which ordinary civil life has to offer. We find pharmacists as municipal deputies, senators, mayors and, later on, as members of parliament. There were three

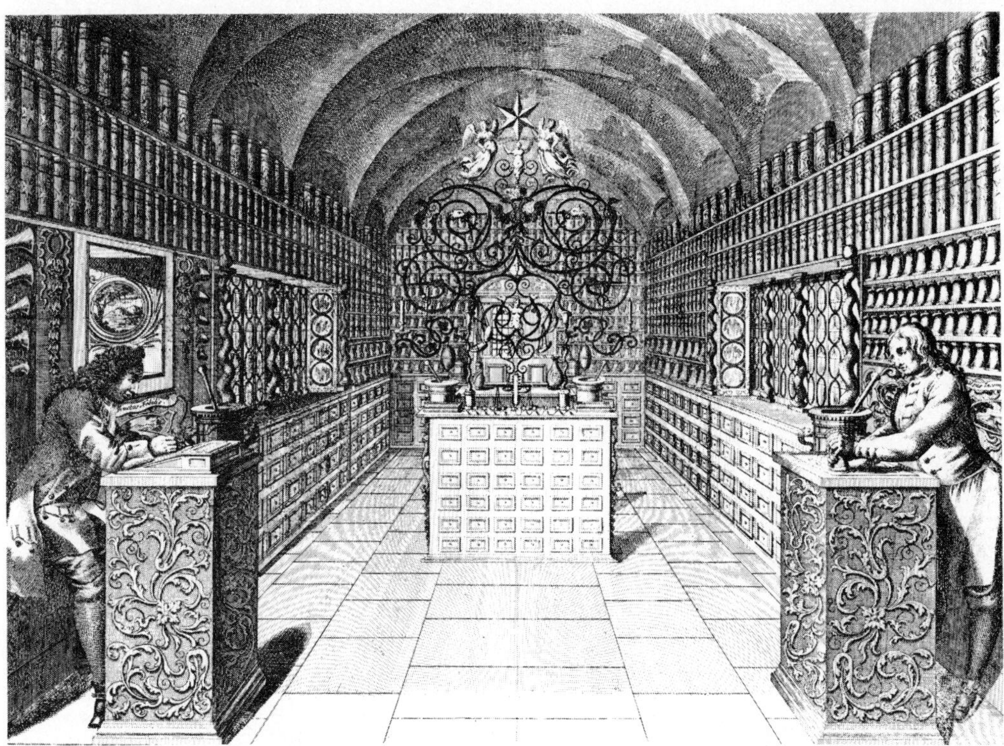

Pharmacy of the Golden Star in Nuremberg as it appeared in the early 18th century may be contrasted with the Angel Pharmacy of Merck (on page 98) as it appeared in mid-20th century. German pharmacies, old or new, set a high standard of professional character.

In the Star Pharmacy, the chief pharmacist (*at the desk on the left*) is bringing his records up to date, while one of his associates (*on the right*) seems to be preparing a dispensing container. The main prescription counter stands in the center of the pharmacy, surmounted by ornamental rococo grillework. Matched sets of stock containers fill the shelves. Below waist-level the pharmacy is lined with small drawers. (Copper engraving by H. Bohrmann, 1710)

reasons for this social esteem: (1) the pharmacist for the most part belonged to the well-to-do class; (2) often there were "dynasties" of pharmacists active for generations in the same place; (3) they were the most available and sometimes the only representatives of natural science within their communities, and their knowledge often benefitted their fellow citizens.[20]

As a classic illustration of the scientific and social standing of German pharmacy at the beginning of the 19th century, one of the greatest Germans, the poet and statesman Goethe, may be quoted. Goethe stated (1822) that "in Germany the pharmacist enjoys a highly esteemed position within society . . . . The German pharmacists cultivate science. They are aware of its importance and endeavor to utilize it in practical pharmacy."[21]

This scientific endeavor of the German pharmacist at times provoked literary derision, as he stood between trade and science.[22] Particularly in Germany, with its precise class distinctions sharply differentiating socially between tradesmen and scientists, this hybrid condition could create tragicomic situations.

In the 17th century the pharmacies began to mirror the social position of their owners. German pharmacists tried to make their homes and shops places of dignity and of artistic culture.[23]

In response to a growing demand, faïence production spread over the whole of Germany after the 17th century; and thus, most pharmacies obtained elegant sets of drug jars for their shelves, which previously had been restricted to the few who could afford to import Italian, French or Delft shelfware.

The fact that, from the beginning of their professional service in the armed forces, pharmacists were given rank and pay comparable with that of commissioned officers testifies to their social as well as their professional level. The German military pharmacists (in rank up to colonel) have been entrusted not only with strictly pharmaceutical work but also with hygienic and chemical warfare tasks, and with the responsibilities of well-educated natural scientists.[24]

## PHARMACEUTICAL LITERATURE

The centuries-old German tradition of painstaking scholarship and scientific competition produced a prolific literature, including a pharmaceutical literature of international influence in every period from the Renaissance onward.

In the century after the invention of printing, when so much of the population did not have professional health services available, a number of herbals appeared that reinforced the therapeutics of folk medicine, as well as serving as an early resource for pharmacists and physicians. Among such books, versions of the "Garden of Health" were particularly of popular renown in the 15th and 16th centuries. In the 16th century encyclopedic books appeared, covering the entire scope of pharmacy, such as J. J. Wecker's *Antidotarium Generale* (1561), which offered a comprehensive formulary, directions for preparing both galenical and chemical remedies of the time, and instructions on the art of compounding and dispensing prescriptions. One of the herbalists, Otto Brunfels, published a specialized work on equipping and managing a pharmacy (*Die Reformation der Apotheken)* already in 1536. It was symptomatic of a maturing European profession that a similar treatise was published in Italy (by Saladin di Ascoli) in the preceding century, and would be published in France (by Jean de Renou) in the next century. Apparently the first book written by a German pharmacist on pharmaco-chemical subjects was J. C. Sommerhof's excellent *Lexicon pharmaceutico-chymicum* of 1701. In this century German scientific pharmacy came of age; and from the mid-18th century on, the number of such books by pharmacists surged upward and set a high standard almost without exception. The laboratories of such pharmacist-authors often were precursors to the later chemical laboratories of universities and to the manufacturing and scientific laboratories of large-scale pharmaceutical industry.

With pharmaceutical services now commonly separate physically, as well as functionally, from the practice of medicine, need was felt by the 16th century in various European centers for more uniform drug products and more uniform prescribing nomenclature for use between physicians and pharmacists. Out of this need grew a special standard-setting literature, often called "pharmacopeias." In Germany the first official pharmacopiea was the *Dispensatorium* published by a physician Valerius Cordus in 1546, and made official for the imperial city of Nuremberg. Probably it should be considered the prototype of all pharmacopeias, in the modern sense of compulsory standards for drugs within a specific political jurisdiction, since Cordus' *Dispensatorium* was enacted as legally binding on all practitioners in the Nuremberg area. (The earlier book in Florence, 1499, had guild authority behind it, but apparently not a documented enactment by civil authorities.)

During ensuing decades, pharmacopeias were compiled for other Germanic areas. The *Pharmacopoeia Borussica* (1799), incorporating the first Prussian standards, was especially noteworthy even beyond the borders of Germany as a work of high quality, as one of the first pharmacopeias to reflect the new chemical theories and as the first one in Germany to be prepared mainly by pharmacists (rather than mainly by physicians). Only a year after the unification of Germany, the first *Pharmacopoea Germanica* appeared and was made official for the entire German Empire.

German pharmacy likewise took the lead in publishing the first periodicals primarily devoted to pharmacy. Beginning in 1780 the pharmacist Johann Goettling edited an annual called the Pocketbook for Chemist and Pharmacist (*Almanach oder Taschenbuch für Scheidekünstler und Apotheker*). Another distinguished pharmacist, J. B. Trommsdorff, began in 1793 to edit his *Journal der Pharmacie*, which in its character as well as more frequent appearance has a claim to being pharmacy's earliest scientific journal. Since then many scientific and professional pharmacy journals have been published in German, some so important as to make a knowledge of the language almost obligatory for pharmacists with scientific pretensions in other countries throughout the decades.

Additional bibliographic notes on representative pharmacopeias, other types of books, and pharmaceutical periodicals will be found in Appendix 6 (p. 425) by those who wish to locate and consult at first hand some works representative of contemporary German pharmacy in various periods.

## ORGANIZATIONS

In German pharmacy the organization of Nuremberg pharmacists in 1632 appears to be the earliest society of some importance. At least three other local societies were functioning by the early 19th century.[25] Regional organizations for north Germany (1820) and south Germany (1848) were formed, then after the federation of the German states, the two amalgamated into a national German pharmacists' society (the Deutscher Apothekerverein, 1872). Specifically to promote pharmaceutical science and research, the Deutsche Pharmazeutische Gesellschaft was organized in 1890.[26]

During the Nazi period (1933-1945) a new totalitarian association was the only one permitted to represent the professional and commercial interests of German pharmacists during those years.[27] Several of the established pharmacy journals also were victims of the regime and had to suspend publication.

Attempts have been made repeatedly, since 1818, to organize separate associations of employed pharmacists. A lasting and active association of this kind was founded in 1904, called after 1910 the alliance of German pharmacists (Verband Deutscher Apotheker). It had grown to represent the majority of employed pharmacists by 1934, when it was absorbed by the new totalitarian pharmaceutical association.

Apart from the voluntary associations mentioned, there have been official bodies. In the initial form of *Gremium* (first organized in Bavaria, 1842), membership was compulsory for all owners of pharmacies in each government district. These were administrative bodies auxiliary to state regulation of the practice of pharmacy.[28] Periodically, the *Gremium* reported to the government about conditions and desirable changes in pharmacy, and it supported social-welfare programs for its members. In more recent decades, the *Apothekerkammern* have served essentially the same purposes, but have additional disciplinary power over unethical acts among pharmacists. During the Nazi period this type of organization was given a totalitarian form that had far-reaching power over pharmacists politically as well as profes-

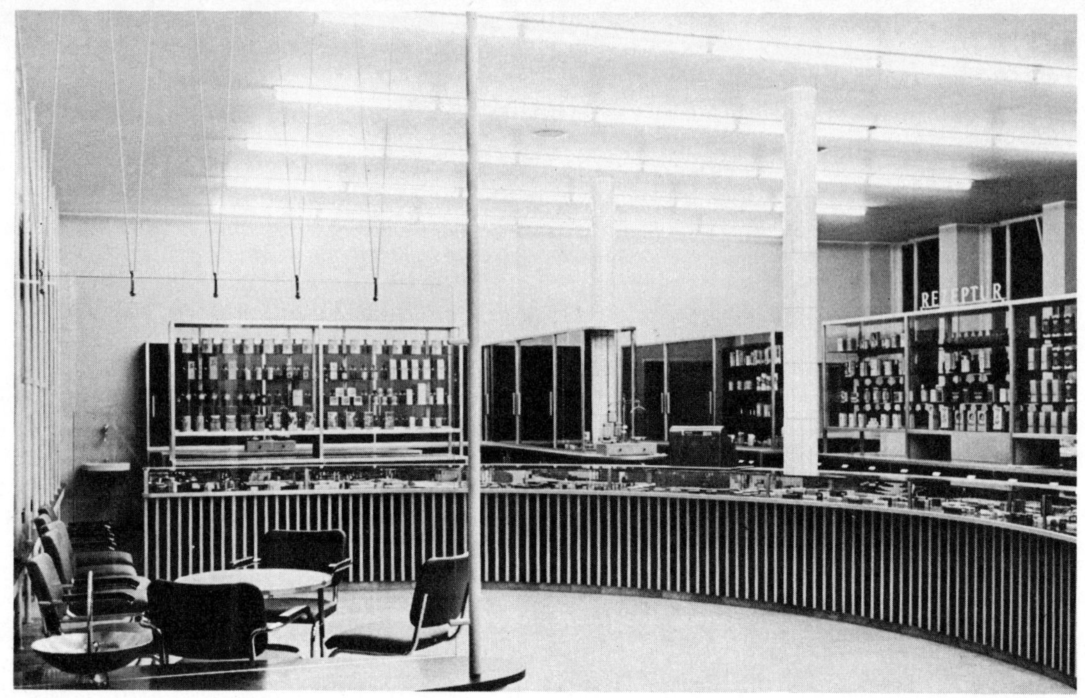

The Merck pharmacy is the modern version of the same pharmacy in Darmstadt out of which grew the great manufacturing laboratory. (The American Merck is an offshoot of the latter, which became independent.) The main area for prescription work in this pharmacy is to the right (*Rezeptur*). The section on the left reflects the curious survival of homeopathy in sufficient strength to warrant a special department. Modern pharmacies such as this one—like those of preceding centuries—have several other rooms besides the public dispensing room shown in these photographs: an office with reference books, a laboratory, a specialties room and stock rooms, including cold storage. (Photograph by Apotheken von Mayer, 1954)

sionally.[29] After World War II these district offices more and more became regulative bodies (*Landesapothekerkammern)* broadly concerned with the supply of medicaments and chemicals in the individual German states.

Each *Kammer* is a corporate body under public law and cannot properly undertake administrative tasks on behalf of pharmacists' private interests. For such a purpose, beside the *Kammer* in each state stands a professional society (Apothekerverein, as a continuation of the earlier Deutscher Apothekerverein and its successors).

As a roof organization uniting these various elements of German pharmacy there was created after 1948 the Arbeitsgemeinschaft der Berufsvertretungen Deutscher Apotheker (often abbreviated ABDA). This ties together and coordinates the management of the Bundesapothekerkammer (regulative affairs) and the Deutscher Apotheker-Verein (professional affairs).[30]

Pharmacy in West Germany since World War II can be seen to unfold facets of fundamental change—unprecedented freedom to open pharmacies, a wider opportunity for the individual mixed with a threat to professionalism (and in East Germany the socialization of the pharmacies); important new laws concerning both the practice of the pharmacist and drug products; and new organizational concepts, as exemplified by ABDA. Thus German pharmacy is forging a new chapter in its history that will be much more than a new expression of the old.

# 7

# The Development in Britain*

## THE PECULIAR BRITISH SITUATION

A striking feature marks the history of British pharmacy: A profession based entirely on the art of pharmacy, with the purpose of developing the professional and social standards of its members, did not exist in England, Wales and Ireland before the 19th century and in Scotland before the 18th century. In this respect Britain differs significantly from the other large European cultural zones—such as the Italian, the French and the German.

Naturally, in Britain as well as on the Continent, there were early dealers in drugs. Moreover, the terms designating them were the same as those used on the Continent. However, while the creation of the calling of the continental pharmacists was based principally on the early separation of the medical and the pharmaceutical professions, either by law or by regulations and privileges, in Britain this separation was not the beginning but a late result of the development.

In all European countries, transgressions of the legal boundaries of both professions were frequent; the complaints on both sides belong to the history of continental pharmacy as well as of medicine. Nevertheless, the principle of separation was in general considered to be beyond all dispute. At times, even in Europe, the transition from one profession to the other was not difficult. In the 17th and the 18th centuries many persons on the European continent had passed the examinations both in pharmacy and in medicine and, therefore, were entitled to practice both professions. Moise Charas, (the author of the famous *Pharmacopée royale,* 1676), Nicolas Lémery (the author of the first *Pharmacopoeia universalis,* 1697) and many other Frenchmen were simultaneously pharmacists and physicians. In Germany this dual education was even more common and caused many conflicts.[1] However, England, Wales and Ireland were the only European countries in which an entire calling gained the legal recognition of its ambition to practice in a neighboring field and became part of another profession without—and this is the irony of the situation—resigning completely the rights of the first profession.

The reason for this peculiarity is found in the insular character of Britain, which isolated it from continental Europe. Of its aboriginal inhabitants, the Celts, only those who lived in Wales and Scotland or were able to flee into these areas survived the conquest of the country by Germanic tribes (about

---

*While an effort has been made to characterize the pharmaceutical development in Great Britain, the limited space available in a textbook, and not historical circumstances alone, places England in the main focus of discussion and prevents all but cursory mention of differences and similarities elsewhere in the British Isles (such as in Northern Ireland and Ireland).

450). Throughout the centuries, there was not much harmony between the people of Wales and Scotland and those of England. The amalgamation between the Anglo-Saxons and the later conquerors of the islands, the Normans, who came over from France (Normandy) and dominated the country after the battle of Hastings (1066), took place very gradually.

Consequently, until the Elizabethan period (in the 16th century), conditions in Britain were not sufficiently stable to cast professional life into uniform and rigid moulds. Even later the proportion of educated people was relatively small. As a result, the way had to be free for each to make the most of opportunity. Indeed, this freedom of every Briton to seek adventure and success inside and outside the British Isles created the wealth and the power of England. On the other hand, this system of *laissez faire*—which found its theoretical basis in Manchester liberalism and was formulated in the thirties of the 19th century by the Manchester school of economics—has often retarded the steady, uniform development and balance within and for the totality of the people. Such may be achieved only by stating and protecting definite principles and regulations.[2]

## PHARMACEUTICAL BEGINNINGS

The social circumstances thus help us to understand the erratic course that must be taken to follow the pharmaceutical path from its faint beginnings in the late Middle Ages onward.

> In Saxon England and in the early Norman period there was no difference between physician, apothecary or surgeon. The practitioners known as leeches performed the functions of all three. During Norman times the trade in drugs and spices was eventually handled by the mercers (a term which originally simply meant a merchant who dealt in small wares).[3]

From France a few spicers and pepperers may have carried their trades across to the British Isles as early as the 11th century. Their number multiplied, and within a century or so they had taken over much of the drug trade—the pepperers as wholesalers, the spicers as retailers. The main stock in trade of both was "spicery," substances "mainly of vegetable or animal origin; almost invariably derived from the East or the Mediterranean; of high value in relation to their weight." This variety of substances of course included spices.[4]

Some of the more knowledgeable and skillful spicers specialized increasingly in dispensing and compounding medicines. By the late 13th century some were being called "spicer" or "apothecary" interchangeably. This was a transitional period, a period of maturing for an ambitious group that would become distinctively "apothecaries."

Meanwhile, the pepperers (wholesalers and shippers of spicery, etc.) changed the name of their guild to the Grocers' Company; in it, at least from the 14th century on, the apothecaries obtained guild benefits as a special section until they finally seceded in 1617.[5] In 14th-century England, Chaucer could write of his Physician, "Ful redy hadde he hise apothecaries to send him drogges."

We are not surprised that, in the absence of legal regulation, the functions of medicine and pharmacy remained poorly separated. The 16th-century "apothecary" has been referred to not only as an assistant to the physician, but also as an independent preparer and dispenser of drugs who not infrequently took a hand in medical practice.[6] In the time of Henry VIII, the long contention between apothecaries and physicians over the division of function of medical care had begun, and in 1511 the king issued the first regulations for the English practice of medicine and pharmacy, ordering that

> . . . no person could lawfully practise medicine or surgery in the City of London, or within seven miles of it, unless he had been first examined, approved, and admitted by the Bishop of London or the Dean of St. Paul's, who were to be assisted

in the examination of candidates by four doctors of physic and of surgery, or other expert persons in that faculty.[7]

This system eventually was extended to the provinces and to Wales. The College of Physicians (later, "Royal" College)—founded soon after the first medical regulation and licensing—was empowered in 1540 to "search, view and see the apothecary wares, drugs and stuffs."

Thereby the continental practice subjecting apothecaries to medical supervision was

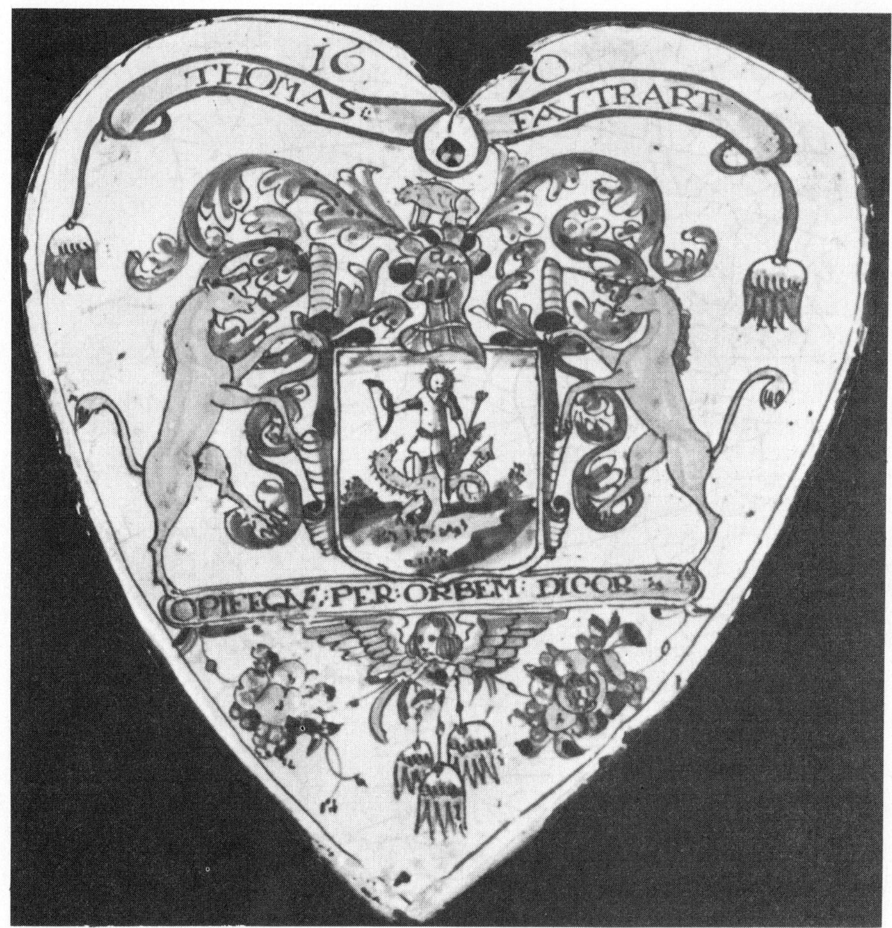


This pill tile bears the coat of arms of the Worshipful Society of Apothecaries of London, with its Latin motto, "Throughout the world I am called help-bringer" (polychrome English delft, 1670). Such tiles perhaps were as much a sign of membership and a symbolic ornament to the pharmacy as they were useful for prescription work. Between the two unicorns in the heraldry, Apollo (the ancient Greek medical god who fathered Asklepios) is vanquishing a dragon. (Original, about 11 inches high x 9½ inches wide, in the collection of the Pharmaceutical Society of Great Britain, London)

introduced into England. In an act of 1618 the new powers of the college were stated more specifically. Four members were authorized to survey and examine the stocks of "apothecaries, druggists, distillers and sellers of waters and oils, and preparers of chemical medicines." This enumeration gives a complete picture of the different groups that were in any way active and officially recognized in the field of pharmacy.

Evolving law tended toward making the practice of medicine the monopoly of physicians licensed as such. But physicians were more zealous in defending their rights than their small number and the urgent need of medical help, especially in the open country, warranted. Therefore, a new act was passed (1543) confirming the right of "every person being the King's subject having knowledge and experience of the nature of herbs, roots and waters to use and minister, according to their cunning, experience and knowledge."[8] This act is a typical instance of *laissez faire*. It paved the way for everyone who had "cunning, experience and knowledge," leaving the decision as to the possession of these qualities entirely to the individual claiming them. However, it related only to medicaments for external application and "Drinks for the Stone, Strangury, or Agues." This act not only protected the numerous irregular practitioners, but encouraged the ambitions of the "apothecaries."

## THE APOTHECARIES—THEIR SOCIETY AND ITS LABORATORY

When King James I first gave privileges to the apothecaries (1607) as a section of the powerful Grocers' Company, he did not give them independence. The more ambitious apothecaries were neither content nor complacent, and, after many dissensions, the King granted them independence in a new charter. Thus was founded on December 6, 1617 a separate City Guild called the "Master, Wardens, and Society of the Art and Mystery of the Apothecaries of the City of London."

This charter conferred upon them the monopoly of keeping an apothecary's shop, and rendered it unlawful for the grocers or any persons, "to make or sell, to compound, prepare, give, apply or administer any medicines or medicinable compositions, viz., distilled waters, compounds or olea chimica, apozemata, sirrups, conserves, eclegmata, electuaria, condita, medicinalia, pilulas, pulveres, troches, olea, unguenta, emplastra, or by any other way to use or exercise the art, faculty, or mystery of an apothecary or any part thereof, within the City of London and the suburbs or within seven miles of the City."[9]

Naturally, the grocers protested. The king held to his original decision, stating that the grocers were but traders, having no professional skill.

During the 17th century, the wealth and the esteem of the calling increased. The guild hall, which the apothecaries acquired in 1632 (rebuilt after the Great Fire, which destroyed the largest part of London) stands even today as a witness of the old glory.[10]

Early in its history, the Society started to manufacture galenic and chemical medicines cooperatively. In 1682 this cooperative acquired the status of a regular commercial company. The laboratory had become a real chemical plant, and in 1703 the Society was granted a renewal of the monopoly of supplying the English navy with drugs. Later (1766) the East India Company also decided to buy huge amounts of drugs and medicines annually from the Society of Apothecaries.[11] The "companies" of the London Society of Apothecaries, organized on a local basis, are the first known example of a pharmaceutical cooperative operated on a larger scale. The Pharmacie Centrale in France (founded in 1852) in contrast consisted of the pharmacists of the entire nation and was the first national cooperative pharmaceutical undertaking.

### Apothecaries Becoming Medical Practitioners

Only a few decades after the founding of the Society of Apothecaries of London the new group found itself in a fight on two

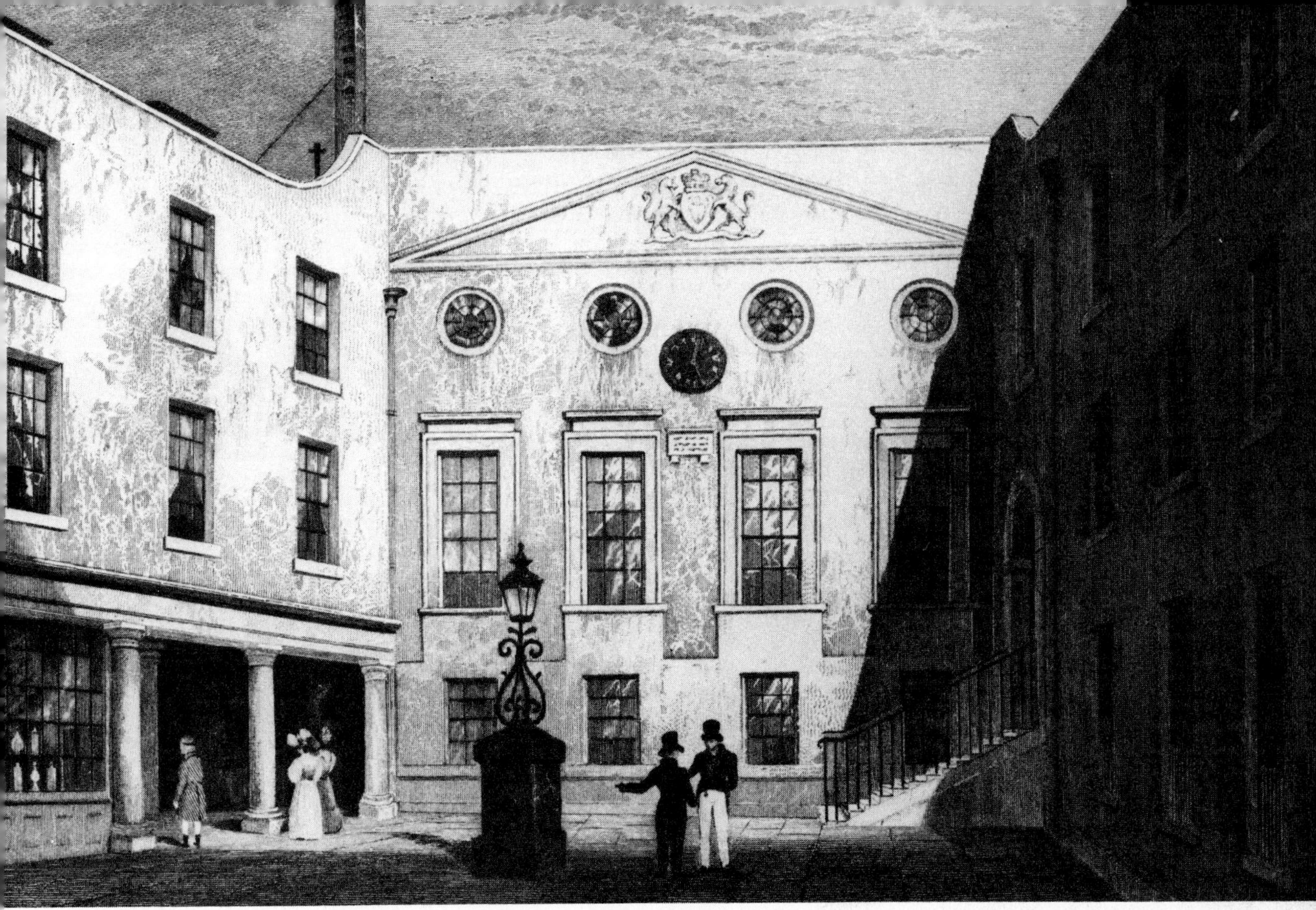

Apothecaries' Hall (Pilgrim St., Blackfriars, London) as it looked in the early 19th century. This building, which still survives, was begun in 1669 to replace an earlier headquarters destroyed in the Great Fire of London. In the early 1670's the Worshipful Society of Apothecaries established both a chemical laboratory and (in Chelsea) a medico-botanical garden. (Drawing by T. H. Shepherd; photograph from The Smithsonian Institution)

fronts: against the physicians, to defend the assumed rights of "apothecaries" as minor medical practitioners, in addition to their pharmaceutical duties, and against the "druggists" and "chemists" who, in spite of the monopoly of the apothecaries, continued to multiply and flourish.

The struggle lasted more than a century. Without any doubt, apothecaries practicing medicine trespassed on territory not belonging to them. Yet, they had gradually gained a large number of clients who depended on them, and they had proved themselves useful in their medical role in a time of need, during the Great Plague (1665–66). At that time, when the majority of the physicians in London either had died or had fled, "the friends of the sick were obliged to call in the aid of the apothecaries, who readily forsook their shops to visit the sufferers at their bedsides."[12]

Even at the end of the 16th century apothecaries in the provinces had begun to give medical advice and prescribe, as well as to run their drug shops. By the late 17th century, the emphasis had been completely reversed, and a majority of provincial apothecaries were engaging almost full time in the practice of medicine, to the neglect of pharmacy. They obviously filled a medical need and were socially accepted in the countryside long before they were legitimatized as general medical practitioners in the London area, the stronghold of the fully qualified physicians.[13]

So far as action was concerned, the quarrel centered on the opening of dispensaries by members of the College of Physicians, and on the prosecution of apothecaries practicing medicine. The dispensaries harmed the apothecaries—for in 1703 they "now make up 20,000 prescriptions."[14] On the other hand, the prosecution of the apothecaries, led to the defeat of the physicians! At first, a judgment of the Court of Queen's Bench decided (November 10, 1703) in favor of the college of physicians and against an apothecary, William Rose, who had been accused of prescribing medicines. However, the House of Lords ordered "That the said Judgement given in Queen's Bench . . . against the said William Rose shall be, and is hereby, reversed." From this time on the apothecaries were recognized medico-pharmaceutical practitioners.[15] One evidence was that, after another quarter century, the terms "apothecary" and "surgeon" were used interchangeably, at least in the provinces.[16]

The battle on the other front, against their competitors, the chemists and the druggists, was not so favorable for the apothecaries.

The "druggists," or "drugsters," and the chemists originally were distinguishable, if overlapping, classes. The English druggist originally emphasized wholesaling, serving, among other functions, "as a middleman in the passing of drug from importer to apothecary." Later, in the 18th century, he seems to have been a rather ordinary sort of storekeeper—at least out in the countryside—ofttimes a grocer who also handled medicines, whether at wholesale or retail.[17] (The 18th-century English druggist and the apothecary both served as prototypes for widespread emulation in early America). The "chemists" were preparers and sellers of chemical substances, with a practical skill in processes employing the use of fire and particularly of distillation. However, they were artisans more akin to the druggists than to the experimental chemists of the time. The historian Leslie G. Matthews has interpreted this development as follows:

> The wider spread of chemicals, as well as the influx of drugs, hitherto unfamiliar, from the newly opened-up countries added complexity to the trade of the wholesaler who had formerly stocked drugs and chemicals as 'grocery.' Some men now began to think that there was sufficient trade to be obtained in these commodities and that concentration upon the apothecaries' demands would yield greater profit. The men who did this styled themselves, or were so styled by others, as 'drugmen' or 'drugsters,' and towards the end of the 18th century they became known as 'druggists' or 'chemists and druggists.'"[18]

It may well be, as Kett concluded, that "the druggist of the eighteenth century was simply responding to demands of poorer people for cheap medicaments by compounding as well as stocking drugs, just as the apothecary had begun to meet demands for cheap medical advice in the preceding century by prescribing as well as compounding medicines."[19]

It will ever be a historical reminder that occupational boundaries are man-made and not divinely ordained that the British apothecary no sooner had become adjusted to his medical function than he was discomfitted by the challenge to his pharmaceutical function from this rising class of chemists and druggists. Probably the pressure hastened the apothecary's transformation into a medical practitioner, over a convoluted historical path, illustrated in rough outline by the chart on the facing page:

After unsuccessful attempts, the apothecaries finally got parliament to pass an Apothecaries' Act in 1815. This gave the London Society of Apothecaries certain powers over professional standards and medical education throughout England and Wales,[20] and forbade "unqualified persons from judg-

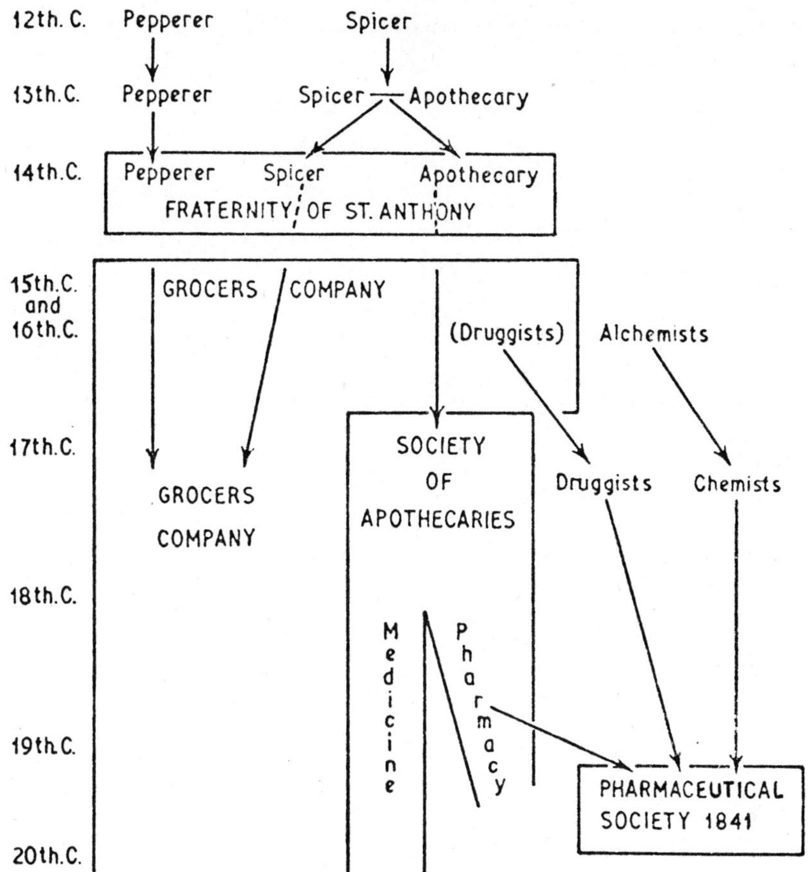

Evolution of pharmacy in England (with special reference to London) from its beginnings to the present day. (Diagram courtesy of Trease, G. E.: Pharmacy in History, p. 32, London: Baillière, Tindall and Cox, 1964)

ing disease by external symptoms (the qualified persons being the physicians, surgeons and apothecaries).

Through an emergency organization the chemists and druggists bid successfully to amend the Apothecaries Act to preserve as rights the pharmaceutical services that it had now become customary for them to render. They defined these rights as consisting of the buying, the compounding and the dispensing of drugs and medicinal compounds, wholesale and retail. With this definition the chemists and the druggists, excluding all medical ambition, drew the boundary between the medical and the pharmaceutical professions. The more the apothecaries became medical practitioners, the more their original tasks passed into other hands.

### The Scottish and Irish Situation

In Scotland and Ireland the pharmacist took a similarly winding historical path. He, too, eventually merged into medicine,

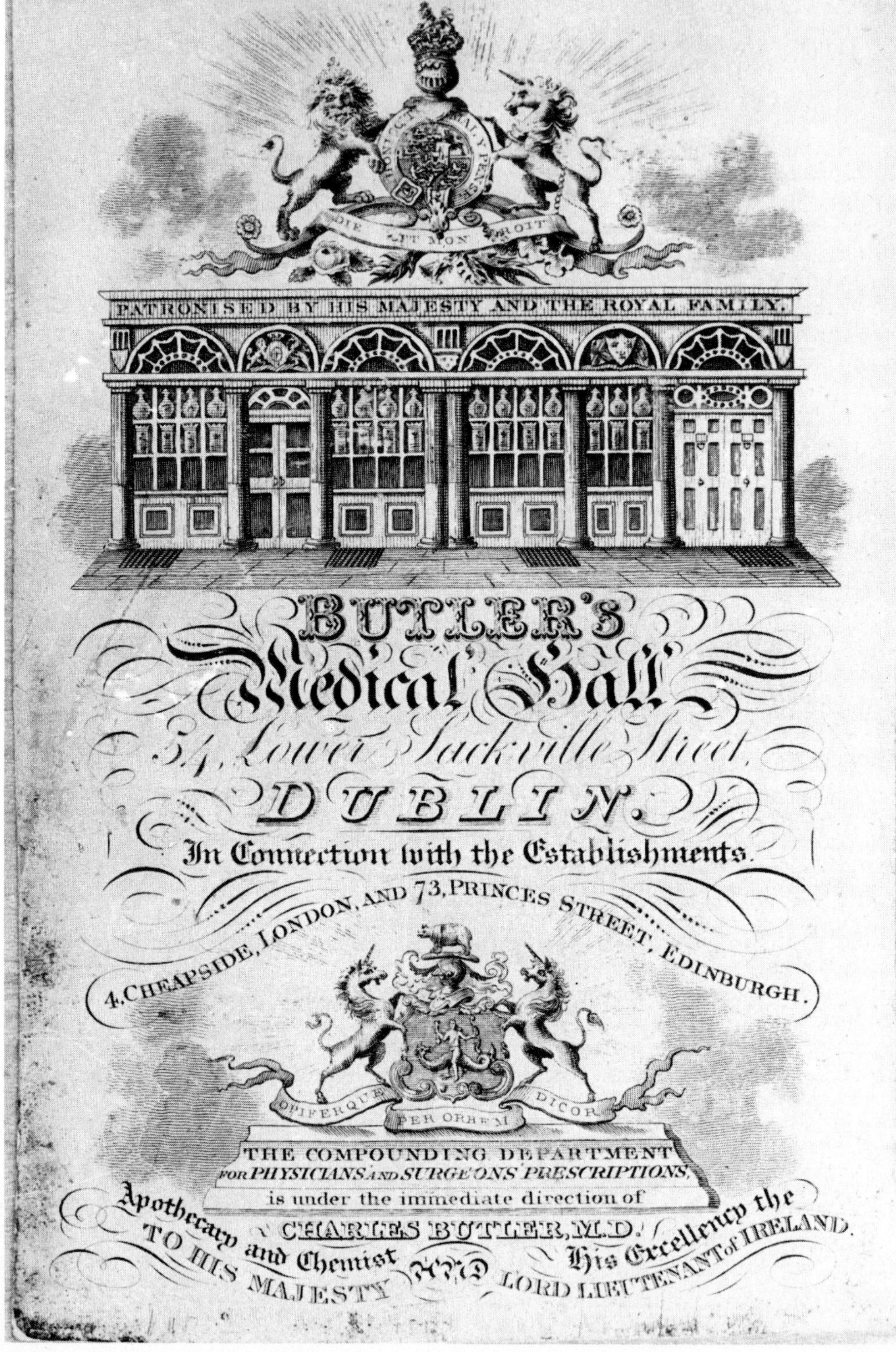
PATRONISED BY HIS MAJESTY AND THE ROYAL FAMILY.
BUTLER'S
Medical Hall
34, Lower Sackville Street,
DUBLIN.
In Connection with the Establishments
4, CHEAPSIDE, LONDON, AND 73, PRINCES STREET, EDINBURGH.
OPIFERQUE PER ORBEM DICOR
THE COMPOUNDING DEPARTMENT
FOR PHYSICIANS AND SURGEONS' PRESCRIPTIONS,
is under the immediate direction of
CHARLES BUTLER, M.D.
Apothecary and Chemist
TO HIS MAJESTY
AND
His Excellency the
LORD LIEUTENANT of IRELAND.

mainly with surgery, rather than with internal medicine as in England. However, the boundaries were drawn loosely, and the surgeon-apothecary came into service as the general practitioner for ordinary folk by the 17th century in some parts of Scotland. Pharmacy now was taught with surgery and, despite divisive tendencies, evenually (1721) all apothecaries were permitted to become members of the corporation of surgeons without examination, on payment of 50 pounds each!

As in England, a new class of practitioners of pharmacy then arose. Unlike their English colleagues, they received immediate and full recognition by physicians; what is more, the College of Physicians in Edinburgh prohibited its members from operating pharmacies.[21]

In Ireland, too, the apothecaries were in a guild with the surgeons (1456); but, after a few centuries, the apothecaries of Dublin were granted an independent charter as the Guild of St. Luke (1745). This guild later amalgamated with the Company of Apothecaries' Hall, whose jurisdiction extended over the whole of Ireland. Like their counterparts elsewhere in the British Isles, Irish apothecaries drifted into the general practice of medicine. The Medical Act of 1858 included Apothecaries' Hall as one of the licensing bodies for medical practitioners, but the Hall has since been closed.

Many medical apothecaries eventually refused to operate pharmacies open to the public, which further stimulated a rising class of "druggists." The Irish "druggist," on the other hand, was blocked from taking a place beside the dispensing "chemist" as a fully recognized pharmacy practitioner (Act of 1875), being held in a subordinate class reminiscent of the German *Drogist*, but permitted a wider scope of function. He has been continually at odds with Irish "chemists" (pharmacists), frequently trespassing illegally on their services. Finally, an enactment of 1951 discontinued any further registration of new druggists, while permitting those in practice who could pass an examination to become pharmaceutical chemists in everything but name.

What became of the apothecaries?

> The Irish . . . , like the English, have passed from pharmacy to medicine, but not so completely. . . . Many own pharmacies as well as medical practices. Some call their pharmacy "Apothecary's Hall" but the term "Medical Hall" is more popular. The latter term is also occasionally used by pharmacists who acquired medical halls from apothecaries. Thus the Irish apothecaries have the best of both worlds, being both physicians and pharmacists; a truly Irish situation.[22]

Although England serves as the main focus of discussion for the present purpose, the British Isles in general illustrate the tangled skein that can result when closely related occupational functions are exercised in a social atmosphere more heavily charged with the idea of "wait and see how it develops" than with preconceived ideas of discipline and planned development of a health system.

## CHEMISTS-AND-DRUGGISTS AND THEIR PHARMACEUTICAL SOCIETY

In the course of negotiations with the College of Physicians in 1841, the members of the board of examiners of the Society of Apothecaries, declared

> . . . that one of the chief evils in the present position of the Apothecary is his name, which has little reference to his actual duties, that he is in fact the Medical Attendant on the larger mass of the community, and should be designated the General Practitioner of Medicine.[23]

That year the Pharmaceutical Society of

←

Professional or trade card of an Irish "medical hall," illustrating the combination of general medical and pharmaceutical practice. The coat of arms (*bottom*, with unicorns rampant) is that of the Society of Apothecaries. (From: American Institute of the History of Pharmacy; gift of T. Douglas Whittet)

Great Britain was founded "to benefit the public and elevate the profession of Pharmacy, by furnishing the means of proper instruction. Jacob Bell felt that he voiced a central idea of the chemist and druggist when he said in 1842 that pharmacy had become so complicated and had embraced so many sciences "that a complete knowledge of the subject can only be acquired by those who devote their exclusive attention to the pursuit."[24]

The Pharmaceutical Society continued on a road diverging from that of the apothecaries, moving slowly toward professional status for a new class of practitioners of pharmacy. The Society's charter (1843) empowered it to regulate the education and the admission of members. The objectives specified were (1) advancement of chemistry and pharmacy; (2) promotion of a uniform system of education for practitioners; (3) protection of "those who carry on the business of Chemist and Druggist"; (4) relief of needy members, associates and their widows and orphans.

The first Pharmacy Act in 1852 empowered the Society to conduct examinations by means of two boards (one for England and Wales and another for Scotland) and to grant certificates of qualification for "pharmaceutical chemists," the title being restricted legally to those so registered. Medical men engaged in practice could not be registered as pharmaceutical chemists, although they could dispense drugs (and a majority did so). The most important change in a new Pharmacy Act of 1868 made qualification and registration compulsory for all members of the profession. In addition, the sale of poisons was henceforth permitted only in pharmacies serving the general public. The Act was a compromise between rival factions of pharmacists, however, and in effect made education secondary to examination. The historian Melvin P. Earles inferred that by thus "failing to safeguard against superficial forms of learning, the Act depressed pharmaceutical education in Britain to a level from which it took more than fifty years to recover."[25]

An amendment passed by Parliament in 1898 extended full membership in the Society—reserved hitherto to the Pharmaceutical Chemists (title of all those who had passed the "major" examination)—to the Chemist and Druggist (title of all those who had passed the "minor" examination). After another decade the law (1908) brought the calling of pharmacy more fully under the control of the Society and gave it power to institute a compulsory curriculum. However, membership was voluntary, and, despite the Society's examination and registration functions, it remained auxiliary to the official authority. The Society became such an authority itself in Great Britain in 1933.

The Pharmacy Act of 1933 made membership in the Pharmaceutical Society *compulsory*. Every person registered as a British pharmacist becomes a member by virtue of his registration. The titles "pharmaceutical chemist" "pharmaceutist," "pharmacist," "chemist and druggist" or "druggist" were protected. The term "chemist" became and remains the most popular designation used by community pharmacists.

The statutory committee of the Society has the power, subject to appeal to the High Court, to remove names from the register. Each registered pharmacist conducting an establishment for the dispensing of drugs is authorized to dispense poisons also. Inspectors, who must be registered pharmacists, are appointed by the Society.

In an editorial explaining the new Act, the Society's journal proclaimed, "Pharmacy is recognized as a self-governing community,

→

Caricature of an English practitioner of pharmacy in the 1820's. The patient already is more than a little impressed by the prescription being handed to him. (Then, and earlier, a prescription label was written on a tag tied to the bottleneck.) A daily task of the pharmacy apprentice *(right)* was to comminute drugs in a mortar. (Engraving by Henry Heath, 1825, in the William Helfand Collection; photo from The Smithsonian Institution)

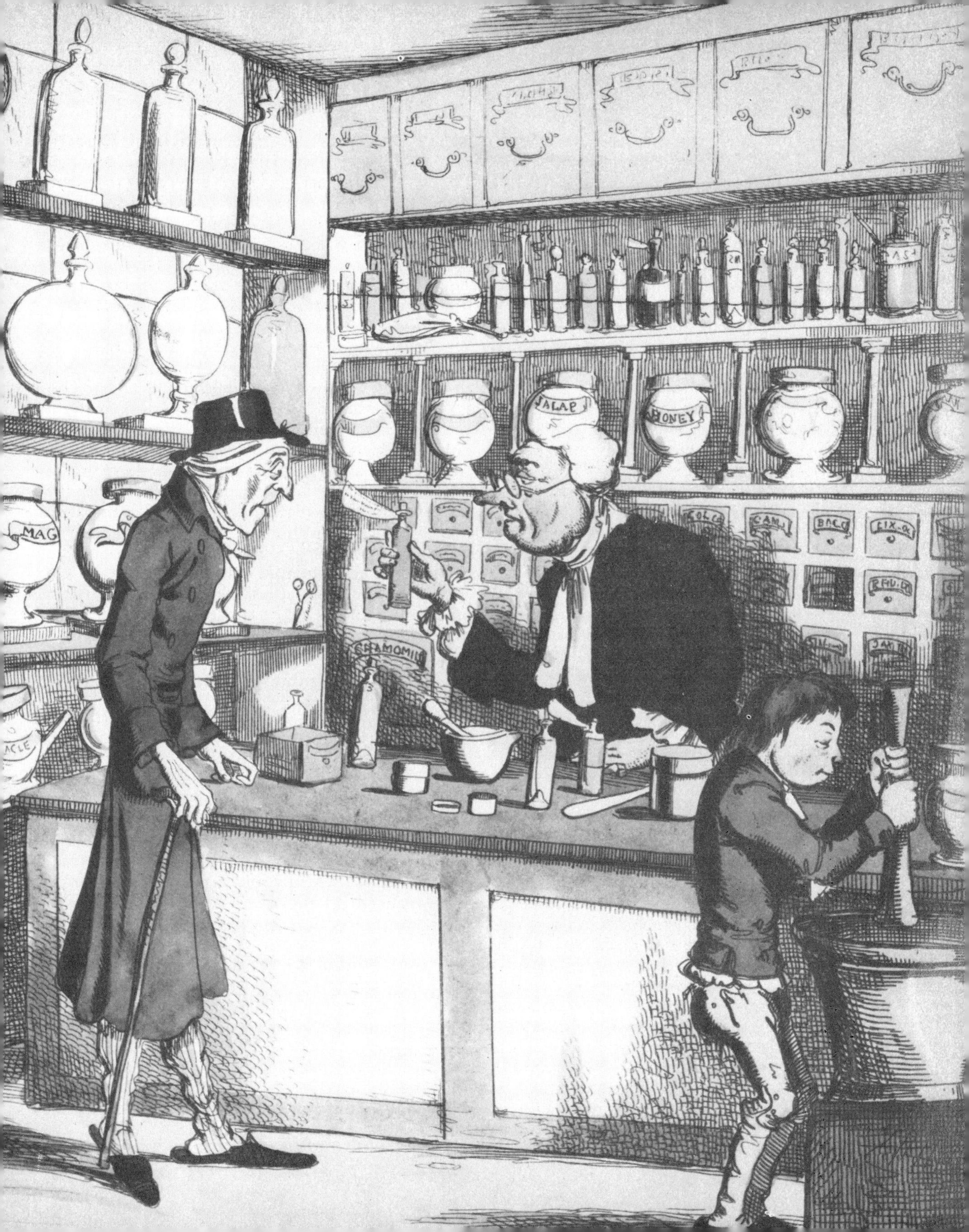
MAG
JALAP
HONEY

free to conduct its own affairs and subjected to governmental control only in those matters where its activities affect the public."[26] "Self-governing community!" The principle employed by England in relation to her colonies (advancing them to dominions if they have proved to be sufficiently mature for self-government) is here applied in internal affairs.

The British have exercised this self-responsibility with the decorum and astuteness that so frequently mark other sectors of British public life. It also has included a strong element of respect for the traditions of the "dispensing chemist." Yet, there have been strong pressures toward change, not arising so much from any internal inadequacies as from outside pressures, from socioeconomic trends in Western societies at large. Three of these particularly have been affecting the "chemist's shop" as a part of medical care.

First, despite the persistence of a variety of small, independent shops—to a far more tenacious degree than in America—the independent pharmacy owner has felt threatened since about mid-century by the encroachment of multiple-unit organizations. Already in the early 1960's about a seventh of the pharmacies in the United Kingdom had become "chain stores." This and other economic pressures, including transfer of some professional functions, decreased the number of chemist's shops in operation by about a fifth between 1955 and 1972.

Second, the availability of medical care to all under the government-operated program has tended to reduce the freedom of action of the pharmacist in professional as well as economic matters. Moreover, the shift of medical services into neighborhood health centers, accelerating in recent years, raises the spector of on-site pharmacy service in competition with the neighborhood "chemist." Provision in the National Health Service Act (1946) to provide on-site pharmacists was successfully blocked by organized pharmacy; although under the expanded construction program for health centers since the early 1960's, an increasing proportion of general medical practitioners were being absorbed into this work-setting. According to one estimate, fewer than 50 of 1300 health centers built or projected by 1972 included on-site pharmacists in their plans. Yet, with the national health program so centralized and integrated, many British pharmacists have considered the future work setting of the average practitioner an open question.

Third, the disappearance of the drug-making function from the pharmacy shop has entered a final stage, as in most highly developed countries. To compensate for this functional loss, the advisory function of the pharmacist has been put forward as a goal by organized pharmacy and has been, to a limited extent, recognized in law. Two factors thus far inhibiting this service (in common with American circumstances) are that the traditional chemist's shop is poorly designed for such a function and that third-party remuneration for pharmaceutical service does not encourage it.[27]

## OTHER ORGANIZATIONS

As a necessary first goal in its early decades, the Pharmaceutical Society gradually formed a class of uniformly and sufficiently educated pharmaceutical practitioners, on whom could be conferred the legal right to supply the people with drugs and medicines. The Society tried to make pharmaceutical science available to the average chemist and druggist, but it could not promote scientific research to the desired extent, since many pharmaceutical scientists were not members.

For this reason the British Pharmaceutical Conference, "an organization for the encouragement of pharmaceutical research," was founded in 1863. The Conference was not connected officially with the Pharmaceutical Society until 1922, when it became an autonomous part of the Society. This close connection between the two associations has continued even though it is not compulsory for a Conference member to belong to the Society.

The founders of the Conference apparently had been influenced by

> . . . the good work done . . . by the American Pharmaceutical Association . . . in the field of pharmaceutical science particularly . . .
>
> Reynolds described the American method of allotting subjects for investigation to individuals for report at the annual meeting, and referred to the inclusion in the published "Proceedings" of the American Association of a section which formed a "Year-Book of Pharmacy" both home and foreign.[28]

The Pharmaceutical Society developed into the administrative and educational body of the profession with the British Pharmaceutical Conference representing its scientific work, supplemented by the Society's Department of Pharmaceutical Sciences (as such since 1959).

During the late 19th century there had been indications that the ordinary "chemist and druggist" seriously doubted, however, that his business interests were being taken care of adequately by the Pharmaceutical Society. This discontent crystallized early in the present century when the dispensing chemists were squeezed economically by unexpected effects from the first government health legislation. In response, a new "Local Executives Association" was organized under auspices of the Pharmaceutical Society to seek redress. A court test case (the "Jenkins judgment") showed that the chemists' business interests lay outside the chartered responsibilities of the Pharmaceutical Society as a professional body. The Society's role being thus defined and limited, a new independent organization of pharmacy owners was set up in 1921, to pursue the business interests of pharmacy under the title Retail Pharmacists' Union (known as the National Pharmaceutical Union since 1932). It was created with the support of the Pharmaceutical Society, since the latter's quite different task was to represent all pharmacists professionally.[29] The new Union mainly served the interests of pharmacy owners as entrepreneurs and has the important duty of representing pharmacy in all affairs concerning national health insurance. In Scotland, similar functions are shared between the Scottish Pharmaceutical Federation (founded in 1919) and the Pharmaceutical Standing Committee (Scotland).

The representative Guild of Hospital Pharmacists (formerly called the Guild of Public Pharmacists) was founded in 1923 by amalgamating the Public Pharmacists Association with members of the pharmacists' section of the Hospital Officers' Association. It includes about 90 per cent of the hospital pharmacists in England, Scotland and Wales and has branches throughout the three countries. The Guild of Public Pharmacists, after a ballot among the membership, joined a trade union, the Association of Scientific, Technical and Managerial Staff. This improved the negotiating power of the Guild with the Department of Health and Social Security, which was reflected in substantial salary increases awarded to pharmacists in the hospital service. (Similar organizations exist in Northern Ireland and the Irish Republic.)

## INSPECTION AND REGULATION

The inspection of the pharmacies reflects the general development of English pharmacy. A royal order of Henry VI first gave the grocers power to examine "anis, wormseed, rhubarb, scammony, spikenard, senna and all sort of drugs belonging to medicine, so as not, in the buying of these to be hurt in their bodily health" (1447).[30] Later decrees (1540, 1553) gave the supervision of pharmacies to the medical profession. However, when the Society of Apothecaries was chartered independently (1617), its master and wardens were empowered to inspect any pharmacy and to burn before the offender's door all drugs and preparations they deemed corrupt or unwholesome.[31]

In the 18th century, power to examine the shops of apothecaries, chemists and druggists was given to the College of Physicians (1723), and cases involving questionable drugs were judged by a court composed partly of physicians and partly of apothecaries (1730).[32]

Scotland also placed inspection of the apothecaries' stock in the hands of physicians in the 17th century, sometimes with assistance from representatives of the apothecaries themselves.[33]

The regulation stemming from the Pharmacy Act of 1933 made the pharmacists throughout England, Scotland and Wales definitely self-governing, under the supervision of their own Society.

The Pharmacy and Medicines Act of 1941, among other changes, relaxed distributive controls on certain poisons, abolished the stamp duty on proprietary medicines and differentiated between pharmacists and other persons distributing them and dealt with the advertising of medicines.[34]

Further legal changes in 1953 allowed everyone on a single register of pharmacists to use the title pharmaceutical chemist (usually shortened to "chemist"), and authorized the Society to register without examination (or with a modified examination) persons granted degrees in pharmacy by universities in the United Kingdom. Additional changes in the operating framework of the Pharmaceutical Society came with a Supplemental Charter granted to it by the government (1954).

The present complexion of British pharmacy has also been shaped during this century by legislation other than the pharmacy acts. The comprehensive Medicines Act of 1968 particularly (in relevant sections of its 165 pages)[35] reaffirmed that the Pharmaceutical Society continue to register pharmacies, maintain discipline over those carrying on pharmaceutical activities, enforce the law relative to substances that could only be sold in pharmacies, and control the use of titles. However, these became powers delegated by the Ministers of Health (who have enforcement responsibility) to the Pharmaceutical Society, yet recognizing the long tradition of self-governance and the responsibility of its exercise by the Society on behalf of the Crown.

The Ministry of Health is also empowered to have its own inspectors, and to instruct the Pharmaceutical Society to withhold licenses in cases of unsuitable premises for the practice of pharmacy, until necessary improvements have been made. This responds in part to the Society's attempt in 1965 to gain control over the nature of the premises for a pharmacy, which was thwarted by the courts.

The terms under which a pharmacy may be conducted are similar to those previously prevailing (and comparable to most of the USA). There has been no legal limitation placed on the number of pharmacies, which in 1972 approached the ratio of approximately 1 per 4000 persons in the United Kingdom. A pharmacy must be conducted by a pharmacist or partnership of pharmacists or a corporate body having a pharmacist as superintedent. And medicinal products must be dispensed under the personal control of a pharmacist, unless it can be shown that they can, with reasonable safety, be supplied otherwise. However safe the products, if sold in an establishment other than a pharmacy they must be formulated elsewhere and sold in sealed containers. One interesting feature of the Medicines Act 1968 permits extemporaneous dispensing in connection with counter prescribing, if the person who will take the medication is present in the pharmacy—the first express recognition of counter prescribing by pharmacists in modern English law.

While the former Secretary of the Pharmaceutical Society, F. W. Adams, concluded that the current legislation would indirectly "improve the status of the pharmacist," it also appeared to entail a "formidable and highly centralised system of wide ranging authority." Certainly it stands a long way from the British conception of *laissez faire* that led to a nation's apothecaries evolving into recognized medical practitioners; or, on another turn of the wheel, led to a large number of druggists becoming dentists (1878)![36] As part of a British trend, pharmacy for more than a decade has been turning away from the degree of *laissez faire* that has long stood in contrast to pharmacy on the European Continent.

This is exemplified by the overwhelming vote (better than 4 to 1) by which members of the Pharmaceutical Society of Great Britain in 1965 approved seeking a limitation on the location and operation of pharmacies. Pharmacists wished to limit the location of new pharmacies to such as would be physically distinct and separate from other types of premises, and wished to limit the function of new pharmacies to the dispensing of drugs and other health-related products, except for a limited number of unrelated items traditionally associated with British pharmacy (e.g., photographic supplies and toiletries). Although not required to change current practices, established pharmacies would not have been permitted to expand further into sidelines principally unrelated to health.

The action seems symbolic of a change in social and professional attitude, but in practice it was frustrated by a counteraction, a successful series of skirmishes fought through the British courts, by the largest British chain store operation (Boots, Ltd.). The Pharmaceutical Society lost the decisive round when the House of Lords decided against the stance taken by the Society members—perhaps partly because it could be interpreted as a move based more on a desire to forestall American-style mass merchandising by chain stores than on public welfare. In any event it seems a landmark decision, since it marked the first time that a charge of "constraint of trade" had been brought successfully against a profession.[37] In effect the Pharmaceutical Society was told that it had no power to decide what a pharmacist could or could not sell from his establishment (apart from medicines and poisons subject to specific regulation).

Another recent tendency of British pharmacy that appears to draw more from Continental models than from its own past has been the consideration of planned distribution of pharmacies. In 1967 the Pharmaceutical Society established a Committee on the Planned Distribution of Pharmacy (renamed the Committee on a Planned Pharmaceutical Service); but did not convince the British government to change from the system of freedom of location of pharmacies. In 1974 the issue was brought up again in connection with a new National Health Services Act, and again did not attract sufficient support.[38]

The universal government health insurance represented by the Act is a British expression of the long-term, worldwide trend in health-care economics that is discussed on p. 128. It merits mention here partly because the British enactment has had an impact on the development of British pharmacy in the 20th century, and partly because it constitutes the health-insurance experience that has been most influential on American thought. The original government health insurance enacted in 1911, which was restricted to lower-income groups, helped British pharmacy by suppressing through restrictions on remuneration the prevalent physician-dispensing of medication, which has been an outgrowth of the old "apothecary tradition." Another salutary effect since health insurance was extended to the entire population in 1948 has been a definite improvement in the status of hospital pharmacists in Britain. The overall impact of government health insurance has been characterized by the historian Leslie G. Matthews as follows:

> This gave the pharmacist opportunity to develop the dispensing side of his business, those in England and Wales being more affected than those in Scotland, where the separation of prescribing from dispensing had long been given greater recognition. From 1912, therefore, the dispensing of prescriptions and the supply of dressings and appliances began to play a much greater part in the daily work of the pharmacist, though it

was not until the National Health Act of 1946, which came into operation in 1948, when the Health Service was extended to the whole population, that the pharmacist became more important to the nation and when, almost without exception, save in some country areas or in emergency, the doctor ceased to dispense the medicaments that he prescribed.[39]

With the reorganization of the National Health Service in 1974 on an area and regional basis, the community pharmacist has become a more integral part of the total complex of health services, at the same time resisting erosion of his independent status or absorption into the NHS area health centers. The actual consequences will of course become clearer after a few decades.

## SOCIAL STANDING

To gain an impression of the social position held by the members of the pharmaceutical calling in England, we must choose as representatives, until the end of the 18th century, the apothecaries. From the middle of the 17th century on, we also must consider the chemist and, from the beginning of the 19th century, the new professional group resulting from the gradual amalgamation of chemists and druggists, which constitutes the rank-and-file of modern British pharmacy.

As in all other countries, the social position of the British apothecary was based, on the one hand, on respect for his professional work and, on the other hand, on the fact that most of the apothecaries were, or at least were considered to be, well-to-do.

Thompson describes two apothecary shops of the 16th century as well equipped with furniture, containers of various kinds and sizes, and weights and balances. The prescriptions of the physicians were copied into a great book which stood on a raised desk or table. As in other countries, the apothecary shops in England in this period had "a windowframe over which canvas was stretched, but when this was rolled up they were open to the street."[40]

The equipment of English apothecaries of the 17th and the 18th centuries—unlike that of their counterparts on the Continent, in general—does not seem to have reflected their prosperity and social position. The fact that the apothecary considered himself to be primarily a medical practitioner probably made it seem unnecessary to strive for a particularly dignified pharmaceutical atmosphere.

> On the wall hang saws, knives, forceps and other surgical instruments; for the apothecary was ready to perform any operation, from the cutting off of a wen to the amputation of a leg. . . . The walls are lined with shelves bearing an array of Delft jars of blue and white for which the Lambeth potters were famous.[41]

Another type of pharmaceutical establishment was represented by the chemist's shops, which are hinted at in 1553 but did not become numerous before the second half of the 17th century.

The most famous of these chemists, the German-born Ambrose Hanckwitz (in England named Godfrey), was brought to England by no less a person than Robert Boyle. Together with Hanckwitz, Boyle found a new method for preparing phosphorus and "for many years the "English phosphorus' supplied by Hanckwitz from his laboratory . . . monopolized the European market.[42]

Around 1800, such manufacturing chemists parted company with the dispensing chemists, although some of them retained both functions and carried on (or, rather, created) the idea of professional pharmacy and, later, became founders of the Pharmaceutical Society of Great Britain. In general, however, little of the old glory of the art of the apothecaries or of the recent fame of chemistry came down to the new combination of chemists and druggists. They practiced pharmacy, it is true, but primarily as merchants like their predecessors, the druggists. This background differentiated the character of their shops and their general social position from those of their continental colleagues, although there were numerous exceptions to the rule. In continental Europe the pharmaceutical profession, as a profession, gave and gives to all of its members a certain traditional reputation. In England, Wales and Ireland most of the tradition and the prestige of pharmacy passed with the apothecaries into medicine. However, the modern calling of pharmacy has done much to regain lost ground and create new prestige—especially as mediated by their prestigious Pharmaceutical Society—even though at times progress has been slow or uneven.

## PHARMACEUTICAL EDUCATION

One of the most important means of building up a professional reputation is, naturally, the education of the rising generation. An examination was required by law for the first time in the British Isles in Glasgow, Scotland. On the basis of the charter granted to the Glasgow faculty by James VI in 1599, the faculty "issued a license to practice pharmacy to candidates who passed its examination in pharmacy."[43] In 1657, in Edinburgh, an examination became compulsory for all those who wished to practice pharmacy within the city.[44] In England the first official requirement of a definite time of apprenticeship and an examination of the presumptive apothecaries is contained in the charter of December 6, 1617, creating the Society of Apothecaries of London, which ordered that:

> No Person or Persons whatsoever may have, hold, or keep, an Apothecary's Shop or Warehouse, or . . . may exercise or use the Art or Mystery of Apothecaries, or . . . may sell, set on sale, utter, set forth, or lend any Compound or Composition to any person or persons whatsoever, within the City of London and the Liberties thereof, or within Seven Miles of the said City, unless such persons or persons have been brought up, instructed, and taught by the space of Seven Years at the least, as Apprentice or Apprentices, with some Apothecary or Apothecaries exercising the same Art, and being a Freeman of the said Mystery.[45]

Botanic courses were organized (1627), which led to the establishment of a famous and still extant "physic garden" at Chelsea (1673).

Apprentices were examined before entering the calling and, on occasion, were rejected "for insufficiency in the Latin tongue." Lectures in materia medica were offered after 1753.

When the first regular curriculum of the Society of the Apothecaries was issued (1827), it was mainly medical. It required 5 years of apprenticeship, including attendance at courses in such subjects as anatomy, physiology and the theory and the practice of medicine.[46]

Real pharmaceutical education began in England only after the founding of the Pharmaceutical Society. One of the fundamental demands in the program of the Society was "the development of scientific acquirements . . . to remove our (the English pharmacists') apparent deficiency as pharmacopolists, when compared with other naions." In 1844-1845, the society's school of pharmacy became the first institution in London to offer laboratory instruction for pharmacy students under proper guidance.[47]

Because of the central importance of education as a tool for shaping a new profession out of the original heterogeneous group of "chemists" and "druggists," the Society consistently fostered and valued the role of education in the life of British pharmacy. The Society's commendable history in this area, says J. W. Fairbairn, "rises up from the past like a signpost pointing out the only way to maintain and improve professional status in an increasingly scientific society is by continually increasing academic standards." However, in view of the various levels and types of knowledge asked for by the complex of pharmaceutical services, how should pharmaceutical education be structured? This question recurs again and again in pharmacy, in various historical contexts.

In England, even after pharmacy proper divorced itself from the "apothecary," two levels of qualification persisted. Originally the Pharmaceutical Society of Great Britain envisaged a society of registered pharmaceutical chemists and registered assistants. Influenced by the relatively undeveloped state of British pharmacy, however, the assistant's examination (Chemist and Druggist's Diploma) by 1869 had become the basic qualification for community pharmacy, while the Diploma of Pharmaceutical Chemist (Ph. C.) became a higher-status qualification for a minority, who tended to enter manufacturing pharmacy, hospital pharmacy, or teaching. "This two-class system of pharmaceutical education persisted for almost a hundred years," Fairbairn points out, "and although the Pharmaceutical Society in 1954 abolished the old chemist and druggist course, the idea of an ordinary and a more advanced pharmacist still persists."[48]

During the 1960's a vestige of this concept remained in the arrangement by which an aspirant might earn either the pharmaceutical-chemist diploma of the Society or the pharmacy baccalaureate of a university. In either case the level of admission to pharmaceutical studies was the same—estimated as perhaps equivalent to one year or more of preprofessional college studies in the United States.

The curriculum for a university degree ordinarily requires three academic years. The alternative non-degree course, which attracted the majority of students, required the same time and covered the same subjects, but tended to be somewhat more practical and less concentrated. Whichever curriculum the prospective pharmacist followed, he also needed one year of practical training under a pharmacist before becoming registered.

Graduates taking a non-degree course were required to pass a comprehensive qualifying (diploma) examination given by the Pharmaceutical Society,) whereas holders of a university degree could become registered by being examined only in the law and practice of pharmacy. Successful candidates were registered to practice as "Pharmaceutical Chemists."

Before 1954 a majority had been registering at the lower level of qualification titled "Chemist and Druggist." This alternative non-degree course for registration as a British pharmacist was phased out in 1967, and one qualifies only by earning a university degree. After graduation from a university or polytechnic college, (ordinarily a three-year curriculum) the candidate enters upon a controlled experience of one year in hospital pharmacy, community pharmacy, or (up to half of the year) in industrial pharmacy.

Just as the Pharmaceutical Society withdrew from teaching—arranging for its famous old school on Bloomsbury Square (1842-1948) to be absorbed by the University of London—now it withdrew as an examining body for licensure, recognizing the university degree itself as a qualification standard (following a Continental pattern, and unlike the USA).

The transition to a single level of qualification, by university graduation, has been facilitated by the establishment of new universities in Britain, as one response to the Robbins Report on Higher Education (1963). Some of these new universities grasped the opportunity to break down some traditional barriers between subject-areas of the curriculum. One university (Bradford) introduced a "sandwich course," where the pharmacy student spends two years in the university, one year in general practice or hospital, then a final year in the university.[49]

Educational standards in Ireland and Northern Ireland are similar, and there are reciprocity agreements with Great Britain.[50]

An examination qualifying for a certificate

can be identified in the development of botany, chemistry and other sciences.

Apothecaries took part in the founding of the Royal Society; T. D. Whittet found that at least 30 British apothecaries and 12 pharmacists have been elected Fellows. The apothecaries contributed many papers to the Society's Philosophical Transactions.

At one time, botanic science in Great Britain was largely the province of apothecaries such as John Houghton (a pioneer of good agriculture), Samuel Doody, William Hudson, James Sherard, Isaac Rand, Phillip Miller, R. Pulteney and Nathaniel B. Ward, all of whom became Fellows of the Royal Society.

Among those who made important contributions to chemistry and were elected Fellows of the Royal Society were Timothy Lane, who made some of the earliest investigations on rusting of iron; Josiah Colebrook, who investigated paints used by the ancients; Thomas Henry, a founder of the Manchester Philosophical Society and of a chemical manufactory, and William Thomas Brande, a pioneer of organic and clinical chemistry, who also conducted important metallurgic investigations.

Sir William Watson, F.R.S., a versatile scientist and apothecary, made significant contributions to botany, chemistry and physics. At least four of the "chemical operators of the Apothecaries' Hall" became Fellows of the Royal Society (Godfrey-Hanckwitz, Henry Hennell, W.T. Brande and Robert Warington).

Six apothecaries or pharmacists associated with the firm of Allen and Hanbury became Fellows of the Royal Society: Silvanus Bevan, William Allen (distinguished as a chemist), Daniel Hanbury (botanist), Luke Howard (botanist and pioneer meteorologist), Richard Phillips (analytic chemist) and William West (chemist and inventor). Luke Howard's son John Eliot Howard, the quinologist, also was honored as a Fellow of the Royal Society—the highest distinction a scientist can be given.

A. W. Gerrard, while chief pharmacist of University College Hospital in London, was the first to isolate pilocarpine and several other plant principles. He later founded the present firm of Cuxson, Gerrard and Co. at Birmingham.

A chemist-and-druggist in community practice, John Walker, invented the friction match. Sir Joseph Wilson Swan, F.R.S., pioneer of photography and electricity and one of the first to produce artificial silk, remained a practicing pharmacist most of his life, as did H. B. Brady, F.R.S., a great naturalist and George C. Druce, F.R.S., the greatest British field botanist of his time.

Sir Robert Kane, F.R.S., a prominent member of the Dublin Apothecaries' Society, became one of Ireland's greatest chemists and a founder of Ireland's chemical industry. William Higgins, F.R.S., who anticipated some of Dalton's atomic theory, was for a few years operator to the Dublin Apothecaries' Hall. Other important names include those of Thomas Johnson, the previously mentioned apothecary and early botanist (d. 1644), and the 19th-century figures Jonathan Pereira, F.R.S., apothecary-physician-professor, William Tilden, F.R.S., organic chemist, Edward Morell Homes, botanist, John Attfield, pharmacist-professor-author, and Edward Frank Harrison, who contributed to the defense of the allied armies against gas attacks during World War I.[56]

## TIES BETWEEN DISPENSING AND PRODUCTION

It is significant that the organizers of the Pharmaceutical Society—William Allen,[57] its first president, and Jacob Bell—were owners not only of pharmacies but also of pharmaceutical manufactories (founded about 1800) that still exist. This union between professional interest and technico-commercial intelligence and activity was not rare in British pharmacy. Of the British pharmaceu-

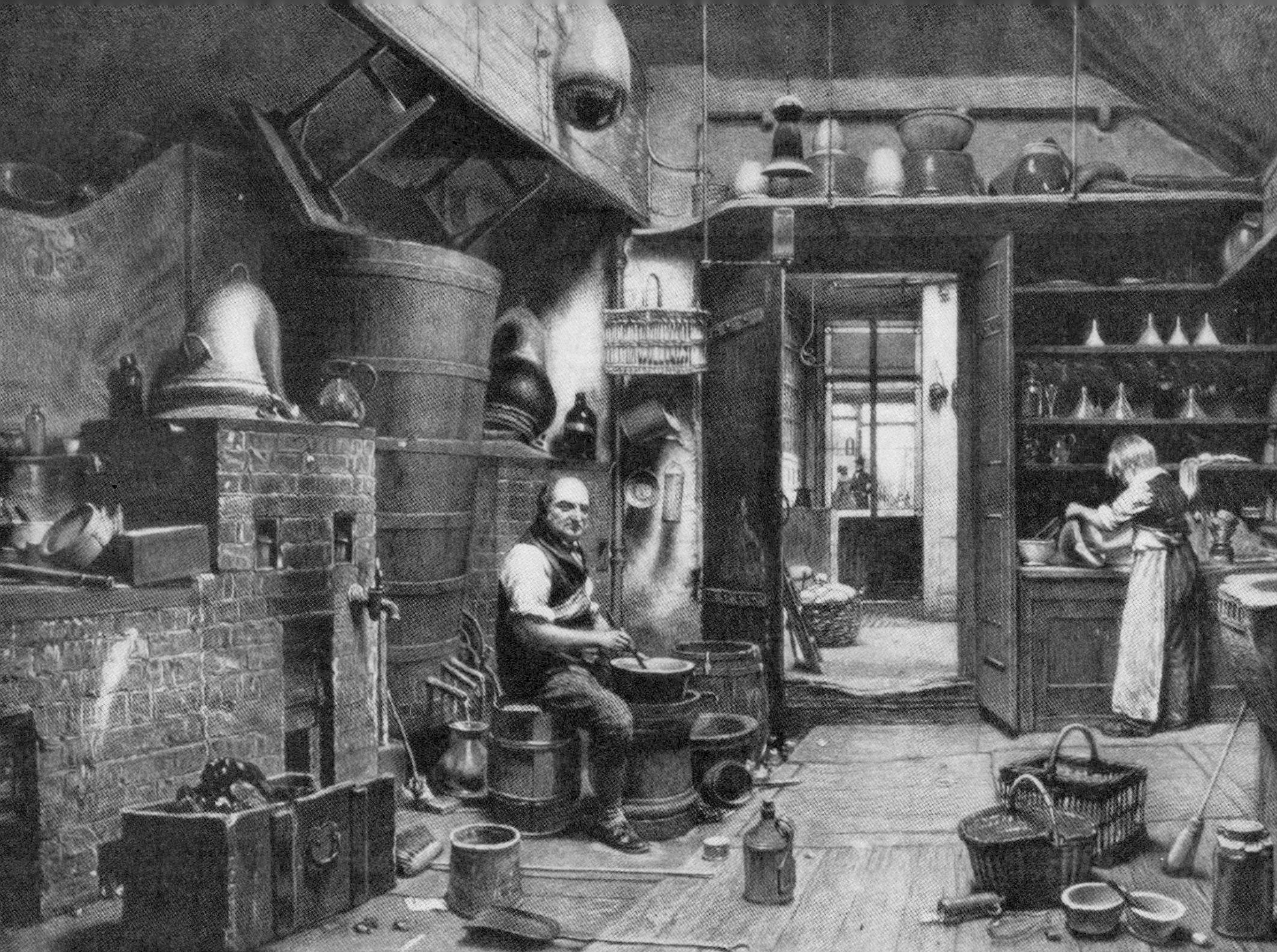

The back-room laboratory of a mid-19th century pharmacy in London typifies practice before large-scale industrialization of operative pharmacy. A furnace *(left)* is fitted at the top with a distillation head, attached to a condensing worm running through the large wooden vat beside it. Through the doorway can be seen a corner of the front dispensing room. A large marble mortar can be seen in the extreme right foreground. Here, at 225 Oxford Street, practiced John Bell, father of Jacob Bell who was a founder of the Pharmaceutical Society, founder and editor of the *Pharmaceutical Journal* and owner of this shop after the death of his father in 1849. The firm later developed into a large-scale manufacturing laboratory. (Engraving from a painting by W. Hunt, 1840; *see* Kassner, E. W.: J. Am. Pharm. Ass. *20*:236–246, 1931)

tical industry in the Manchester area, in Scotland, London and Leeds, a number of the industrial pharmaceutical laboratories, wholesale drug houses and several non-pharmaceutical establishments [58] originated in the shops of dispensing "chemists" and often can be traced back a century and more. Several of the founders of the Pharmaceutical Society extended their pharmacies to make them industrial or wholesale establishments. To the names of Allen and Bell there should be added those of John May, Thomas Morson and John Savory, all of London, and those of F. B. Benger of Manchester and Richard Raimes of York—founders of firms still serving British medical care. The chemist John Fletcher Macfarlan of Edinburgh was one of the pioneer British manufacturers of alkaloids, at first in the laboratory of his pharmacy and later on in the manufactory that grew out of it. The fact that some of the same people in England who, in the beginning of the 19th century, created anew the profession of pharmacy, simultaneously took an important part in the development of the British pharmaceutical industry is a further proof of the intimate historic ties between dispensing and production in pharmacy, which one finds internationally.

One of the largest pharmaceutical concerns in England, with headquarters in London and with associated houses across the world, was developed by men with American pharmaceutical education. S. M. Burroughs as well as Henry Wellcome, the two late founders of Burroughs Wellcome and Company, were graduates of the Philadelphia College of Pharmacy. Although Henry Wellcome became a naturalized British subject and later on an English knight and Fellow of the Royal Society, he never lost his connections with his native country and, through life membership in the American Pharmaceutical Association, he maintained his relations with American pharmacy. Perhaps this is symbolic.

## CONCLUDING REMARKS

The long-term relations between British and American pharmacy have had consequences, on both sides of the Atlantic. In American history we will meet again the "apothecary," the "druggist," the shopkeeper tradition and outlook, the lingering devotion to occupational independence and self-determination. Under specifically American conditions and a new time, these traditions have been modified, renamed, or hybridized with other influences; but so, too, have they in Britain. The 20th-century dispensing "chemist" or pharmacist feels the tightening circle of regulation within the concept of the welfare state; and he feels the dilemma of having so much spiritual and capital investment in the corner "shop,' while a new role and status for the profession may be slipping from his own control into the developing plans and rising health centers of the National Health Service across Britain. Yet, any professional group that has survived such an erratic history seems likely to continue to prosper in some setting—and to continue its interactions with the former American colonies.

# 8

# Some International Trends

European peoples have been so interrelated that most developments within individual countries since the Middle Ages can be considered as a national reaction to general European trends. Naturally, special conditions and the character of the people concerned often yield interesting differences. In one sphere national trends may predominate, while in another we may find them submerged by trends that meet common needs and cannot long be barred by boundaries. The powerful thrust of science and its technologic applications are in this category, as are movements that facilitate trade and commerce, sometimes followed by the spread of democratic-humanitarian ideas in their wake.

For the purposes of this discussion, examples of such international trends will be considered in three categories: (1) commercial (2) social and (3) pharmaceutical.

## TRENDS OF INTERNATIONAL COMMERCE

The development of drug manufacture by use of power machinery on a large scale was accompanied and promoted by legislation that created an exclusive right to exploit new products or processes. These patent and trademark laws exerted a great and growing influence on the practice of pharmacy.

Large-scale production, though by hand methods, existed for certain drugs already in Greco-Roman antiquity and in the Middle Ages. For example, the tablets consisting of a special clay found on the island of Lemnos (and elsewhere) were sold over the entire known world up to early modern times. There was large-scale manufacture of distilled waters and perfumes in some monasteries of Italy, France and Germany[1] in the 13th century and later, and of troches of vipers in Venice. However, these early precursors of pharmaceutical mass production were commonly an accident of circumstance—the local raw material granting, in effect, a monopoly to the producers.

In other words, with few exceptions (for instance the preparation of corrosive sublimate, cinnabar, sugar of lead, borax, etc., at Venice around the year 1300) quantity manufacture of pharmaceuticals was incidental and conservative. Modern mass production has been systematically planned and progressive.

Drug manufacture in the United States began to convert to mass production technics in this sense after the middle of the 19th century and, within a century, transformed not only the pharmaceutical industry but also the practice of pharmacy. In industries based on science and elaborate technology, the vigorous, steady thrust of this development scarcely could be expected without a two-pronged legal support that society gave to the massive investment ordinarily demanded by mass production. This support consisted of the legal definition and protection of the *patent* and the *trademark,* two quite abstract forms of property that have had far-reaching—and sometimes controversial—effects in the pharmaceutical field.

In general, when a government grants a patent, it intends to protect the rights and the rewards of discovery. If a drug product represents nothing particularly new, or if, for some other reason, it is not patented, the government may grant registration of an exclusive trademark. This helps to protect the rewards that accrue from the public's belief in the merits of the manufacturer or of his product (merits that may be real or, on occasion, largely imaginary).

Linked to this development in the early modern period were the nostrums, fancifully promoted to physicians and laymen alike. Lacking legal and scientific means to expose and curb extravagant claims, the responsible drug maker and medical practitioner often were no match for the impostor and charlatan.

**Patents**

Reigning princes, as part of their prerogatives, granted special privileges—whether for safe passage, for a trading monopoly, or for exploiting invention—to anyone who had gained their favor or had paid the rather considerable amounts asked for. Here we find the beginning of "patent" legislation in most countries. Such privileges for the production and the sale of nostrums were granted by the German emperors and princes, as well as by the French kings until the end of the 18th century and by the English kings until the first third of the 17th century.

Many drug products that were granted the early and rather arbitrary "letters patent" held too little that was original to be considered for a patent today. Today's so-called "patent medicines" commonly are *not* in fact patented, but rather derive their misnomer by lineal descent from this class of early English nostrums.

Some nostrums prepared in the 17th and the 18th centuries were so highly regarded that rulers bought the formulas from their inventors and published them for the supposed benefit of their people. Here are several famous examples: The formula for a decoction of cinchona bark was sold (1680) by the Englishman Talbor to Louis XIV of France, for an extraordinary price.[2] The English parliament (1739) permitted the payment of 5,000 pounds to Joanna Stephens for her remedy (alicante soap and burnt eggshells) for vesical calculus.[3] Frederick the Great of Prussia (1775) gave the inventor of a nostrum against tapeworm (consisting of filix, jalap and scammony) not only an annuity but also a noble title.[4] Similar "bargains" are reported elsewhere.[5]

Such remedies, cleverly promoted into high esteem, came to represent large enterprise and high monetary value. Purveyed with an air of mystery, and often actually secret in composition, they pretended to represent some unique virtue or invention. This circumstance gave such drugs a role in bringing about legal rights that formed the basis of modern patent legislation.

England was the first country to establish governmental regulation in lieu of princely arbitrariness. A statute of King James I (1624) declared all monopolies that were grievous to the subjects of the realm to be void, except privileges for the

> sole working or making of any manner of new manufacture within the realm to the true and first inventor of such manufacture, which others at the time of making such letters patent or grants should not use, so they be not contrary to law nor mischievous to the state by raising of the prices of commodities at home or hurt of trade or generally inconvenient.[6]

On these words rests the modern legal concept of patents for inventions.

The first real medicinal patent was granted in England in 1698 for Epsom salts (Patent

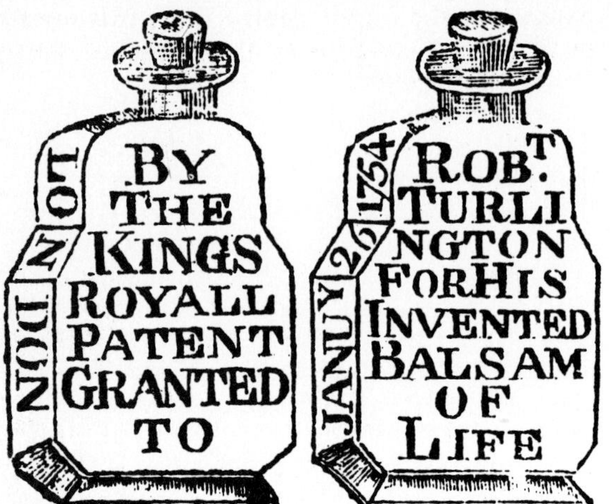


Turlington's Balsam of Life received one of the early medicinal patents in England, under government regulation that began to move "patents" away from the old arbitrary privileges by whim of a monarch, toward the modern system of granting protection only for a novel invention and only for a stated length of time. Turlington's Balsam became popular in both England and America during the 18th century. (From the Smithsonian Institution; original at the Pennsylvania Historical Society)

No. 354). Subsequent patents included *Sal oleosum volatile* (1711), Stoughton's elixir (1712) and Turlington's balsam (1744). The patent granted to the London pharmacist Thomas Wilson for his Patent Ague Drops (1781) evolved into the famous "Fowler's Solution," which had lasting usefulness in therapeutics.[7]

Thus, patent legislation and its application to the pharmaceutical field, as we know it, was born in England. In the American colonies, the British monarch or his governors granted letters-patent of the old type for exclusive privilege (land, trading companies, manufacture), but this practice never was more than casual. The explanation lies in a combination of circumstances: the colonial preoccupation with agriculture, the restrictive policies of the Crown concerning dissemination of industrial information and enterprise in the colonies and the sheer red tape in which patent grants were entangled.

Apparently the Colonies had no concept of patenting inventions on a systematic basis and thereby lagged behind the mother country's marked shift toward emphasizing patents of industrial or inventive purpose. This was rectified rather suddenly after the Revolution, when "between 1790 and 1836, five major statutes were enacted in pursuance of the constitutional provision of the granting of patents."[8]

That this American development was part of an international trend of the 19th century—a concomitant of the rise of large-scale industry—may be seen in the emergence of modern patent laws elsewhere (e.g., France, 1844; England, 1852; Italy, 1864; Germany 1877). In the United States, the modern regulation of patent rights is based on the patent law as revised by an enactment of 1870.

It is noteworthy that the patent law for a federated Germany (supplanting earlier laws for the separate German states) adopted the English concept that only a new method of manufacture—not the product itself—is patentable for medicines, foodstuffs and substances prepared by means of chemical processes. This stand was taken to avoid the granting of monopolies on such vital necessities of daily life. The idea raises a complicated social issue that meanwhile has been much debated internationally. It has not been adopted in the United States, where drugs as well as the processes for making them can be patented.

The development of the patent system provided a legal property of far-reaching importance to pharmaceutical industry (and industry at large). This international trend came to maturity in 1883 with the signing in Paris of an International Patent Convention. Its provisions, as meanwhile amended, are adhered to by nearly all of the principal countries.

The strength of patent laws protecting inventors and their inventions in the individual countries seems to have some correlation with their contribution to the progress of applied science in all fields, including pharmacy.[9] The extensive development of large pharmaceutical firms, based on research, could not have occurred in the same way without patent laws. The fact that the industry, the ingenuity and the money invested in the discovery of new drugs and processes have been rewarded by a temporary monopoly (17 years in the USA) has helped to stimulate the startling advances since the last quarter of the 19th century.

## Trademarks

Because of the limited term of patent protection, and the requirement of full disclosure of what is being patented, most pharmaceutical manufacturers have preferred to reinforce the property value of a new product by trademarking. An important advantage to be gained was well summarized by R. P. Fischelis when he said:

> If the individual who registers a trademark for a patented product is careful enough to apply his trademark in such a manner that it will indicate the brand of the patented product rather than the patented product itself, he can acquire unlimited exclusive rights to the brand name and by clever advertising he can continue to enjoy a virtual monopoly on a given product even after his patent rights have expired.[10]

Historically, the "trade mark" has been a mark—such as a sign or a symbol—used to identify the origin or the ownership of the goods to which it is affixed. The mark of ownership (such as a cattle brand) has a history interwoven with the mark of origin (such as the design embossed on a medicinal tablet), which is today the primary function of trademarks. At first such marks generally were not adopted in the makers' own interest

> . . . but were imposed upon them in the interest of the public, in order to locate responsibility for short weight, inferior material or poor workmanship. Like the finger prints taken today by the police, they established a liability rather than a right. But since this liability tended to secure honest and efficient workmanship, the trade-mark came to be regarded as an assurance of quality, and the confidence of the public in the quality of wares bearing a trade-mark of good repute became an asset.[11]

The use of a "mark of origin" in pharmacy may be traced back into classical times. For example, when Lemnian clay was processed into pastilles (as early as the 5th century B.C.) each pastille was stamped with a seal to indicate its authentic origin (hence called Sealed Earth). In early modern therapy, when such pastilles were made from earths of varied origin, each was "sealed" with a distinctive design.[12]

By the 17th century, the use of trademarks had been systematized and regulated to a certain extent by the guilds, such as those that gave European pharmacy its first organized and regulated form. These old guild provisions were transformed into common law and, hence, given their modern meaning as trademarks—a process that involved a particularly tangled legal history. Suffice it to say that adequate legal recognition came, concomitant with the rise of large-scale industry and patent legislation. The two-part modern British legislation was inaugurated in 1862 and 1875.[13] In the United States a statute was enacted in 1870 (superseded currently by the Lanham Act of 1946).[14] The fundamental enactments came in France beginning in 1857 and in Germany in 1874. Events in other countries likewise give evidence that this international trend was in floodtide during the late 19th century, culminating in an international trademark agreement of 1883 at Paris, which was signed by 25 countries.

As long as the pharmacist prepared most of his own drugs, guided by a pharmacopeia or a formulary, and using raw materials gathered locally or bought from men whom he knew, the system of trademarking could not have seemed as important to him professionally as it has since the development of remote mass production. Thereafter, his prescription ingredients passed through the hands of many he would never meet, under conditions he could not know. This half-blind dependence on the identity and the responsibility of the pharmacist's remote suppliers helped to catapult pharmaceutical trademarks into modern importance, especially under American conditions that prevailed between the end of the Civil War and the passage of the first Federal food and drug legislation (1906).

Intensifying the pharmacist's dependence and perplexity was a disturbing circumstance. At the very time when more potent drugs were being marketed—and in more concentrated forms—the changing character of drugs and drug tests made it impracticable for the community pharmacist to verify personally the quality of drugs he dispensed. Therefore, a drug guaranteed by its maker's mark gained an enhanced practical value in the professional practice of both pharmacists and physicians.

The emphasis on trademarking drugs, which once had served mainly to tout nostrums and quack remedies, thus in the 20th century came to dominate the field of prescription drugs likewise. This second line of development in pharmaceutical trademarking was encouraged by a growing realization among marketing experts that physicians are readily influenced by advertising technics coupled to easily remembered trademarks (when choosing between drugs of similar quality and effectiveness), even as human beings in general are influenced in other kinds of choices.

As refinements in mass marketing and promotional psychology magnified the commercial effectiveness of trademarks internationally, so the proliferation of improved, privately controlled medications expanded the area of the application of trademarks. In the United States soon after the turn of the present century, programs of industrial research increasingly generated products the distinctiveness of which could be maximized by reliance on trademarks in the form of product names ("trade names"). In the struggle for markets, less creative manufacturers often used the same trademarking weapon of distinctive trade names to obscure their paucity of distinctive products, by applying a new tradename to, basically, an old remedy. Trademarks used as manufacturers' "house marks" signifying reputation or quality began to be subordinated to trademarks used as a primary system of nomenclature for prescription drugs.

Arguments about what seemed to be a needlessly irrational system of nomenclature (i.e., fanciful trade names) applied to a professional-scientific area were already old in 1903, when one of the distinguished American pharmacists of his time, M. I. Wilbert, commented:

> The nuisance arising from this self-evident right [to trademarks] is that we, particularly in connection with the medical and pharmaceutical professions, are being overwhelmed with a multitude of meaningless and in many cases misleading names. Many of these names are dangerously similar, and are likely to lead to serious misunderstanding and possibly fatal mistakes. The injustice to the public, as well as the pharmacist, is evidenced by the unnecessary duplication of names and titles for substances or mixtures that are not themselves covered by patents.[15]

In America the validity of the trademarking system has never been seriously challenged, but the question of its appropriate limits came back into pharmaceutical focus with Congressional hearings on policies and methods of drug pricing, which have been recurrent since the late 1950's. In this context, emphasis centered on the possible exploitation of the patient that may occur if the value of product trademarks should be unduly inflated. Additionally, the scientifically oriented segment of the medical profession continued to feel uncomfortable with what one medical editor called

> . . . the peculiarity of the present system of drug terminology whereby the number of names that

can be given to a product is limited only by the number of manufacturers that are producing it . . . a system that is confusing and irritating and should be to a degree humiliating to the presumably intelligent members of a profession that is forced to conform to it.[16]

Apprehensive that the patent system alone would not assure adequate protection to investments in research and promotion, manufacturers tended to construe such attacks as attacks on the trademark system itself—perhaps, even on the system of free enterprise—and as fostering a market for substandard drugs. Speaking on behalf of American pharmaceutical manufacturers in the early 1960's, the National Pharmaceutical Council termed the prescribing of drugs by nonproprietary names "second-class medical care" and proposed that "the crux of the controversy is whether all drugs with the same generic name even when they bear U.S.P. on their label are equivalent therapeutically."[17]

Two questions underlying this statement would be raised repeatedly in the ensuing years, by those arguing from the viewpoint of prescription-drug manufacturers. First, if drugs are prescribed by a system of standardized names more rational than the fanciful trade names, then could the average pharmacist be trusted to select a drug product having therapeutic effects as predictable as the physician had a right to expect? A second question lurked behind the first: Even if pharmacists proved to be sufficiently knowledgeable and ethical, did differences of effect among various brands of the same drug occur so often that patients ordinarily should receive prescriptions specified by brand names (i.e., product trademarks)?[18]

These were not burning issues before the 20th century, either for the public or for the health professions. Traditionally, most drugs had been prescribed by other than trademarked names (e.g., see prescriptions p. 314; today commonly miscalled "generic drugs"). If a prescriber had strong preferences among various manufacturers of a drug, he might add a company name or "house mark," but routinely left the product selection to dispensing pharmacists. Since American pharmacists then had limited and variable professional training, such confidence might be misplaced; but the tendency was to rely upon a miscreant losing his clientele through the purifying forces of a free marketplace or (by the late 19th century) upon his being legally penalized.

Ironically, as American pharmacists became better prepared educationally to protect the public from questionable prescription products the need became less obvious, as prescribers followed the lead of drug manufacturers in a massive shift toward use of product trademarks as the primary system of drug nomenclature in medical care during the first half of the 20th century. There were several reasons, although this development has never been carefully analyzed historically. Perhaps above all, as the processing of the final dosage forms moved into remote mass-production laboratories (as the processing of individual prescription ingredients had moved during the 19th century), manufacturers introduced into therapeutics new combinations and new proportions of ingredients. These myriad variations helped to justify a myriad of new trademarked names for medications (sometimes to the patient's advantage, sometimes not). Moreover, manufacturers came to see more clearly that a distinctive trade name could give a prescription product a distinctive aura in the minds of prescribing physicians, whether or not it had a distinctive advantage over the same product made by a competitor (just as in earlier centuries a distinctive name for routine self-medication products had given them a distinctive aura in the minds of laymen). By the 1960's a more compelling factor reinforced the trend. At an earlier stage pharmaceutical science and technology commanded general confidence that the standards it proposed and the tests it devised could assure therapeutic equivalence if a medication were made by several different manufacturing laboratories. By the end of the 1960's some demonstrable examples to the contrary (e.g., Chloramphenicol) had challenged the old assumption,[19] as a more quantitative pharmaco-therapeutic science made product differences more measurable. If a drug from two different makers met required standards, but might not be acceptably equivalent therapeutically, many physicians inferred that a medication should be prescribed consistently by a product trademark. However convincing the victory and the rationale of trademarks as a system of drug nomenclature seemed, the scientific community of medical care without industrial ties continued to feel uncomfortable with its implications.

In the United States, counteractions arose here and there by the 1970's and gathered support among pharmacists and laymen alike. The American Pharmaceutical Association reaffirmed its decades-old stance favoring noncommercial prescription nomenclature.[20] Several agencies of Federal government, through their regulatory or purchasing policies, further undermined the pedestal upon which trademarks had been placed. Further, the Department of Health, Education and Welfare set up the Task Force on Prescription Drugs, whose report in 1969 fueled as well as clarified the controversy.[21] Efforts expanded to define and minimize the problem of assuring acceptable equivalency between lots of a drug coming onto the market from different production laboratories. Senate committees probed for evidence of abuses of the trademark privilege in the field of medical care,[22] and muckraking journalists escalated concern among the public and health professions.

In this sensitive and complex field, a permanent solution seemed unlikely, even after a century of sporadic controversy about the appropriate role of trademarks in the field of therapeutics. At least a new balance of contending interests was being struck, as critics continued to insist that what had begun as a social invention to protect an intangible form of property was sometimes being turned back upon society as a weapon of commercial exploitation.

## INTERNATIONAL SOCIAL TRENDS

Modern social legislation has been one consequence of the change in the structure and the living conditions of human society produced by industrialization and mechanization of life.

A harbinger of later social welfare legislation were the laws (1802–1847) by which the English administrative policy of *laissez-faire* received its death sentence. These factory laws were born out of the necessity of protecting working people, women and children especially, from exploitation by industry.

One of the most characteristic expressions of social-welfare legislation, meanwhile, has been a world-wide trend toward paying for medical care on the insurance principle.

### Compulsory Health Insurance

In ancient Rome, as well as in the Middle Ages, organizations built on compulsory membership had been devoted to the care of the sick. This care became the required or the self-imposed duty of almost all guilds.

Particularly in mining (the first European large-scale industrial undertaking) there were early institutions of a rather modern character, requiring periodic payments and affording medical care. However, the change from private cooperative assistance in cases of sickness to authoritative institutions introduced by law and guaranteed by the government was begun during the middle of the 19th century, in Germany. The laws were perfected by social legislation introduced in 1881 by a special public message of the German Emperor. They were intended to make the agitation of the German socialists ineffective by countering with a well-planned, government-fostered social welfare program.[23] A publication of the International Labour Office (1925) claimed that

> the motive of the reform was a desire to improve the living conditions of the workers in order to reconcile them with the state as an institution defending the capitalistic organization of [paternal] protection, and at the same time to deprive the workers' occupational organizations of the potential weapon they possessed in numerous mutual aid and provident bodies attached to the trade unions.

A disadvantage of the original German system—not only for the physician and the pharmacist but for the insured as well—were the contracts concerning medical and medicinal care. These were negotiated, not by a centralized governmental authority, but by individual representatives of local independent health insurance bodies. Frequently, these representatives tried to deprive the physicians of their liberty of action by prescribing detailed rules for the medical treatment of the insured. Moreover, they endeavored to limit the role of the pharmacist—for example, by delivering bandages and many remedies directly to the insured; and they produced drugs in laboratories conducted by or affiliated with individual health insurance bodies or their central organizations, rather than in the pharmacies. Restrictions placed on both physician and pharmacist in the providing of medicaments for the insured were numerous.[24] From the beginning, the remuneration of the pharmacist was based on government price lists issued annually, less discounts to insurance agencies of 10 to 20 per cent. The final objective was socialization of the health profession.[25] The contributory principle of paying for health insurance had already been established in the final form of the German plan. Both worker and employer contributed, but under certain circumstances the government would pay a worker's share. Manual workers were insured no matter what their income; others could participate on a voluntary basis.[26]

A number of social circumstances[27] united to carry the idea of social insurance around the globe and, with it, provision for health insurance, usually under government supervision or sponsorship. Within 70 years after the German innovation, 44 countries had a social security program, all but 5 including health insurance. Most programs with health benefits included a pharmaceutical component. By the early 1960's 59 nations were providing health benefits.[28] In most later versions of health insurance, the goal of providing primarily for low-income classes has never been far out of sight, although the appeal of health insurance eventually tends to broaden benefits and expand the occupational strata covered.

It was in England that this tendency first reached its culmination in providing compulsory health insurance for an entire population. But there, too, the original provision was only for lower-income classes. This provision was effective from 1912 until 1948, when parliament placed all citizens under a government health insurance plan (National Health Service). After a penetrating historical study of the British plan, Eckstein concluded that "In a very real sense the institution of the [British] Service marks a triumph of non-socialist over socialist ideas, however much we have become used to calling systems like the National Health Service 'socialized' medicine."[29] Nevertheless, with this popular and far-reaching move, England went far toward realization of the "welfare state" idea.

Although British pharmacists remained private entrepreneurs (as in other non-socialist states), most of their prescription practice fell within the National Health Service. As such, it has been paid for through government-collected funds. Prescription orders, for which medication has been dispensed, are sent periodically to a bureau that prices them according to a negotiated schedule of fees covering ingredients, professional service and other costs. To discourage the careless use of pharmaceutical services that was encountered, since 1952 a token payment from the patient's pocket is required in England, as in France and some other countries.

A steady rise in the cost of pharmaceutical

service has attracted the government's attention repeatedly over the years. In 1962 the Secretary of the Pharmaceutical Society of Great Britain, Sir Hugh Linstead, interpreted this circumstance as follows:

> The number of prescriptions has remained fairly steady—about 210 million annually for 50 million people. But the cost of each item has steadily risen owing to the increasing use of new and more expensive drugs . . . about three times the cost in 1948 when the service started, and it has only been kept down by the most strenuous efforts with what we call the *British National Formulary*, which gives recipes for non-specialty medicines and advice about equivalent preparations for expensive [trademarked] specialties . . . In consequence about 60 percent of the medicines prescribed under the National Health Service are for specialties and the remainder are not. On the European continent 90 percent or more prescribed medicines are for specialties, and I suspect that in the United States and Canada the percentage is even higher.[30]

Until the introduction of health insurance, England was the only one of the larger European countries in which the physicians had full liberty to dispense and deliver medicines. After adoption of the English health insurance plan the physician was forbidden to do so, the dispensing of medicines being restricted to pharmacists.[31] In France and Germany, where the separation of functions between physician and pharmacist has been compulsory for centuries, such a clause was not necessary.

Another danger to the orderly development of a profession of pharmacists serving the public at large, emerged under compulsory health insurance plans: a tendency toward the dispensing and the delivery of medicaments and medicinal supplies by the health insurance bodies themselves, and the establishment of special pharmacies for the insured. Clauses within the insurance act itself in France, or in other laws as in Germany, excluded such possibilites, at least to a great extent. In Poland before socialization, where a similar precaution was not taken, the local health insurance bodies established their own pharmacies (numbering 200 in 1925) and deprived private pharmacies of a great part of their legitimate field. As a consequence, "many private pharmacies, especially in highly industrialized centers, became completely ruined and had to be closed."[32] Meanwhile, sickness-benefit agencies in at least five other countries have tried to operate some pharmacies of their own.[33]

In a majority of countries, pharmaceutical and other health services remain in traditional and private channels. However, the amount of government regulation and compensation for insured services varies. One study showed that under social-security plans, the share of total medical care paid on the insurance principle varied widely, from about 25 per cent to as high as 95 per cent.[34]

The circumstance has been quite different in the Soviet Union and in other communist countries, as the People's Republic of China and Yugoslavia. There, pharmacists and other health practitioners are socialized and employees of the state. Under socialistic arrangements the patient may, however, be asked, just as in other countries, to pay for part or all of his pharmaceutical service out of his own pocket or obtain government-paid services, depending on particular regulations.[35]

The concept of paying for medical care on the insurance principle slowly took root in the United States, likewise, although with strong resistance to the international trend toward compulsory government-administered plans. Americans became fully conscious of the issue just before World War I, when the British parliament and public were considering their first health insurance plan for lower-income groups. It was a time when early social-welfare measures were being considered here, encouraged by the Progressive movement. When workmen's compensation laws were being passed in state legislatures, several states were also confronted by bills proposing health insurance, but none were passed.

The American Medical Association awakened to the implications and passed a policy resolution in 1920, the fundamentals of which have survived the ensuing decades:

> . . . The American Medical Association declares its opposition to the institution of any plan embodying the system of compulsory contributory insurance against illness, or any other plan of compulsory insurance which provides for medical service to be rendered contributors or their dependents, provided, controlled, or regulated by any state or the Federal government.[36]

During the prosperous years before the Great Depression the principle of insurance applied to medical care persisted mainly as a matter of social study rather than political action. With the depression, problems of medical care became more acute, and a broader segment of the American public became acutely aware of the issues of medical economics.

In an influential and privately sponsored study, the Committee on Costs of Medical Care recommended in 1932 that "the costs of medical care be placed on a group payment basis," whether by insurance or taxation or both—a conclusion at that time still controversial. Interest in such social-welfare proposals tended to gain a broader base as the United States gained experience with its social security system, newly adopted in 1935. The first serious bid for compulsory national health insurance came in 1939 with the Wagner bill; and other bills went into the Congressional hopper sporadically during the ensuing decades.

Even voluntary group insurance had been considered an unacceptable alternative to traditional fee-for-service by many American physicians and other conservatives until a few years after the adoption of the social security system. However, in the other direction stood a threat of government-sponsored health insurance, against which the voluntary insurance movement was thrust as a counterforce by many who originally opposed or ignored it.

Pharmacists in the American Pharmaceutical Association maintained a low profile on the issue during the 1940's, perhaps partly because health-insurance proposals ordinarily did not cover their services, partly because organized pharmacists seemed readier to concede that some change would be in order to "make more adequate medical care available to all our people." At the same time, the A.Ph.A. supported the A.M.A. (1949) in "opposing compulsory national health insurance," which seemed "unsuited to the American way" and threatened "socialization."[37]

By the late 1940's insurance as such no longer was controversial in America as a device for reducing the economic risks of illness. After another decade the voluntary movement, aided by contributory plans of both employers and unions, which blanketed large groups from all economic classes, was keeping pace with the hopes of its most optimistic advocates.[38] Compared with health insurance plans in some countries, the American voluntary coverage remained more limited in scope of benefits, but it mushroomed in the proportion of Americans voluntarily insured. About 169 million Americans were protected to some degree by private health insurance in 1968, compared with about 12 million in 1940.[39] Three main types of insuring organizations responded to this basic shift in medical economics occurring within less than three decades: 1. Nonprofit corporations largely under medical control (about 150 Blue Cross and Blue Shield organizations); 2. Private insurance companies entering the field of health risks (about 1000); 3. Prepaid group-practice plans (of which Kaiser-Permanente became one of the most influential prototypes, with perhaps 200 other consumer-oriented, group-practice plans initiated by the end of the 1960's).[40]

Like the citizens of many other countries, Americans thus indicated their preference for escaping some of the uncertainties and financial threat that the costs of modern medical care entail. Also paralleling the international trend has been a tendency since the 1950's to broaden insured coverage, and to include pharmaceutical services. Although added most often as an integral feature of basic medical-care coverage, some early prescription-insurance plans were developed separately, such as the "Green Shield Plan" of Windsor, Ontario, in the 1950's and the plan of the Bricklayers Union of New York in 1961. Both of these early plans provided prepaid prescription service through existing community pharmacies. The subsequent development of varied agencies to administer prescription-insurance programs led, in 1969, to the establishment of a National Pharmacy Insurance Council to provide a unifying and liaison function. Growth of pharmacy coverage has been steady, but one estimate for 1971 suggested that only about 18 per cent of the total cost of prescribed drugs and medical supplies in the United States was being paid by third parties.[41]

During this complex growth of private health insurance after mid-century, sporadic debate has continued nationally on the extent to which the problems of pharmacomedical economics should be met through government regulation and administration. Several partial measures were authorized by Congress during the same period. Through Social Security, benefits were provided after 1950 for certain categories of the medically indigent (e.g., the aged and disabled), culminating in the Kerr-Mills amendment of 1960, which aided individual states with matching funds, but achieved only limited effectiveness.

In 1965 American society made a major decision in health care when two major amendments to the Federal Social Security Act set up "Medicare" (title XVIII) and "Medicaid" (title XIX). Medicare proved to have the greater social import and success, by providing a wide range of health and medical services to Americans 65 years old or older (utilizing some of the private experience with health insurance in constructing the government model). The other program (Medicaid) was another medical assistance plan (not insurance) through which the Federal government aids financially a variety of state programs for the medically indigent; it has been complicated to administer and periodically has come under critical fire. Under Medicaid a state may include prescription service, while Medicare does not include it except within a hospital or an authorized "extended care" facility.[42]

Despite the consensus that government health insurance for older citizens has been well accepted—or partly because of it—the American debate about major reform in the financing and delivery of medical care has continued into the last quarter of the century. During nearly a century after the German chancellor put forward government-supervised health insurance to ameliorate the workers' plight, the socioeconomic landscape of medical care over much of the world had been transformed. The historical trend found its American expression, but a question still remained: What would be the final relationship between private and governmental arrangements, for the health care of the public at large?

### Opium Treaty; Narcotic Controls

The introduction as well as the scope of health insurance, while an international trend, has remained strictly a separate national decision of the individual country. However, the trade in opiates and other "narcotic" drugs became a matter of international cooperation and decision. For no boundaries or informal arrangements could prevent the spreading of drug addiction, with all its demoralizing consequences, from one country into the other. Nevertheless, it was the second half of the 19th century before the great European trading nations and the United States of America became aware of the threat to themselves of what originally was considered to be peculiarly an Eastern vice.[43]

In the early 19th century the English government, in order to retain the profitable trade in opium, overcame by force of arms attempts of the Chinese government to eliminate the import of the drug from English-dominated India. Defeated in two so-called opium wars (1839–1843 and 1856–1860), the Chinese government—to the lasting discredit of the English—had to compensate the traders for their losses and withdraw laws prohibiting the trade in opium. It is an irony of history that the rapidly developing cultivation of the poppy in China itself soon turned the tables, making opium a Chinese export to India.

All over the world, medicine and pharmacy came to place opiates high on the list of the drugs most useful to mankind, because of their unmatched analgesic power. Then the isolation of narcotic alkaloids and the development of hypodermic injection by the mid-19th century formed a two-edged sword that on one side enhanced medicinal use and, on the other, intensified widespread abuse.

As both the character and the dimensions of the addiction problem were perceived more clearly, West European and American interest in some form of cooperative control came to a focus early in the present century. This culminated in an international treaty agreed on at The Hague in 1912. Eventually, most governments of the world signed the agreement in some form, which stimulated corresponding legal restrictions in the individual countries. (The Single Convention on Narcotic Drugs signed in 1961 superseded all but one of the multilateral treaties negotiated on the subject during the intervening decades.)

The United States of America was among the very first to implement her moral and legal obligations, by Congressional enactment of the Harrison Narcotic Act in 1914. Earlier legal concern with the problem could be seen in the prohibition of nonmedicinal imports (1877) and of nonmedicinal use (1908). However, it was the Harrison Narcotic Act (see p. 223) that gave American expression and force to the far-reaching control envisioned by The Hague Convention.

After World War I, supervision of the international agreement was given to the League of Nations, through its Opium Advisory Board. Since World War II the functions once performed by the League of Nations have been continued by the United Nations, in several constituent bodies: 1) A Commission on Narcotic Drugs, a policy-making body, makes recommendations to improve control of narcotic drugs. 2) The Permanent Central Opium Board collects and studies global statistics on the movement of medicinal narcotics, and recommends ways to minimize diversion into illicit smuggling. 3) The World Health Organization of the U.N., through its Expert Committee on Addiction-Producing Drugs, contributes counsel on medical and pharmacological aspects of controlled substances and evaluates drugs considered for addition to the controlled group. 4) The U.N.'s Drug Supervisory Body, a joint commission drawn from the three other bodies, annually assesses the legitimate needs of each member-nation and negotiates with the country concerned a fixed allocation from the world supply of addiction-producing drugs.

Such a complex system can be attributed partly to the unexpected complexity of international control. Moreover, several types of expertise and interests must be accommodated: administrative, legal, scientific, commercial, economic, and governmental. A further complication is the periodic appearance on the world market of new examples of drugs that produce harmful dependencies. The degree of harm attributed is itself partly culturally conditioned, so that classifying drugs in this category becomes at least as perplexing internationally as it has been in the U.S.A.

The problem of discussing all such drugs within the twin concepts of "addiction" and "habituation" increased with the increase in the types of illicit drugs and in the social and scientific understanding of their effects. Under this pressure the old concepts had fragmented by 1964, and the term "narcotics" itself as commonly used became misleading and outmoded. In their place the World Health Organization put a whole series of well-characterized types of "drug dependencies."[44] One of these is the classic dependency, opiate addiction ("morphine-type"), whose ravages had evoked so early a demonstration of the possibility of international cooperation for seeking a common solution to a common problem.[45]

If the solution proved to be uncommonly elusive, yet the World Health Organization could point to constructive results that illuminate and make safer the complex relationship between man and drugs. It is understood that the regulation of dependency-producing drugs places a special responsibility on international pharmacy, emphasizing its importance from the point of view of public health. It might even be doubted that the satisfactory enforcement of the laws would be possible without the strategically distributed pharmacies, with their professional standing and their fixed place within health administration, all over the civilized world.

## INTERNATIONAL PROFESSIONAL TRENDS

In the development of industrial pharmacy, of health insurance under governmental control and of laws controlling dependency-producing drugs, the pharmacist had to adapt as best he could to a given situation. However, there was a wide field left to the initiative of the members of the profession that could be cultivated fruitfully on an international basis.

It was the old pharmaceutical dream of an international pharmacopeia which may be regarded as the main incentive for the creation of organized international intercourse. The General Association of German Pharmacists took the initiative to convene an International Congress of Pharmacy to exchange information, internationally, but primarily to plan an international pharmacopeia and to tackle the problem that quackish self-medication represented for the public and for pharmacy—a concern that would recur perennially at future congresses. At this first Congress, convened in Germany in 1865, international drug standards proved to be too difficult to accomplish. But the usefulness of such conferences was so obvious that the international congresses, once started, became a standing feature of the life of the profession.

### Fédération Internationale Pharmaceutique

International Congresses of Pharmacy continued to be held every few years in various countries,[46] but there was no continuity through year-around organization or support of services through regular membership fees. Participation in a Congress was open to everyone interested in the pharmaceutical topics to be discussed, regardless of the type of affiliation with pharmacy or with a national pharmaceutical association. When each Congress adjourned, the international cooperation and communication thus established risked disruption.

These handicaps of the occasional Congresses led the Dutch Pharmaceutical Association to propose (in 1908) that professional pharmaceutical associations in Europe be circularized to interest them in organizing a permanent international association of pharmacy. Two years later, at the Tenth International Congress of Pharmacy, when the Dutch suggested the founding of such an association, the suggestion won approval. It was decided to place the headquarters and the secretariat at The Hague, where it has since remained. During 1911, promises of collaboration were gained from pharmaceutical societies around the world, culminating in an organizational meeting of delegates that summer.

The new International Pharmaceutical

Federation became a federation of the important national pharmaceutical associations, dedicated to the furtherance of the profession and of pharmaceutical knowledge, and seeking better collaboration and understanding on issues of common concern.

The federation of national associations represented a new concept of international cooperation, but it was decided to continue the old International Congresses of Pharmacy for all interested pharmacists, within the framework of the Federation. From the beginning, the Federation has published some type of periodical, not only for member-associations but for interested pharmacists.[47]

The First General Assembly, convened at The Hague in 1912, gave a new expression to pharmacy as a world-wide brotherhood dedicated to providing the same responsible services wherever civilization thrives. After the Third General Assembly, and before the Federation had matured, World War I and its aftermath reduced activities largely to keeping a foundation intact for survival.

Between the two World Wars, the International Pharmaceutical Federation came of age. Its assemblies were increasingly well-attended and productive. It gave pharmacy an organized link with international bodies of related professions and with intergovernmental agencies. It continued to foster efforts toward unifying drug standards in-

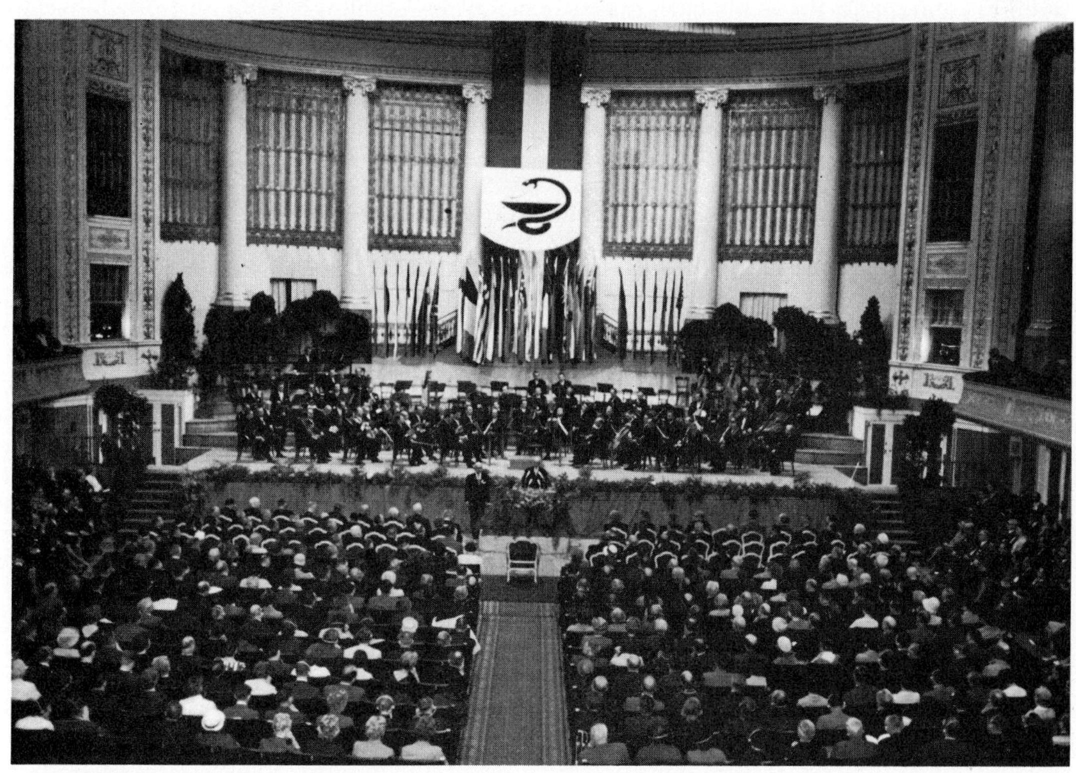

Beneath the symbol of the profession and a panoply of national flags, the opening session of the 19th General Assembly of the International Pharmaceutical Federation, at Vienna, is addressed by the President of the Austrian Republic. (From the American Pharmaceutical Association and Foto Schikola, 1962)

ternationally. A Federation commission studied the control of medicaments aboard ships at sea and, in 1934, issued its first International Ships' Formulary. A Scientific Section was established (1926), and the later development of other sections permits special-interest meetings and studies that, for Americans, resemble the modern structure of the American Pharmaceutical Association. Pharmacy leaders were gaining new insight into the varied national guises in which common problems could be posed and could be attacked.

Then a harbinger of catastrophe appeared in 1939 when the General Assembly scheduled for Berlin had to be abandoned. In the following year the Germans overran Holland, and the Federation headquarters there had to go underground. With the war's end, the records were pulled back together and the representatives of the Federation were recalled, activities were revived (such as the International Commission on Specialties), and the revival was completed with the staging of the Twelfth General Assembly (Zurich, 1947).

The American Pharmaceutical Association became a member of the Federation in 1925, although the United States had been represented recurrently at the International Congresses since 1867. After sharing with the country at large a period of relative isolationism, American pharmacy entered the present period of active collaboration and support of the International Federation during the early 1950's, under the leadership of Don E. Francke, a distinguished editor and practitioner in hospital pharmacy. A growing group of American pharmacists linked themselves with other pharmacists internationally through Associate Membership, and a number of them attend each biennial General Assembly, as do the delegates officially representing the American Pharmaceutical Association. Two American pharmacists have achieved sufficiently central roles in the Federation during its history to be recognized with Vice Presidencies, Don E. Francke (1958–66) and William S. Apple (1974– ).

A junior counterpart of the Federation, the International Pharmaceutical Students' Federation, was organized in 1949 by 24 students from 11 countries meeting in London. The national organizations of pharmacy students are federated into the "IPSF" as full members; individual pharmacy students of the world may affiliate as associate members. In 1973 there were 27 member nations, including the United States.

The Students' Federation promotes the interests and international cooperation of pharmacy students, holds a study-tour in a different country every year and publishes an IPSF *News Bulletin*. One of the most significant accomplishments has been a developing exchange program which permits selected pharmacy students and young graduates to experience life and pharmaceutical work in another country for a time, at low cost.[48]

As the International Pharmaceutical Federation itself has continued to evolve, it reflects periodically some tensions between the disparate elements and concerns within pharmacy that could be observed in individual countries. Questions of science and technology tended to dominate the Federation, for example, during its first quarter-century. The essentiality of the interaction between the science and the profession of pharmacy has never been lost sight of , but especially since the 1950's there have been more insistent calls for dealing more explicitly in the General Assembly with concerns of the practitioner. Some delegations, perhaps particularly the United States, have pressed the Federation toward more emphasis on the changes faced by community pharmacists everywhere, toward expanding its membership around the world and, in the process, toward becoming less European-oriented.[49] In 1975, 62 national organizations of five continents comprised the Ordinary Membership, representing a majority of the world's pharmacists. During the early 1970's a special commission generated proposals for changes in operating structure and policies.[50] If a more pluralistic organization has been emerging, it has also expressed a renewed vitality. The Federation can be expected to continue to produce worthwhile results from the international forum of pharmacy that has been ongoing for more than a century. By representing and expressing a pharmaceutical world ideology, it has brought the concept of pharmacy as a profession, and the importance to public welfare of its professional status, to the knowledge and the appreciation of all governments of the civilized world.

## Unification of Drug Standards

To unify standards for drugs internationally has been a goal to which pharmacists and others in the health sciences return again and again. Why has this been so? The British pharmacopeial expert, C. H. Hampshire, once replied:

> Differences in national standards for widely used materials are a hindrance to the spread of medical knowledge, an inconvenience to pharmacists who have to dispense prescriptions brought from various countries, a source of trouble and possibly of danger to travellers. . . . An International Pharmacopoeia will help to resolve these difficulties, will tend to economy of production and will facilitate commerce in drugs between the nations.[51]

From the beginning the International Congresses of Pharmacy showed concern about the international tangle of diverse names for medication of the same specification, and about diverse specifications for medication of the same name. A draft of an international pharmacopeia came before the Congress in 1885, but never found acceptance. After that, efforts to achieve effective influence concentrated on standardizing the strength of the more potent drugs.

At the international pharmaceutical congress held in Chicago in 1893 (the first on American soil) the American Pharmaceutical Association pressed for practical steps toward making more uniform at least some of the potent drugs listed with different strengths in the various national pharmacopeias. The idea of an international code of potent medicaments, supported by the American Pharmaceutical Association, was backed by delegates of 18 countries who agreed on the principles of such a code.[52]

In 1906 the first intergovernmental convention concerning the unification of potent medicaments met and signed the *Protocole International* (also called "P.I." and "International Formulary"). An enlarged revision of this formulary was drafted by the Federation's committee for pharmaceutical nomenclature and accepted by the second international conference on the unification of potent medicaments. The final protocol was signed in 1925 on behalf of 26 governments, including the signature of the pharmacist Andrew G. Du Mez on behalf of the United States of America.

These efforts were disrupted by two World Wars. Although the agreement (completed 1929) had a constructive influence, it seemed not to have the far-reaching influence that sanguine proponents had expected.

The second agreement had applied mainly to standards for 27 potent drugs and preparations, methods of preparation, nomenclature and maximum doses. Other important clauses proposed to continue such endeavors and called "for the creation of an international body for the unification of pharmacopoeias." For this purpose it was later proposed that a permanent secretariat be established within the League of Nation's Health Organization. As a consequence, the League of Nations set up, in 1937, a Technical Commission of Pharmacopoeial Experts, which held its first meeting the next year.

World War II shattered this promising new medium of collaboration, as it did much else in European life. Some technical work of the Commission was kept alive through the war, especially by British and American representatives.[53] Postwar work built on the foundation from previous decades, finding a new home within the World Health Organization that emerged in 1946 as a part of the United Nations. Several previous members of the defunct Commission could be called on to help to form the W.H.O. Expert Committee on the Unification of Pharmacopoeias. It first met in 1947 and, "by all odds, has been the most active of all such W.H.O. expert groups ever since." This Committee is aided (since 1950) by an Expert Advisory Panel on the International Pharmacopoeia.

The American pharmacist and then U.S.P. chairman, E. Fullerton Cook of Philadelphia, served as a member of the small expert committee that held the main responsibility for pharmacopeial work in the League of Nations and later in the United Nations (W.H.O.). His contribution has been carried forward by other Americans.

As a fruit of this work there appeared the first edition of *Pharmocopoea Internationalis,* published by the World Health Organization, Geneva (Volume I in 1951, Volume II in 1955) in English, French and Spanish; and other translations were published in German and Japanese.

In accord with a resolution of the Third World Health Assembly, the International Pharmacopoeia ("Ph.I.") was presented as "a collection of recommended specifications, which are not intended to have legal status as such in any country, but are offered to serve as references so that national specifications can be established on a similar basis in any country." Thus, the International Pharmacopoeia is not a pharmacopeia in any legal sense. When W.H.O. published a second edition (1967), this limitation was reflected in the title, *Specifications for the Control of the Quality of Pharmaceutical Preparations.*

In this work the W.H.O. Secretariat had the voluntary cooperation of scientists from more than 30 countries, with assistance from a large number of laboratories, both governmental and private. To help implement the standards, the W.H.O. arranged to provide reference samples of authentic chemical substances (for comparative checking) from a center in Stockholm and reference samples of biological products from laboratories in Copenhagen and London. To buttress the standards further, the W.H.O. has issued a separate volume on *Specifications for Reagents Mentioned in the Interational Pharmacopoeia.*[54]

The World Health Organization of the U.N. developed a supplementary project through a Subcommittee (of the Expert Committee) on International Non-Proprietary Names. The Subcommittee mainly tries to attain international agreement on public names for new drugs (trying to avoid conflict with trademarked names) and to publicize their selections, with the aim of fostering a more standardized and rational pharmaceutical nomenclature. This has been a significant modern response to the concern among pharmacists, on record since 1892, about the multiple nonproprietary names for drugs in use internationally. The program is said to have met with "universal approval" except for the United States, where there is an unusually intense fear that scientific names may dilute the benefits of brand-name advertising.[55]

The tendency toward international cooperation may be affected by regional as well as national differences. This has found expression in the effort toward unification of standards for drugs when the "Common Market" countries decided to develop a multivolume *European Pharmacopoeia* (Vol. I, 1969). These standards are intended to replace, eventually, the individual national pharmacopoeias, just as the regional *Nordic Pharmacopoeia* has in pharmaceutical service to 20 million Scandinavians.[56] Regional affinities likewise have affected the international groupings organized by pharmacists.

### International Groups of Specialized Scope

Fully developed professions and sciences are predominantly international, rather than national, in their knowledge, ethos, technics

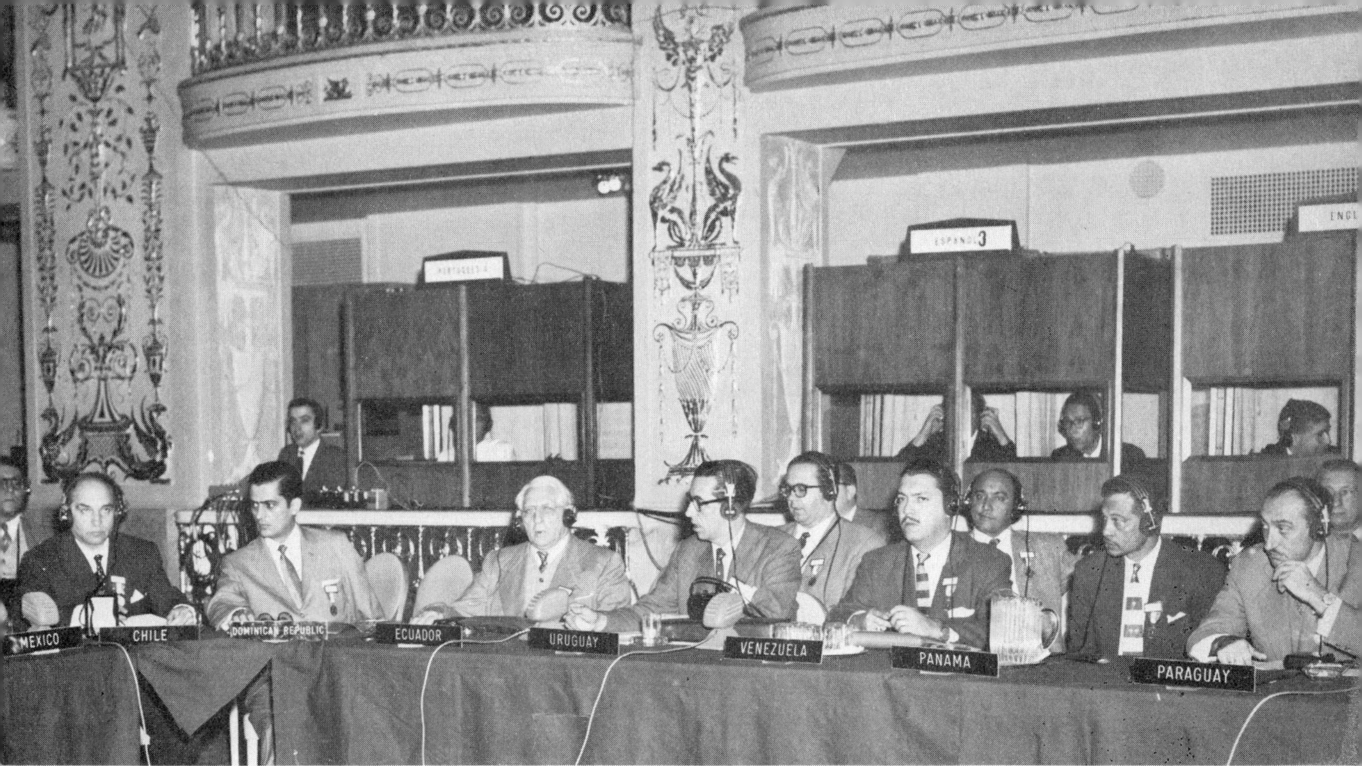


A Pan-American Congress of Pharmacy and Biochemistry convenes each triennium in a different country. At sessions in Washington in 1957 *(above)* simultaneous translation from three booths in the background permits heads of delegations in conference to select the language of their choice on headphones. (From: Reni Photos, *Drug Topics* Collection, A.I.H.P., Madison, WI)

and services. Therefore they tend to ignore artificial political boundaries in spheres of specialized interest. Countertendencies are the cultural (including linguistic) differences and the fact that while the "space age" has banished the handicap of time, it has not banished cost in spanning great distances. For such reasons, pharmaceutical workers have established supranational assemblies that are limited to a specific cultural region of the world rather than being global—perhaps encouraged by the circumstance that the International Pharmaceutical Federation itself has tended to be more European in cast than is suggested by its global concept. The Federation itself has been cooperating in the programs of pharmacists organized on a regional basis, and has been considering in the 1970's to what extent to organize even its own activities around such regional affinities of peoples.

Among the periodic regional congresses, the nations of the Americas find common pharmaceutical ground in a triennial Pan-American Congress of Pharmacy and Biochemistry. The first such Congress in 1948 was attended in Havana by delegates from most of the countries in the Western Hemisphere, including the United States. By 1975 ten such Pan-American Congresses of Pharmacy had been held.[57] As Alejandro Orfila of the Pan-American Union pointed out on the occasion of the Fourth Congress, at Washington, D. C.:

> This Congress—by its very name and composition—is a living example of the broad, all-inclusive scope and influence of the Pan American movement of the 20th century. We can multiply this example many times; for this Congress is only 1 of 12 inter-American conferences that will take place during the present month in 10 different countries of the Western Hemisphere.[58]

Bylaws revised at the 1957 Congress provided a continuing agency between meetings called the Pan-American Pharmaceutical and Biochemical Federation, of which the American pharmacist George B. Griffenhagen has served as first Vice President. The biochemical link with pharmacy can be understood here mainly in terms of the clinical chemistry that has been so closely associated in South America with pharmaceutically-trained personnel.

Similar regional congresses have been staged by countries of the Near and the Middle East, for both professional and scientific interchange. The first Middle East Pharmaceutical Conference was held in Lebanon in 1956, with 11 nations represented.[59] The Federation of Asian Pharmaceutical Associations was organized in 1963 and has staged a number of general assemblies and scientific congresses. A Commonwealth Pharmaceutical Association was founded (under British aegis) in 1969. An Organization of Pharmacists of the European Community arose from the six countries of the European Economic Community; and with the growth of the "Common Market" countries conceivably might develop as another full scale regional organization of pharmacy.

Other series of international congresses that are part of the organized development of pharmacy have been given a scope restricted by the specialized subject rather than by geography. These have included an International Congress of Military Medicine and Pharmacy (first meeting in 1921, at Brussels), an international union of pharmaceutical employees (first meeting in 1925, at Vienna), International Congress for Hospital Pharmacy (first meeting in 1953, at Basel), and international congresses for the history of pharmacy (first meeting in 1934, at Basel) sponsored biennially by the International Society for the History of Pharmacy. In addition, since 1952, international historical meetings also have been staged by the World Union of Societies for the History of Pharmacy in conjunction with General Assemblies of the International Pharmaceutical Federation. A complete listing of the specialized international relations of the profession would be still longer, not to mention those of individual sciences underlying the progress and practice of the profession.

Speaking of this development before American pharmacists, as President of the International Pharmaceutical Federation, Sir Hugh Linstead observed:

> In spite of the special example of some of the newly born countries, it is broadly true to say that the 19th century was a century of nationalism while the 20th century is a century of internationalism. We in Europe are moving fairly rapidly towards the integration of that continent just as you in the Americas are groping towards closer unity between the United States and Central and Southern America. Similar tendencies are showing themselves in embryo in Africa and among the Arab States.
>
> Within these large international movements there are moves to secure closer cooperation and understanding between professional groups. You have your Pan-American Congress of Pharmacy, we have in Europe a committee representing the pharmaceutical organizations of the six countries of the European Economic Community. I have only this month had the privilege of attending the Eighth Pan-Arabic Congress in Cairo. The oldest organization in this field is of course the International Pharmaceutical Federation . . . ; [and though we have not] yet found the answer to the coordination of professional pharmacy internationally . . . our problems are essentially the same in every country; our ideals are the same; all of us are bound to profit from an increasing interchange of experience and ideas which modern communications make possible.[60]

This uniting tendency, leaping national boundaries, thus finds roots in a community of tasks among pharmacists, in a common professional idealism, and in common problems (especially those created by industrialism, state control, and commercialism impinging upon medical care). At another level, however, it can be seen as a pharmaceutical expression of a broader trend developing during the past century or so. At diverse levels of human thought and activity, a revolution in transportation, communication, and socioethnic attitudes has progressively broadened the sense of community from being predominantly local, to sectional, to national and, finally, to international in contact and cooperation—despite disruptive wars and conflicting social philosophies. Pharmacy has participated in this development and has been affected by it. The grave need of our century to give substance to the old dream of a one-world brotherhood of man probably means that the pharmaceutical segment of international trends—of which only some examples have been mentioned—will continue to gain in significance.

PART THREE

# Pharmacy in the United States

Section One

## The Period of Unorganized Development

# 9

# The North American Colonies

## THE SPREAD OF EUROPEAN CIVILIZATION

Pharmacy develops as an integral facet of the whole history of mankind, and there is no better illustration of this relationship between the microcosm that is the history of pharmacy and the macrocosm that is the history of civilization than in the explosion of Renaissance Europe into a world civilization. This explosion was a Commercial Revolution—a tremendous industrial and commercial expansion, but also concomitant discovery and exploration (from about 1400 to 1700). New routes opened to the Orient, and a whole new world in the Americas.

The age of discovery and exploration was sparked by the desire of the Spanish and Portuguese to circumvent the monopolies in Oriental and Near Eastern trade that were held by the Turks and the Venetians. From the Orient and the Levant came drugs and spices in great demand in Europe—and extremely expensive because of the monopolistic controls. The trade and trade routes in drugs from Venice into Western Europe have been thoroughly investigated;[1] for example, most drugs at the Nördlinger Fair in 1477 "were imports that had probably all been brought there from Venice."[2]

The close connection between drugs and spices and between the spicer and the apothecary (already noted in the history of French pharmacy) is evident also from price lists such as that of the Nördlinger Fair. Pepper, ginger, nutmeg, cinnamon, and sugar, as well as camphor and alum, were to be found. No wonder that French and Spanish terms like "épicier" and "especiadors" and the Italian term "speziali" have historic associations with "pharmacist"—the etymologic relationship between these terms and "spices" is obvious.

It is therefore not surprising that the zeal of explorers and adventurers, first for gold and silver, and later for indigo, tobacco, naval stores and furs, included also an interest in drugs and spices. Sir Humphrey Gilbert, in seeking a northwest passage in 1576, for example, promised not only a "great aboundance of gold, silver, precious stones, Cloth of Gold, silkes," but also "all maner of Spices, Grocery wares and other kinds of merchandise." In 1585 Richard Hakluyt placed "men skilful in all kinds of drugs" second only in importance to "men skilful in all mineral causes" on his list of the sorts of men he wanted for a forthcoming expedition.[3]

## COLONIZATION OF NORTH AMERICA

With the beginning of the 17th century, North America gradually became a land for colonization, instead of a collection of colonies destined for exploitation by European sovereigns.

Among the European colonizing nations, Spain*, France and England particularly left their early political impress on the civilization that developed within the territory that has become the United States of America. Spanish influence was felt in the area now included in Florida, Louisiana, Texas and the Southwest, and it is still dominant in Puerto Rico.

Relatively small attention was paid to North America by European governments during the first century after its discovery, as evidenced by the lack of permanent settlements until St. Augustine, Florida, was settled by the Spaniards in 1565. It remained the only such abode of white men in this vast area until Spaniards from Mexico settled in New Mexico in 1598.[4]

French influence manifested itself north of the St. Lawrence river and along the Great Lakes, penetrated the wilds of Michigan and Wisconsin and the prairies of Illinois, and drifted down the Mississippi to Louisiana, which was originally a French territory named in honor of Louis XIV.

English civilization remained the dominant factor in the thirteen original colonies and throughout the vast domain west of the Alleghenies, and later beyond the Mississippi and the Rockies.

Dutch influence acquired an early footing in New Amsterdam and continued to play an important part there long after this city had become New York. Although the German states do not figure among the colonizing nations, Germans contributed a considerable number of colonists to Penn's woods (shown, for example, by the name of Germantown, now a part of Philadelphia).[5] To a slight extent, Swedish influence had gained a footing on the Delaware even before the Dutch and William Penn's coreligionists, the so-called Quakers, took possession.

## DRUGS IN THE NEW WORLD

The search of the flora of the New World for aromatics, spices, and medicinal plants started immediately after discovery in South America and not long thereafter in North America. Out of it came the introduction into the European materia medica of a host of new drugs of botanical origin. As a few examples may be mentioned guaicum, introduced by the Spanish from the West Indies; sassafras, first noted by the French in Florida; copaiba, introduced by the Portuguese from Brazil; the balsam of Peru and the balsam of Tolu, introduced by the Spanish; winterian, introduced by the British from the Straits of Magellan—all introduced within the period 1517–1579. Simarouba and Canadian balsam are examples of drugs introduced by the French from Guiana and Canada in the eighteenth century.

Most important of these drugs, of course, was cinchona (or "Peruvian bark"). Cinchona illustrates that these drugs, new to Europeans, were introduced mainly as a consequence of an interest in medical botany, rather than because these drugs were used by the natives. It seems improbable that cinchona was used by the indigenous peoples. Alexander von Humboldt and other explorers did not find the bark in the medicine bags of Indian medicine men. Credit for discovering the specific value of cinchona in treating malaria, it is now assumed, probably goes to the Jesuits.[6]

This is not to say that the drugs used by American Indians were not of value to the

*For an excellent summary of the Spanish contribution to the history of pharmacy, of particular interest here because of its influence on Spanish-held territories of America, see Chapter 6 of the Second Edition (p. 97), which may be consulted in most pharmacy libraries. The chapter was prepared by the distinguished pharmacist-historians at the University of Madrid, Professors Guillermo Folch Jou and Rafael Folch Andreu. To restrict the present textbook edition to a scope feasible for the usual instructional program, it has been expedient to omit the chapter.

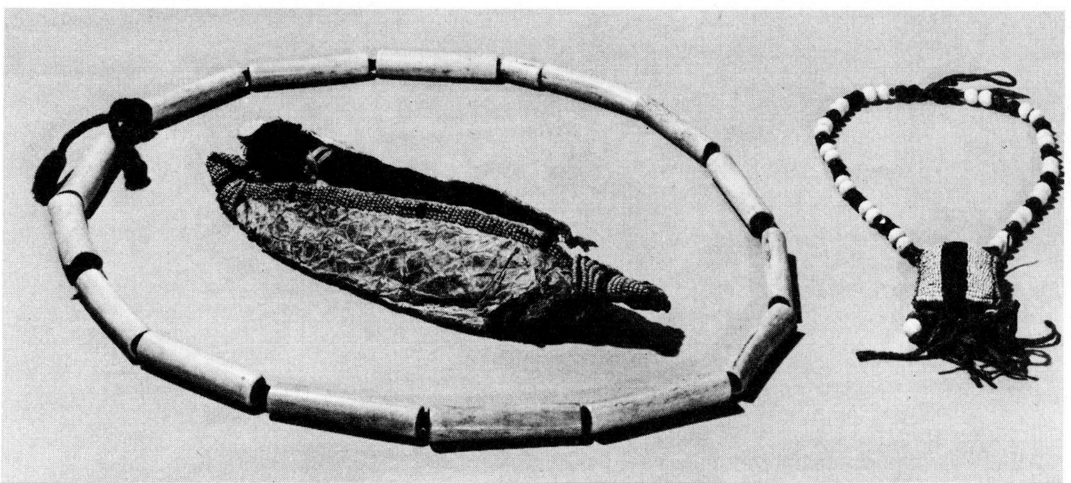

The medicine man of the American Indians relied heavily on his command of the spirit powers–although Europeans on both sides of the Atlantic found therapeutic activity, real or imagined, in various botanic substances which he used. In the photograph, three aspects of Indian medicine are illustrated: *(1)* The individual bone tubes in the necklace *(left)* could be used by the medicine man (Chippewa "juggler") to suck disease-causing foreign matter or spirits out of the body. *(2)* Lying within the necklace is a diuretic device (Menominee) consisting of a wood twig covered with blue cloth, which is encased in a bladder ornamented with beadwork. The patient drinks hot water in which this device has been boiled. *(3)* The amulet bag on a beaded cord *(right)* could be worn to fend off or help overcome disease. (From the State Historical Society of Wisconsin; Joan Freeman, Anthropologist)

European; and it is of pharmaceutical and medical interest to learn which indigenous drugs were used by the natives.

The knowledge of drugs varied with the cultural levels of various Indian tribes. Several lists of drugs have been made on the basis of research and inquiry among these tribes[7] (see the tabulation in Appendix 1). The Maya Indians had extensive botanic knowledge and more than four hundred uses for botanic drugs.[8] An Aztec, Martin de la Cruz, compiled a herbal in the 16th century, which another Aztec, Juannes Badianus, translated into Latin (1552). The original "Badianus manuscript" (as it is now called) became one of the treasures of the Vatican Library, and a facsimile has been published in an annotated American edition.[9]

The knowledge of drugs used by the Indians of northern America comes from a different kind of source, the accounts of explorers of the new continent, and also from early medical practitioners.[10] About 170 drugs used by the Indians of the United States and Canada, and perhaps 50 used by the Indians of the West Indies, Mexico, and Central and South America, became official in the *United States Pharmacopoeia* or the *National Formulary* at one time or another.[11]

An organized endeavor was made, during the early part of the 18th century, to transplant valuable medicinal herbs from Spanish Central and South America to Georgia. James Oglethorpe, founder of the colony, secured the patronage of influential British friends, particularly Dr. Hans Sloane, who, together with the Worshipful Society of Apothecaries of London, lent financial support to the

Trustees of the colony. The botanist Robert Miller (following the death of the first appointee, William Houston) travelled through the Caribbean area and worked for 5 years diligently searching for ipecac, jalap, sarsaparilla, contrayerva, cochineal, cinchona trees (producing "Jesuit's bark"), copaiba, and balsam of Tolu. However, Miller was sickly, was opposed by the Spanish, and often seemed more interested in science than in practical agriculture. When he died in 1740, the Apothecaries Society withdrew further support, and this first activity undertaken in North America by organized pharmacy came to an end. The Botanical Garden in Savannah, which had been established as something of an experiment station had ceased operation the year before.[12]

A more literary attempt in the same direction was made by John Ellis, a member of the Royal Society and the agent for West Florida. His "Catalogue of Plants That May be Useful in America" appeared first in William Stork's *A Description of East Florida* (London, 1769) and then again in Ellis' own copious *Directions for Bringing over Seeds and Plants from the East Indies* (London, 1770). He listed 82 plants, about 50 of which were medicinal. In America, the *Transactions of the American Philosophical Society* (1771) included not only Ellis' "Catalogue of such FOREIGN PLANTS as are worthy of being encouraged in our American Colonies, for the Purpose of Medicine, Agriculture, and Commerce," but also large extracts from his "Directions." Ellis' efforts, however, seem to have had no more practical results than similar suggestions made at least as early as 1682.[13]

Much more significant was the introduction of America drugs into the European materia medica, already alluded to. The first treatises on American drugs were published by Nicolas Monardes, a physician in Seville (1574).[14] It is significant of the great interest in the medicinal and the botanic treasures of the New World that new editions soon followed. Carolus Clusius published a Latin translation, which in turn was translated into other languages.[15] The excitement of the new drug discoveries is revealed in the title of the English translation: *Joyfull Newes out of the New Founde Worlde.* Monardes himself (1493–1578) never had been in South America, but, living in one of the principal ports for imports from the "Occidental Indies," he collected much information about exotic medicinal plants and secured samples.

Other such works followed, for example, from publishers in Mexico, Amsterdam, London, and Paris.[16] The German materia medica likewise absorbed medicinal plants brought from the New World, particularly after the publication of Johann D. Schöpf's *Materia Medica Americana Potissimum Regni Vegetabilis* (Erlangen, 1787). Throughout Europe, hope for a new therapeutic resource spawned optimistic reports.[17]

## New Spain

Columbus and those explorers of the new continent who succeeded him could be expected to pay attention to the medicinal uses of plants, and their special interest in the spice trade is well known.

During his first voyage (1492–1493), Columbus was accompanied by a surgeon, but neither his name nor his journal has been preserved. The admiral himself diligently wrote a journal until the day of his return to Palos.[18] The second expedition of Columbus included a surgeon and a physician. The latter wrote (1493) a letter in which he mentions cotton, turpentine, tragacanth, nutmeg, ginger, aloes, cinnamon, mirobalans and mastic.[19]

The works of Badianus, Monardes, Hernandez and others show that the Spaniards were interested in pharmaceutical matters throughout the colonial period. However, their greatest impact on the pharmacy of North America came during the 28 years that Spain controlled the vast territory of Louisiana.

Don Alexandre O Reilly, governor of

Louisiana, issued an edict (in French) that demarcated the areas of medicine, surgery, and pharmacy (February 12, 1770). It contains the first legal definition of pharmacy, as a separate branch of medicine, to be issued in North America:

> Medicine . . . embraces three parts, namely: medicine proper, which is the science of recognizing diseases and the relation which they have with remedies, and of prescribing the latter together with the diet. The other two parts, which are surgery and pharmacy, are its attendants and have their special field. Surgery includes the use in general of hands and of external remedies. Pharmacy is concerned, generally speaking, with the preparation of remedies.[20]

O Reilly's interest in pharmacy was not fortuitous, *The Rudolph Matas History of Medicine in Louisiana,* under the editorship of John Duffy, reveals. The Spanish regulated medicine and pharmacy more strictly than did the French who preceded them in Louisiana. They required that a chief pharmacist be responsible for compounding prescriptions in all colonial hospitals. More important, in 1769 a colonist (Jean Peyroux) was examined in materia medica by the Royal Physician and was given a certificate to operate a pharmacy. He is the first pharmacist known to have been examined and licensed within the territorial limits of what is now the United States.

Certification was based on his acceptance of seven conditions: to maintain what might be called a poison register; to notify the authorities of drugs purchased by him; to dispense them at honest and reasonable fees; to compound prescriptions exactly as written; to submit to the "code of Paris"; to compound medicines on prescription but not prescribe them himself; to agree to inspection of his stock by the Royal Physician. These requirements—so reminiscent of professional oaths often required of European pharmacists—were intended by Don Alexandre to apply to all pharmacists. The names of four additional pharmacists who submitted to examination during the Spanish period are known. In one instance (1792) examination was by a board of two pharmacists, in others, by a board of from one to three pharmacists, together with physicians and surgeons (or at least in their presence). Probably more pharmacists than the five now known were examined and licensed under the Spanish regulation.

## New France

From the time Cartier sailed up the St. Lawrence (1535) until the first family effected permanent settlement (1617), New France was visited by explorers, fur traders and missionaries, seeking glory, wealth and the extension of Christianity. The credit of being the first real French settler in America belongs to a pharmacist, Louis Hébert.

Samuel de Champlain saw the necessity of establishing homes if the French settlement was to be permanent. It was he who finally induced Hébert, who had been with him on his first trip to New France (1604), to establish his home in the new country. It shows the pioneer character of Hébert that he again and again left security and his regular profession, following the voice of what he considered to be his proper vocation.

He had been born in Paris, the son of a well-known pharmacist; he possessed a pharmacy of his own on the banks of the Seine, but he sold it[21] to go to Port Royal (now Annapolis Royal, Nova Scotia) with the expedition of De Monts. Hébert arrived there with 50 other colonists in 1606. When the English destroyed the place and took over the land, Hébert returned to Paris and reopened his pharmacy. However, when his friend Champlain decided to establish a new colony, to be called Quebec, and asked Hébert to accompany him, the courageous pharmacist sold his possessions once more and migrated to Quebec in 1617 with his family, his household goods and a small store of drugs. Hébert well knew from his previous experience that he would have to devote himself to

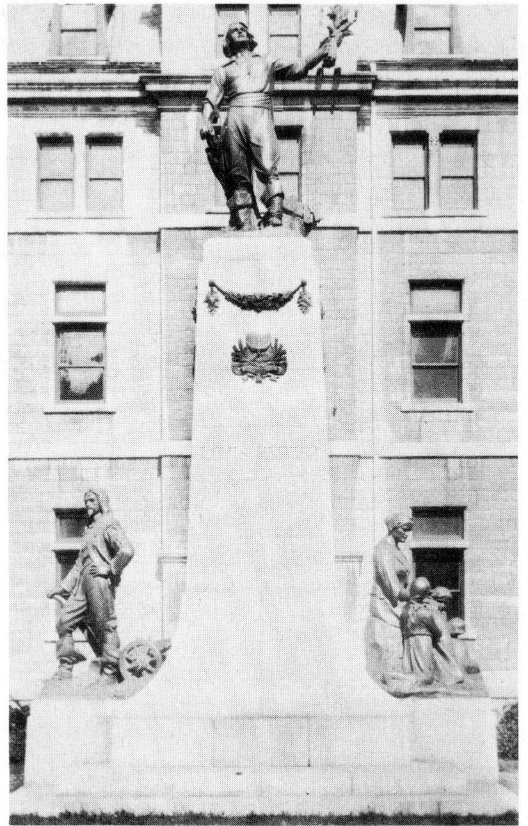

This bronze monument to Louis Hébert in the city of Quebec (between City Hall and Saint Anne Street) shows the French pharmacist holding aloft the first sheaf of wheat harvested from Canadian soil. At the right, his wife is teaching the children of the first colonists, while a statue of Hébert's son-in-law stands on the left. The sculptor was Alfred Laliberté, 1917. There is also a commemorative tablet at Annapolis Royal that honors Hébert.

husbandry. We are told of his cattle and his apple trees, "the first to be planted in America."[22] He also made a study of the indigenous grapes, which he cultivated and improved.

On the other hand, the fur company, which had been induced by Champlain to support Hébert and his family for 3 years, had required his bond for free medical attention at all times to the settlers and the clerks employed by the company. Thus, while devoting his time primarily to the cultivation of the soil and to the study of the native plants of his new home, Hébert put to good use his pharmaceutical skill as well as his supply of drugs brought from France. With and without contract obligation, he tried to help in Quebec as he had previously helped in Annapolis (Port) Royal. The activity of the first pharmacist to settle in North America was cut short after 10 years by an accident which caused his death.[23]

The activity of the Sisters of Charity and of the Jesuit missionaries was important in developing early medicine and pharmacy in New France, and record survives of two apothecary-brethren (*pharmacopoles*) there as early as the mid-18th century. Four of the important documents connected with the early history of pharmacy consist of lists of drugs and medicaments, which were sent to Paris by the sisters of the hospital at Quebec (1664 to 1668) with requests for new supplies. These lists reveal a rather extensive materia medica for so early a period in the development of a distant colony.[24] It may be assumed that the colonists also were supplied from any surplus in the medicine chests of vessels from French ports.[25]

The itinerant missionaries made the best use of such medical and pharmaceutical knowledge as they possessed in befriending the Red Man. In the instance of Father Hennepin, who was a member of La Salle's party which explored the Great West in 1680, specific examples of such practice are recorded.[26] In their reports to superiors, these Jesuit missionaries also occasionally mentioned the use of drugs by the Indians. During one expedition south of the Great Lakes, the Father was taken by his Indian guides to a spring that was not only salty but had a film of oil on its surface. The salt water was used by the Indians as a purgative, the oil as a remedy against rheumatism. Another Jesuit,

Father Lafitau, found ginseng in Canada and wrote a detailed account of this plant and drug.[27]

In French Louisiana a "physic garden," growing imported herbs mainly, was begun as early as 1724 in New Orleans. Its overseer, Sieur Dameron, also had charge of a "laboratory" in which medicines for the garrison and the hospitals were produced. At least two surgeon-apothecaries are known to have been in New Orleans at this time, and one of them may have first suggested establishment of the laboratory, which probably was in the Royal Hospital. In general, hospital pharmacy became the responsibility of the Ursuline Sisters and remained so until after the arrival of the Spanish.[28]

In 1763 Canada passed from the French to the British, and in 1803, the territory of Louisiana—which included much more territory than the present state of Louisiana—became by purchase a part of the United States of America. Thus ended New France as a political unit, though the romantic history of the French settlers and *coureurs de bois* continued on the St. Lawrence, throughout the Great Lakes region and down the Mississippi.

## New Sweden and New Netherlands

The political units of New Sweden and New Netherlands were short-lived on the North American continent.

On board a Dutch vessel, Henry Hudson had sailed up the river that now bears his name in the same year (1609) that Champlain penetrated to the lake named after him. It was nearly three decades before the founding of New Sweden.

Dutch settlers followed the early explorers and fur traders and, in 1626, Peter Minuit transacted the real estate deal in which he bought Manhattan Island from the Indians for about $25. The colony was prosperous and an example of tolerance, permitting the settlement of persons of all nationalities and faiths.

Sweden's colony on the Delaware by 1654 comprised the territory of the present state of Delaware and parts of Pennsylvania, New Jersey and Maryland. The settlers were Finnish rather than Scandinavian.[29] In 1655 New Netherlands captured New Sweden and united it with the Dutch colony. A few years later this greater New Netherlands had to suffer a like fate at the hands of the English. It was captured by an English fleet with the Duke of York on board, and thenceforth the former New Amsterdam was called "New York." Intermarriage of both Dutch and Swedes with the English settlers eventually blended the three peoples.[30]

At least one medical person is known to have come over from Sweden to the new colony, the barber-surgeon Hans Jancke.[31] The first known surgeon in New Netherlands was Herman Meynders van den Boogaerdt (1631),[32] who was appointed commissary of stores at New Amsterdam and later at Fort Orange. It is not reported whether or not he dealt in drugs. Another surgeon, Gysbert van Imbroch (van Emburgh, d. 1665) "kept a shop at New Amsterdam" in 1653.

> Besides being the local physician and pharmacist, he kept a general store, and the inventory of his estate includes a wide variety of objects, from high priced books down to the commonest necessaries of life.[33]

Was Imbroch's "shop" at New Amsterdam a drugstore? It may have been a surgeon's and barber's shop. However, the "general store," which from 1663 to 1665 he carried on in Wildwyck (since 1669 called Kingston) may be considered one of the first drugstores in North America.

Another medical person of pharmaceutical interest in New Netherlands was the surgeon Hans Kiersted from Germany, who

> came to New Amsterdam with Governor Kieff (1638). For a long time he was in the employ of the Dutch West India Company. While nothing is known about a pharmacy kept by him, some of his drug formulas have survived.[34]

## New England

In British North America pharmaceutical activity began in 1602. In that year Bartholomew Gosnold and his crew landed in Massachusetts to load the first cargo of New England's exports. "It consisted of the bark and pith of the sassafras tree."[35] In that year, too, Sir Walter Raleigh returned from the vicinity of Cape Fear with a cargo of timber, sassafras, china root, benjamin, sarsaparilla, cassia lignea, and an unknown "strong bark."[36] When the colony of Virginia was founded, seamen and settlers stampeded in what must be called a sassafras rush, and even though the price of it fell as it became plentiful, sassafras was exported throughout the colonial period; in 1770 alone England imported over 76½ tons of it.[37] Indeed, the collection, cultivation, and exportation of plant drugs—ipecac, Virginia snake root, and ginseng became especially important—was of considerable economic significance in the colonies.[38]

In 1606, King James I granted the London corporation a charter which gave to it the ownership of Virginia, at that time including all the unoccupied country between the settlements of the Spanish in Florida and those of the French in Canada. In 1607 the first English colonists sailed into Hampton Roads, and the very next year two "apothecaries," Thomas Field and John Harford, arrived. There are no records of their fate.[39] Two years later a "Table of such as are required to this Plantation" was sent by the settlers to their "Virginia Company" at London, asking for "foure honest and learned Ministers, two Surgeons, two Druggists." Letters sent to London by the settlers requested "that the Company would send them some Phisitians and Apothycaries of which they stand much need off."[40]

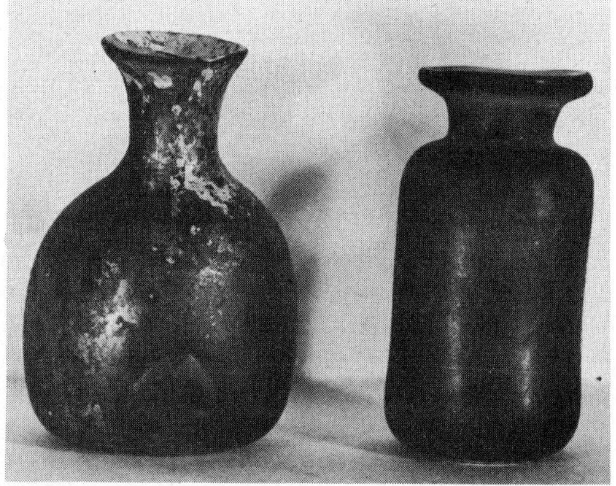

Medicine vials used by the American colonists, as unearthed by the National Park Service. A glass-bottle factory established in the woods near the Jamestown settlement (1607) has been considered to have been the earliest industrial enterprise within present United States territory. (From the National Park Service, Jamestown, Va.)

Whether these "Phisitians and Apothycaries" ever arrived, history does not record. However, there is an entry in the Records of the Virginia Company (1621) reading:

> It was signified unto the Court that an apothecary offered to transport himself and his wife on his own charge to Virginia if the Company would please to give them their transport of two children . . . which offer the Council did very well like of in respect of the great want of men of his profession, and being put to the question did agree thereunto; provided that the Apothecary at his coming over did exercise his skill and practise in that profession.

According to Blanton, "there is no further record of apothecaries living in the colony in this [the 17th] century, the physician being 'for the most part his own apothecary.' "[41]

The records as yet unearthed prove only that in the early days of the Virginia Settlement need was felt for the presence of "druggists" and "apothycaries." They do not mention the establishment of pharmacies or of general stores dealing in drugs and emphasizing pharmaceutical activities.

As important as the early Virginia Settlement was, as the first English foothold on the American continent, the decisive dates for English colonization are 1620 and 1628. In 1620 the Pilgrims sailed on board the

Mayflower from Plymouth, landing by accident not within the limits of Virginia as they should have done according to their patent, but at a place they called Plymouth in remembrance of their English port of embarkation. In 1628, the Puritans founded Salem; they were followed a year later by 400 additional colonists and, in 1630, by the main group with Governor John Winthrop, who founded Boston in the same year. This man and this town became the two most important landmarks of early American cultural life, including medicine and pharmacy.

"Medicine was promulgated, for the first hundred years of colonial America, by three types of individuals: the governors, the churchmen, and the educators."[42] As always in primitive and in pioneer society, it was practiced to a large extent by the housewives. The housewives of the early English emigrants brought their peculiar kind of knowledge and practice over from their native country. Books giving advice for self-treatment, as well as for the cultivation of herbs furnishing the drugs recommended, were much cherished and used by the English emigrants. The most important of these books were Gervase Markham's *The English Housewife* and *The English Husbandman* (1613). Another was Nicholas Culpeper's *The English Physician* (London, 1652) which was reprinted again and again and used for more than a century. (In 1708 an unrelated work of the same title and attributed to Culpeper was published in Boston, a tribute to the work's popularity.[43]) Culpeper's title page spoke of "such things only as grow in England [as] being most fit for English Bodies," and the colonists transplanted herbs from England into their gardens. They were certain that the mysterious mutual reaction between English plants and English bodies would continue in the New World.[44]

In addition to these European plants, the New England housewives and others practicing medicine within the colonies used a gradually increasing number of native herbs. Of the 56 Indian drugs still holding official recognition in 1925, 30 of them had been used by the Indians of New England.[45]

The first governor of Massachusetts Colony, John Winthrop, and his son John Winthrop, Jr. first governor of Connecticut Colony, are the most outstanding examples of North American governors interested in and practicing medicine. They apparently often asked friends in England for advice on medical topics. In 1643 one of them received from London a list of "Receipts to cure various disorders."[46] These "receipts," mostly of household character, show us something of the pharmaceutical resources used. They had been drawn "from John Gerard's herbal."[47]

The younger Winthrop was a political leader of importance and at the same time an outstanding figure in the history of science in North America during the 17th century. His great interest in chemistry makes understandable his use of many medicinal chemicals—such as saltpeter, preparations of antimony and mercury, tartar, copperas, white vitriol, sulphur and iron—in addition to red coral, powdered ivory, rosin, some American and European vegetable drugs and several galenics. He prepared some chemical compounds and galenics himself.[48] Thus, he was one of the first to do real pharmaceutical work in North America.

George Starkey, a Harvard College graduate (1646) was a protégé of Winthrop. He won a great reputation as a chemical practitioner and invented numerous remedies, of which his oil of sulphur was best known. Having built a furnace in Boston, he wrote to Winthrop asking for "a little mercury and antimony." These two substances, of which especially the latter had been the subject of many a quarrel in Europe about this time (see p. 72), became "principal bases of the chemical remedies used in America for the next two centuries."[49]

A year before the death of John Winthrop, Jr., the so-called King Philip's War broke out. The Indians, under their "King" Philip, fought desperately, and there was much need of medicaments among the troops from the Bay Colony. A letter, written (1676) by a surgeon who had joined the troops, to the secretary of Massachusetts Bay Colony contains a list of medicaments that the writer urgently demanded. Most of these items were from the London pharmacopoeia of 1650, and probably imports.[50]

There were few physicians in the New England colonies until 1700. The first apothecary who entered New England came to die rather than to live there. This Englishman, Giles Firmin of Sudbury, arrived at Boston probably toward the end of 1632 and died in 1634. Nothing is known of Firmin's opening a shop in Boston. Presumably he practiced medicine "as one of Boston's few physicians. His son became a physician as well as an apothecary."[51] It may be recalled that during this period the apothecaries in England became, more and more, general medical practitioners (see p. 103). However, the primary occupation of the first English apothecary on North American soil seems to have been preaching, and that by vocation as well as by necessity. Even the younger Firmin is quoted as having written to Governor Winthrop: "I am strongly set upon to study devinitie, my studies else must be lost, for physic is but a meene helpe."

Indeed, most of the male medical practioners of the early colonial days seem to have resorted to other callings for a livelihood.

> [Among 134 medical practitioners who settled in Massachusetts Colony before 1692] twelve and probably many more, practiced surgery: three were barber-surgeons. . . . Six or seven, probably a larger number, were ministers as well as physicians. . . . One was not only a doctor, but also schoolmaster and poet. One was a butcher, but called himself a surgeon in his will, a union of callings which suggests an obvious pleasantry.[52]

Whatever else the early medical practitioners may have done to earn their livelihood, in one particular they were no doubt alike: With few exceptions they dispensed their own medicines, unless they directed the relatives of the patient to prepare potions from indigenous or cultivated herbs or roots.

The apothecary shop, as it existed at a later period in the larger cities of the American colonies, was thus a kind of dispensary attached to the office of a medical practitioner.[53]

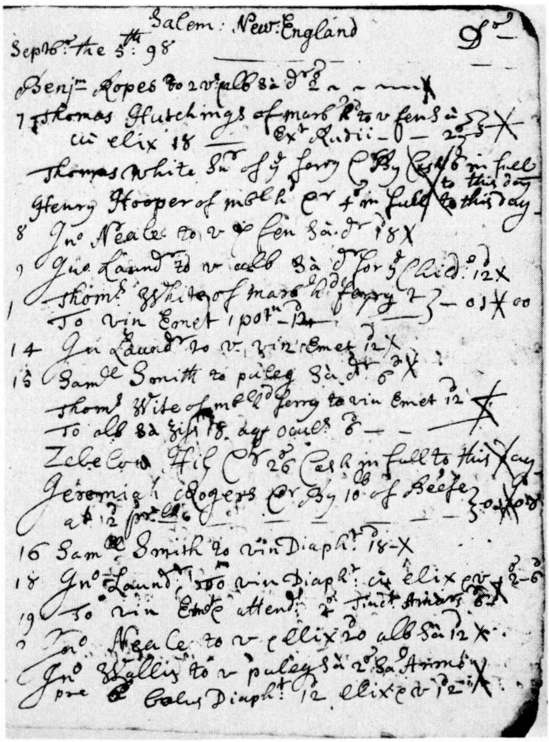

One of the earliest financial records of an American pharmacy was kept by a dispensing "pharmaceutical chemist," Bartholomew Browne. The excerpt *(left)* from his 90-page account book was written September 5, 1698, at Salem, New England. "White Samech" was the drug most frequently dispensed. (Original in the Essex Institute, Salem, Mass.; from Griffenhagen, G.: Essex Institute Historical Collections, pp. 19–30, January, 1961)

The "general store" of the surgeon Gysbert van Imbroch at Wildwyck (Kingston), mentioned above (see p. 151), was doubtless an enlarged dispensary. The earliest owner of a pharmacy in British North America is usually considered to have been William Davis (Davice) of Boston. An official record of 1646 indicates that the Selectmen of Boston ordered that a fence be erected before his hall window for the benefit of the apothecary Davice.[54]

The earliest known written record of the day-by-day operations of an American colonial pharmacist is an account book of Bartholomew Browne of Salem, Massachusetts, begun in 1698. George Griffenhagen, who has studied this manuscript,[55] referred to Browne as a "pharmaceutical chemist" because his medical armamentarium "was uniquely chemical in nature." However, although Browne's income was derived mainly from dispensing, he occasionally charged for "attendance." That is to say, he was practicing medicine to a limited extent, like the British apothecary. In fact Browne turned to the practice of medicine entirely and exemplifies the casual migration from one profession to another and the particular lack of separation or definite standards with regard to the practice of pharmacy of the times.

As was common then (and long afterward) among practitioners of the health professions, Browne took a considerable amount of produce and merchandise in exchange for his services, spent a great deal of time collecting, and still had time and need to work his own farm.

The remedy most widely used by the 200 or so patrons identified in Browne's accounts was White Samech, the neutral salt of potassium tartrate made by adding potassium carbonate to cream of tartar (335 pots). In addition, 104 pots or vials of other types of Samech (tartar combined with herbs) were dispensed. Second in popularity was an unidentified "Elixir" (326 pots). A cordial powder was dispensed on 145 occasions.

## EIGHTEENTH CENTURY PHARMACY

The modern American drugstore developed from four roots in the 18th century, a century of population expansion in America that brought with it increasing need for systems of delivery of medicine. These four were the dispensing physician and the dispensary or "shop" of such physicians, the apothecary shop, the general store, and the wholesale druggist. The first, which had its beginnings, as just noted, in the 17th century was common throughout the colonies in the 18th century and was to continue down to very recent times. In Boston, for example, Zabdiel Boyltson, reportedly the first medical practitioner to inoculate against smallpox and "most meritorious physician of his day in America"[56] industriously advertised his drugs in the *Boston Gazette* (1723–1724). In New Jersey, the fee schedule issued by the New Jersey Medical Society—the first provincial society of its kind—in 1766

> provided no charge for visits in town but gave a long list of medications and the prices the doctor was to charge for them. These were not simples that the doctor dispensed: the list included boluses, decoctions, electuaries, draughts, elixirs, essences, emulsions, plasters, powders, pills, ointments, and tinctures. . . . [Moreover] the office equipment of the doctor makes it clear that he, or his apprentice, was a compounder of medicines.[57]

In Charleston, South Carolina, a similar situation prevailed, although there the Faculty of Physic had already rejected (in 1755) the system of their New Jersey colleagues. They did not believe the "Payment of an Apothecary's Bill a sufficient Reward to him who acts in the three distinct offices of Physic, Surgery, and Pharmacy."[58]

In all the colonies, probably only about a ninth of the established medical practitioners had some formal medical training (estimated at 400 of 3500 before the Revolution; and only about 200 held medical degrees).[59] Even these academically educated physicians usually played a dual role as pharmacists. For example, Silvester Gardiner of Boston, who had studied at London and Paris, was so successful in pharmacy that his stock of drugs filled more than twenty wagons when it was sold after he fled to England during the Revolution.[60] Another medical practitioner, Hugh Mercer, who had been educated at Aberdeen (and later died a hero as a General in the Continental army), conducted a pharmacy from 1771 to the start of the Revolution as part of his services to the people of Fredericksburg, Virginia.[61] Even John Morgan of Philadelphia, a medical educator who became Director-General of the Hospital and Chief Physician of the Continental Army (see p. 164), found himself forced to operate a public drug shop or pharmacy late in his career. Such "doctor's shops" often were indistinguishable from "apothecary shops." The situation was succinctly summed up when Dr. William Douglass observed in 1722, "We abound with Practitioners, though no other graduate than myself, we have fourteen Apothecary shops in Boston; all our Practitioners dispense their own medicines."[62]

Whereas the doctor's shop was run by a practitioner of medicine who also performed pharmaceutical functions, the apothecary was a genuine pharmaceutical practitioner specializing in the collection, preservation, dispensing, and compounding of drugs, who might secondarily engage in a limited practice of medicine. Such a man was Bartholomew Browne mentioned above (see p. 155). Such also was Robert Talbot who was operating a shop in Burlington, New Jersey in the 1720's. Talbot's broadside *Catalogue of Medicines* was the first separate publication by an American pharmacist. This Catalogue and the inventory of Talbot's estate (taken after his death in 1725) tell us a great deal about the colonial apothecary shop. In the first place, Talbot carried a stock of chemicals and galenicals characteristic of European pharmacy of the time. Some, like Venice treacle, hartshorn, ambergris, sealed earth, and "crab's eyes" were hoary with tradition. This European rather than American materia medica, it must be noted, was generally to be found in the American apothecary shops, to judge by newspaper advertisements of the time. Talbot's inventory also tells a great deal about the operation of an apothecary shop:

In his Burlington establishment there were four mortars and pestles. One was glass, another was lignum vitae and two were 17-pound "Bell Mettle" mortars with iron pestles. Talbot's laboratory was equipped with one "Chafin dish" weighing about 100 pounds, two small copper stills, 17 "Cedar Drugg Tubs," 27 small "Cruciples mostly odd Ones," one four-pound infusion pot, two copper pans weighing together 22 pounds, one copper funnel and three glass ones, and miscellaneous "Receivers," "Upright Bodys," "Crook Necks," and "Blind heads." There were, of course, the inevitable scales (two pairs), brass weights, and apothecary "tyles." [There were also] 57 galley pots, five large earthen jars, and 15 "oyle Potts & Electric [electuary?] ditto." The tally of round bottles indicated 18 one-gallon, 22 quart, eight more quart with ground stoppers, ten pint, eight half-pint,and 18 smaller such bottles. He also had 25 "half pints with Covers," and 12 "Painted Labell'd Pill Potts." He kept his drugs in 96 large and 48 small drawers.[63]

Pennsylvania was the first American colony to have a pharmacy conducted according to the German model and designated *Apotheke*. Germanic pharmacy in Philadelphia (around 1780) supplied the German farmers and settlers in Pennsylvania with all the domestic remedies to which they had been accustomed in the old country.[64]

The third root of the American drugstore was the general store. The merchant, who laid no claim to medical or pharmaceutical knowledge, found drugs a profitable commodity in his business. The process was hastened and strengthened by the enormous popularity in the colonies of proprietary remedies. These, sometimes called "patent medicines," had had an astounding rise in England early in the 18th century. To the busy settler with little time and small means, these ready-made and not too high-priced remedies seemed to solve at once, conveniently, all the problems of medical and pharmaceutical aid—and even of finance—arising in sickness; the daring advertising appealed to his plain and optimistic turn of thought. Bateman's "Elixir," Godfrey's "British Oyle," Daffy's "Elixir" "Scotch Pills" and others were advertised in Colonial newspapers almost immediately after their appearance on the English market and were sold everywhere.

The merchant carried a vast array of sundries as well as drugs. Mary and Sarah Barnes, of Trenton, New Jersey, in a rare instance of women associated with pharmacy in 18th-century United States, advertised in 1781, along with a long list of crude and proprietary drugs, "painted silks and gauze, china, sewing silks, thread, needles, orris of different kinds, brass furniture for carriages, and sundry other articles."[65]

Printers often resorted to the sale of sundries and drugs (and advertised them in their newspapers).[66] Foremost among them was none other than Benjamin Franklin. About the time of his marriage (1730), Franklin opened a store and advertised in his *Pennsylvania Gazette* all "commodities varied from needles and pins to horses and slaves." Among these "commodities" we find advertised coffee, tea, chocolate, palm oil, saffron, spermacety, crown soap, powdered mustard, linseed oil, patent medicines and "seneca rattlesnake root, with directions how to use it in pleurisy." Franklin doubtless prescribed over the counter.[67]

For pharmacy this dabbling in drug dispensing by one of the most eminent and influential Americans during the 18th century had its favorable consequences. Franklin retired from business in 1749, but never lost his interest in medicine and pharmacy. It was he who, having dabbled in both professions without being educated in either helped bring about the first obvious practical example of the separation of pharmacy and medicine in America. In the Pennsylvania Hospital, in whose founding he was a prime mover, it soon found necessary to appoint "an Apothecary to attend and make up Medicines only, according to the Prescriptions."

There are several other proofs of Franklin's interest in pharmacy. From London, he sent his friend John Bartram, the famous American botanist, "some of the true rhubarb seed" (1770). This reportedly was the first attempt on American soil to cultivate Chinese rhubarb, which yields the medicinally-used rhizome.[68]

The fourth root of the American drugstore was the druggist, to use that term in its 18th-century sense of a wholesaler in drugs. One such wholesaler, the Smith, Moore & Co. of New York, advertised in 1784 (in verse!) that they had for sale "At the Medical Pillar," "a general collection of the materia medica, botanical, chemical, and galenical," as well as proprietary remedies, confections, groceries, chemicals, sundries (leather, tinfoil, oil-cloth), perfumes, paints, and medical and pharmaceutical equipment. Their clientele were "Practitioners" who could "command/Supplies of drugs for sea or land."[69]

It should already be obvious that there were no clear-cut distinctions between the physician, apothecary, merchant, and wholesale druggist. We have already noted the interchangeability of medical and pharmaceutical functions between physicians and apothecaries. By the same liberty in practice, the doctor and the apothecary dealt with proprietary medicines just as did the general store. Moreover, they took on sidelines, sometimes books as in New England, but more generally materials needed for the building and upkeep of homes in rapidly growing communities—such as paints, oils, varnishes, brushes, wallpaper, and glass. By the same token, the merchant dealing with drugs and the wholesale druggist prescribed over the counter, and probably were not backward about compounding remedies. The apothecary also acted as wholesaler, especially to physicians, and physicians themselves were not above establishing a wholesale-druggist business, supplying their colleagues as a sideline to their practice.[70]

Yet, although their number was small,[71] a number of shops did develop that we could call drugstores owned by men who could be considered pharmacists. These shops often carried distinctive names: in Boston, Sylvester Gardiner's shop was "At the Sign of the Unicorn and Mortar" (1775);[72] in New York, Richard Speaight's shop was "At the Sign of the Elaboratory" (1776),[73] and also in New York, G. Duyckinck's, "At the Sign of the Looking Glass and Druggist Pot" (1769);[74] in Philadelphia, Evan Jones' "At the Sign of Paracelsus' Head;"[75] and in Charleston, William Brisbane's "At the Sign of the Eagle."[76] In Charleston also, Phillip Moser was at the "Sign of the Man and the Mortar" (early 1790's)."[77] In Philadelphia, the "apothecary, druggist, botanist, and chemist" Christopher Marshall established himself in 1729, the first in a family line of Philadelphia pharmacists.[78] In Williamsburg "druggist and chymist" Thomas Wharton kept a shop for 11 years (before 1746).[79]

## COLONIAL LEGISLATION RELATED TO PHARMACY

The English colonies, influenced by the initiative of private individuals and not by governmental actions, enacted laws dictated by immediate needs of these individuals. It is but natural that the laws mirror English custom and spirit. Not until 1736 did an English-American colony deal legislatively with pharmacy. So far as is known, the first North American law concretely mentioning the apothecary and having a direct bearing on pharmacy is the Virginia "act for regulation of the fees and accounts of the practicers in physic," passed in 1736. As David L. Cowen points out, this act has no "direct relation to the pharmacy laws of today," but it reveals much about the pharmaceutical situation in colonial America and deserves to be quoted:

I. WHEREAS the Practice of Physic, in this Colony, is most commonly taken up and followed, by Surgeons, Apothecaries, or such as have only served Apprenticeships to those Trades, who often prove very unskillful in the Art of a Physician; and yet do demand excessive Fees and exact unreasonable Prices for the Medicines which they administer, and do too often, for the Sake of making up long and expensive Bills, load their Patients with greater Quantities thereof, than are necessary or useful, concealing all their Compositions, as well to prevent the Discovery of their Practice, as of the true Value of what they administer; which is become a Grievance, dangerous and intolerable, as well to the poorer Sort of People, as others, and doth require the most effectual Remedy that the Nature of the Thing will admit:

II. Be It therefore Enacted, by the Lieutenant-Governor, Council, and Burgesses of this present General Assembly, and it is hereby Enacted, by the Authority of the same, That from and after the Passing of this Act, no Practicer in Physic, in any Action or Suit whatsoever, hereafter to be commenced in any Court of Record in this Colony, shall recover, for Visiting any sick Person, more than the Rates hereafter mentioned.[80]

(In the list the "Rates" allowed "those Persons who have studied Physic in any University, and taken any Degree therein" are about twice as high as the fees allowed "Surgeons, and Apothecaries, who have served an Apprenticeship to those Trades.")

III. AND to the End the true Value of the Medicines administred by any Practicer in Physic, may be better known, and judged of, Be it further Enacted, by the Authority aforesaid, That whenever any Pills, Bolus, Potion, Draught, Electuary, Decoction or any Medicines, in any Form whatsoever, shall be administred to any sick Person, The Person administring the same shall, at the same Time, deliver in his Bill, expressing every particular Thing made up therein; or if the Medicine administred, be a Simple, or Compound, directed in the Dispensatories, the true Name thereof shall be expressed in the same Bill, together with the Quantities and Prices, in both Cases. And in Failure thereof, such Practicer, or any Apothecary making up the Prescription of another, shall be nonsuited, in any Action or Suit hereafter commenced, which shall be grounded upon such Bill or Bills: nor shall any Book, or Account, of any Practicer in Physic, or any Apothecary, be permitted to be given in Evidence, before a Court; unless the Articles therein contained, be charged according to the Directions of this Act.

IV. AND be it further Enacted, by the Authority aforesaid, That this Act shall continue and be in Force, for and during Two Years, next after the Passing thereof, and from thence to the End of the next Session of Assembly.

Influenced if not drafted by an academically educated and graduated physician, this act reflects the attitude of London physicians of this period toward the medical ambitions of the apothecaries. On the one hand, it is deprecating in its judgment of both surgeons and apothecaries who have only served an apprenticeship and is, in a way, an answer to the denial by London apothecaries (1724) of the necessity of academic education for engaging in the practice of medicine. On the other hand, the act reluctantly recognizes the apothecary as a medical practitioner. Since only the fees of graduate physicians and those of surgeons and apothecaries who had "served an apprenticeship" were enumerated, the conclusion seems justified that only such skilled apothecaries as were eligible to practice in Virginia could legally demand remuneration for services mentioned in the act.

Of special importance is Section III of the act. Cowen states that "the bill of particulars took the place of the practitioner's oaths of the earlier laws, and such particularization often became an integral part of later medical legislation throughout the country."

The reference to "dispensatories" is new and perhaps indicates European academic training of the author of the act. According to Cowen, "this is the first legal recognition of such compilations" in the colonies. (The only such work that had been published in British America by that time was a reissue in Boston, in 1720, of Culpeper's *Pharmacopoeia Londinensis* of 1653, which apparently attained no professional status.)

Pharmacopœia Londinenſis ;
OR, THE
London Diſpenſatory
FURTHER
Adorned by the *STUDIES* and
*Collections* of the *Fellows* now living,
of the ſaid *COLLEGE*.

*In this Impreſſion you may find,*

1. Three hundred uſeful Additions.
2. All the Notes that were in the Margent are brought into the Book between two ſuch Crotchets as theſe [ ]
3. The Virtues, Qualities, and Properties of every *Simple*.
4. The Virtues and Uſe of the *Compounds*.
5. Cautions in giving all Medicines that are dangerous.
6. All the Medicines that were in the *Old Latin Diſpenſatory*, and are left out in the *New Latin* one, are Printed in this Impreſſion in *Engliſh*, with their Virtues.
7. A *KEY* to *Galen* and *Hippocrates*, their *Method* of *Phyſick*, containing Thirty three Chapters.
8. In this Impreſſion, the *Latin* name of every one of the Compounds is Printed, and in what Page of the new Folio *Latin* Book they are to be found.

By *Nich. Culpeper*, Gent. Student in Phyſick and Aſtrology.

*Boſton*, Printed by *John Allen*, for *Nicholas Booone*, at the Sign of the Bible in *Cornhill*; *Daniel Henchman* over-againſt the Brick Meeting-Houſe; and *John Edwards*, at the Sign of the Light-Houſe 1720

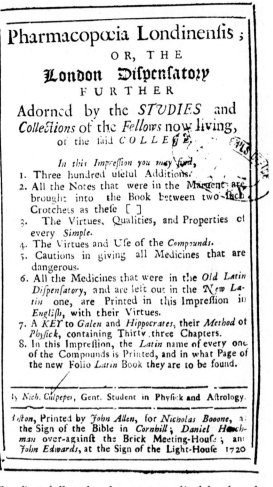

The first full-scale pharmaco-medical book published in British North America was introduced by this title page, dated 1720, Boston. It is an American edition of an English work written by the controversial Nicholas Culpeper, who was introduced to medicine through his apprenticeship to apothecaries. (From the National Library of Medicine)

Another reference in the act to which attention should be directed refers to "any apothecary, making up the prescription of another." This is the first official statement implying that medical practitioners, at least at times, wrote prescriptions instead of dispensing their medicines themselves. Hence, it may be assumed that the most significant pharmaceutical task, the dispensing of the prescriptions of medical practitioners, was carried out by some apothecaries in North America before 1736.

The first legal mention of the term "druggist," as well as "apothecary," appears in an "Act for the better Ordering and governing Negroes and other Slaves . . .", promulgated in South Carolina (1751), prohibiting "any Physician, Apothecary, or Druggist" from employing any slave "in the Shops or Places where they keep their Medicines or Drugs."[81]

## ATTEMPTED SEPARATION OF PHARMACY FROM MEDICINE

The above-quoted Virginia act of 1736 contains a general confirmation of the fact that apothecaries in Colonial America sometimes must have had the opportunity to "make up prescriptions" brought or sent to them by medical practitioners. However, a specific record of the appointment of an individual apothecary to fill prescriptions, other than his own or those of his preceptor, is to be found in the *Account of the Pennsylvania Hospital, from Its Rise To the Beginning of the Fifth Month, called May,* 1754, written by Benjamin Franklin, then the clerk or secretary of the board of trustees of this institution. In this interesting account we find the following paragraph:

> The practitioners charitably supplied the medicines gratis till December, 1752, when the managers having procured an assortment of drugs from London, opened an apothecary's shop in the hospital; and it being found necessary appointed an apothecary to attend and make up the medicines daily, according to the prescription, with an allowance of fifteen pounds per annum for his care and trouble, he giving bond, with two sufficient sureties, for the faithful performance of his trust.[82]

Jonathan Roberts, who was warmly recommended by Dr. Thomas Bond, was appointed as the first apothecary to the hospital and served the institution well until the spring of 1755, when he resigned to accept more remunerative employment. John Morgan, an apprentice of Dr. John Redman, became the second apothecary at the Pennsylvania Hospital (1755–56), resigning after a year to complete a medical education.

A decade later (including 5 years' study and experience in European medical centers) this former hospital pharmacist, John Morgan, was attempting to make the Continental practice of writing prescriptions, "the regular mode of practicing physic" (as he called it in his *Discourse upon the Institution of Medical Schools in America*[83]) a generally recognized American custom. In his *Discourse*, which he wrote during his residence in Paris and in Italy, then gave as an introductory lecture at the inauguration (1765) of a medical school in connection with the College of Philadelphia, he recommended the complete separation of pharmacy and surgery from the practice of medicine. "We must regret," he said, "that the very different employment of physician, surgeon, and apothecary should be promiscuously followed by any one man: They certainly require different talents." Morgan's prime object in advising the separation of the several branches of medical practice was doubtless to improve the entire profession by having each department cultivated successfully. "The knowledge of medicine will then be daily improved," he pointed out; "and it may be practiced with greater accuracy and skill."

To objections that were raised to this idea, which was strange and, from a business point of view, inconvenient to most American medical practitioners of this time, Morgan made the following reply:

> Practitioners in general business never do, or can do, the business of an apothecary in this place themselves. They have apprentices for the purpose. After visiting the sick, do not their apprentices make up their prescriptions? I should ask, is

not an apothecary acquainted with the art of compounding and making up medicines as skillful in it as an apprentice? Is not a man educated in the profession to be trusted in preference to one who is only learning the business?

Morgan's probable acquaintance with the 1754 statute of the Edinburgh Royal College of Physicians "that prohibited their Fellows and Licentiates from taking upon themselves to use the employment of an apothecary, or to have or to keep an apothecary shop,"[84] and his observations in Edinburgh and on the continent, together with his experience as "apothecary" in the Pennsylvania Hospital, undoubtedly account for his advocacy of "the regular [European] mode of practicing physic." Furthermore, there is hardly any doubt that Morgan would be familiar with the famous *Elémens de pharmacie théorique et pratique*, by the French pharmacist Antoine Baumé. If so, he would have read this statement in the introduction:

Those who in the early times devoted themselves to the art of healing, practiced simultaneously medicine, pharmacy, and surgery; but gradually it became obvious that each one of these different branches requires the entire devotion of an individual person.

Some physicians here and there adopted Morgan's recommendation of sending prescriptions to a pharmacy. Others eventually became public advocates on principle—for example, Dr. Abraham Covet, in Philadelphia (1774), and Dr. John Jones, the first professor of surgery in the New York Medical School.[85] But the time was not ripe for effective separation of the professions of medicine and pharmacy in America. Morgan himself, because of financial need or "local prejudice" had to withdraw "from the high position he had taken in 1765. . . . He kept a shop and sold to anyone."[86]

English spirit and English customs, the philosophy of *laissez faire,* dominated pharmacy in Colonial America despite the sometimes large influx of people of other nationalities. This influence was not to be neutralized easily by ideas brought from the European continent or by such men as Morgan, who had been influenced by the progressive University of Edinburgh.

Like English pharmacy during that period, American pharmacy showed little scientific life of its own. The earliest publications in North America that were devoted substantially to pharmaceutical information were written characteristically as much for physicians and for "home doctoring" as for practitioners of pharmacy—books such as the Culpeper books mentioned above (pp. 153 and 159); *The Husbandman's Guide: In four parts . . . Part second, Choice physical receipts . . .* (Boston, 1710); and a tract by the Reverend Thomas Harward, *Electuarium novum Alexipharmacum* (Boston, 1732). Later in the century William Buchan's *Domestic Medicine* was so popular as to be published at least 15 times in the colonies and the new United States between 1771 and 1799, and many times thereafter. After 1784 this work included a "Dispensatory for the Use of Private Practitioners" directed especially to "the ladies, gentlemen and clergy who reside in the country." Popular, also, was the aptly named *Primitive Physic* by the Methodist theologian, John Wesley. It was printed in America at least seven times between 1764 and 1795.[87]

The first teacher of pharmacy and pharmaceutical chemistry was the oft-mentioned physician John Morgan, who also taught materia medica and the theory and the practice of medicine in the first medical school in America. The school had been founded partly at his initiative, as part of the College of Philadelphia (later the University of Pennsylvania).[88] Morgan, like his successor Benjamin Rush, taught pharmacy, pharmaceutical chemistry and materia medica to medical students, as a part of the medical curriculum.

It remained to be proved that pharmaceutical knowledge as a basis for pharmaceutical practice separated from the practice of medicine was important for public welfare. Only then could professional pharmacy be established firmly in America. Despite a decided impetus by the Revolutionary War, this proof did not become convincing until well into the 19th century.

# 10

# The Revolutionary War

To what extent was the American Revolution in fact a revolution that radically altered the fabric of American society? Historians do not agree, and similar uncertainty faces the historian of pharmacy. For, although evidence shows that changes in American pharmacy were quickened and brought to a head by the Revolution, still there persisted a confusion with respect to pharmaceutical practice among physicians and apothecaries and merchants in the post-Revolutionary United States.

After the Revolution as before, if there were any notable differences between the kinds of health-care practice, they were voluntary or dictated by the given circumstances. They were not the result of special education or examination. It was up to practitioners themselves whether they preferred to act as physicians, surgeons or apothecaries—and to choose their titles accordingly. In their apprenticeship they could learn to practice all these branches of medical care. More often than not, they tried to make the best of all of them.

## MILITARY PHARMACY IN THE REVOLUTION

Pharmaceutical services for the several forces fighting in the Revolution reflected their respective civilian practices. For example, the medical service in the British army accorded with the situation in the mother country, where physicians had to be examined and graduated; and apothecaries, although entitled to attend the sick, considered themselves to be also the legitimate representatives of the art of pharmacy.

So only a graduate of one of the great universities or a licentiate of the College of Physicians of London could become an army physician.[1] The surgeons and the apothecaries had to prove that they had a professional education. Their service in the army was restricted to their special field. Within the Hessian corps of the British North American Army, a distinct separation between the different branches of medicine reflected the German authoritarian system.

The medical staff of the British army on American soil consisted of physicians and surgeons, purveyors, apothecaries, and mates. The names of 13 men who served as apothecaries in the British forces in the Revolution are known.[2] Similarly, the medical staff of Hessian troops in the British service included pharmacists, and the names of at least four of them are known.[3]

The French auxiliary army fighting on the side of the Americans likewise had its own medical staff, consisting of well-educated physicians, surgeons, and pharmacists. The chief pharmacist C. H. Ferrand, after his return to France, received the honorary title "Apothecary Major of the Battlefields and of the Armies of the King," in acknowledgment of his services.[4]

> There were French pharmacists among the civil personnel, the military service, and the surgeons of the navy and even among the soldiers. Ten French pharmacists—Augé, Chefdieu, La Chesnaye, La Crampe, Métayer, Rollandeau, Rosancelin, Souchet, Tarrault, Tual—died for the noble cause which they defended.[5]

## THE AMERICAN MEDICAL MILITARY ESTABLISHMENT

The Continental Congress, using the British army for a model,[6] passed a resolution (1775) establishing an "Army Hospital" (i.e., a Medical Department) with a staff consisting of a director-general and chief physician, 4 surgeons, 1 apothecary, 20 mates, and others. According to this resolution, it was the duty of the "Surgeons, Apothecaries, and Mates to visit and attend the sick, and Mates to obey the orders of the Physician, Surgeons, and the Apothecary."[7]

Shortly after the resolution went into effect, Dr. John Morgan, a man who knew and understood the special tasks of pharmacy, became Director-General and Chief Physician (the second of four in that post[8]). It was Morgan who pointed out, as the Congressional resolution had not, the specific responsibilities and scope of activity of the apothecary. He did this in a letter to Dr. Jonathan Potts (then at Ft. George; later Purveyor-General), dated July 28, 1776: Morgan wrote that he had given, "a Warrant to Mr. Andrew Craigie, to act as an Apothecary" under Potts and expressed the opinion that Potts will find this appointment "particularly useful," because the necessity of experience in the apothecary business. "Without such a one I know not how you could either procure sufficient Medicine for your Department or dispense them when got." Morgan admonished Potts "to make it a part of the Duty of the Mates to assist the Apothecary in making up and dispensing Medicines." He stated that "the Apothecary. . . to all intents is to be looked on in Rank as well as pay in the light of a Surgeon and respected accordingly and if he is capable he should in return do part of the Surgeon's Duty."[9]

The making up and dispensing medicines was, according to Morgan, the prime task of the apothecary in the army. When Congress passed a resolution effecting the reorganization of the medical department of the army (1777), the plan, for the first time in the history of American pharmacy, officially stated the duties of the apothecary and restricted him exclusively to professional pharmaceutical tasks. The paragraphs concerning pharmacy read:

> That there be one apothecary general for each district, whose duty it shall be to receive, prepare, and deliver medicines and other articles of his department to the hospitals and army, as shall be ordered by the director general, or deputy directors general respectively;
>
> That the apothecaries [general] be allowed as many mates as the director general, or respective deputy generals shall think necessary.[10]

The country was divided into four districts. Each district—Northern, Eastern, Middle, and Southern—was to have an "Apothecary General" and the names of five or six men to whom that title has been applied (officially and unofficially) are known: Andrew Craigie and John B. Cutting of Massachusetts, Henry C. Flagg of South Carolina, a "Dr. Giles," and Israel and/or Josiah Root of Connecticut. Even in the Southern Department, which had an administration of its own and where no "Apothecary General" was appointed, that title was applied to Dr. Flagg. In addition, the appointment of subordinate apothecaries was authorized until 1782 when Congress "discontinued" the office of Assistant Apothecary, except for the Southern Department.[11] Altogether we know the names of 24 or 25 men who served in the American Revolution as an apothecary or assistant apothecary.[12] In salary, the apothecaries-general ranked between the senior surgeons and the second surgeons.

A further reorganization of the military medical department (1780) abolished the different departments and concentrated all authority in one medical staff. The title "apothecary general," borne by several persons of the same rank, disappeared. There was now one "apothecary," with five assistants, to be appointed, like the other principal officers, directly by Congress. Andrew Craigie became this "apothecary" and kept the position until the end of the war.[13]

An equivalent rank of "Deputy Apothecary" was established for the Southern Department (just as the head of the Southern Medical Department was called "Deputy Director General") in 1781, and John Carne was appointed to the post.[14]

Through a resolution of Congress, a "continental druggist" was "appointed at Philadelphia whose business it shall be to receive and deliver all medicines, instruments, and shop furniture for the benefit of the United States."[15]

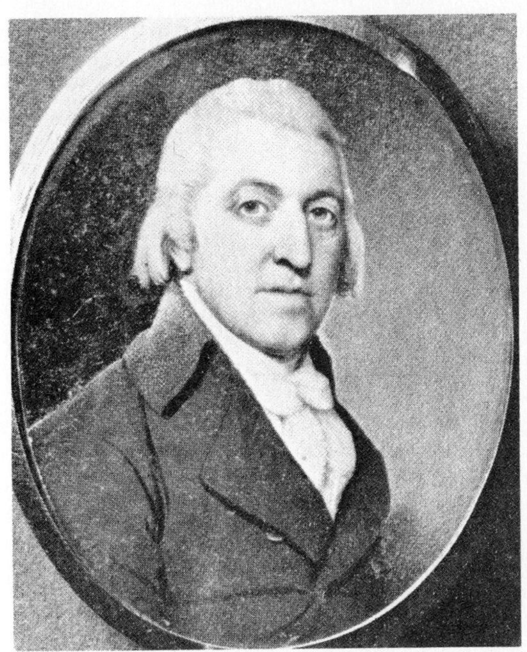

Andrew Craigie, patriotic Whig and prosperous druggist, who became Apothecary General during the Revolution. (Miniature painted about 1791; reproduced from Pratt, F. H.: *The Craigies*, Cambridge, 1942)

## APOTHECARY-GENERAL ANDREW CRAIGIE

There is some mystery surrounding Andrew Craigie, the apothecary-general. Nothing is known of his professional training or of what his proper profession was. On May 14, 1775, "Mr. Andrew Craigie, who had been made commissary of medical stores, was directed to impress beds, bedding, and other necessities for the sick."[16] A few months later the Massachusetts Provincial Congress appointed Craigie, "being informed of his skill in medicine . . . to be medical commissary *and apothecary* to the army raised by this Congress."[17] Although restricted to the Massachusetts troops, this was the first official appointment of an army apothecary in America.

There can be no doubt that Craigie was efficient in fulfilling his duties and, also, had a talent for making friends. His reappointment after the radical reorganization of the military medical department ( resolutions of Congress of October 7, 1780) was certainly helped by the mentioning of his name by General Washington in a letter written to an influential member of Congress. In this significant letter, after referring to several physicians and surgeons as having "a just claim to be continued, from their abilities, attention, and other considerations," General Washington wrote, "Dr. Craigie, the present Apothecary General, a gentleman not personally known to me, has been reported as very deserving of the appointment." The concluding lines read: "The reason of my mentioning these [gentlemen] particularly proceeds from a hint given to me, that the new arrangement might be influenced by a spirit of party out of doors, which would not operate in their favor."[18] Washington was well aware that politics could play havoc with the medical service.

## MILITARY DRUG SUPPLIES

Shortages of drug supplies, market speculations, and uncertain transport were problems that continually plagued the Continental armies. At first, the Revolutionary Army drew on the stocks of private pharmacies such as the Greenleaf shop at Boston, where at least five of fifteen medicine chests wanted by the Provincial Congress of Massachusetts (1775) were assembled, and the pharmacy of Christopher Jr. and Charles Marshall at Philadelphia where medicine chests authorized by the Continental Congress (1776) were prepared. The contents of these field chests[19] provide concrete evidence of the drug therapy available to the wounded and the afflicted under the conditions of the revolutionary years.

Private drug stocks became totally inadequate for medical needs in the war that ensued. Imports were cut off from England, and channels for medicinal supplies from other countries did not develop effectively until late in the war and afterward. The most immediate relief from drug shortages, George Griffenhagen concluded, came from American privateers who preyed on British shipping. "Drug cargoes from British prize ships, many of which were en route to New York, served as a most important source of supply, particularly in 1777 and 1778."

The place of purging and emesis in therapeutics of the late 18th century is reflected in the drugs most in demand, although cinchona headed the pharmaceutical needs of military medicine. In discussing the drugs in most critical supply, Griffenhagen also mentions that prices had skyrocketed:

Jalap, ipecac, and rhubarb were the botanical favorites, while bitter purging salts (Epsom salts) and Glauber's purging salts were the chemical choices for purging. Tartar emetic (antimony and potassium tartrate) was the choice for a vomit, and cantharides (Spanish flies) was the most important ingredient of blistering plasters. Gum opium was administered for its narcotic effects, while gum camphor, nitre (saltpetre or potassium nitrate), and mercury (pure metal as well as certain salts) were employed for a variety of purposes. Lint, a form of absorbent material made by scraping or picking apart old woven material, also often was short in supply.

Equipment shortages included surgical instruments and mortar and pestles for pulverizing the crude drugs. Glass vials for holding compounded medicines were also a supply problem, especially after essential drugs were again available.

## THE RESPONSIBILITIES OF THE APOTHECARIES

Medical procurement in the American army often reflected the disorganization and confusion of the entire medical service. The Director-General,[20] the Purveyor-General,[21] Congressional committees[22] and various "Commissaries" and Quartermasters[23] were at one time or another, and sometimes at the same time, involved in getting medicines and medical supplies. The Continental Congress even appointed special agents to procure drugs for the navy.[24] But the procurement of drugs became one of the responsibilities of the Apothecaries-General. In fact, at one time in 1777, both Craigie and Cutting were in Boston competing with each other for drugs (and competing with Congress' agents for the Navy).[25]

It did not take too long for the responsibilities of the apothecaries to be broadened to encompass the preparation of medicines and the putting up of medicine chests for the general and regimental hospitals. Just where and when the idea originated is not known, but by February 24, 1778 Director-General Shippen and Purveyor-General Potts were informing the Board of War that "Our laboratory for ye reception of medicines, etc . . . cannot possibly be finished without we obtain assistance," and requested such "assistance as from time to time shall be required by the Apothecary General of the Middle Department at Carlisle."[26]

A few months later Craigie characterized the department as "in chaos." He felt threatened by his former assistant and now rival, Cutting, who was in charge of the main store of drugs that had been moved from Mannheim to Yellow Springs, Pennsylvania.[27] In May, 1778 Craigie expressed his concern to Purveyor-General Potts:

> I beg leave to query whether this will not be the plan. To have the principle store at Carlisle where all the medicines shall be prepared and the chests completed. Under the supposition that the general hospitals will be more collected and the number lessened, I would propose that an apothecary attend each with a complete chest of medicines; that the surgeon and physician general of the army be attended by an apothecary with a good chest . . . I would have an issuing store at a convenient distance from the army, from which the hospital and regimental chests might occasionally be replenished.[28]

That Craigie's proposal found acceptance and support is confirmed by a later report "that hospital drugs were prepared and compounded mostly in Apothecary General Craigie's shop at Carlisle, Pennsylvania."[29] However, for a time at least, a "dispensing store" (i.e., storehouse) was maintained at Yellow Springs under Cutting as well.[30] Pharmaceutical needs were also met by establishing new local manufacture. "Lint was produced in large quantities, and glass vials were manufactured in numerous glasshouses. Even local manufacture of the purging salts and nitre aided in eliminating shortages of these essential items, and at the same time initiated the first large-scale pharmaceutical manufacturing in America."[31]

The army apothecaries' responsibilities of procurement and large scale production of medicines extended over into making up medicine chests, as already noted. The Director-General himself had originally undertaken this task on orders from General Washington, and he continued to keep a watchful eye on the chests thereafter.[32] Craigie had suggested a procedure for the provision and distribution of medicine chests (letter to Dr. Potts cited above), and Cutting recommended a similar procedure.[33] In any case, Craigie at Carlisle and Cutting at Yellow Springs were both putting up chests in 1778, not always rapidly enough to meet the army's needs.[34]

The general military hospitals were supplied with large chests "too capacious for field service" and smaller ones were issued to the regimental surgeons.[35] The regimental chests, sometimes referred to as "the Apothecary Ration,"[36] were replenished as needed from the large chests at the general hospital or other depot. "Such of the Regimental Surgeons as have not had a fresh supply of Medicines are Immediately to send their Chests to Mr. Cutting, Apothecary General to the Army, at his Store near Paramus Church where they will get a Supply," ordered Major General Nathaniel Green on September 24, 1780.[37]

Late in the war, (1782), Congress spelled out the responsibilities of the apothecary in some detail. Among them were:

> The apothecary shall be accountable for all articles in his department to the purveyor throughout the states, until they come into the hands of the prescribers; and all deputies, assistants, and mates, shall make returns and be accountable to the apothecary for the medicines, instruments and other property. . . .
>
> The hospital prescribers shall be supplied, upon their own application, with medicines and instruments. . . .
>
> Every regimental surgeon shall receive yearly from the apothecary, a supply of medicines to such amount . . . as . . . necessary.
>
> Every prescribing surgeon or physician, either in hospital or with the army, shall be supplied by the apothecary with such a set of capital instruments as . . . necessary.[38]

In addition to these duties, the army apothecaries, particularly the assistants,

PHARMACOPOEIA

SIMPLICIORUM

ET

EFFICACIORUM,

IN USUM

NOSOCOMII MILITARIS,

AD EXERCITUM

Fœderatarum *Americæ* Civitatum

PERTINENTIS;

HODIERNÆ NOSTRÆ INOPIÆ RERUMQUE ANGUSTIIS,

Feroci hoſtium ſævitiæ, belloque crudeli ex inopinatò patriæ noſtræ illato debitis,

MAXIME ACCOMMODATA.

PHILADELPHIÆ:

Ex Officina STYNER & CIST. M DCC LXXVIII.

A modest military formulary was the first publication compiled on American soil to be termed a "pharmacopeia." It is commonly called the Lititz pharmacopeia, after the Pennsylvania town of that name, which was the site of an army hospital for wounded patriots. The reproductions show the title page *(left)* and sample pages *(opposite page)* of text. The annotations in this copy by "BR" are those of Benjamin Rush, one of the most competent American physicians of the 18th century. (From the Library Company of Philadelphia)

served as hospital pharmacists. It is evident that the general army hospital usually had an apothecary's laboratory attached, to which an apothecary and/or assistant apothecary were assigned. On March 11, 1778, Dr. William Brown, then a Physician-General, requested from the Purveyor-General for use in the hospitals, quantities of small apothecary's weights and scales, bolus knives, spatulas, mortars and pestles, measures, earthen or copper vessels and delft tiles, obviously intended to outfit hospital "laboratories."[39] On July 22, 1778 the "Elaboratory" of the Pennsylvania Hospital, used then by the Army in part, "was turned over to the medical department for use as a pharmacy for the preparation of medicines for the army hospitals."[40] At the Basking Ridge hospital (a part of the Morristown encampment) a small school house was "converted into an apothecary shop;[41] Apothecary John Hay served in the hospital at Williamsburg, Virginia;[42] and "Apothecary's Mate" Evan Lewis served at the Continental Hospital at Charleston, South Carolina.[43] The importance of the work of these men, and others like them, was pointed up when, upon Lewis' capture by the British, Deputy Director-General Oliphant, of the Hospitals of the Southern Department, eagerly sought to make a new appointment because Lewis' duties were being "performed by a mate unequal to the task."[44]

Finally, it should be noted that it frequently devolved upon the regimental surgeon and mates to do their own compounding. "Dr. Howell [the surgeon] came up . . . and after putting up a quantity of medicines, we rode off . . . to visit our sick," Surgeon's Mate Ebenezer Elmer noted in his diary in 1777.[45]

Although most of the men whose work has just been described were not considered and did not think of themselves as "pharmacists," it is manifest that the Revolutionary War pointed up the necessity for specialists concerned with the procurement, preservation, compounding, and dispensing of drugs. Pharmacy's special tasks and professional skills were being recognized, if only because of military necessity.

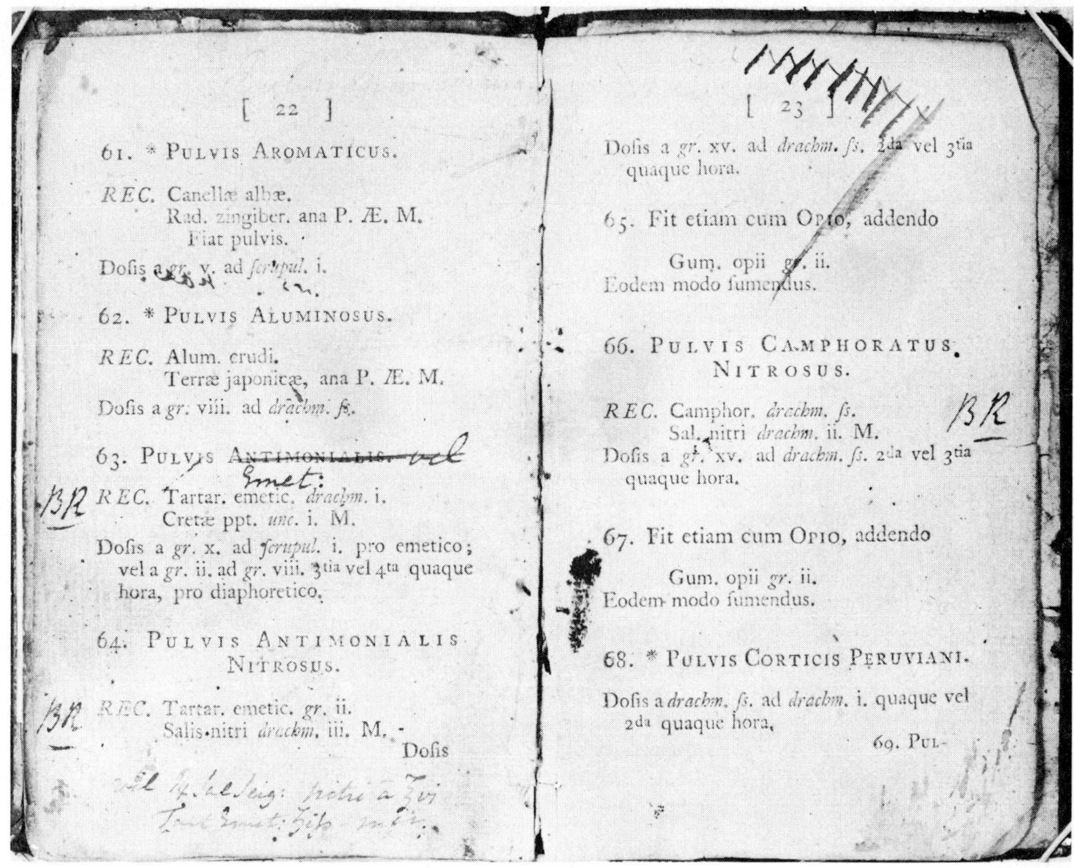

[ 22 ]

61. * PULVIS AROMATICUS.

*REC.* Canellæ albæ.
Rad. zingiber. ana P. Æ. M.
Fiat pulvis.

Doſis a *gr.* v. ad *ſcrupul.* i.

62. * PULVIS ALUMINOSUS.

*REC.* Alum. crudi.
Terræ japonicæ, ana P. Æ. M.

Doſis a *gr.* viii. ad *drachm.* *ſs.*

63. PULVIS ~~ANTIMONIALIS.~~ vel Emet:

*REC.* Tartar. emetic. *drachm.* i.
Cretæ ppt. *unc.* i. M.

Doſis a *gr.* x. ad *ſcrupul.* i. pro emetico; vel a *gr.* ii. ad *gr.* viii. $3^{tia}$ vel $4^{ta}$ quaque hora, pro diaphoretico.

64. PULVIS ANTIMONIALIS NITROSUS.

*REC.* Tartar. emetic. *gr.* ii.
Salis-nitri *drachm.* iii. M.

Doſis

[ 23 ]

Doſis a *gr.* xv. ad *drachm.* *ſs.* $2^{da}$ vel $3^{tia}$ quaque hora.

65. Fit etiam cum OPIO, addendo

Gum. opii *gr.* ii.
Eodem modo ſumendus.

66. PULVIS CAMPHORATUS NITROSUS.

*REC.* Camphor. *drachm.* *ſs.*
Sal. nitri *drachm.* ii. M.

Doſis a *gr.* xv. ad *drachm.* *ſs.* $2^{da}$ vel $3^{tia}$ quaque hora.

67. Fit etiam cum OPIO, addendo

Gum. opii *gr.* ii.
Eodem modo ſumendus.

68. * PULVIS CORTICIS PERUVIANI.

Doſis a *drachm.* *ſs.* ad *drachm.* i. quaque vel $2^{da}$ quaque hora.

69. PUL-

**Lititz Pharmacopoeia**

As time went on, both the medical organization of the army and the drug supply situation improved. One indication of this improvement and a basis for its continuance was the publication of a military formulary in 1778, the so-called "Lititz pharmacopoeia." This small booklet, modest in appearance, proved to be a landmark in the history of American pharmacy.

The Lititz pharmacopoeia illustrates in a most remarkable way the choice of items suggested by the medical knowledge (particularly English medical knowledge) that was current, the results of the American experience, and, finally, the difficulties arising from the actual situation of a nation at war, which was restricted in its imports. The Lititz pharmacopoeia is thus called because the booklet was written, at least in part, in the Moravian village of Lititz (preface dated at Lititz, March 12, 1778). It was first used in the military hospitals of Lititz and Bethlehem, Pennsylvania. The actual title (see p. 168) may be translated, "Formulary of simple and yet efficacious remedies for use of the military hospital, belonging to the army of the Federated States of America. Especially adapted to our present poverty and straitened circumstances, caused by the ferocious inhumanity of the enemy, and the cruel war unexpectedly brought upon our fatherland." The author of this "pharmacopoeia"—or, more truly, emergency military hospital formulary— was, in all probability, Dr. William Brown, an American graduate of the University of Edinburgh.[46]

About half the formulas listed seem to stem from the experience of the author and his American colleagues. The most important overseas source for this first book of its kind in America was the *Pharmacopoeia Edinburgensis* (1756), which was official when Brown himself was studying at Edinburgh. Other sources of formulas, in order of importance, were the *Pharmacopoeia of the Royal Hospital of Edinburgh*, the *Pharmacopoeia Londinensis* (1746) and the *Pharmacopoeia contracta* of *Beth Holim* in London.[47]

Because of perplexing and unpredictable drug shortages, the Lititz pharmacopoeia followed an old pharmaceutical tradition of permitting official substitution of therapeutically equivalent substances for drugs in uncertain supply. In official European drug books of the 16th and 17th centuries, when imports were irregular, lists of authorized substitutes were sometimes annexed under the heading *Quid pro quo* or *De succedaniis*. The earliest known list of this kind goes back 1800 years to Galen.[48]

Another feature of the military formulary was indicated in its introduction by the statement:

> There are distinguished by an asterisk the formulas of medicaments which must be prepared and compounded in a general laboratory; the others are to be mixed, as needed, in our hospital dispensaries.[49]

This remark is the first official mention of large-scale manufacture of pharmaceutical products in America. The purpose was to relieve the apothecary in the hospital of the preparation of compounded medicines which could not be made quickly or without special effort and unnecessary waste of time and material. A comparison of the preparations with and without asterisks shows that the differentiation was not according to the professional skill required.

The Lititz pharmacopoeia was published about the same time that Apothecary-General Craigie's proposed "principle store at Carlisle" was established. This "principle store" was, in all probability, the "general laboratory" mentioned in the Lititz pharmacopoeia. Thus, officially recognized American manufacture of pharmaceutical products on a large scale—the first we know of—was established according to the proposal of an apothecary, under his direction and for the public welfare.

## Coste's Compendium

Two years after the issuance of this formulary "for the use of the military hospitals belonging to the army of the Federated States of America," there appeared a "Pharmaceutical Compendium compiled for the French military hospitals in North America" *(Compendium pharmaceuticum militaribus gallorum nosocomiis in orbe novo boreali adscriptum,* 1780). It was compiled by Jean-François Coste, Chief Physician to the French army fighting with the American patriots against the British. This booklet, limited to the use of the comparatively small French contingent on American soil, did not gain the practical or the historical significance of the Lititz pharmacopoeia.

Necessity had stood godfather to both books. "The incertitudes of war, of the sea and of a long voyage," says Coste in his introductory remarks to his formulary, "called for the employment of a few remedies," i.e., of a selected number. While the Lititz pharmacopoeia is based on Scottish and English sources, Coste's book naturally follows French patterns (especially the *Codex medicamentarius seu pharmacopoea Parisiensis,* 1758). A significant difference lies in the fact that the Lititz pharmacopoeia makes use of indigenous North American drugs, such as sassafras and serpentaria, while Coste's formulary does not.

The exigencies of war are well illustrated by the *Compendium* and the medicines used by the French. "Few or no chemical remedies are employed by them. . . . Their hospital pharmacopoeia consisted chiefly of potions, decoctions, and watery drinks," commented a prominent American army physician, in 1781. Coste himself was to comment later that "we did not call into practical use a tenth part, perchance, of the approximately 100 formulae."[50]

## IMPORTANCE OF THE REVOLUTION FOR PHARMACY

When we try to understand the significance of the Revolutionary War for pharmacy as a profession, the following seem to be especially prominent: (1) Eight years of successful pharmaceutical activity, separate from medicine but equally recognized and given the same official status; (2) the first known American manufacture of pharmaceutical products on a large scale, initiated by an apothecary in order to meet national needs; and (3) the first practical attempt at a uniform and obligatory formulary as a basis for satisfactory and reliable pharmaceutical work (in this case, military pharmacy). The importance of pharmacy for the public welfare had been proved by the experiences of the Revolution.

# 11

# Young Republic and Pioneer Expansion

The Revolutionary War was over. The American people were free. The question then was, free from what and for what? The first part of this question may easily be answered. The American people had severed their connection with Great Britain and, hence, with Europe. They had gained the liberty to work out their own destiny. This destiny was not apparent at the time, although it had found its basic expression in that declaration of the inborn and eternal rights of men—the first amendment of the Constitution of the United States.

The United States was a nation founded not on the organization of kindred tribes or on dynastic imperialism, but as the result of the free decision of peoples of varying descent. It had won a victory, but simultaneously a task had been assigned to it. This task was to prove that liberty of the individual was within, not beyond, the limits of human nature and political wisdom.

After the war, among the immediate necessities of the new nation were to find as firm a basis for the life of professions and trades as for the individual, and to derive the greatest possible benefit from the natural resources of the country.

## INDIGENOUS MATERIA MEDICA

This War of Independence and the new nation emerging from it not only had a special and alluring ideology but seemed to open up a limitless country to all peoples. It awakened the interest of the whole civilized world. Many former enemies, especially German soldiers in English service, remained in America. Others stayed for a while to explore the country and to study its resources and possibilities. One of the latter, the physician-botanist Johann Schoepf, traveled through the country for more than a year and published (1787) a book about the indigenous American materia medica (*Materia Medica Americana Potissimum Regni Vegetabilis*). Schoepf's journey was only one of the successful botanic and medicobotanical expeditions by foreigners following the Revolutionary War. They were supported and supplemented by intensive research on the part of American botanists.

Botany, and especially medicinal botany, had been cultivated in North America during early Colonial times. Thus there was a fund of experience on which to build.[1] Schoepf's *Materia Medica Americana* is based largely on the observations of the excellent American botanist G. H. E. Muehlenberg and the work of Bartram, Clayton, Colden, Kalm, Catesby and others.[2] To Muehlenberg, Schoepf wrote from Baireuth, Germany:

> My lists [describing about 400 North American plants] make it certain that North America owns a rich indigenous materia medica in her plants and can find all she needs, apart from a few East Indian spices and plants, on her own soil . . . I almost may flatter myself in writing this little book

to have rendered sufficient services to America to be pardoned for my assistance in combatting her.[3]

Schoepf was not the only one who took advantage of the diligent, comprehensive and unselfish work of Muehlenberg. Numerous European and American botanists, among them Benjamin Smith Barton, author of the *Collections for an Essay Towards a Materia Medica of the United States,*[4] and Manasseh Cutler,[5] author of the first scientific treatise on New England botany, were in close scientific contact with Muehlenberg.

Barton's treatise on American materia medica (two parts, 1798 and 1804) was the first of its kind in English and simultaneously was a critique of the work of Schoepf. Evidence of the inspiration that Barton imparted to research on the medicinal value of American plants can be found in a good number of theses of medical graduates of the University of Pennsylvania, where he taught natural history and botany.

Muehlenberg considered the pharmacist an authority to be consulted for information about indigenous medicinal plants in regard to their strength as well as their common names. Twice in his notebook he mentions the necessity of consulting a pharmacist for this purpose.[6]

All this valuable scientific work, besides enriching American medical and pharmaceutical science and practice, added to the international materia medica. It was supplemented by the observations of unscientific empirics. These observations of laymen formed the basis of sectarian movements and, later on, were subjected to scientific evaluation. Coupled with the results of early research work previously mentioned, they played an influential part in American medicine and pharmacy.

These scientific interests had their practical application in the botanical gardens devoted to the cultivation and study of medicinal herbs. The first of these was probably established in Philadelphia early in the 18th century in connection with the Friends' Almhouse there.[7] In the mid-eighteenth century, Drs. David and Jonathan Lathrop, who have been said to "dominate the apothecary trade of southern New England" and who once imported a single shipment of drugs worth £8,000, were "growing herbs in huge gardens and greenhouses" in Norwich, Connecticut.[8] Early in the 19th century, the religious communities of the Shakers in New York state began to cultivate medicinal herbs on a

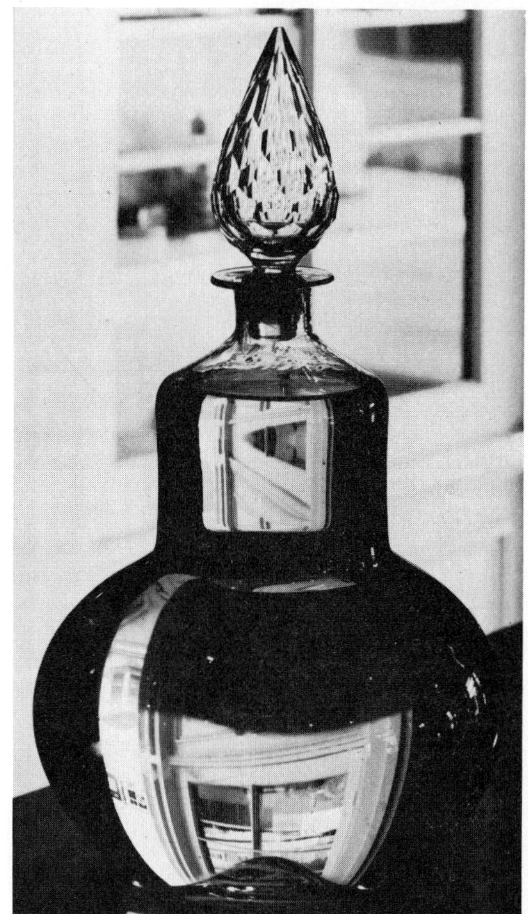

An early type of show bottle (or "show-globe") of the 19th century, brought to America from England, is similar to the carboys that contained stock solutions, which became symbolic of pharmacy (see Glossary, p. 486). (Specimen owned by The Upjohn Company)

large scale. Their enterprise—which extended to the packaging, the making up of extracts, and the marketing of the drugs—was so highly successful, at least to 1875, that it attracted commercial imitators.[9]

## THE "THOMSONIANS" AND THE "ECLECTICS"

About 1800, Samuel Thomson entered the scene. His personality and work gained nation-wide recognition in spite of the simplicity and the lack of originality of what he called his "system"—or, perhaps, because of these characteristics. Thomson was an uneducated man, the son of a farmer, and originally a farmer himself. His early desire to become an apprentice to a doctor could not be fulfilled because of his almost complete lack of education. In 19th-century America he rediscovered the fundamentals of the ancient theory of Galen (see p. 19) and used them for his own theory, the "Thomsonian system." His doctrine reads like a slightly modified abstract from Galen's writings when he states:

> I found, after maturely considering the subject, that all animal bodies are formed of the four elements, earth, air, fire, and water . . . that a state of perfect health arises from a due balance or temperature of the four elements.[10]

Before Thomson there had been so-called botanic physicians and herb doctors, the latter strengthening their offerings with supposed medicinal "secrets" of the American Indians; but they remained individualistic practitioners, local or itinerant in their practice. Unlike them, Samuel Thomson systematized his crude teachings, patented his therapeutics, and propagandized his band of rabid followers, who launched a movement

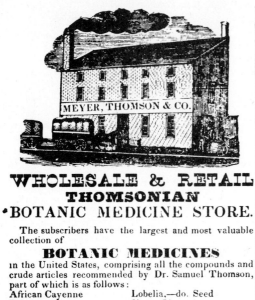

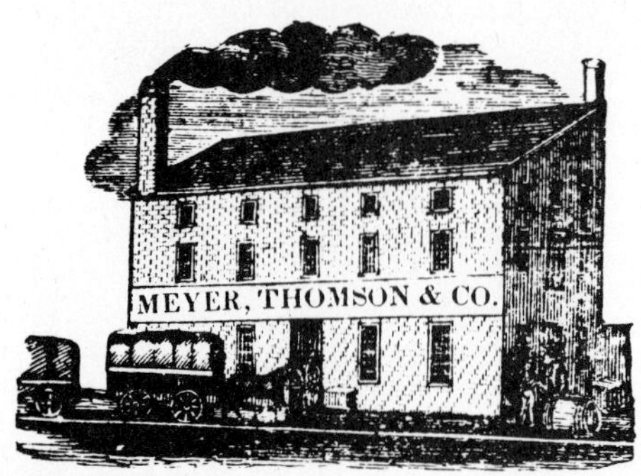


**WHOLESALE & RETAIL**
**THOMSONIAN**
**BOTANIC MEDICINE STORE.**

The subscribers have the largest and most valuable collection of

**BOTANIC MEDICINES**

in the United States, comprising all the compounds and crude articles recommended by Dr. Samuel Thomson, part of which is as follows:

African Cayenne — Lobelia,—do. Seed
Balmony — Nerve Ointment
Barberry — Nerve Powder
Butter Nut Syrup — Pond Lily
Cancer Plaster — Poplar Bark coarse and fine
Clivers — Prickly Ash
Composition — Raspberry Leaves
Conserve of Hollyhock — Slippery Elm
Cough Powder — Woman's Friend or Females' Bitters
Ginger — Unicorn Root
Golden Seal — Wake Robin, &c. &c. &c.
Gum Myrrh

**SUPERIOR WINE BITTERS**

For the Dyspeptic. This valuable article has been found highly beneficial in restoring the natural tone of the stomach of weak and dyspeptic patients.

**DYSENTERY SYRUP.**

This article is a new invention of Dr Thomson, and has seldom failed in curing the Dysentery. It needs but a single trial to recommend it.

**PEPPER SAUCE.**

The subscribers have a superior article of Pepper Sauce, prepared after a plan of Dr Thomson, and for family use is far superior to that sold at the shops. It is excellent to give a proper tone to the stomach, and excite the digestive powers.

**FAMILY RIGHTS.**

We keep constantly for sale Dr Thomson's Family Rights both in the English and German languages, and all other works connected with the Thomsonian System.

**STEAM MILL.**

Having built an eight horse power Steam Mill, expressly for grinding the Thomsonian medicines, they are enabled to sell on the most favorable terms, and warrant their medicines to be genuine and pure, and clear of any deleterious or poisonous qualities, put up in the best condition. All orders punctually attended to.

GODFREY MEYER & CO.
Gen. Agents for Dr Samuel Thomson,
Near Pratt st. Bridge, Baltimore.

Advertisement of 1835, by a drug depot serving the botanic system. Thomsonian Manual, V. 1, p. xvi (from A. Berman).

accepted by large segments of the American public.

The appeal of these "irregular" practitioners undoubtedly drew strength from therapeutic excesses of regular practitioners, who were still bloodletting with abandon and giving massive doses of cathartic and emetic as veritable cure-alls. Thomsonians played openly on the citizen's fears that the "heroic" treatments might be worse than the disease. They offered to substitute "milder" and "safer" botanic remedies for the "harsh minerals" of the orthodox school. However, their "less lethal remedies" could be characterized as "frequent lobelia emetics, scalding capsicum and herb teas, medicated enemas, and parboiling steam baths—all built around a distinctive monistic pathology."[11]

The founder of the sect divided the main part of his materia medica into six classes, each based on the properties of the drugs. The original Thomsonians usually prepared and dispensed their own medications, based on drugs marketed by special manufacturers through authorized botanic drug depots. Georgia, in 1847, created a special Botanico-Medical Board of Physicians that was empowered to examine and license "Botanic or Thomsonian apothecaries." There is, however, nothing to indicate that this legislation seriously affected the practice of pharmacy.[12]

Thomson's policies and attitudes eventually generated schisms in the ranks of the movement that produced the Neo-Thomsonians and various Botanic splinter groups. Most important were the Eclectics and the Reformed Practice of Medicine. The name *Eclectics* was put forward earlier in the classification of medical practitioners by C. S. Rafinesque, the prominent botanist, in his *Medical Flora; or a Manual of Medical Botany of the United States of North America*. The Reformed Practice of Medicine had its basic impetus in Dr. Wooster Beach's *The American Practice of Medicine* which appeared in 1833. The Eclectics and the Reformed Practitioners—their concepts are difficult to distinguish—were significant parts of American medicine in the 19th century, eventually establishing medical schools and attaining a considerable professional respectability.[13]

Rafinesque had described Eclectics as "those who select and adopt in practice whatever is beneficial, and who change their prescriptions according to emergencies and acquired knowledge."[14]

This definition holds true for classical eclectics who did not recognize any dogma. However, the American eclectic medical practitioners did cling to one dogma, namely, the rejection of a large number of remedies of mineral origin, particularly all mercury compounds. Nevertheless, compared with the Thomsonians, they were liberal.[15]

The Eclectics and their associates had greater scientific pretensions than their predecessors. Rafinesque, who thought of himself as belonging to the Reformed Practice,[16] intended his *Medical Flora* to serve the daily use of medical students, physicians, druggists, pharmacians [a term revealing the French origin of the author], chemists, botanists. He stated that "pharmacy, by the aid of botany and chemistry, has become a science," and that "druggists and chemists" must be able "to distinguish the genuine kinds and detect the frauds of the collectors and herbalists."[17] Rafinesque also laid down rules for the pharmaceutical manipulation of plants in order to get efficient medicaments.[18] Moreover, he believed that "The active principles of medical plants may be obtained in a concentrated form by chemical operations" and he urged American research in plant chemistry, particularly praising the work of the Society of Pharmacists of Paris.[19]

However, although "the Botanic practitioners as a group evinced a marked disinclination and a lack of ability to conduct phytochemical work"—John Uri Lloyd was a notable exception to this—"a number of drug plants employed exclusively in Botanic practice eventually entered the general phar-

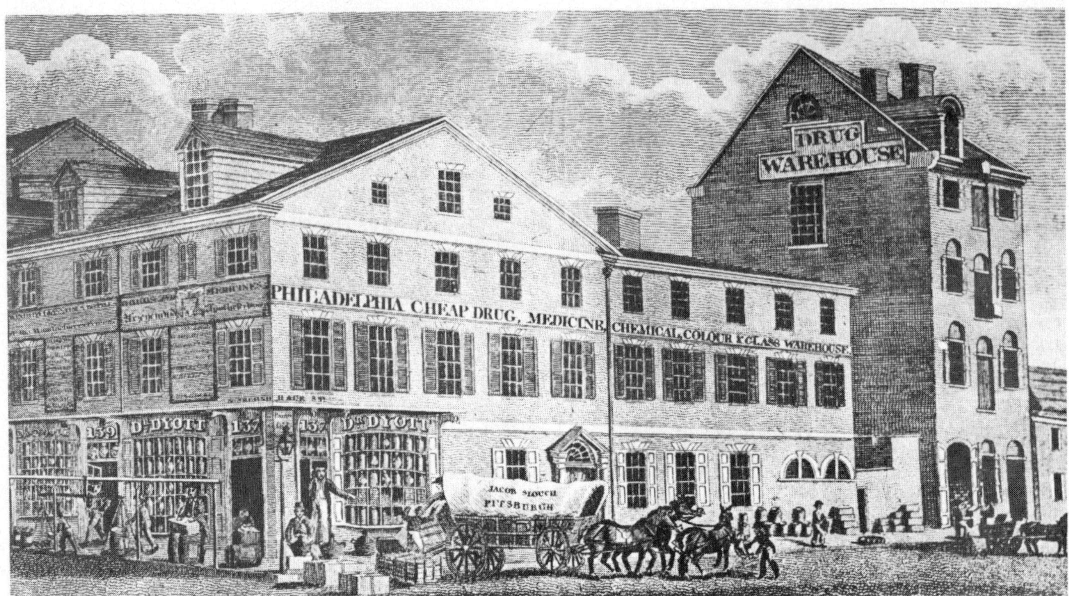


Crates and barrels of drugs are being loaded onto a Conestoga wagon before the door of one of the first American druggists to develop a national wholesale trade. Excessively shrewd and unusually successful financially, Thomas Dyott was operating his "Drug Warehouse" in Philadelphia as early as 1807 and, later, manufactured his own line of household remedies. (Young, J. H.: J. Am. Pharm. Assoc. ns *1*:290, 1961; illustration from Porter, T.: The Picture of Philadelphia, 1831)

maceutical literature and the official compendia."[20] Through the efforts of William S. Merrell the large and unpleasant doses of Eclectic remedies gave way to their concentrated "resinoid" botanic medicinals (e.g., resin of podophyllum). This development stimulated Eclectic optimism that they could match the alkaloidal pharmacy of the regular practitioners and that the "designation of 'unscientific' could no longer be applied" to them.[21]

The Thomsonian, Botanic, Eclectic, and Reformed practices of medicine contributed more to American medicine and pharmacy than their additions to the official compendia and the "resinoids." It soon became obvious that the gentler therapeutics of the botanics seemed no less successful than the forceful therapeutics of the "regulars." Thus they served to moderate the use of the huge dosages and powerful medicines that the regulars were prescribing as part of their "heroic" approach to therapeutics.

## HOMEOPATHY

The impact on the regular practice of medicine by Thomsonianism and its successors was supplemented from another sectarian quarter, that of the homeopathists. Homeopathy and its ideas of *similia similibus curantur* and of infinitesimal doses (see p. 47) were introduced into the United States in 1825 by Hans B. Gram, a Danish immigrant who had returned to Copenhagen for his medical education. He, and his disciples in New York, were followed by German-speaking practitioners in Pennsylvania whose knowledge of homeopathy came through reading and correspondence.[22] Constantine Herring, a German homeopath arrived in Pennsylvania in 1835 and established an academy at Allentown to teach homeopathy. Graduates of the academy were to spread the doctrine through the East and Midwest, aided by a steady influx of European homeopaths.[23] In the 1840's, translations of homeopathic literature from the German spurred the growth of the sect in America. By 1850 a homeopathic medical college had been founded at Cincinnati.[24]

Homeopathy had a strong appeal, not only to the public but to many regular ("allopathic") physicians. It had the virtue of relying largely on the healing power of nature, perhaps unintentionally, to be sure, and soon demonstrated that it, like the Eclectic and Reformed systems, had no worse and perhaps better success than the allopaths. The American Institute of Homeopathy, founded in 1844, was the country's first national medical society; by 1900 there were 22 homeopathic medical schools in the country;[25] and in 1897 the first edition of *The Homeopathic Pharmacopoeia of the United States* appeared (see p. 281).

Homeopathy proved more objectionable to regular medicine than Thomsonianism, and by the 1830's a fierce campaign of disparagement and discrimination against the homeopaths began that did not abate until the final decades of the century. To the regulars the homeopaths were charlatans with whom professional ethics would permit no intercourse.

Eventually, the education of homeopaths came somewhat closer to that of the allopaths (materia medica and pharmacy constituting major points of departure); homeopathic physicians often found themselves practicing much like allopaths; regular physicians were influenced to use smaller doses (although by no means homeopathic). However, new scientific developments greatly undermined the rationale of the homeopaths; and by 1923 only two homeopathic medical schools remained in the country (and they were to disappear in the 1950's).[26]

Pharmacy was affected by homeopathy. Although the homeopaths included "pharmacists" (six of the twelve men on their original pharmacopoeial committee intentionally were pharmacists[27]), it is not likely that these were ordinary pharmacists. The homeopaths did not acknowledge the ability of the allopathic pharmacist to prepare homeopathic remedies. Some pharmacists did become "the professional pharmacist who understands the preparation of remedies for homeopathic use,"[28] and, in the larger cities special "homeopathic pharmacies" came into existence. For the most part, however, the homeopathic physician provided his own pharmaceutical services. Later, prepared and pre-packaged proprietary homeopathic remedies were marketed and the regular pharmacy often carried a "homeopathic cabinet" from which remedies were dispensed by number.

In the original Hahnemannian system, the pharmaceutical resources used would seem without value in modern pharmacologic terms. Yet, it was a relatively harmless alternative compared with orthodox therapeutics of the time. Lacking firm ties to the mainstream of "scientific" medicine or pharmacy, homeopathy remained a cult of dwindling public support, without significant place in American pharmacy during recent decades.

## INDIVIDUAL LIBERTY VS. PROFESSIONAL RESPONSIBILITY

Sectarianism in medicine became a touchstone for the meaning of constitutional "liberty." This question had to be answered: Which was of greater importance and broader general consequence, the recently acquired and legally guaranteed "liberty" of the individual to take up any profession, or the protection of the people from dangers arising, particularly in the field of medicine, from the unchecked activity of individuals practicing their profession by no other standard than their own belief in their ability and a modicum of experience?

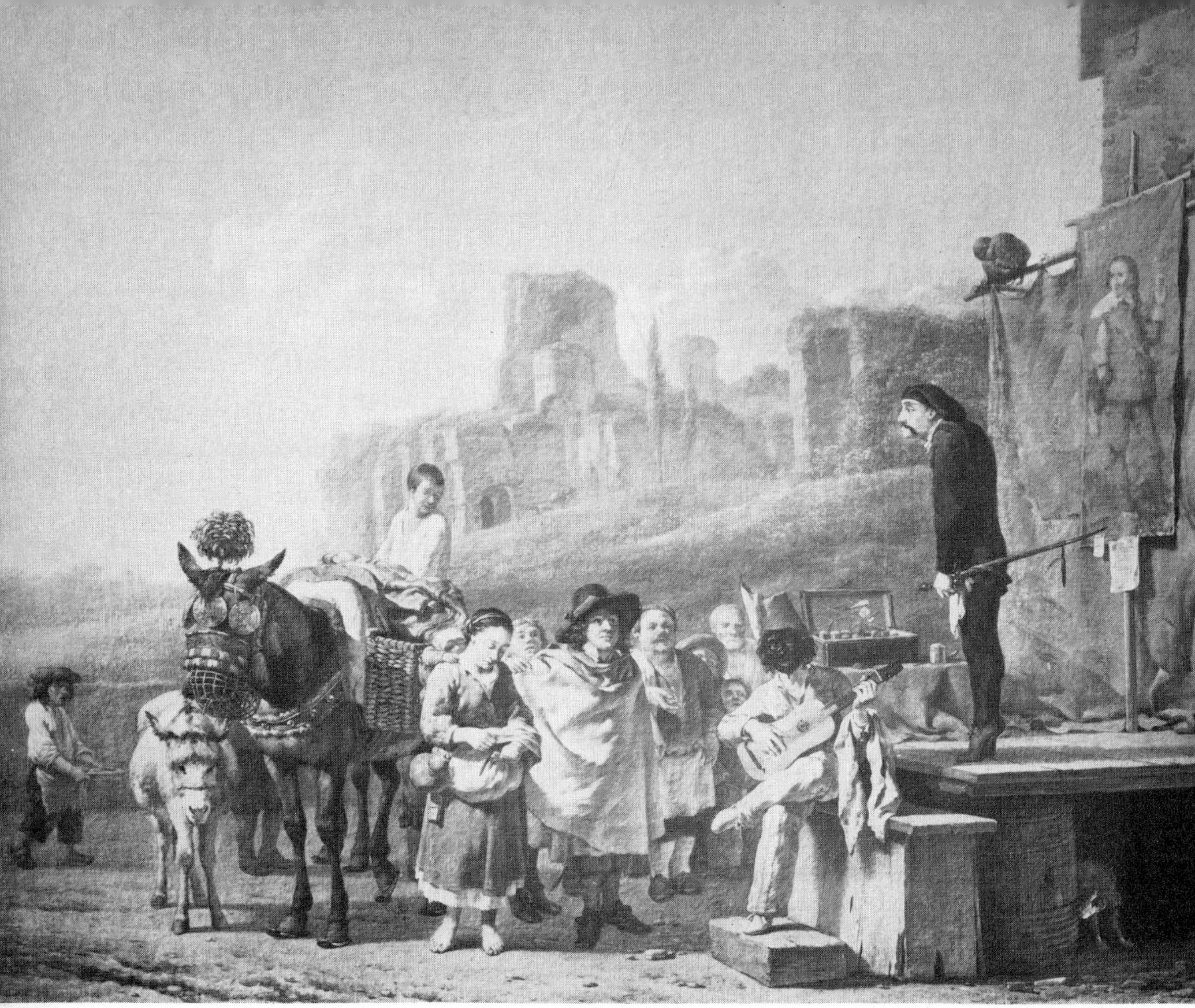

*Above,* a European prototype of the itinerant American "medicine show" is vividly portrayed in the 17th-century painting, "The Italian Charlatan" by Karel Dujardin. (From the Louvre, Paris, through Pharmaceutical Library, University of Wisconsin)

*Opposite, top,* an American counterpart of Dujardin's scene is the photograph of "Doctor" Matthews' medicine show as it toured Wisconsin in the early 1890's. His troupe included elements of the earlier European tradition: a spieler (Dr. Matthews in top hat, *far right*), an acrobat *(left foreground),* musicians to attract a crowd, and of course a chest of prepackaged medicines. Some purported Indians are included to reinforce the banner's imperative: "Use Umatilla Indian Hogar for Long Life and Good Health." It represents a tradition extending from the street-corner quacks of antiquity up to the 20th-century examples of medicinal exploitation (whether through peddling in person or by television). Drug shops or stores did not have to be much more than a permanent habitation for such itinerant quackery until, through a publicly defined level of education and responsibility, a class of "pharmacists" was created that could be expected to protect the public against it. (Photos on opposite page by C. J. Van Schaick through State Historical Society of Wisconsin)

*Opposite, bottom,* "Dr." Matthews poses in top hat with (?) "patient." (The skulls on the table in the tent no doubt remind the gullible of their need for the "Doctor's" aid to preserve their health.)

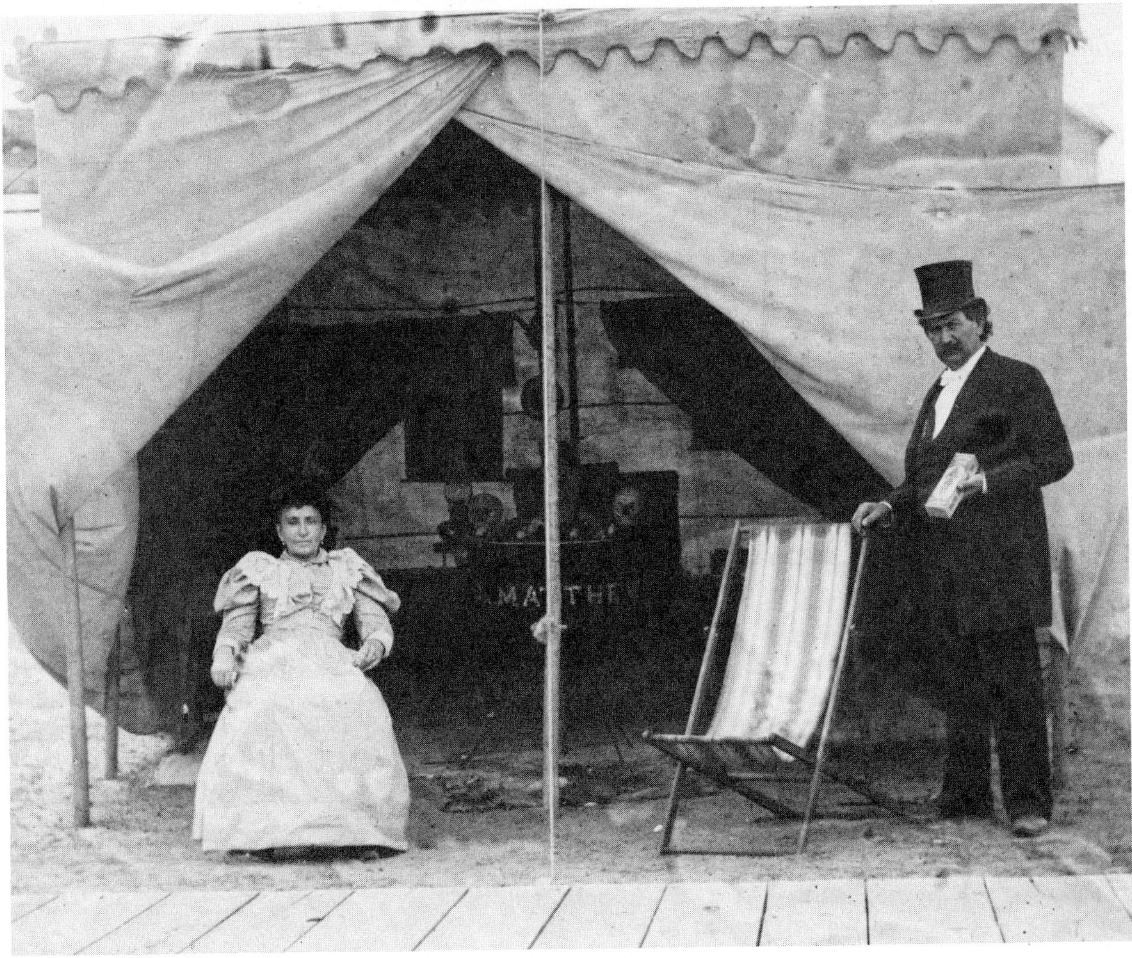

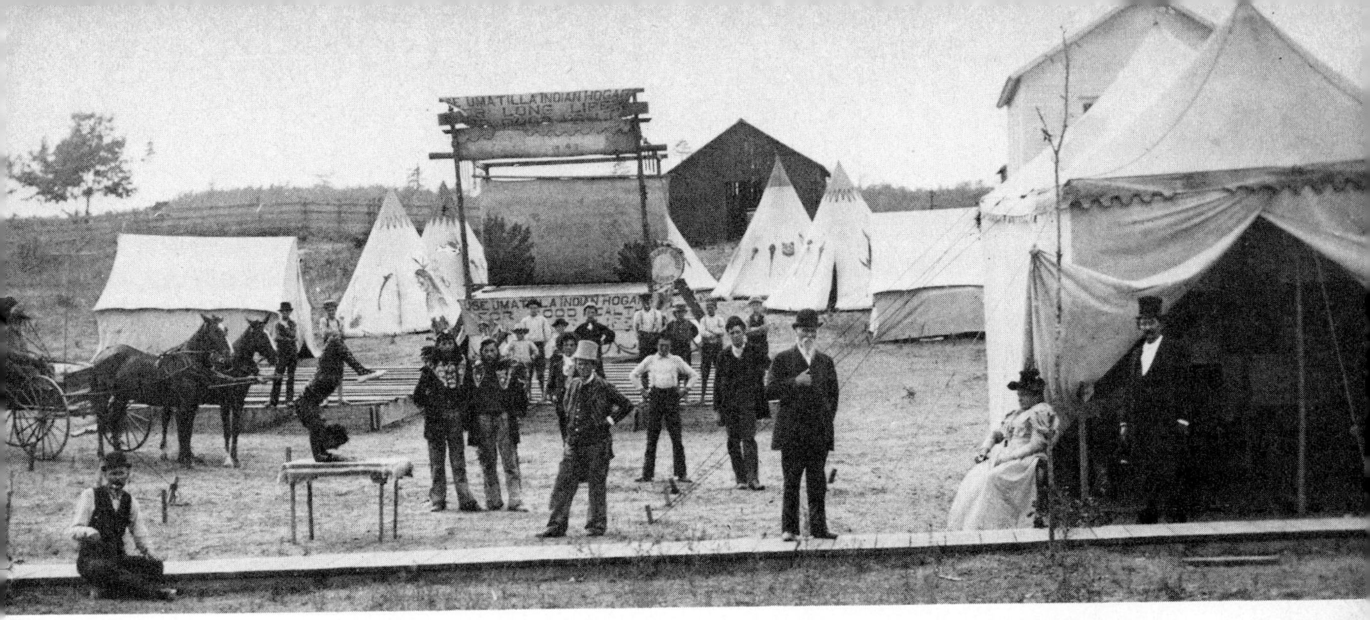

This question always becomes acute and must be decided whenever and wherever "liberty" is introduced as the inborn right of the individual. This happened in France after the great revolution and in Germany (Prussia) with the introduction of the so-called "liberty of trades." In both countries the idea of protection of the people proved to be stronger than the dogma of liberty. The attempts made in France (1791) to introduce unrestricted liberty to practice pharmacy without educational requirements were short-lived. This was true also in Germany (1810 and 1811). Even the customary English *laissez-faire* attitude, although confirming the right to practice medicine and pharmacy to persons who had previously practiced these callings, did not recognize the liberty of anyone to claim to be a physician or pharmacist who had not been duly examined and licensed.[29] The Americans were too practical and equalitarian a people to follow even British examples.[30]

What this meant to the formation and the development of the health professions becomes evident from the fact that for decades the attempts by physicians to regulate the practice of medicine—through educational requirements, examinations and licenses—and to control the professional conduct of practitioners proved to be futile. True, regulations requiring the licensing of medical practitioners had been issued before the Revolutionary War in New York, New Jersey and, soon afterward, Massachusetts and New Hampshire. True, also, that by the 1830's almost all the states had statutes requiring examination and licensing of physicians, but thereafter the laws were repealed: in 1849 only New Jersey and the District of Columbia were said to retain any real control over licensure.[31] The powerful impact of the individualism, the anti-intellectualism, and the abhorrence of monopoly during the period of "Jacksonian democracy," the attacks of the empirics and sectarians, and the realization by the profession of the futility of regulation, all combined in the repeal or emasculation of the legislation.[32]

If such was the situation for medicine, what had pharmacy to hope for in recognition and protection of its professional aims? The same forces, it will later be seen, influenced the pattern of legislative control of pharmacy (see p. 213).

The lack of enforceable standards in the health field left the way open for unbridled and profitable promotion of drugs—whether patented medications administered by irregular practitioners such as the Thomsonians, or preparations for self-medication.

In early America even regular medical practitioners made liberal use of the so-called "patent" medicines. Later, as the growth of newspapers developed a nation-wide medium of promotion and as improved transport could place the promoted remedies in stores available to all and without legal hindrance, the trade in medicines flourished in all sorts of unlikely places. Imitations of English patent medicines, prepared on a large scale by American wholesale druggists, evolved into independent large-scale enterprises.[33] Thus, the trade in English and American patent medicines became the backbone of many American "drugstores" that came to make drugs something of a specialty and often vied successfully with the waning drug shops operated by physician-apothecaries.

In the young republic there were no effective definitions of a pharmacist or pharmacy to guide the erratic course of such establishments, in the majority of which the professional and scientific pharmacy of older European countries was not merely a strange but probably even an unknown way of life.

*The origin and development of European pharmacy was, in general, parallel with professional medicine, as a profession concerned with public health, the nonprofessional aspects being incidental. To a very great extent, nonprofessional medicine was responsible for the development of American pharmacy as an independent calling, the professional aspects being incidental.* Many of the peculiarities in the evolution of American pharmacy can be explained by this fact. Fortunately, however, a group of individuals who fought for higher aims in time created professional American pharmacy. These people came, for the most part, from the wholesale drug field.

## BEGINNINGS OF AMERICAN PROFESSIONAL PHARMACY

As long as the dispensing of medicine was primarily in the hands of the physician-apothecary, the only domain of the "chemist and druggist" proper was the wholesale distribution of drugs. The wholesale druggists provided the country physicians with the imported or indigenous drugs and chemicals needed by physicians in their practice, and they naturally were held responsible by their clients if the expected effects of the drugs were not realized. Furthermore, the Revolutionary War had taught wholesale druggists the advantage of domestic manufacture of products previously imported. Thus, to be able to detect adulterations and to do their own manufacturing, they became highly interested in a better knowledge of drugs and chemicals. The interest in real pharmaceutical activity had begun.

Advertisements of the period immediately after the Revolutionary War reveal this active interest in professional pharmaceutical knowledge. Thus the owner of "Atwood's medicinal store" in New York, announced (1784) "the latest arrivals from Europe" in the *New York Packet* and simultaneously made known that he would like to engage a partner. "The want of capital, with good security, will be no objection to a man of abilities. He must understand pharmacy thoroughly, and he should be grounded in chemistry."[34] Effingham Lawrence in New York advertised the receipt of "a large and general assortment of genuine drugs and medicines from London and Amsterdam" and asked for "a person well acquainted with practical chemistry."[35]

During the early national period wholesale druggists began to issue printed lists enumerating the goods they had in stock. The title of one of these lists (Boston, 1795) reads: "Catalogue of drugs and medicines, instruments, and utensils, dyestuffs, groceries, and painters' colours, imported, prepared, and sold by Smith and Bartlett at their druggists store and apothecaries shop." This title is the best possible illustration of the combination of importing with manufacturing, of wholesale business (the "druggist's store") with dispensing (the "apothecary's shop"), operated in this period by prominent American "druggists." A remark at the end of the catalogue of 22 pages states that "physicians' prescriptions will always meet an exact and particular attention."

Some of the wholesale druggists very early started to manufacture chemicals, thus establishing a basis for large American chemical and pharmaceutical industries.[36] Again the name of Marshall of Philadelphia appears. The firm of Christopher Marshall, Jr., and Charles Marshall (sons of and successors to the druggist Christopher Marshall, Sr., the founder of the venture) "had, as early as 1786, entered quite extensively into the business of making muriate of ammonia and Glauber's salt." The Philadelphia druggist, John Harrison, began (1793) to manufacture various chemicals, notably sulfuric acid. Other druggists took up similar lines of manufacture.

People working as apprentices or clerks in such establishments of necessity acquired pharmaceutical knowledge and skill and, finally, professional pride and aims.[37] The number of apprentices was large, at Marshall's pharmacy ranging from six to twelve. These men, who were accustomed to real pharmaceutical work, later became pioneers in the professional practice of pharmacy in the United States and, to some extent, the first teachers of pharmacy for pharmacists.[38]

A parallel with the development in England is evident. There, too, wholesale druggists initiated professional pharmacy during the first half of the 19th century, filling, in this way, the gap left by the transformation of the apothecaries into medical practitioners. The main difference was that the establishment of the Philadelphia College of Apothecaries (1821) represented the first ob-

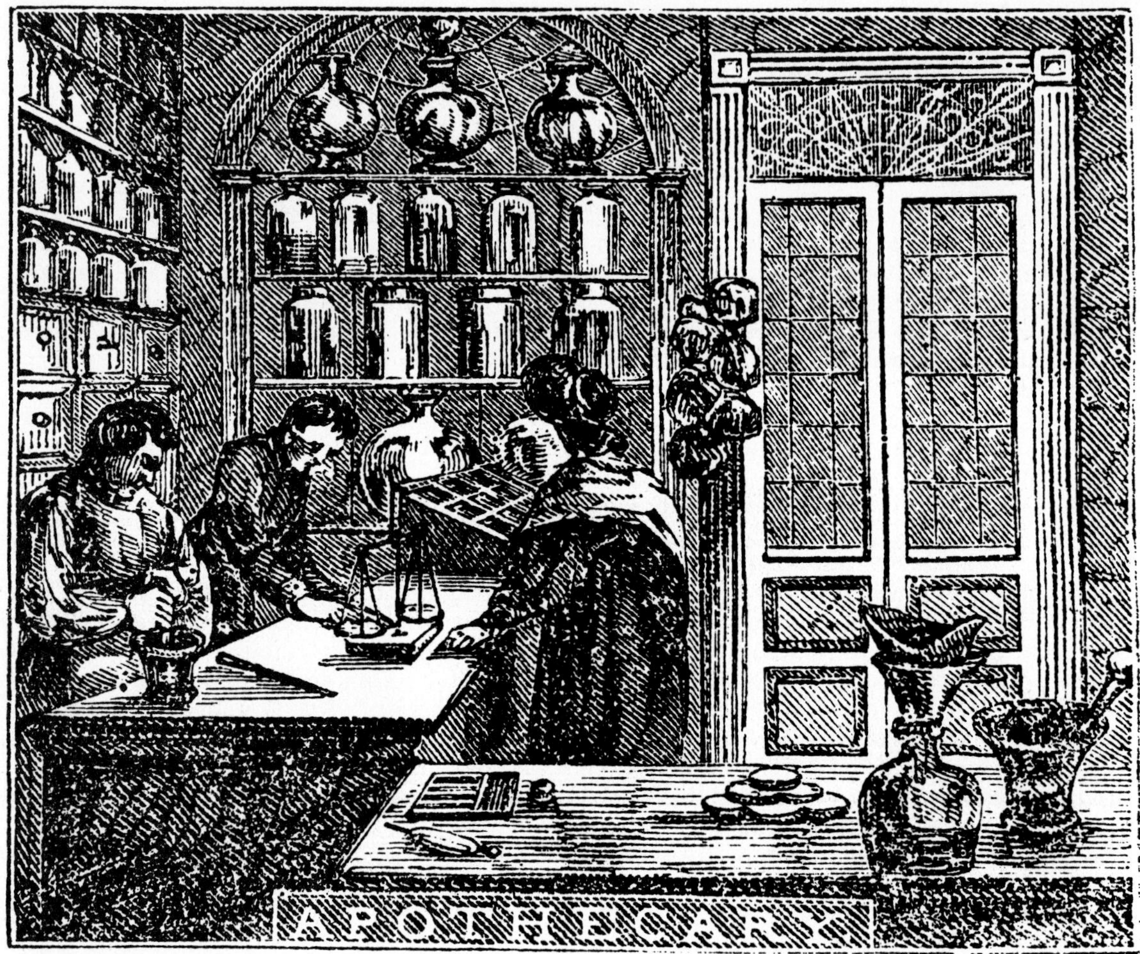


This interior of an American pharmacy is one of the earliest depicted in literature. It appeared in a book of vocational guidance, first published in 1836. (Edward Hazen: Popular Technology; or, Professions and Trades, vol. 1, New York, 1841, p. 236; photograph from the University of Wisconsin)

vious manifestation of a pharmaceutical profession in America, whereas the organization of the Pharmaceutical Society of Great Britain (1841) implied a revival.

In 1808 the legislature of the Territory of Orleans (Louisiana), apparently for the first time in the United States of America, made a diploma and an examination prerequisites for "practice . . . as . . . apothecary," as well as for practice as a physician or a surgeon. In spite of this law, no record of such an examination of an "apothecary" has come down to us. When the legislature of the new State of Louisiana (1816) revised the law, "one apothecary" was added to the four representatives of medicine and of surgery, who were entrusted with the examination of applicants for licensure in one of the health profes-

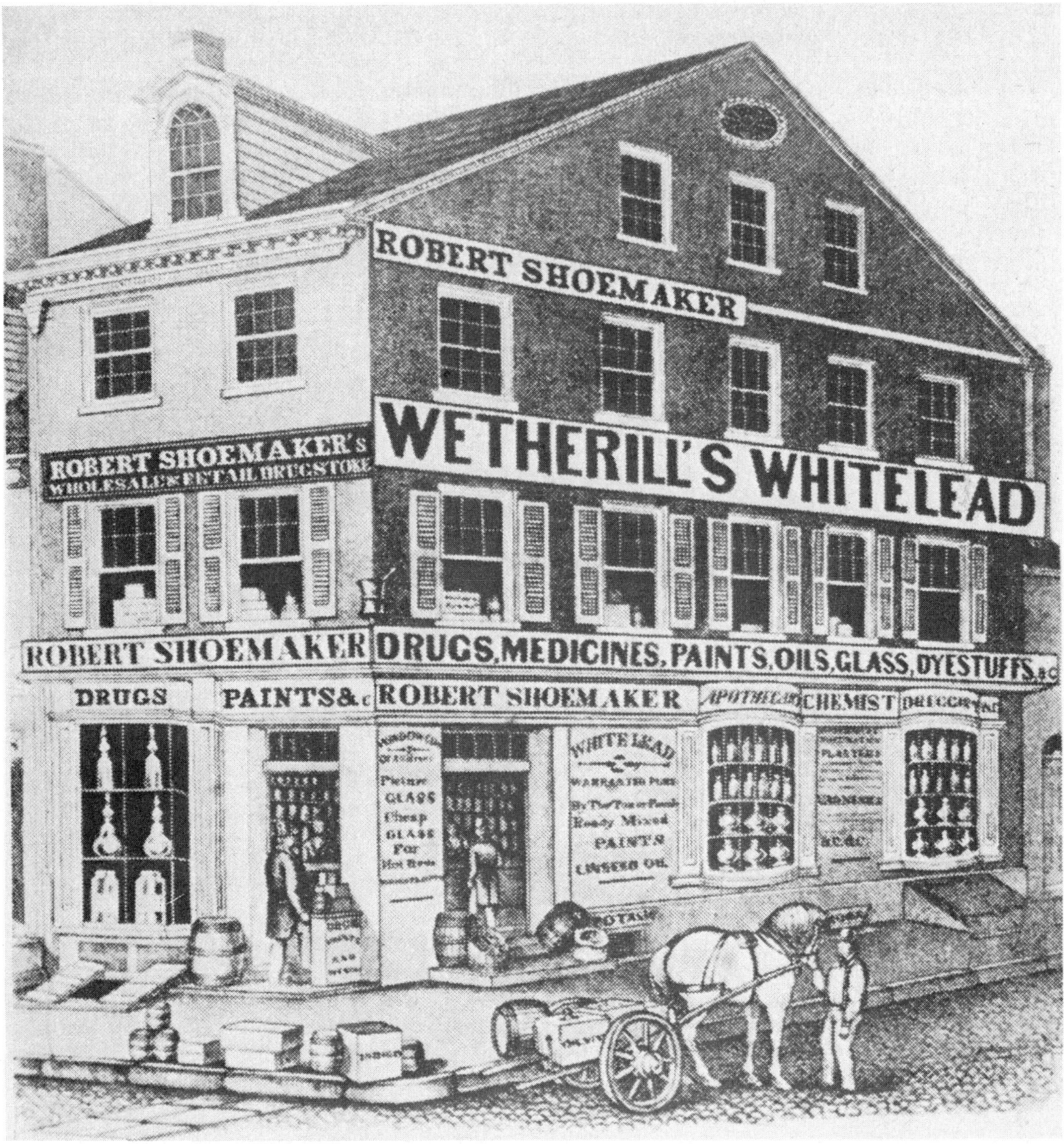

This Philadelphia establishment, depicted about 1850, exemplifies the combining of retail and wholesale functions in early American pharmacy. Glycerin manufacture in a back-room laboratory by Robert Shoemaker (1817–1897) may have been the first in America on a larger scale. The "show" globes and bottles filling the display windows reflect British custom. (From: American Institute of the History of Pharmacy)

sions.[39] Although a committee of the Louisiana House of Representatives preferred not to "insist on the examination of apothecaries which had been urged in the law submitted to us," two gentlemen of New Orleans, F. Grandchamps and L. J. Dufilho, became the first pharmacists known to have been licensed within a political jurisdiction of the United States.[40]

The State of South Carolina was the first of the former British colonies for which there is undeniable evidence of a pharmaceutical examination (1818) as a prerequisite for a pharmaceutical license. The legislature had passed an act (1817) obliging every apothecary to obtain a license from "the medical society of South Carolina or board of physicians," thus empowering these bodies "to examine any apothecary, who may apply to them for a license." In 1818, a Richard Johnson was granted the license "to pursue the business of druggist," after being examined:

> 1. on the definition of chemistry and pharmacy, 2. on the preparation of mercury and phosphorus, 3. on the preparation of phosphate of antimony and tartar emetic, 4. on the doses of Laudanum, tartar emetic, ipecac, and Fowler's mineral solution of arsenic, 5. on the mode of making the common plaster and mixing the ol. ricini with water.[41]

Thus, after the Revolutionary War, the groundwork was laid for a system to certify the competency of American society's pharmacists. The groundwork also had been laid—by previous decades of unstructured, divergent developments—for a large proportion of commercially oriented drugstores, and for some establishments with professional aims, such as we viewed earlier in the West European development of pharmacy.

These drugstores signalled a trend toward the separation of pharmacy from medicine, increasingly from the last quarter of the 18th century on.

For example, in place of the six drugstores in Philadelphia not owned by physicians about 1750, there were twenty in 1785.[42] At that time the population numbered 40,000. In 1786, when New York City had a population of 23,600, six "druggists and apothecaries," are mentioned besides one "physician and apothecary" and one "surgeon and apothecary."[43] Medical men operating public drug shops were listed separately from the "druggists and apothecaries" proper. In 1821, in Philadelphia and its outlying districts with a population of 137,000, there were about 130 stores "identified with the trade in drugs."[44] In Boston at the same time with a population of 43,000, there were 7 wholesale and 23 retail establishments,[45] the wholesale druggists also dispensing directly to the public.

The public drug shops of the physicians, although not disappearing entirely until the end of the 19th century, were definitely on their way out. However, few of the medical practitioners surrendered the *dispensing* of medicines within their practice. As late as 1819, this custom was taken for granted by physicians to such an extent that the president of the New York College of Physicians and Surgeons argued that it was unnecessary for the students of medicine to attend a course in materia medica, because before entering the school the candidate was required to have "studied three years with some regular practitioner." In this time, he claimed, the medical candidate would learn "better than in any other school, the nature, powers, and doses, of all the remedies in common use, by daily handling and preparing them in putting up the prescriptions of his teacher."[46]

The importance of pharmacy in times of emergency, which had been demonstrated during the Revolutionary War, was soon to be re-emphasized. In 1793, the first plague —believed to have come to the city with refugees from Haiti—broke out in Philadelphia, then the seat of the national government. It is said that 5,000 died and 17,000 left the city. "The national government removed its offices; papers stopped publication; business, except dealing in drugs, almost ceased to exist."[47]

This availability of drugs in time of great public need must have increased both the general respect in which the apothecaries of Philadelphia were held and their own professional self-esteem—the two bases on which the first American professional association was later founded. It may here be recalled that a similar event occurred in the history of English pharmacy (see p. 103).

The period of reconstruction after the Revolutionary War was a time of ferment. Some problems were touched on, ways of clarification were attempted, many a beginning was made. While all of this was necessary and not in vain, nothing assumed definite shape. The first attempts at regulation of medical and pharmaceutical practice failed. America was not yet amenable to the firm regulation and limitation of professional activity that are considered necessary in more densely populated countries, but impracticable in a continent with vast undeveloped areas.

The rapid conquest of these areas for civilization, and for developing them commensurately with the progress in the older parts of the United States, would not have been possible without giving the pioneers all possible "liberty" to do what the actual circumstances demanded of them. Thus, for a long time regulation was left to self-discipline and initiative by the professional groups.

## WESTWARD MOVEMENT OF THE FRONTIER

The "westward movement" before the Revolutionary War had been, in large part at least, a movement to the south—down the fertile valley of the Shenandoah, for example. After the Revolution the mountain barriers were overcome, and the movement west of the Alleghenies became one of the dominant factors of American national life. As a result of the Revolution, all the western areas that had been partly ceded to the province of Quebec by England shortly before the war were transferred to the United States. Furthermore, the war necessitated a rapid westward development for both political and financial reasons.

"As early as September, 1776, Congress tried to encourage enlistments by offering bounties of land—500 acres to a colonel, 100 acres to a private, and other ranks in proportion."[48] After the war, George Washington gave his officers the parting admonishment that "The extensive and fertile regions of the West will yield a most happy asylum to those fond of domestic enjoyment, and seeking for personal independence."[49] Many people poured across the free land that held promise of this "personal independence." With every wave of this movement, extending westward the boundaries of the United States, pioneer scenes of the Atlantic coast were re-enacted.

In 1800, it was estimated that there were a million people inhabiting the area west of the Alleghenies. Ten years later, the number had risen to two and a half million; by 1830, to three and one-half million.[50]

As the West became more populous, the frontier medicopharmaceutical scenes described in such works as Cooper's *The Pioneers* and Gestäcker's *Die Regulatoren von Arkansas*,[51] and others,[52] gave way to practices that were hardly different from those of the East. The advertisements in a Milwaukee journal, for example, could just as well have appeared in a seaboard newspaper: "Higby and Wardner, dealers in drugs, medicines, paints, oils, dye-woods & stuffs" recommended (1841) an extensive assortment of these goods, listed as "just arrived," together with "brushes, perfumery, patent medicines and a general assortment of physician's and chemist's preparations, among them Corrosive Sub, Red Precip, Opium, etc." In

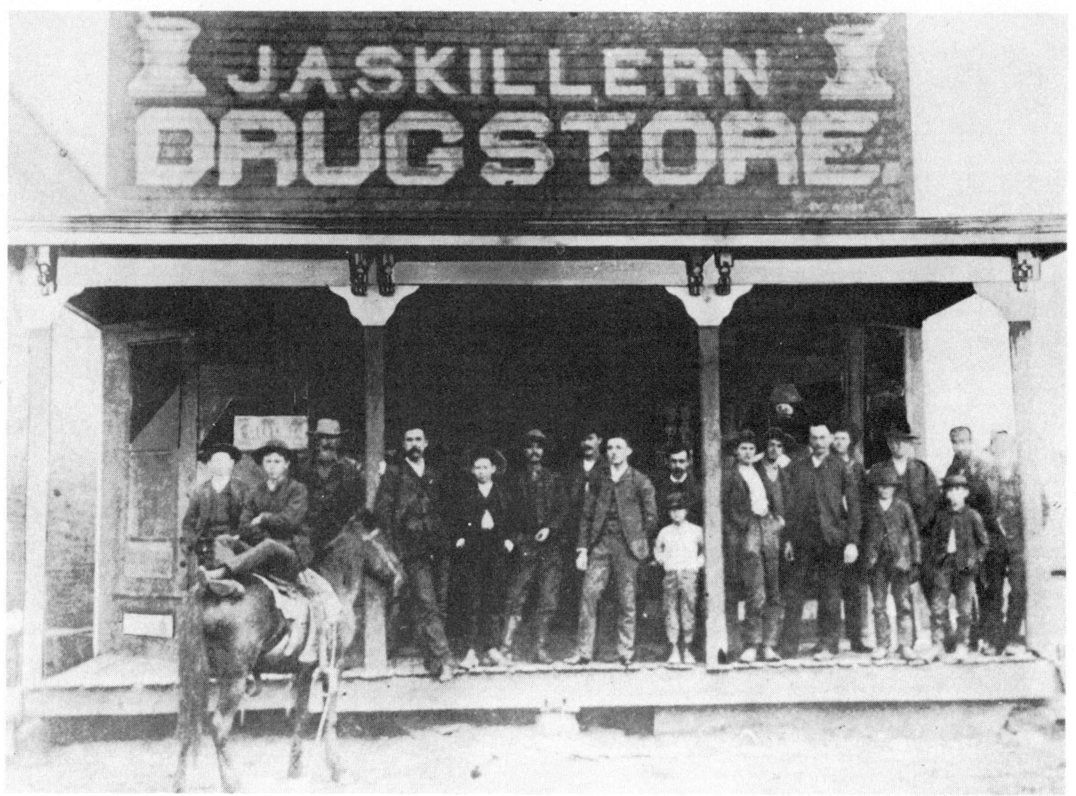


A drugstore in a Texas town of the 1880's reminds us that those practicing pharmacy faced the same rude conditions of life and work as did most people who migrated Westward. Uneven development of the country long hindered attempts to establish national standards for pharmacy and other occupations with professional aspirations. (Photograph of first drugstore in Lewisville, Texas; from Chain Store Age)

another advertisement, Fred Wardner announced a most varied line of goods (steel, stoves, glassware, etc.) as well as drugs and medicines.[53]

It would be a mistake to conclude from some crudities that the pioneers had only material objectives. Already in 1787, the charter of the settlements in the old Northwest Territory stated that "religion, morality, and knowledge, being necessary to good government and the happiness of mankind, schools and the means of education shall forever be encouraged."[54] In its contract with Congress the Ohio Company provided, on its own initiative, two entire townships for a university. "Under this provision Ohio University was established at Athens in 1808 as the first state university in the world under democratic government."[55]

In these new states, after the period of infancy, ideas of importance for pharmacy developed. In the recognition of pharmaceutical education as a valid function of a university, the state universities of the Midwest were to assume a role of leadership in American pharmacy. (See p. 232)

PART THREE

# Pharmacy in the United States

Section Two

## The Period of Organized Development

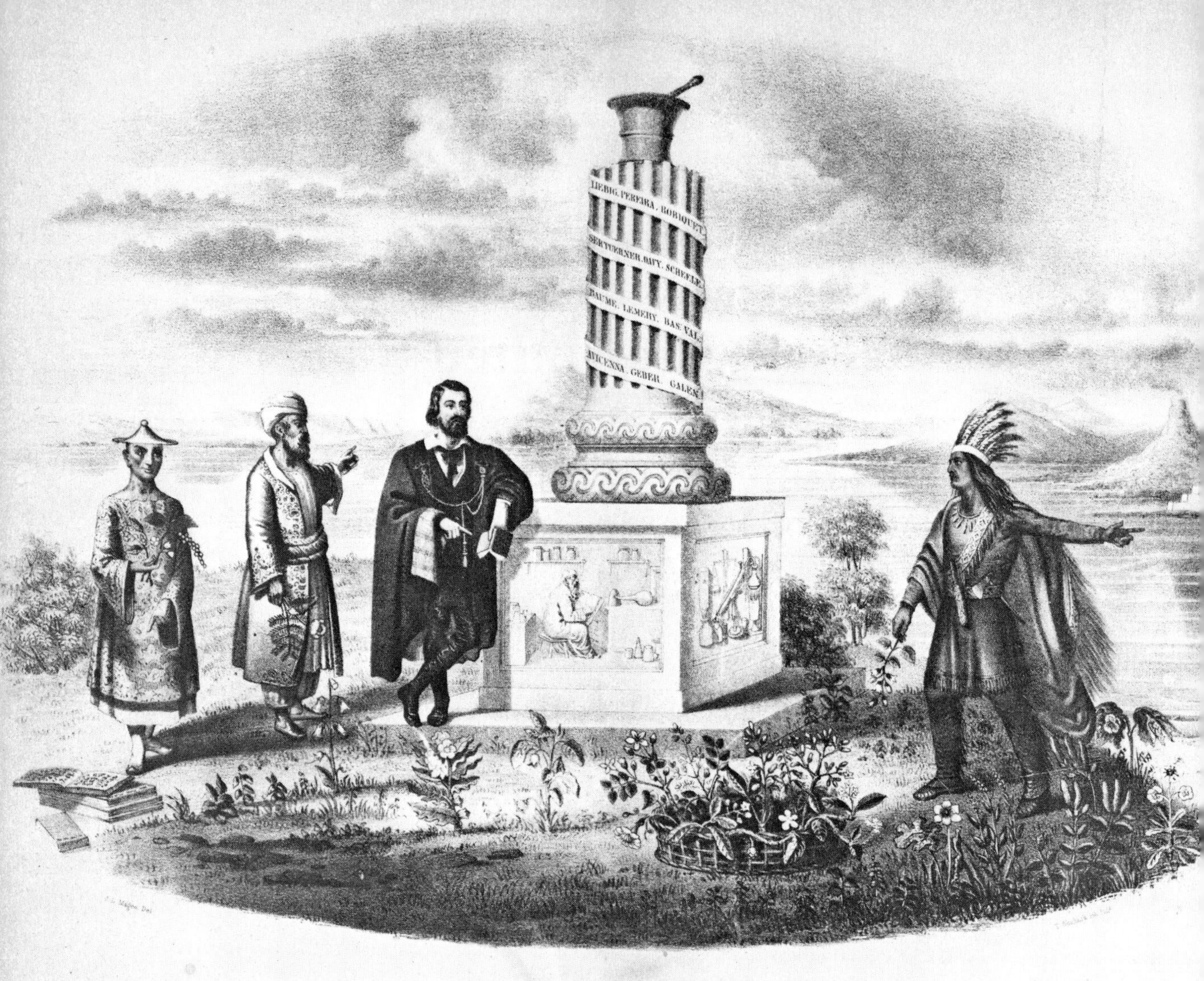


# AMERICAN PHARMACEUTICAL ASSOCIATION.

**FOUNDED A.D. 1852.**

*This is to Certify that* John F. Hancock *has been elected a* Contributing *Member of the American Pharmaceutical Association*

ATTESTED this Ninth day of September 1863. *In Testimony whereof are hereunto affixed the names of the proper officers.*

William Evans Jr. SECRETARY

J Faris Moore PRESIDENT

J. M. Maisch V. PRESIDENT

# 12

# The Growth of Associations

## LOCAL ORGANIZATIONS

The preceding chapter pointed out how the restrictions and regulations necessary to raise American pharmacy to the status of a profession were, for a long time, left to the initiative of individual pharmacists. This initiative was not always taken spontaneously.

On the one hand, the few people who combined professional vision with pharmaceutical education and skill prospered, requiring no regulations for the proper conduct of their establishments. On the other hand, the uneducated merchants who called themselves druggists did not want regulation. This merchant class may be divided into two groups. One was worried about its ability to meet regulations requiring even a modicum of knowledge. The other group conducted an unscrupulous business, possible only because there was no regulation and control.

Pressure from outside pushed pharmacists and druggists in the United States toward organizing their first associations. This pressure came from the medical profession. During the first half of the 18th century, the situation within the medical profession was not much better than that of pharmacy. However, one center of American cultural and scientific life had the oldest American school of medicine and the greatest number of well-educated physicians: Philadelphia, where a proper separation of pharmacy and medicine already had been undertaken by the founder of its medical school. So it is not surprising that the next step in the direction of professional pharmacy was taken in Philadelphia, originating in the proposal of a Philadelphia professor of medicine. In response to the implied challenge, pharmacists organized the first pharmaceutical association striving to attain professional aims, based on adequate education.

This undertaking was not the first attempt by physicians to secure better regulation of the drug trade. Shortly after the Revolutionary War the Massachusetts Medical Society petitioned the legislature to prohibit the sale

←

Ornate and symbol-laden, the original membership certificate of the American Pharmaceutical Association was based on the certificate of the Pharmaceutical Society of Great Britain. ". . . Objections were made to the adoption of any part of the English certificate, desiring a picture suggestive only of American ideas, but the Committee very properly pointed to the universality of Pharmaceutic Science . . . " The classic column represents the old and solid foundation of the profession; on it a winding scroll lists some of the great names out of its history. Every region contributes to pharmacy and the materia medica (note medicinal plants and books), as suggested by the four figures representing, *left* to *right*, the Far East, the Middle East, Europe and the Americas. (See Am. J. Pharm. *27*:483, 485, and *28*:187–188.)

of bad or adulterated drugs.[1] Early 19th-century laws in Louisiana and South Carolina, under medical impetus, established the principle of examination and licensure as prerequisites for the practice of pharmacy.

A difference between these movements and the one in Philadelphia is noteworthy: In their earlier efforts, the medical societies in Massachusetts and the legislators in Louisiana introduced measures affecting future druggists. In the attempt at Philadelphia (March, 1820), all shopowners in the city who called themselves apothecaries, chemists or druggists were affected directly and immediately. J. Redman Coxe, with the support of the University of Pennsylvania, made a "suggestion" to which 16 prominent Philadelphia druggists affixed their signatures:

> It is suggested that by a close attention for at least three years in an apothecary's shop to the practical part of their duties and after two courses of lectures on the subject of chemistry, materia medica, and pharmacy, such persons may be subjected to an examination by the professors of those branches in the University, and if found qualified, may receive a degree under some appropriate denomination which, being publicly known, may ensure them a greater chance of popular favor than will probably be granted to those who are neglectful or indifferent to the high responsibility they are invested with.[2]

There was a general outcry against the plan among Philadelphia druggists, opposition fanned by a proposal of the medical faculty to offer honorary degrees initially to a select few. Those not distinguished by the proffered degree of "master of pharmacy" and not able or willing to obtain it by passing the examination inferred that they were to be branded as "neglectful or indifferent." However, the same statement which caused Philadelphia druggists to resent the action of the medical faculty also suggested the proper way of counteraction. The medical leader of the University of Pennsylvania plan, having referred to the English Society of Apothecaries, remarked that the pharmaceutical progress (in Philadelphia) which he had in mind could not be achieved in any "other way than by the measure proposed," because "such an incorporated association does not exist here."

Apothecaries and druggists organized their first meeting only four days after the board of trustees of the University of Pennsylvania published its resolution concerning the examination (February 1821). This was the first united action known in the history of American pharmacy. A committee was appointed to determine whether it might not be "preferable to adopt a plan as a substitute, distinct from the one proposed."[3] This committee, led by Henry Troth[4], consisted of nine men, among them the most prominent Philadelphia wholesale druggists. "It was an enterprise of youth, for the average age of the five whose ages we know was but 28 years at the time of the founding.[5]

The report of the committee, delivered at a second meeting, admits that "medicines of inferior or sophisticated qualities" were "too often introduced into the shops," due to "the want of proper pharmacological information on the part of some druggists and apothecaries who vend" and also "of physicians who buy." One passage frankly states that it was the "happy effect" of the action of the University to rouse the druggists "to a sense of the propriety of placing their business on the respectable footing it ought to possess as a branch of the science of medicine." As the best method "to effectuate the reformation generally desired in the business," the committee recommended "the establishment of a College of Apothecaries, the attention of which will be constantly directed to the qualities of articles brought into the drug market," and furthermore of "a school of pharmacy."

Despite that, the University of Pennsylvania carried through its arrangements, conferred the honorary degree of a Master of Pharmacy on 16 Philadelphia pharmacists, and opened a course in pharmacy. Yet, "not a single student ever attended the lectures in the Medical Department with the view of

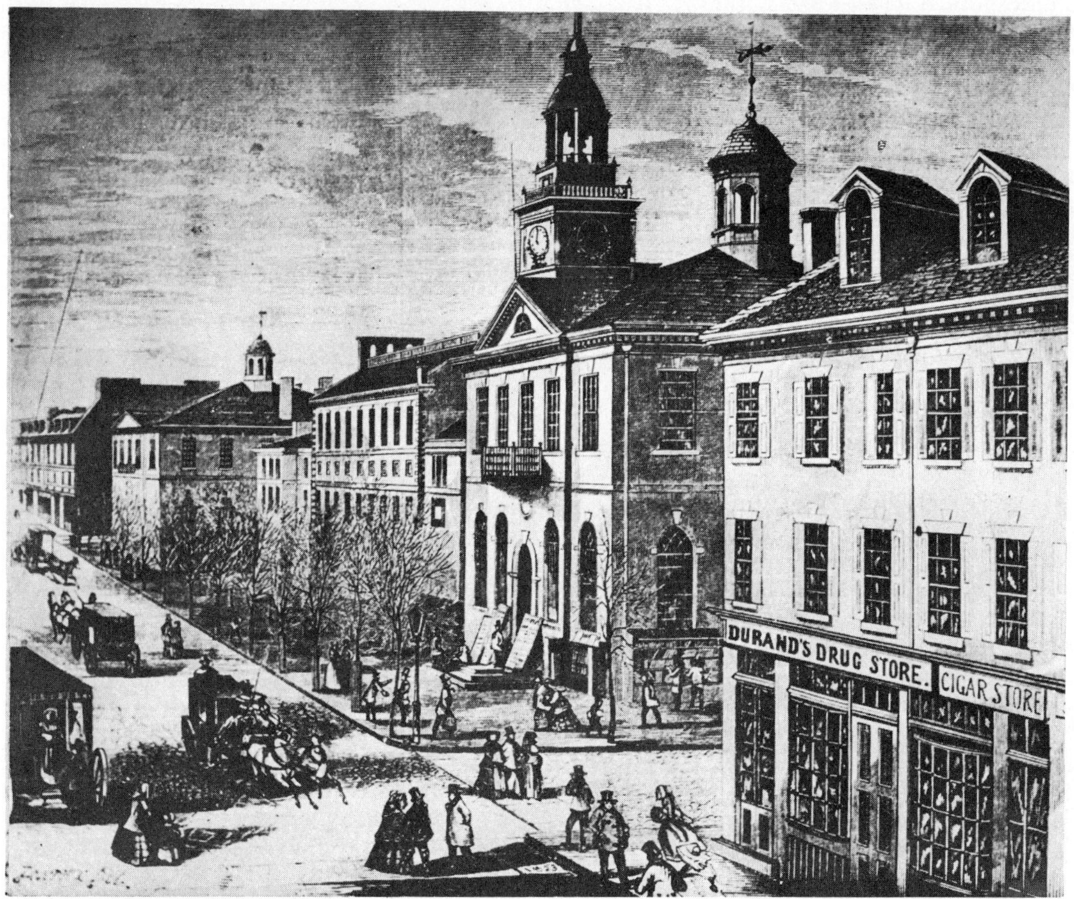


Many contributions to American pharmacy during its formative period stemmed from this corner pharmacy at Chestnut and 6th Streets in Philadelphia, shown as it appeared in the 1850's. It was outfitted in the most elegant French manner by a French immigrant pharmacist, Elias Durand. Durand and his chief staff pharmacist, Augustine J. L. Duhamel, kept American pharmacy in touch with pharmaceutical developments in France, published investigations of their own in American pharmacy's first journal and were active in the first association (Philadelphia).

securing the degree of Master of Pharmacy."[6]

The "College of Apothecaries,"[7] established after the hearing of the report by those present at the meeting of March 13, 1821, changed its name about a year later to "College of Pharmacy." This term was to be applied later to other early American pharmaceutical associations but eventually became restricted largely to pharmaceutical schools.

The designation "College" was chosen with the intent of placing the new organization on the same footing with its well-known medical sister, the Philadelphia College of Physicians. This in turn had been named in accord with an old English custom. (The English "Royal College of Physicians," for example, was founded in 1518.) However, the change in the College title, from "apothecaries" to "pharmacy," shows an understanding of the situation in the world of pharmacy at this time.[8]

The English "apothecaries" had become medical practitioners to an increasing extent and could no longer be considered as typical representatives of the profession of pharmacy. Hence, the designation "apothecary" could be misleading. The more recent English terms "chemist" and "druggist" did not solve the dilemma, for neither had yet achieved the status of a profession.

France and, to a certain extent, Germany offered a solution. Almost half a century earlier, the French term *apothecaire* had been replaced by the term *pharmacien.* A *Collège de pharmacie,* an association of Parisian pharmacists had included members of the highest scientific attainment. This made the word *pharmacie* a recognized European designation for the entirety of professional pharmaceutical activity. Even in Germany, where the pharmaceutical practitioner still called himself by the old term *Apotheker,* the word *pharmacie* had replaced the expression *Apothekerkunst* to designate the profession as a whole. The two pharmaceutical journals of international fame were the French *Bulletin* [later *Journal*] *de pharmacie* and the German Trommsdorff's *Journal der Pharmacie.* Hence, "College of Pharmacy" was the term of choice for an association of practitioners who were eager to conduct their activities on the basis of scientific knowledge and professional ideals.

A French pharmacist in Philadelphia, in connection with the Philadelphia College of Pharmacy, immediately exerted a strong foreign influence on American pharmacy. This was the former *pharmacien* of the Grand Army of Napoleon I, Elias Durand, who established a pharmacy in Philadelphia (1825). William Procter, Jr., his famous contemporary, describes Durand's importance as follows:

> His [Durand's] store became an important center of pharmaceutical information, which directly and indirectly had much to do with the introduction of scientific pharmacy into Philadelphia, and through this college, its Journal and graduates into the United States. Many of the finer medicinal chemicals were made in this country first by Durand. . . .[9]

A young Philadelphian, born of French parents, Augustine J. L. Duhamel, had learned pharmacy under Durand's tutelage, and strengthened the French influence on American scientific pharmacy. By the age of 33, he had published 34 papers in the *American Journal of Pharmacy.*[10]

Since the Philadelphia College of Pharmacy had been founded as an association (like the early colleges of physicians and the French *Collège de pharmacie*), its professional activity was by no means restricted to the establishment and the administration of its school. Its constitution provided for "a committee of inspection" for the examination of drugs "brought into the market and submitted to them," and a "committee of equity, to settle any disputes that may arise in the transactions of the members of the college." The constitution stated that members "guilty of adulterating or sophisticating any articles of medicine or drugs or of knowingly vending articles of that character, or of deteriorated qualities may be expelled."[11]

The leaders of the College maintained a balance between the scientific and the commercial interests of the calling which they represented and tried to promote. One of the first steps was the publication (1824) of carefully determined formulas for the imitation of secret-formula "patent medicines" hitherto imported from England.[12]

The leaders of the College founded the first American pharmaceutical journal (1825), the *Journal of the Philadelphia College of Pharmacy,* to disseminate current scientific and professional information.[13] The College also issued (1826) *The Druggist's Manual,* "a price current of drugs, medicines, paints, dyestuffs, glass, patent medicines, etc., with

Latin and English synonyms, a German, French, and Spanish catalogue of drugs, tables of specific gravities, etc., etc., and a variety of useful matter."[14]

Having laid down in its constitution the fundamentals of professional pharmacy and having tried to realize them partially, it is not surprising that the Philadelphia College of Pharmacy became the model and sometimes the advisor of other local American pharmaceutical associations founded between 1821 and the Civil War—that event which so greatly changed the political, economic and spiritual life of the United States. The following list shows the spread of the early pharmaceutical associations:

- 1821 Philadelphia College of Pharmacy
- 1823 Massachusetts College of Pharmacy
- 1829 College of Pharmacy of the City (and County) of New York
- 1840 Maryland College of Pharmacy
- 1850 Cincinnati College of Pharmacy
- 1859 Chicago College of Pharmacy
- 1864 St. Louis College of Pharmacy (precursors in 1854 and 1857)

Boston and New York were the first American cities to follow the example of Philadelphia in organizing pharmaceutical associations. These three cities were at that time not only leaders in general cultural standards but the most important ports for the entrance of drugs from overseas, and the sites of the three oldest medical schools in the country. The medical associations of these three cities took the first steps toward the establishment of uniform drug standards, which finally brought about the first *United States Pharmacopoeia* (1820).

Repeating an earlier attempt to bring about legal regulation of pharmacy, the Massachusetts Medical Society petitioned the legislature (1823) to give the Society, "together with an association of apothecaries for all parts of the Commonwealth, if such an association should hereafter be incorporated," the power to appoint "Boards of Examiners," to examine all people "who may hereafter wish to compound or retail medicines in small quantities or to put up the prescriptions of physicians," and to grant licenses. In justifying the interest of the physicians in this regulation, the petition stated that:

> physicians are daily discontinuing the practice of compounding or preparing the medicines which they use, and have therefore become in a great measure dependent upon the druggists and other retailers of medicine.[15]

This separation of pharmacy from medicine had been advocated as a desirable goal, and noted as partly achieved in the big cities, in the *Pharmacopoeia* of the Massachusetts Medical Society 15 years earlier (1808).

The attempt of Boston physicians to play a decisive role in pharmaceutical affairs suffered the same fate as that of their Philadelphia colleagues. As a result of the opposition led by several wholesale druggists, it was defeated.[16] However, the pharmaceutical association recommended in the medical petition was founded (December 26, 1823) in accordance with advice asked of the Philadelphia College of Pharmacy.[17] The constitution of the new Massachusetts College of Pharmacy emphasized the same points as its Philadelphia model. In the activity of the two first American pharmaceutical colleges, the main difference was that in Philadelphia lectures were provided continuously from the year of founding, whereas in Boston no serious attempt at regular instruction was made until 1867.

The early drug lists published by the Massachusetts College (e.g., 1828) may be considered the first American attempt to fix the prices for drugs and medicines on the basis of associative agreement.[18] The "Catalogue of the Materia Medica and of the Pharmaceutical Preparations with the Uniform Prices of the Massachusetts College of Pharmacy" gives in classic brevity the motives for the "uniform prices":

> . . . A judicious arrangement as to prices is no small means of adding support and dignity to the

business. . . . One evil where there is a difference in price is, that the purchaser either thinks that the one who charged high wronged him as to price, or that the one who charged low wronged him as to quality. . . . A competition as to prices must be eventually ruinous to all; but a competition as to the quality of the medicines and attention to business will add to the respectability and standing of the profession.

Significantly, this preface still appears with exactly the same wording in the price list published in 1854.

The list of founders of the College of Pharmacy of the City of New York shows that here, too, the wholesale druggists were instrumental in promoting American professional pharmacy.[19] These proud and self-conscious men, like their colleagues in Boston and Philadelphia, wished to regulate their affairs according to their own ideas and not under the supervision of the medical profession. The College was founded as "an association of pharmacists, druggists, and others interested in the progress of the profession, for purposes of mutual instruction, protection and assistance in all matters pertaining to their professional welfare; the school for undergraduates forming merely the teaching department of the institution."[20]

The Maryland College was founded, not in counteracting some action or demand on the part of physicians, but as a fruit of friendly understanding. The Maryland medical and chirurgical faculty initiated a meeting with representatives of Baltimore pharmacists "with the idea of elevating pharmacy." At this meeting, a committee of five pharmacists was appointed, which undertook all further steps leading to the founding, in 1840, of the Maryland College of Pharmacy. This association was more or less active until 1847, "but thereafter languished until 1856, when . . . it was thoroughly reorganized."[21]

The founding of the Cincinnati College of Pharmacy was more indirectly influenced by the sister profession of medicine, when "The meeting of the American Medical Association in Cincinnati in the year of 1850 . . . was so fraught with the high ideals in medicine that the founders of the Cincinnati College of Pharmacy were stimulated to greater effort in the accomplishment of their plans.[22]

After the St. Louis Medical Society in 1854 protested against the "habit of prescribing for and administering medicines" by druggists and the refilling of prescriptions without authorization by the physician, the pharmacists founded the St. Louis Pharmaceutical Association for promoting a more brotherly feeling among the members of the profession of pharmacy . . . and [for] the improvement of the educational status of the apothecaries and druggists."[23]

This association was not very active. It was reorganized in 1857 but died during the Civil War.[24] Finally, on November 11, 1864, the St. Louis College of Pharmacy was founded, not in defense against but in close harmony with the medical profession. Like the older associations, this new St. Louis pharmaceutical organization was influenced by Philadelphia, for example, adopting for its own use the constitution and by-laws of the Philadelphia College.[25]

The foundation of the Chicago College of Pharmacy, in 1859, was influenced by the American Pharmaceutical Association,[26] which had been established in 1852 and gradually became inseparable from each progressive step in American pharmacy. The constitution, the by-laws and the code of ethics of the Chicago College were unmistakable offspring of those of the Philadelphia College and of the American Pharmaceutical Association.

All the local organizations noted above developed into institutions in which the educational branch (i.e., the school) became dominant. There were some other early local pharmaceutical associations that did not.[27]

As demonstrated, the rise of early local pharmaceutical associations was due to outer circumstances more than to professional enthusiasm of member druggists. Even the Philadelphia College of Pharmacy, the early and consistent herald and standard-bearer of

American professional pharmacy, experienced times in which indifference among the passive majority of practitioners became threateningly obvious in the decrease of its membership.

The general American appetite for independence expressed itself both in the formation of the early American pharmaceutical associations and in their decline when the independence of the drug trade no longer seemed endangered. The average American of this period did not want any restrictions, whether by a special group thinking itself superior to him (in this special case the medical profession), by his own associations, or even by laws that tried to regulate his conduct. Legislators respected this sentiment. This same typically American spirit had defeated early medical endeavor to regulate legislatively the practice of medicine in all its branches, including pharmacy, by forcing it under the control of legally authorized and chartered medical associations.

**German Influence**

On the other hand, there were pharmacists in America imbued, because of their origin and education, with an appreciation for authority. These were pharmacists of German descent who came to the United States in the turbulent years before the German Revolution (1848) or in its wake. Often ambitious and competent, they gained a steadily growing influence over the development of American pharmacy.

In early colonial times the German pharmacists in North America were neither numerous nor ambitious enough to exert lasting influence. Rather, the early development of American professional pharmacy found its model more in the French pharmacist, whose native country was America's ally in the struggle for independence. Had the later period (1830 to 1860) brought as many French pharmacists to the United States as it did of German pharmacists, the development of American pharmacy might have taken other directions. But in France, the July Revolution of 1830 (as well as that of 1848) was successful and hence caused no emigration. The German upheaval of 1848 failed, and the stern measures of the German princes against the revolutionaries forced thousands of the best-educated Germans to seek refuge in the United States. This fact has been important in American cultural life. The fact that German physicians and pharmacists had played an important part in the German political movement of 1848 brought a great number of them to America.[28]

These German pharmacists spread over the country. All of them possessed practical and scientific training and a professional standard which at that time could not be equalled either by the English chemists and druggists or by the few graduates of early American colleges of pharmacy, not to mention the druggists without college education. As a result, their pharmaceutical practice was recognized as exemplary and was imitated. In some cities, such as St. Louis, Cincinnati and Milwaukee, a great number of the genuine pharmacies were for a long time in the hands of such "'48ers" or of German immigrant pharmacists following them. Others were owned by American-born citizens trained by German immigrants; occasionally they completed their pharmaceutical education in Germany. These people were inclined to foster professional ideals and to endeavor to promote them by means of associations.[29]

A group of such German pharmacists founded (1851) the *New Yorker Pharmaceutischer Leseverein* (New York Pharmaceutical Literary Society), the first American pharmaceutical group formed with the purpose of improving the scientific, cultural and professional standards of its members without any regard to business affairs. Furthermore, it was the first to obligate its members to notify the board of the society when taking an apprentice, to fix the period of apprenticeship, and to make the examination of apprentices obligatory.[30]

In the first years of its existence the members of the New York German Pharmaceutical Society sent their apprentices to the New

York College of Pharmacy. When the College became dormant in the late 1850's, the German Society filled the gap by instructing apprentices until the College revived.[31]

The two German immigrants who exerted the greatest influence on the development of American pharmacy were John M. Maisch, the first general secretary of the American Pharmaceutical Association, and Charles Rice, the creator of the modern American pharmacopeia. They did not come to America as German pharmacists but became pharmacists after their immigration. Perhaps that fact helped them to give more to American pharmacy in general. The danger of isolation because of special professional education and traditions acquired abroad did not exist for them. They thought in terms of American pharmacy and tried to improve it in accord with their general background. A third man who should be named together with these two great American pharmacists of German birth is Frederick Hoffman. He was a German pharmacist, having passed all German pharmaceutical examinations, but, nevertheless, one of the greatest journalists and the most stimulating spirits that American pharmacy has had.

Some of the later local pharmaceutical associations have been branches of national organizations, e.g., the American Pharmaceutical Association branches (after 1905)[32] and the Greek-letter chapters of academic fraternities and sororities in pharmacy.[33] Of a different type are the alumni associations of the colleges (the first, in Philadelphia, f. 1864).

It required a central, nation-wide organization, which fostered the founding and growth of state organizations, in order gradually to develop a general professional feeling among pharmacists in America. With this came (as will be shown later) a greater willingness on the part of individual pharmacists to give up part of their independence for the benefit of all, to submit themselves to legal restrictions, and even to ask for them. However, this central organization, the American Pharmaceutical Association, originated not so much in a growing understanding of the necessity of professional solidarity among pharmacists as in pressure from outside, which also had brought into existence the early local associations. This pressure arose from bad conditions in the drug trade.

## STATE ORGANIZATIONS

Fifteen years after the founding of the American Pharmaceutical Association, the first state association, that of Maine, was founded (1867). Significantly, the establishment of this association coincided with the appointment of a "committee on legislation regulating the practice of pharmacy" by the American Pharmaceutical Association and was welcomed by the *American Journal of Pharmacy,* whose editors were among the most active leaders of the American Pharmaceutical Association.[34] However, the *Journal* apparently did not recognize at this time that the Maine association of pharmacists, representing an entire state, was not merely another local group, but the beginning of something entirely new.

The fate of the Maine association is obscure, but it had faltered, lay dormant until 1890, then revived and developed into the present association of pharmacists in that state.[35] Such was the fate of several state pharmaceutical associations. But their necessity had become so obvious that none disappeared permanently, as so many local associations had done. As John M. Maisch saw the main task of the state associations:

> A few subjects that ought to claim their attention are the enactments of laws for the regulation of pharmacy where none exist, and the amendment of those now in force where they are inadequate to the public or oppressive to those engaged in the practice of pharmacy. The cooperation of these various societies ought to be secured in an endeavor to modify the laws and rulings of the general government where they oppress the true liberty of those engaged in business.[36]

C. Lewis Diehl called these state pharmaceutical associations "the children of the American Pharmaceutical Association,"[37] and indeed, the Association inspired their founding wherever and whenever it could. "Thus we often find, that the early officers of the state organizations are also active members of the American association, and that the organization of a state body followed a meeting of the American association near the birth place of the new society."[38]

However, the medical influence, which had been so decisive in the formation of early local pharmaceutical societies, was sometimes an impelling force also in the establishment of state associations. For instance, it was only after steps by the Medical Society of New Jersey to force legislative measures on "all dispensers of medicines" in the state, that the New Jersey Pharmaceutical Association was founded (1870) "to establish the relation between them [the pharmacists] and physicians, and the people at large, upon just principles . . ."[39]

The State Medical Association of Mississippi resolved (1871) "that the druggists, pharmacists, and chemists of the State of Mississippi be requested to call a convention at an early day, and organize a State Pharmaceutical Association, to meet annually at the same time and place that the Medical Association does, and cooperate with it in any and all measures of mutual interest and importance."[40] Only a month later, the Mississippi Pharmaceutical Association was founded. This new organization tried to stabilize the good relations with its older medical sister, adopted the constitution of the American Pharmaceutical Association and urged "all pharmacists in the State to join" the national representative of American professional pharmacy.[41]

Yet, the founding of state pharmaceutical associations soon became a self-propelled and independent movement. At least potentially, these associations gave pharmacists a more effective medium for organized cooperation, but until the present century they usually represented—as did the earlier local associations—only a small ambitious minority of pharmacists. How the organization of pharmacists into state blocs spread through the country may be perceived from the chronologic list of the founding of the state associations (see Appendix 2).[42] That more than half of them were organized in little more than a decade, centering in the 1880's, gives striking evidence that the "time was ripe" for pharmacists to put their group efforts on a wider stage. During this period, also, most of the state pharmacy acts came into existence. Both lines of activity were stimulated by the American Pharmaceutical Association and, more particularly, by its general secretary, John M. Maisch. The desire to secure a pharmacy law, or amendments to a law considered unsatisfactory, caused most of the revivals of early and inactive state associations.[43]

While pharmacists themselves, through their associations, often were responsible for establishing schools and even operating them, by the turn of the century the associations and the schools tended increasingly to go separate ways. The influence of the local associations dwindled as state associations became dominant, and pharmacy schools, following an example set in some of the midwestern state universities, gradually associated themselves with general colleges or universities.

For a long time state pharmaceutical associations strongly reflected the business orientation and the limited education of the average American practitioner. They only slowly gathered support and more adequate staffs (even as late as 1947, of 39 associations reporting, 15 had no full-time executive officer)[44]; and their programs tended to be dominated by commercial concerns. But by midcentury, state associations in general were gaining wider support (partly by giving employee-pharmacists a status more nearly comparable with that of pharmacy owners), enlarging administrative facilities, and sharing more fully in the professional as well as economic concerns of pharmacy.

Symptomatic of the change was the increasingly widespread debate on how

American pharmacy might be organized for more effective action. In 1962, first in Michigan, then in Virginia, Delaware and Wisconsin, the state associatons voted to integrate more closely with the American Pharmaceutical Association at the national level and, at the same time, to try to revivify local associations. This became an "affiliation movement," which by 1975 had linked 20 of the 50 states into a more integrated structure—linking local, state and national levels through concurrent memberships and more effective lines of administration and communication on behalf of practicing pharmacists. It was a debatable trend, after decades of divided allegiances and disparate viewpoints. Probably it was the changes in the pharmacist's function and work setting, the shifting structure and economics of medical care, the inroads by crassly commercial interests after World War II that combined to convince large numbers of independent pharmacists that their professional heritage and prerogatives must be safeguarded cooperatively. In that cause, the American Pharmaceutical Association already had invested more than a century of consistent thought and endeavor. For, paradoxically, the Association was not erected on the foundation of an established professional pharmacy; rather, it had largely created American professional pharmacy.

## NATIONAL ORGANIZATIONS

### The American Pharmaceutical Association

The American Pharmaceutical Association was the first national pharmaceutical organization. For a long time it was the only one. During the decades in which the calling gained its distinctive shape, it represented, defended and promoted all fields of pharmaceutical enterprise and interest—the scientific and educational as well as the commercial, ethical and the legal. It always has been the guardian, although not always the initiator, of progressive movements concerning American pharmacy.

Until 1852, the concept of professional pharmacy was only a dream of the few colleges of pharmacy. Even if their influence extended beyond local boundaries, as that of the Philadelphia College of Pharmacy did, no means was available to promote the concept of professional pharmacy on a larger scale, to bring this concept to the presumptive members of the should-be profession, the general public, and especially the legislators. The American Pharmaceutical Association was founded by the early colleges of pharmacy to provide this means.

The immediate incentive for the founding of the American Pharmaceutical Association lay elsewhere, in the bad conditions of the drug market, whose dangers were accidentally made evident once again.

In New York, Ewen McIntyre, at that time a pharmacist for George D. Coggeshall, discovered that a portion of supposed calcium carbonate, imported from England, was in fact calcium sulfate. Coggeshall and his friend John Milhau brought the matter before the New York College of Pharmacy. Other preparations were examined and likewise proved to be substituted, adulterated or deficient in strength. Protests to British exporters brought a significant reply from one Englishman who stated that the products were "as good as the Americans would pay for."[45]

A petition to Congress, signed by pharmacists as well as by physicians all over the country, resulted in the subsequent passage of a law requiring the observance of certain standards for imported drugs, which went into force in 1848. The effect was unsatisfactory.

> This failure to secure the desired results was attributed to the lack of fitness on the part of the inspectors installed at the several ports of entry, who were appointed for their political affiliation rather than for their ability, although they were to some extent handicapped by the lack of clearness in the wording of the law in regard to standard books.[46]

In the mid-19th century there was still no strict borderline between medicine and pharmacy in the United States. Many men with medical degrees made their living chiefly, if not exclusively, by operating pharmacies. One of these, a doctor of medicine and a practicing pharmacist in the city of New York, requested (following the advice of the New York College of Pharmacy) that the American Medical Association act against drug adulteration. As a delegate of this pharmaceutical group, he presented a proposal (1851) concerning standards to be used by drug inspectors at the ports of entry.

The result was illuminating. The physicians attending the meeting doubted whether this proposal of a local group of pharmacists represented the opinion of American pharmacy as a whole. As the report in the *American Journal of Pharmacy* puts it, "the sentiment of the [American Medical] Association was evidently in favor of such a tariff of standards, but they wanted it to be more fully matured by a convention of Colleges [local associations] of Pharmacy."[47]

What a striking demonstration of the necessity for a national pharmaceutical organization, which would be representative of American pharmacy and could speak for the whole profession. Four months later (September 9, 1851) the New York College of Pharmacy invited the sister Colleges (that is, the local associations) in Philadelphia, Baltimore, Boston and Cincinnati to send delegates to a convention, with the restricted purpose of complying with the medical demands made at Charleston for united action of medicine and pharmacy in the question of drug adulteration. As the invitation put it, the convention was convened "for the purpose of considering the propriety and practicability of fixing a set of standard strengths and qualities of drugs and chemicals for the government of the United States Drug Inspectors."[48]

However, there was a strong feeling, at least among the members of one local group (the Philadelphia College of Pharmacy), that the time had come to consider, not one individual problem of American pharmacy, but the all-comprehensive problem of an American profession of pharmacy and its adequate and permanent representation. In the *American Journal of Pharmacy*, William Procter, Jr., then the Editor, gave the following account of their goal:

> When the invitation . . . was received by the Philadelphia College of Pharmacy, several of the members expressed the opinion that, although the call was for a special object, the Convention might take a wider range in its influence, and form a *point d'appuï* from which the pharmaceutical profession of the whole country may be reached, and a course of action instituted, which eventually would revolutionize the condition of Pharmacy in the United States.[49]

Coming to the "Convention of Pharmaceutists and Druggists" at New York in 1851 with such definite views, the Philadelphia delegation—particularly its most important member, William Procter, Jr.—imbued the minds of the participants from Boston and New York with a broader aim. (There were no delegates from Baltimore and Cincinnati.) It decisively shaped the unanimous adoption of the memorable resolution recommending

> that a Convention be called, consisting of three Delegates each from incorporated and unincorporated Pharmaceutical Societies, to meet at Philadelphia, on the First Wednesday in October 1852, when all the important questions bearing on the Profession may be considered, and *measures adopted for the organization of a National Association,** to meet every year.

When William Procter, Jr., stated that with the unanimous adoption of this resolution "the most sanguine hopes of these members [of the Philadelphia College of Pharmacy] were gratified," he was referring to a success which, to a very great extent, was won as a result of his personal insight and endeavor. As Procter declared "Fewness of numbers should not deter pharmaceutists from associating. A dozen well-disposed men can accomplish wonders when enlisted in a

*Italics added.

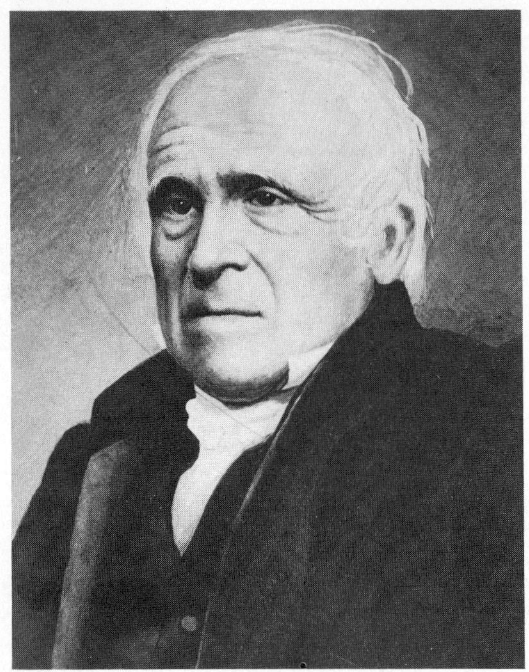

Presiding over the founding meeting of the American Pharmaceutical Association in 1852 was one of the most respected American pharmacists of his time, Daniel B. Smith, a practicing pharmacist of Philadelphia whose name is associated with diverse civic enterprises. For example, he was one of the organizers of Haverford College as well as the Philadelphia "House of Refuge" and the Apprentice's Library. He was the first President of the American Pharmaceutical Association, the first Secretary of the Philadelphia College of Pharmacy and the first Corresponding Secretary of the Historical Society of Pennsylvania. (From a portrait by John Collins, Philadelphia)

common cause and animated by a single interest."[50]

When the founding convention met the next year, October 6 to 8, 1852, in the Hall of the Philadelphia College of Pharmacy, probably 20 men from various parts of the country actively participated (including several officially seated although not bearing credentials as delegates of a society).

The venerable Daniel B. Smith, who 31 years earlier had been one of the founders of the Philadelphia College of Pharmacy (and its president from 1829 to 1854) was made the first president of the new national association. William Procter, Jr., of the same College, was elected corresponding secretary. The other officers were residents of Baltimore, Boston, Cincinnati and New York. The only other states represented at the founding convention were Virginia, California and Connecticut. There is no doubt that the early American Pharmaceutical Association was essentially an Eastern affair. Yet, at this time, so was the whole idea of pharmaceutical education and professionalism. The *aim* of these pioneers of American pharmacy, however, was a truly national and all-embracing one.

The preamble of the constitution admitted that "a large portion of those in whose hands the practice of pharmacy [in the United States] now exists, are not properly qualified for the responsible offices it involves, chiefly by reason of the many difficulties that impede the acquirement of a correct knowledge of their business."[51] How could this lack of education be remedied if those who needed it most were excluded instead of taken in? Hence the doors were thrown open to "all pharmaceutists and druggists who shall have attained the age of twenty-one years, whose character morally and professionally is fair, and who, after duly considering the obligations of the Constitution and Code of Ethics of this Association, are willing to subscribe to them." [Constitution of 1852]

Yet, this opening of the doors to "all pharmaceutists and druggists" seems more symbolic than actual, as the applicants were to subscribe to a "Code of Ethics" advanced far beyond the realities of common practice. This Code of Ethics, modeled after the one accepted by the Philadelphia College of Pharmacy (1848),[52] asked those who honored it "to discountenance quackery," which would include giving up the sale of nostrums regarded as "quackery" by organized medicine. This obligation, said Edward Parrish, "has never impressed itself as a duty upon many whose aid we desire to invoke in our earliest efforts. It is mainly by the sale of quack medicines that many druggists subsist, who yet desire a reform in their business, and would be glad to cooperate in the laudable objects of the Association . . . "[53] In his opinion, these ethical norms had to be the goal but not the condition for membership, while the new national organization was in its embryonic stage. Assenting to this view the Association dropped the obligation to subscribe to the Code of Ethics as a prerequisite of membership only three years after the founding.

The Code of Ethics disappeared from the literature of the American Pharmaceutical Association until its modified revival in 1922. At the instigation of Charles La Wall, the Association adopted a new and rather comprehensive code, stating in three sections the duties of the pharmacist (1) in his services to the public, (2) in his relations to the physician and (3) in his relations to other pharmacists and to the profession of pharmacy at large.[54]

In consequence of the shelving of the code of ethics, the goals of the Association, insofar as they were to be formalized and accepted by the members, had to be included in the Constitution. Therefore, Article I, which originally stated only the name of the organization, read as follows in the form adopted in 1856:

Article I. This association shall be called the American Pharmaceutical Association. Its aim shall be to unite the educated and reputable pharmaceutists and druggists of the United States in the following objects:

1st. To improve and regulate the drug market, by preventing the importation of inferior, adulterated or deteriorated drugs, and by detecting and exposing home adulteration.

2nd. To establish the relations between druggists, pharmaceutists, physicians and the people at large, upon just principles, which shall promote the public welfare and tend to mutual strength and advantage.

3d. To improve the science and the art of pharmacy by diffusing scientific knowledge among apothecaries and druggists, fostering pharmaceutical literature, developing talent, stimulating discovery and invention, and encouraging home production and manufacture in the several departments of the drug business.

4th. To regulate the system of apprenticeship and employment so as to prevent as far as practicable, the evils flowing from deficient training in the responsible duties of preparing, dispensing and selling medicines.

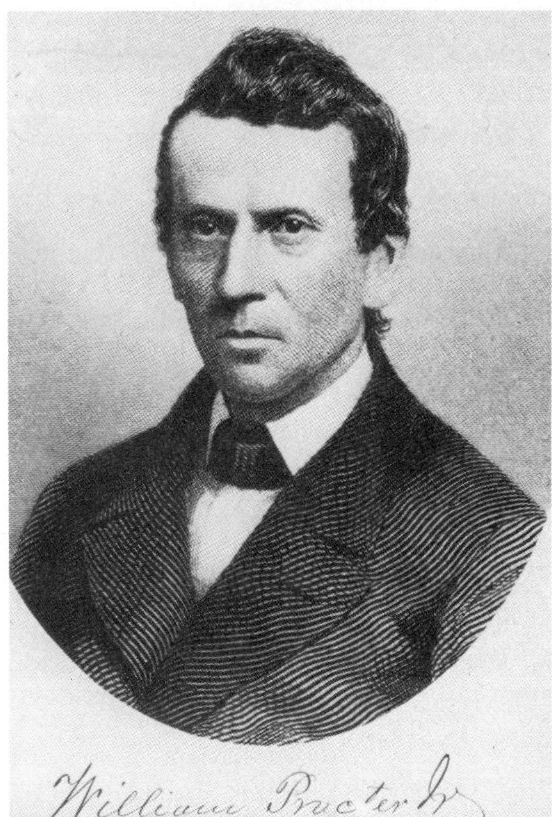


William Procter, Jr. (1817–1874), one of the most admired of all American pharmacists, depicted while a young, vigorous leader. An unruffled and unpretentious "Quaker" of integrity, Procter was astonishingly productive (about 550 articles) and versatile (practitioner, experimenter, editor, association leader, professor). "The favorite child of his genius was the American Pharmaceutical Association," said a contemporary, Albert Ebert.

5th. To suppress empiricism [i.e., quackery] and as much as possible to restrict the dispensing and sale of medicines to regularly educated druggists and apothecaries.

The 1856 constitutional revision required that each "pharmaceutist or druggist of good moral and professional standing" who became a member consider these objects and be "willing to subscribe to them." A member could be expelled "for improper conduct" by a vote of two-thirds of the members present, just as provided in connection with the earlier code of ethics.

An amendment adopted in 1870 implied that it no longer seemed appropriate to concede that "a large portion" of the pharmaceutical practitioners were "not properly qualified." The words "as much as possible" therefore, were dropped from clause 5 above, thus making it the unconditional task of the American Pharmaceutical Association "to suppress empiricism and to restrict the dispensing and sale of medicines to regularly educated druggists and apothecaries." Finally, two new clauses were added to Article I:

6th. To uphold standards of authority in the education, theory and practice of pharmacy.

7th. To create and maintain a standard of professional honesty equal to the amount of our professional knowledge, with a view to the highest good and greatest protection to the public.

The wisdom with which these constitutional purposes were originally written (1856) is evidenced by the Associations's "Objects" today. For although the phrasing has been modernized extensively (revision of Constitution and By-Laws, 1951), the fundamentals have changed little.[55]

The fact that the early colleges of pharmacy were associations of practicing pharmacists, which maintained educational institutions, was of the highest importance for the development of the new organization. The leaders of the colleges, who shaped the work of the American Pharmaceutical Association, had experienced in their local districts all the problems faced by pharmacy in this period and therefore were able to deal with them efficiently and realistically within the national organization.

Indeed the original constitution entitled each local society to five delegates at the annual meeting. Other individual pharmaceutists and druggists could be certified as voting participants under stated conditions, to give the Association a broader base of operations. After all, most drug dispensers were not organized into local societies, and no statewide organization yet existed.

Throughout its history the Association has tried to be representative of all pharmacists nationally who shared its professional aims. Since only a minority of those eligible have held personal membership at any given time, the Association has been careful to try to strike a balance between direct democracy and a representative form of decision-making that could claim to speak for the American profession at large.

The idea of adequate representation of all groups within American pharmacy, coupled with the growing complexity of reaching decisions in general sessions of accredited individuals participating in the annual meeting, led in 1911 to the establishment of the House of Delegates within the Association, a mechanism originated and promoted by the pharmacist-lawyer James H. Beal of Ohio.[56]

This policy-making body until the present day has consisted of delegates formally representing not only substituent groups within the Association itself, but delegates formally representing other local, state and national organizations. For several decades now, the controlling vote has lain, collectively, with delegates from each of the state pharmaceutical associations.

Since the 1950's there has been a spirit of growing professional independence among practicing pharmacists, particularly to avoid having their policies and values as a part of health care shaped or prefabricated by "drug groups" not consisting predominantly of pharmacists (e.g., manufacturers' organiza-

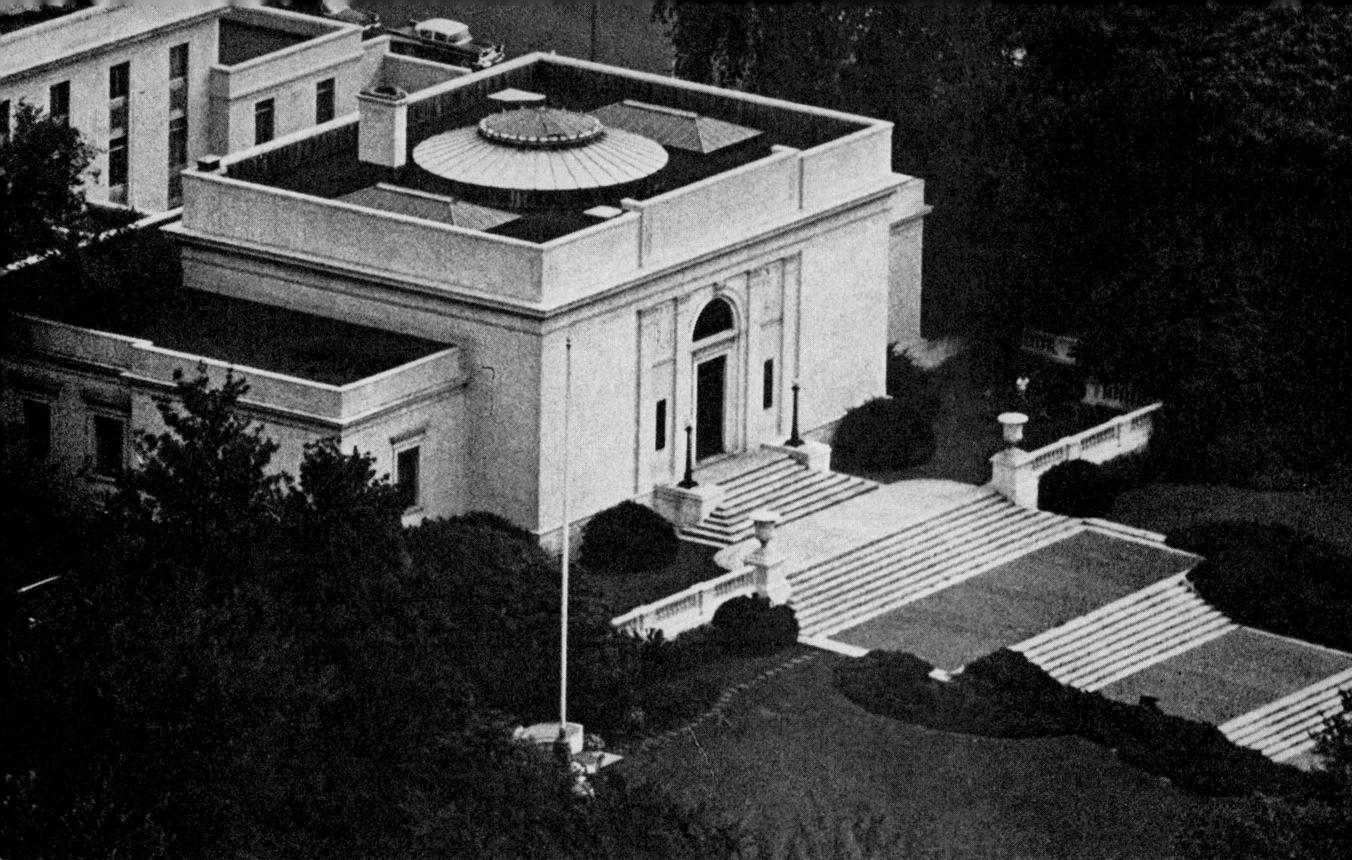

Professional representation of organized pharmacists centers in this headquarters building of the American Pharmaceutical Association in Washington. The first phase was dedicated in 1934, with an addition in 1961. Nearby are the U.S. Department of State and the Lincoln Memorial. (From Pharmaceutical Library, University of Wisconsin; A.Ph.A. photo)

tions). For example, full membership in the A.Ph.A. since 1960 has required that the applicant be a pharmacist or at least a graduate in pharmacy. A few years later the Association moved to assure that policymaking, in the House of Delegates would be more representative of this category of membership. This was accomplished by changing the structure and complexion of representation in the House, first (1963) in relation to its own subdivisions and the affiliated and recognized organizations and, second (1965), by a decision that recognition in the House "should be limited to groups or organizations the majority membership of which is composed of individual pharmacists." Conversely, as each state pharmaceutical association affiliated with the Association (implying concurrent membership in both organizations by the individual members, see p. 211), it received a more commanding voice and vote in the House.[57]

These years constituted in a sense a declaration of independence on the part of professionally organized American pharmacists, as demonstrated by a sense of self-determination in subsequent years that repeatedly has produced friction but also respect in A.Ph.A relations with agencies of government, medicine, and industrial producers. In its manner and in its continuing claim as "the most representative body" of professional pharmacy, the A.Ph.A has fostered the aspirations of the American pharmacist in the face of industrializing, commercializing, and bureaucratizing tendencies affecting the structure of pharmaceutical services during the 20th century.

The other large national pharmaceutical associations in the United States, have been, in some sense, specialized outgrowths of the American Pharmaceutical Association. They rarely lost their connection with the mother organization, since the latter, while recognizing the specialized functions of the younger societies, has maintained its position as the highest court within the profession for all matters pertaining to pharmacy proper.[58]

Wherever continuous systematic work or propagandistic action in a special field was required, specialized organizations have tended to crystallize out. But wherever special interests could be served by an occasional forum and channel for policy formation, these have tended to find expression within the American Pharmaceutical Association itself. Responding to these needs in 1887, the Association established 4 sections "to expedite and render more efficient the work," apparently using the American Medical Association as a model.

Said Joseph P. Remington, chairman of the Committee on Management, ". . . We believe that a National Association should be so comprehensive in its scope that every important interest should be effectively represented."

Thus arose the "Sections"—annual forums in which specialized pharmaceutical questions could be discussed and whence came many of the policy proposals debated in the House of Delegates of the American Pharmaceutical Association.

Through the decades the structure of the Sections at annual meetings changed occasionally as pharmacy or the outlook of the Association changed, or as a new specialized association made one of the old separate sections of the A.Ph.A. less essential. Of the original four sections, only the Scientific Section remained unchanged in its scope, reflecting the steadfastness of the Association in trying to represent adequately the scientific basis on which pharmaceutical practice rests. The old Sections on Commercial Interests (called Pharmaceutical Economics after 1937), on Pharmaceutical Education and on Legislation merged into a Section on General Practice of Pharmacy. The concerns of these former Sections became largely the responsibility of "daughter" associations—respectively, the National Association of Retail Druggists, the American Association of Colleges of Pharmacy, the National Association of Boards of Pharmacy and the American College of Apothecaries. The Section on Historical Pharmacy, an annual forum for historical papers since 1904, became in 1968 one of the functions of the separate society, the American Institute of the History of Pharmacy.

For the specialized subdivisions remaining within the A.Ph.A., a revised structure was activated in 1966 to accommodate evolving functions and ambitions. The present Academy of Pharmaceutical Sciences (with a full-time secretariat at A.Ph.A. headquarters) absorbed three of the old subdivisions: Scientific Section, Section on Pharmaceutical Technology (which before 1961 had been practitioner-oriented, under the title Section on Practical Pharmacy), and Section on Industrial Pharmacy (which had been founded in 1960). At the same time, with coordinate status, an Academy of Pharmacy Practice (also having a full-time secretariat) was formed out of the old Section on General Practice of Pharmacy. A semi-autonomous national society, the Student A.Ph.A., emerged three years later (1969) from the parent body's Student Section (which had represented local chapters of student members in the schools since 1954). By 1974 it contained about two-thirds of all pharmacy undergraduates. Temporarily, this left the Section on Military Pharmacy in the old format, which in 1973 had been rechristened the Section on Federal Pharmacy. It formalized a broader scope that includes the interests of all pharmacists in federal services, not in the armed forces alone.[59]

Other special interests, though distinguishable from the profession as a whole, have not found permanent expression through a distinct Section or separate affiliate (e.g., the Woman's Section, 1914–1923).

Some of the specialized organizations that have grown out of activities of the American Pharmaceutical Association, under diverse circumstances and retaining varying degrees of coordination or affiliation with the "mother association," are listed below. (The sequence is according to the founding of the initial organization in a field, even though it died and was later reborn in a new form.)

Conference of Teaching Colleges of Pharmacy[60] (1870–1884), the first organization of school representatives, was succeeded by the present American Association of Colleges of Pharmacy (1900), at first called (before 1925) the Conference of Pharmaceutical Faculties[61] (see p. 248)

National Retail Druggists Association (1883–1887), the first organization devoted mainly to the business and financial interests of the owners of pharmacies or drugstores, was succeeded by the present National Association of Retail Druggists (1898; see below)[62]

Association of Boards of Pharmacy and Secretaries of State Pharmaceutical Associations (1890–?1892),[63] which soon faded away, was succeeded by two separate organizations of today, the National Association of Boards of Pharmacy (1904; see p. 218) and the National Council of State Pharmaceutical Association Executives (1927), at first (before 1949) called the Conference of Pharmaceutical Association Secretaries[64]

Conference of Pharmaceutical Law Enforcement Officials, founded (1929) under the aegis of the A.Ph.A. but since 1944 a component of the National Association of Boards of Pharmacy as a forum on methods and problems[65]

American College of Apothecaries (1939), the first organization for exclusively professional pharmacies, was called during its first year the Conference of Professional Pharmacists[66]

American Institute of the History of Pharmacy (1941),[67] society and year-round center for research, information, publication and other sociohistorical activities.

American Society of Hospital Pharmacists (1942; see p. 208), an offshoot of a former Sub-Section on Hospital Pharmacy established 1936 in the A.Ph.A.

Three of the organizations mentioned that serve practicing pharmacists merit further comment: the principal organizations for pharmacy owners, for hospital pharmacists, and for pharmacies mainly devoted to prescription service.

### National Association of Retail Druggists

The National Association of Retail Druggists is to the business sphere of pharmacy what the American Pharmaceutical Association is to the professional and scientific sphere. In the early 80's of the 19th century, a strong feeling existed among community pharmacists that their business interests could not be taken care of adequately within the framework of the American Pharmaceutical Association. This feeling was strengthened when the Western Wholesale Druggists' Association (founded in 1876) was transformed into a national organization under the name of "National Wholesale Druggists' Association."

One year later, in 1883, the "National Retail Druggists' Association" was founded. The name itself intimated a close analogy between the two groups. The wholesale druggists as well as the retail druggists felt endangered by a growing tendency toward a direct connection between manufacturer and consumer of home remedies and by rapid expansion of ruinous price cutting. Nevertheless, it soon became obvious that the wholesale druggist and the retail druggist did not have identical interests, and that no quick and sweeping results could be expected, especially with regard to price cutting.

Consequently, the National Retail Druggists' Association was dissolved, and the "Section on Commercial Interests" was created within the American Pharmaceutical Association (1887). The last president of the N.R.D.A., A. H. Hollister, served as the first chairman of the Section. It soon became evident that, while the Section on Commercial Interests, with the weight of the American Pharmaceutical Association at its command, could *help* protect the business interests of pharmacy owners, it could not watch the situation adequately and *initiate* and pursue consistently the actions and the counteractions required.[68]

Again frustrated in dealing with commercial economic forces generated outside their own ranks and not easily controlled, pharmacists decided to begin anew an organization devoted to their business interests. On the initiative of the Chicago Retail Druggists' Association, and with the approval of a committee of the Section on Commercial Interests of the American Pharmaceutical Association, headed by J. P. Remington, "The National Association of Retail Druggists" was founded in 1898.

It had the encouragement of initial success when it won repeal of the tax imposed on proprietary medicines and toiletries after the Spanish-American war. Thereafter, the National Association of Retail Druggists embarked upon its decades-long campaign to popularize the concept and then to secure and defend the laws of "fair trade" (see p. 295), as the most effective weapon yet devised against ruinous price cutting. After the 1911 Miles case before the Supreme Court, "vertical" agreements for price maintenance (between vendor and distributors) became legally questionable, as "horizontal" agreements (among distributors) had been before. The issues at stake have been, in some form, a matter of legal and legislative controversy ever since. Since attempts to protect the prices of branded products had met with repeated failure into the 1920's, the effective leadership exercised by the Association in obtaining valid "fair trade" legislation commanded loyal support, especially among the pharmacy owners who constitute its regular membership.

In this and other ways the "N.A.R.D." has demonstrated the compelling need for organized cooperation on questions of business and finance, just as the "A.Ph.A." has done in the professional and scientific sphere.

## The Problem of Coordination

Cooperation between these two great national associations long has been an accepted principle and goal among many American pharmacists. There even have been periodic calls for merger of the N.A.R.D. and A.Ph.A., in the hope of avoiding representation working at cross purposes and avoiding duplication of resources. For example, in 1935 the former Secretary of the A.Ph.A., James H. Beal, observed that "periodically during the past quarter of a century" there had been suggestions that by consolidation "a single great organization . . . would then be able to speak with a single voice for all the scattered units of the drug world."

The powerful American Medical Association often was cited as an example of the advantages to be gained. Beal, who was widely respected for his experience in the politics and diplomacy of pharmacy, could not see the analogy. The pharmaceutical field, he argued, had a vertical division of separate groups (e.g., manufacturing, wholesaling, dispensing) with "separate and sometimes conflicting interests [that] grows out of the nature of things, and consequently it can be expected that there will always be questions between them upon which there will be differences of opinion. . . . In medicine no such inter-relationships exist," Beal contended. The specialized medical groups instead tend to be horizontally structured, bearing a common relationship to each other and to the public.

Beal probably was speaking for a large constituency in pharmacy when he went on to maintain that merger of the A.Ph.A. and N.A.R.D. would destroy the distinctive character of membership of each organization and the strikingly different focus of effort, which he felt would be a loss to American pharmacy. "The functions of the two organizations are not incompatible but they are different. . . ."[69]

These differences had been traditionally viewed, since the turn of the century, as the A.Ph.A. promoting the pharmacist's professional and scientific interests and the N.A.R.D. promoting the pharmacist's business and economic interests.

This neat division of function did not always work out in practice, and at their points of collision, the differences sometimes seemed more understandable in terms of the classical antipathy between professionalism and commercialism.

In the decade after Beal spoke, the antipathy and lack of cooperation between the two powerful organizations led the Conference of State Pharmaceutical Association Secretaries to request peace negotiations between the executive secretaries (E. F. Kelly for the A.Ph.A. and John W. Dargavel for the N.A.R.D.), which culminated in a combined meeting of the executive boards in 1943. Out of these sessions grew one mechanism for more effective coordination and communication. The two boards "provided for annual conferences between the executive bodies to be held in the fall of each year," for the purpose of "surveying and studying the resolutions adopted by the A.Ph.A. and the N.A.R.D. and by the state and local associations during the year; and for a competent study of mutual problems of recognized pharmaceutical importance and significance, and for the purpose of each group dealing with these matters as circumstances may indicate."

The following year "plans were made to coordinate future activities of the two organizations in meeting the developing problems of American pharmacy," and a continuing joint committee was named to function, between joint conferences, the year round (consisting of the president, the secretary and the board chairman of both the American Pharmaceutical Association and the National Association of Retail Druggists).[70] Moreover, cross representation was provided on key committees of the two associations.

This productive mechanism disintegrated by the 1950's for a complex of reasons never fully evaluated, including disagreement on legislative issues (such as the Durham-Humphrey bill), overlapping functions, personal incompatibilities and, not least of all, a question of primacy between professional and commercial values among practitioners. The chronic disharmony that ensued[71] revived old ambitions and efforts to give the practicing pharmacist a more unified voice and a more effective medium of organized endeavor.

This culminated in 1971 with a tripartite conference being projected (A.Ph.A., N.A.R.D., A.S.H.P.) concerning the "organizational needs of the profession of pharmacy." The N.A.R.D. balked at sitting down at a conference table, however, when it became known that the A.Ph.A. and A.S.H.P. intended to give emphasis to "unifying organizational structure."[72] Although the old bugaboo of trying to "integrate" American pharmacy had aborted the heralded tripartite conference, persistent pressures from the grass roots brought about discussions between A.Ph.A. and N.A.R.D. representatives on more limited grounds.

The most visible result was formalized in 1973 as a joint body for continuing cooperation, called the "Committee on Pharmacy Economic Security" (C.O.P.E.S.). The rationale for its name lay in the announced central purpose, "to identify courses of action that the A.Ph.A. and N.A.R.D. collectively and individually pursue to help pharmacists gain a reasonable return on their education, professional and capital investment."

A wave of optimism among organized pharmacists followed this accord, as had followed the movement of the early 1940's toward joint meetings of the two executive boards. The N.A.R.D. president expressed conviction that "there is a way and a place for these two great national associations to work cooperatively, confidently and effectively for the profession."[73] The A.Ph.A. president affirmed that, through C.O.P.E.S., a mechanism had been found to "discuss the differences their [two] associations have and attempt to suggest how these differences can best be resolved in the interest of our profession." Thus a measure of diplomacy had been restored by the mid-70's, even if it stopped short of moving toward an integration of organizational structure at the national level, which some constituents had been calling for.[74]

### American Society of Hospital Pharmacists

As the National Association of Retail Druggists had drawn strength from the business problems and economic ambitions of pharmacy owners, so the professional ambitions of hospital pharmacists carried them beyond the family circle of the American Pharmaceutical Association into a separate society that developed vigorously.

Until the 1920's American hospital pharmacists had been a subordinate group, in organization as well as in the institutions where they practiced. In a "classic paper" that Alex Berman has called the manifesto of the hospital pharmacy movement, E. C. Austin, Cincinnati hospital pharmacist, spoke of the appalling lack of well-trained hospital pharmacists and of the apathy of the pharmaceutical profession toward its hospital specialty.[75]

That same year the A.Ph.A. Secretary, William B. Day responded that he would like to see established "a sub-section of the Section on Practical Pharmacy and Dispensing where the hospital pharmacist would have part in the program each year. . . ." However, it was not until 1936 that the upsurge of participation by hospital pharmacists brought about such a sub-section. One of the early leaders of American hospital pharmacy saw it as "a turning point and milestone in the development of hospital pharmacy practice," although in retrospect a modest start toward group consciousness.[76]

Increasingly dissatisfied with the limited status and sphere of activities provided by a Sub-Section on Hospital Pharmacy within the American Pharmaceutical Association, the professionally ambitious hospital pharmacists struck out on their own as the American Society of Hospital Pharmacists during the 1942 meeting of the American Pharmaceutical Association. Like the American College of Apothecaries before them, the hospital pharmacists made membership in the parent Association a prerequisite to membership in their own Society.

The first two chairmen of the Society were especially influential in maintaining its high level and progressive direction: H. A. K. Whitney (in the formative period) and Don E. Francke. The Society and the American Pharmaceutical Association set up, in 1947, a Division of Hospital Pharmacy with headquarters in the A.Ph.A.'s building in Washington, D.C. This strengthened the Society's base of operations; and during the 1950's it entered upon a period of sustained professional growth and enthusiasm that meanwhile has brought American hospital pharmacy into favorable comparison with its best European counterparts. When the A.Ph.A.'s Division of Hospital Pharmacy was discontinued, the A.S.H.P. had become self-sustaining. In two decades the membership had grown from 150 to more than 3,000. By 1970 the Society had outgrown the quarters that the A.Ph.A. could provide, and moved into its own headquarters building in nearby Bethesda, Maryland. The stepwise evolution toward independence from the parent Association culminated in 1972 when the A.S.H.P. ceased to require dual membership in the A.Ph.A., after the two organizations could not agree on "a more equitable and viable affiliation agreement." Pending renewed negotiation, relations between the two professional bodies were continued through a board-level joint committee.[77]

With an esprit de corps often unmatched by their colleagues in community practice, hospital pharmacists in the A.S.H.P. gave their society a remarkable vitality, producing such activities as the first minimum standards for hospital pharmacies, early establishment of short postgraduate courses or "institutes" (in cooperation with the American and the Catholic Hospital Associations and the A.Ph.A.), the setting of standards for internships and residencies in hospital pharmacy, the substantial *American Journal of Hospital Pharmacy* (f. 1943), the *American Hospital Formulary Service* (f. 1959),[78] the *International Pharmaceutical Abstracts* (f. 1964), and the far-reaching Audit of Pharmaceutical Service in Hospitals (jointly sponsored with the A.Ph.A.). Hospital construction on a large-scale since the 1940's, the mushrooming growth of prepaid medical care, and steadily increasing drug distribution through hospitals, all favored the Society's program. "When all is said, however," concluded the historian Alex Berman, "the most important single historical event for hospital pharmacy in this country has been the appearance on the scene of the American Society of Hospital Pharmacists."[79]

## American College of Apothecaries

The American College of Apothecaries (f. 1940), a selective society consisting basically of community pharmacists whose establishments meet defined standards, organized about the same time as the hospital pharmacists. Both groups emerged from the ranks of the A.Ph.A., and the members of both have shown exceptional dedication and enthusiasm.

As early as 1914 the pharmacist-educator H. V. Arny of New York had advocated an "American Institute of Prescriptionists" that would have been similarly selective in concept and membership. An A.Ph.A. study committee examined the concept and, in effect, concluded that the objective instead should be to upgrade all of pharmacy and make it more scientific. In practice this upgrading proved to be too slow and spotty for Arny and his supporters, and in 1928 he returned to the idea of organizing "prescriptionists" who met certain criteria. Other proposals and conferences during the 1930's matured the idea, as the pharmacist-historian Ernst W. Stieb has shown; and at the A.Ph.A. meeting of 1940 the American College of Apothecaries was born.[80] Adopting terms already old fashioned—"College" for their society, and "Apothecaries" for themselves as practitioners—may seem to imply a nostalgia for the traditions and controls that gave European pharmacy at its best the professional dignity and homogeneity toward which A.C.A. members aspired, a model they hoped would be emulated by all of American pharmacy eventually. There was nothing old fashioned, however, about the progressive program of mutual support mounted by the A.C.A. to make their pharmacies viable, which mainly depended upon health services for income.

The A.C.A. appears to have been particularly influenced during its first quarter century by its two Secretaries, Charles V. Selby of St. Louis and Robert A. Abrams of Philadelphia. Since then (1965), the College has had a salaried, full-time executive director.[81] Its publications have been persistently outspoken in support of a more independent and professionalized pharmacist, an independent voice that members safeguarded by paying relatively high dues rather than accept advertising or other substantial subsidies.[82]

"No feature of the American College of Apothecaries has so distinguished it from other organizations," Stieb points out, "as its stringent requirements of membership.

. . . The decision in favor of high quality at the expense of quantity was made as the constitution and bylaws were forged at Chicago in April 1940 and have been maintained since."[83] The actual requirements have been changed repeatedly in detail; but the general concept of a full Fellow of the A.C.A. ("F.A.C.A.") has implied a pharmacist who has owned, for a prescribed period, a pharmacy that complies with specified standards of specialization and dignity (e.g., no soda fountains, no blatant advertising, etc.). For retaining membership in good standing there has been, since 1959, a point system that stimulates members to various types of activities on behalf of the profession and the organization (e.g., civic activities, public addresses, volunteer professional service, etc.), although assuring full compliance has been difficult. The idea of A.C.A.-accredited pharmacies was extended, during the 1960's, to include periodic inspection for compliance with standards.[84] The A.C.A. always has required dual membership in the A.Ph.A. as an affiliate.

Although never exceeding a thousand in membership, this unique organization of community pharmacists (plus associate members who share their goals) often has achieved a constructive effect "out of proportion to the size of the organization," through interaction with other professions, public bodies and with other segments of pharmacy itself.[85]

## Other National Organizations

After the turn of the century the pharmaceutical personnel of America became increasingly segmented under the growing influences of specialization, differences of function and objective, divergent educational backgrounds and socioeconomic circumstances. The deeply probing national "Pharmaceutical Survey" of 1946 to 1949 concluded that

> American pharmacy is represented by a wide range of professional and commercial associations and their publications. However, their aims and activities are uncoordinated, ofttimes in conflict, and therefore tend to produce a low rate and quantity of professional accomplishment.[86]

This diagnosis by an outside analyst helped to stimulate efforts within organized pharmacy toward better coordination after World War II. At the same time there seemed to be a clearer recognition that the profession of pharmacy was by no means co-extensive with the pharmaceutical field, a field whose varied, vertically structured components have not favored a stable entente concerning policies and programs.

The tendency toward fragmentation has produced so many temporary organizations during the present century that there would be little use in reviewing them all even if space permitted. Some organizations repeatedly encountered in pharmaceutical literature are listed below by date of founding. (Unlike associations previously discussed, these did not arise, historically, within the A.Ph.A. framework.)

*Owners and Employees of Pharmacies:*

National Drug Clerks Association (1910–1934)[87] served employed pharmacists seeking better salary and hours, but also better standards of practice generally and national reciprocity of licenses; before 1912 called the National Association of Pharmacologists.

National Association of Chain Drugstores (1933), basically a trade association of owners of multiple-unit organizations to help improve the merchandising operations of its members and represent them, including liaison with other segments of pharmacy.

National Pharmaceutical Association (1949), for the Negro pharmacist "to improve himself and his economic position"; an outgrowth of two pharmacy seminars for Negroes, 1947 and 1948[88]

National Catholic Pharmacists Guild of the United States (1962), for promoting dedication to Catholic principles and missions, particularly in terms of pharmacy, and for fostering diocesan pharmacists' guilds.

American Society of Consultant Pharmacists (1970), serves the interests of practitioners providing service to nursing homes, and aims to establish certification standards.

*Pharmaceutical Manufacturers:*

Proprietary Association of America (1881),[89] for makers of home medications, home medical supplies and cosmetics.

American Pharmaceutical Manufacturers Association (1908; known before 1921 as the American Association of Pharmaceutical Chemists) and the American Drug Manufacturers Association (1912; known before 1917 as the National Association of Manufacturers of Medicinal Products) merged in 1958 to form the Pharmaceutical Manufacturers Association, like its predecessors consisting of makers of prescription drugs.[90]

Parenteral Drug Association (1946), consisting of makers of injectable pharmaceutical products, to deal with the specialized technical and regulatory requirements.

*Wholesale Druggists:*

National Wholesale Druggists Association (1876); before 1882 called Western Wholesale Druggists Association[91] (what would be now known as "Midwestern")

Drug Wholesalers Association; between 1974 and 1976 called International Pharmaceutical Distributors Association, which merged the Federal Wholesale Druggists Association[92] (f. 1916, originally for "mutual" houses or cooperatives) and the Pharmaceutical Wholesalers Association (f. 1957, originally mainly Western wholesalers).

The length of such a list could be multiplied in a specialized account of all relevant organizations in the American past and present.[93] This historical circumstance suggests not so much a highly organized profession as it does a profession that has not been as effectively organized and unified as analogous professions such as dentistry, law and medicine have been.

A movement to surmount this handicap by a federation of associations, through the medium of the A.Ph.A.'s House of Delegates found some support during the decade following its establishment.[94] This movement never became a tightly structured, unifying force, partly because many state associations felt a competing owner- and business-oriented kinship with the N.A.R.D. A renewed interest and sustained effort arose in the 1950's following the collapse of hopes that the activities of the pharmacist's professional society (A.Ph.A.) and the pharmacy owners' association (N.A.R.D.) could be coordinated or at least better harmonized. One of the most effective spokesmen for the "federation" movement was J. Curtis Nottingham of Virginia, although his proposal (1954) at first received scant support.

This movement culminated in the American Pharmaceutical Association's action (1962) to create a new basis for unified professional action among pharmacists. In its fundamentals, the plan has permitted local, state and national organizations of pharmacists to link themselves together as affiliates of the Association. All who join an '"affiliate" must also belong to the American Pharmaceutical Association. An affiliate gains a commanding voice in the policy-making House of Delegates of the Association without yielding its local powers or authority in its specialized field.

Since the 1950's affiliation has been controversial in state after state, but the trend was clear. By 1974 the twentieth state pharmaceutical association had voted to affiliate (thereby requiring dual membership in the American Pharmaceutical Association). In other states, pharmacists were continuing the debate, which was complicated by deeply divided views about some of the important pharmaceutical issues of the time. If the "one voice for pharmacy" continued to be elusive, the determination to achieve more effective local-state-national professional organization continued to gain ground after mid-century. Some saw the issue as a crucial one. Said the distinguished pharmacist and editor Don E. Francke,

Despite the existence of a plan for the federation of American pharmacy with its inherent program for developing a closely knit integrated county-state-national membership structure, the big question remains: Will American pharmacy, and particularly the state associations, become an integral part of it through direct affiliation? We dare not hope otherwise.[95]

# 13

# The Rise of Legislative Standards

Any movement contains the seeds of its own destruction. Gradually they may grow until the movement itself is overshadowed, until its originators find themselves in the uncomfortable position of condoning what they had condemned, and of following what they had organized to oppose. Thus, too, in pharmacy. Some organizations dedicated to avoiding legal restrictions became the initiators and, subsequently, the guardians of American pharmaceutical legislation. Legally enforced standards and controls in any profession often have an ambivalent quality in the public mind: whether in the long run the assurance of more predictable and effective professional services will outweigh the risk of fostering special privileges and restrictive practices that may not be in the public interest?

Since the late 19th century, however, an increasingly complex network of regulatory standards has governed the practice of pharmacy and the supply of drugs and other health resources, drawing strength from several circumstances: inherent safety risks that are hard both to assess and control; an American trend toward welfare capitalism; and, more recently, a new "consumerism" that spurs government toward maximizing public safety in all fields, despite economic costs.

Various types of laws have affected the pharmaceutical field in some way; but for the present purpose we are mainly interested in the evolution of legislation that either has created the American structure of pharmacy or at least has influenced it decisively.

## LOCAL LAWS

Special legislation that covers pharmaceutical activities comprehensively did not become common in the United States until after 1870. Before that time, American democratic and laissez-faire ideology, frontier conditions and lack of pharmacy schools made any systematic attempt at regulating pharmacy the exception rather than the rule.

Local attempts at regulation sprang up here and there between 1804 and 1870, mostly in cities, since pharmacy tends to be an urban institution: New Orleans tried briefly (1804) to require dispensers of drugs to register their diplomas or to be examined.[1] New York City asked for a diploma from a college of pharmacy or an examination by the county medical society (state statute of 1832), but legal controversies led to modified requirements after only seven years.[2] In Natchez and Adams County, Mississippi (1884), an apothecary or vender of medicines was to be licensed and inspected periodically by a Board of Medical Censors.[3] The General Council of Louisville, Kentucky, had been empowered (1851) to establish a Board or Institute of Pharmacy to examine and license apothecaries and "to regulate the trade of retail Apothecaries in the business of making up prescriptions, and vending poisonous substances"[4]—provisions apparently not enforced.[5] A Pennsylvania statute required (1866) that in Williamsport and Lycoming County only "licensed druggists" be permitted to practice, but established neither criteria nor procedures for licensing.[6]

Thus, under urban conditions, there was some public response to the risk of having a health service without any established standards. But these few local regulations seem to have been more important in principle than in practice; and no others before 1870 are known, even after authoritative studies by the historian David L. Cowen. Between 1870 and 1876 the licensing of pharmacists in at least six additional cities was authorized by state legislatures (for Baltimore, San Francisco, Philadelphia, St. Louis, Cincinnati, and Milwaukee). In New York City, an attempt to impose the "Irving Law" became distasteful when it appeared to make pharmacy subservient to the politics of Tammany Hall, and pharmacy groups unified in opposition. In consequence, a new pharmacy law (1872)[7] placed control of the local Board of Pharmacy in the hands of the College of Pharmacy of the City of New York.[8]

This trend toward local regulation of the practice of pharmacy was cut off, and eventually outmoded, as the country developed and state-wide pharmacy laws were enacted.

## STATE PHARMACY LAWS

The establishment of state statutes to set standards for pharmacists and pharmacies has remained the traditional American pattern until the present time because of the Constitutional delegation of policing powers to each state, concerning activities within its own borders. Apparent exceptions (discussed later) arise from what can be construed as activities across state borders (i.e., interstate commerce), thereby subject to Federal control.

The first four states that required the licensing of pharmacists (in the period 1808–1851) all were in the deep South and all made the regulation of pharmacy part of the regulation of medicine.[9] These beginnings were so early, so dependent upon particular local conditions, that—as shown below—the pattern of present day pharmacy laws finds its prototype instead in a new line of development after about 1870.

Earlier regulatory efforts first found some success in the Territory of Orleans (1808; Louisiana after 1812), which was influenced by Franco-Spanish traditions. Not only were apothecaries required to exhibit proof of qualification and to be examined by a board of physicians, but it banned the sale of deteriorated drugs and restricted the sale of poisons. In 1816 Louisiana became the first state to pass a law regulating pharmacy. An apothecary was added to the old Territorial examining board (a second was added in 1840), thus creating not only the first state board of pharmacy, but the first such board in the United States to have a pharmacist as a permanent member (1838, the apothecary A. Delpeuch). The Louisiana statute existed until 1852, when, due to a resurgent spirit of laissez-faire coupled with the persuasiveness of quacks, all medical legislation was repealed![10]

The second statute, that of South Carolina in 1817, provided for examination and licensing of apothecaries by a medical body, until it was replaced by a "modern" statute (1876). However, the act had been emasculated (1838) by repeal of its penalty provisions.[11]

In Georgia the statute of 1825 repeated almost word for word the first statute for South Carolina. Although the penalty provisions were later removed (1836 to 1839), the act remained in force until it, too, was replaced by a "modern" statute (1881).[12] In Alabama, the licensing of pharmacists provided by the Code of 1852 remained in effect until replaced by a "modern" state pharmacy law (1887).[13]

For some time these statutes were not the "dead letters" that they later became. In

Louisiana, records indicate that licensing began as early as 1816, and by 1847 no fewer than 124 apothecaries had received licenses.[14] In the French quarter of New Orleans a pharmaceutical museum is located at the site of the original pharmacy of L. J. Dufilho[15] (licensed in 1816). In South Carolina between 1818 and 1836, the Medical Society of Charleston licensed 17 apothecaries and the Medical Society of Columbia one. The Medical College of South Carolina licensed four more before the Civil War and an additional 51 by 1876.[16] (See also p. 184).

When John M. Maisch presented his influential report on legislation to the American Pharmaceutical Association in 1868, he believed that only Georgia had a statewide statute. Among those practicing pharmacy in Georgia in 1868 only five were known to be formally licensed. In Alabama there is only presumptive evidence that the law there had ever been enforced.[17] South Carolina did not respond to his inquiry. This suggests that under the double impact of the growth of medical laissez-faire and of the Civil War, the laws—to use a phrase applied to the New York City statute—had become "dead letter[s] upon the statute books."[18]

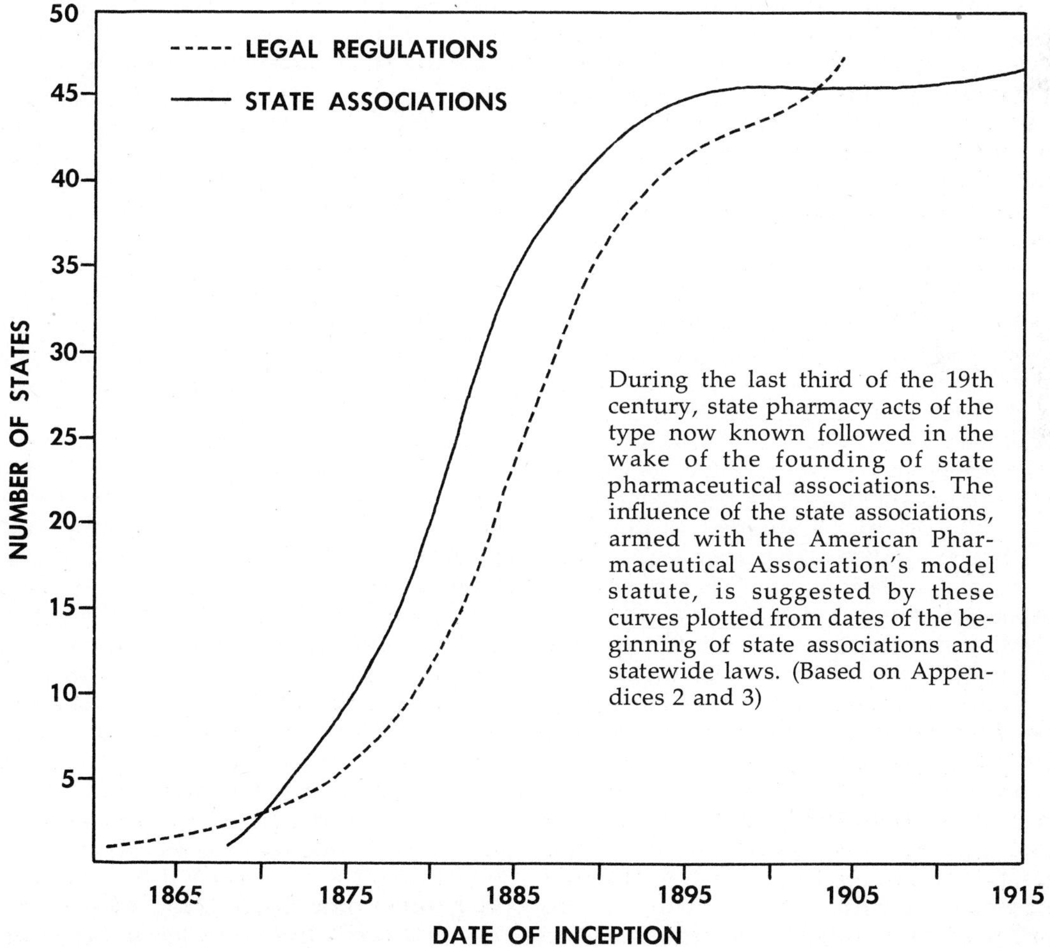


During the last third of the 19th century, state pharmacy acts of the type now known followed in the wake of the founding of state pharmaceutical associations. The influence of the state associations, armed with the American Pharmaceutical Association's model statute, is suggested by these curves plotted from dates of the beginning of state associations and statewide laws. (Based on Appendices 2 and 3)

Despite prevailing concepts of laissez-faire in the first seven decades of the 19th century, laws regulating pharmacy were not uncommon where public safety or questions of ethical practice appeared to be at stake. Before 1870 at least 25 states or territories had some statutory provisions against drug adulteration, and a few more had some statute concerning poisons.[19] These statutes affected the pharmacist directly. Typically, the sale of "pernicious and adulterated . . . drugs and medicines" was forbidden on the penalty of fine or imprisonment. Poison legislation requiring labeling, frequently enumerated a poison schedule, detailed special care to be taken in dispensing poisons, and, toward the end of the period, required a poison register to be kept (e.g., Pennsylvania, 1860; Wisconsin, 1862).[20] In addition, David Cowen found, over 25 states had laws on abortion, some specifically prohibiting the advertising and the sale of abortifacients by pharmacists (e.g., Indiana, 1859).

All this legal activity did not yet add up to much effective support for the development of professional standards in American pharmacy in general. In particular, the pharmacy practice acts—following some initial enthusiasm—commonly offered only weak penalties for violations and equally weak budgets to apply the laws. After the Civil War it became evident that the key to effective legislation lay in organizing those practicing pharmacy. Thus it is not surprising to find that state pharmaceutical laws and state pharmaceutical associations have been closely related, most associations having been organized partly for the purpose of fostering legislation. Once an association had succeeded, there often has been a consistent fatherly interest in helping to assure proper administration of a state's pharmacy law.

The American Pharmaceutical Association, which had fostered the organization of state pharmaceutical associations, did not send her children into legislative battle without providing them with a weapon. This weapon was the model "draft of a proposed law to regulate the practice of pharmacy and the sale of poisons and to prevent the adulteration of drugs and medicines."[21] The draft was prepared by a special committee (more particularly by John M. Maisch) and presented to the American Pharmaceutical Association meeting in 1869. The history of this model law shows the transitional character of this period. "The draft was liberally discussed and finally ordered to be printed in the proceedings but without the formal endorsement of the association, as many of the members doubted the advisability of encouraging pharmaceutical legislation."[22]

Inner resistance against legislative restriction, by some of the best men in American pharmacy of that time, had its origin partly in the circumstances described by John M. Maisch 3 years later when he said:

> We must remember that in thinly settled districts, where frequently for many miles no drugstore can be found, physicians are compelled to dispense medicines and carry them in suitable forms in their saddle bags, while the sale of popular remedies is usually in the hands of country storekeepers who make no pretensions as to any acquaintance with drugs and their preparations. Hence the necessity which exists in the larger cities to confine the practice of pharmacy to pharmacists alone is not felt there, and the opposition to general laws came, in most cases, only from the representatives of such districts.[23]

An additional reason lay in the deep mistrust for state administrations. "If we propose a law," said Dr. Squibb during the discussion of the draft, "that makes a whole train of offices and office holders, we are simply establishing another political engine in each state that will soon become corrupted to political ends."

The knowledge that some states were about to adopt pharmacy laws without guidance, and thus might produce quite undesirable regulations, made the model draft the lesser evil. Therefore, a pamphlet was printed, containing the model bill together with the somewhat lukewarm resolutions and conditional recommendations of the American Pharmaceutical Association. Ten copies were sent to the governors and to the speakers of the legislatures of each state in the Union.

The results confirmed the need for a model law. It became the basis of a majority of the early laws, some of which were rushed through legislative committees of the state associations and through the legislatures.[24] The first success was in Rhode Island, where a statute quite close to the model law was passed (1870). But in at least seven other states proposed laws failed to pass by 1871.[25] Still the young state pharmaceutical associations persisted in their efforts: in eight other states and the District of Columbia statewide statutes had been adopted by 1878; at least 21 more states and territories added laws in the 1880's, 12 more in the 1890's. (Appendix 3 tabulates the passage of these pharmacy laws chronologically.)

In 1900 an updated model law—of which the pharmacist-lawyer James H. Beal was the spiritual father—was adopted by the American Pharmaceutical Association, this time unanimously, without long debate and without any reservations.[26] Like its older brother, this model law was sent to the various state governments.

These laws legally defined the difference between a pharmacist and a mere merchant; they established professional pharmacy as a distinct entity, existing for the public good.[27] The first model law suggested that . . .

> the incorporated Colleges of Pharmacy and Pharmaceutical Societies of this State shall submit to the Governor the names of twenty pharmacists or professors in Colleges of Pharmacy, out of which number the Governor shall appoint seven persons who shall constitute the Pharmaceutical Board of the State of . . . , who shall hold office for the term of three years and until their successors shall have been appointed. . . .

This part of the model law has been adopted and retained (with changes by individual states as to the number of the names submitted, the ineligibility of professors and the term of office of the State Board members).

The duties of these pharmaceutical law enforcement agencies, as described in the model law, were "to examine all candidates presenting themselves; to direct the registration . . . of all persons properly qualified or entitled under this Act; to cause the prosecution of all persons violating its provisions."

The expansion of state as well as federal legislation pertaining to drugs, within and without the profession of pharmacy, has considerably expanded the general law-enforcing duties of the State Boards of Pharmacy. For example, during the 1950's a majority of the states enacted "antisubstitution" measures to assure that the brand of a drug dispensed to a patient would always be the one specified by their physician. A counteraction in the name of health-care economy began to reverse this trend and became a national controversy, however, after the American Pharmaceutical Association launched a policy (1970) aimed at modifying such laws to permit the pharmacist to select the brand to be dispensed (e.g., Michigan, 1974).

Still, the main task of the Boards consists in examining, licensing and registering pharmacists: *the guardianship of the identity and the integrity of a well-defined profession of pharmacy.* Without a legally recognized and effective pharmaceutical profession, the important national laws adopted early in the 20th century to control drugs and cosmetics moving in interstate commerce would have lacked a fundamental base upon which their effectiveness rests. These national laws, to be discussed later, do not deal exclusively with pharmacy, yet have affected it substantially.

### States Boards Organize

The new state boards of pharmacy often were not well equipped, by experience, knowledge or budget, to meet the heavy responsibilities thrust upon them. Legal provisions varied widely enough across the country to make reciprocity of a pharmacist's license, from one state to another, more a wish than a goal. By the late 19th century these conditions made clear the place and the purpose of cooperation among the state boards of pharmacy.

At meetings of the American Pharmaceutical Association after 1887 the Section on Education and Legislation helped to pull together and guide the efforts of board members. From the beginning, it was understood that state board affairs and legislation would be perennial topics in the Section. But this annual open forum and meeting ground for pharmacists on state boards soon proved to be too cramped as a medium for dealing with such specialized problems, especially with the impasse on interchange of pharmacists' licenses between states ("reciprocity").

Therefore, in the same year that a rather ineffectual National Confederation of State Medical Boards came into existence (1890), there was born a short-lived joint organization between state boards of pharmacy and state association secretaries. The principle and the need that gave birth to this ill-fated association did not die with it.

Speaking before the American Conference of Pharmaceutical Faculties (1903), Edward Kremers of the University of Wisconsin suggested that it would be desirable for members of the faculties and the boards to meet together nationally. His Conference colleagues agreed and invited the Boards to a joint conference proposed as part of the next annual meeting (held, by tradition, in association with the meeting of the American Pharmaceutical Association). Six days later, the Association's Section on Education and Legislation heard Henry Whelpley of St. Louis refer to the invitation from the Conference of Pharmaceutical Faculties and again propose, as he had in 1901, that the boards of pharmacy organize.

At the next meeting of the American Pharmaceutical Association (1904), in the Section on Education and Legislation, Dr. Murray Galt Motter, one of the key figures, announced that representatives of 16 boards had just participated in an organizational conference for a "National Association of Boards of Pharmacy."

Then as now, the autonomy of individual states and their constituent agencies in the control of professions barred any national compulsory standards or uniform patterns of administration, from whatever quarter this might be attempted. Yet, there has been a wide area where interchange of views and agreement on *recommended* practices and minimum standards affecting pharmacists and the public can be largely effected through the informal federation of state board members represented, still today, by the "N.A.B.P."

A common desire for reciprocity of licenses strongly motivated the founding; and this keystone of the Association's program long remained a persistent problem. Some boards stood defiantly on "state's rights." Others insisted that their own, and naturally "best" methods be adopted by other boards wanting to reciprocate. After the 1940's, the Association also encouraged the constituent boards to overcome deficiencies that were bluntly pointed out by The Pharmaceutical Survey. Despite these circumstances, a functioning system of reciprocity was evolved by the National Association of Boards of Pharmacy that commands the allegiance of all but a few states. Corollary activities have been the encouraging of more valid and uniform state-board examinations, especially through the program for a Standard Examination in Pharmacy (issued first in 1970), which subsequently has been used at least in part by nearly all states; encouraging meaningful standards of pharmaceutical internship; and promoting required continuing education (postgraduate) as a qualification for continuing licensure.[28]

Effective communication and cooperation with the schools of pharmacy has been especially important, since legal authority over the qualifications of a pharmacist rests with the boards, but the educational authority rests with the schools. Therefore, joint conferences between the respective associations of boards and schools have been traditional.[29]

Misunderstandings and dissension limited the effectiveness of this relationship until about the time of the first World War. Then, in 1921, boards of pharmacy convened in nine district meetings across the country for the first time, supplementing the annual national meeting. Within a few years these meetings were functioning effectively as joint sesssions of the boards and the faculties serving each group of states. Thus a new channel for regional cooperation emerged that still retains a significant place in American pharmacy.

The concern of the National Association of Boards of Pharmacy for the welfare of the American Council on Pharmaceutical Education finds a fundamental basis in the tenet that "all member Boards recognize only such colleges and schools of pharmacy which are on the accredited list of the American Council on Pharmaceutical Education."[30] (Concerning the Council, see p. 250.)

## FOOD AND DRUG LAW

The Constitution of the United States and court decisions left police power largely with the individual states. However, there are activities for which uniform national regulation has been found both Constitutional and

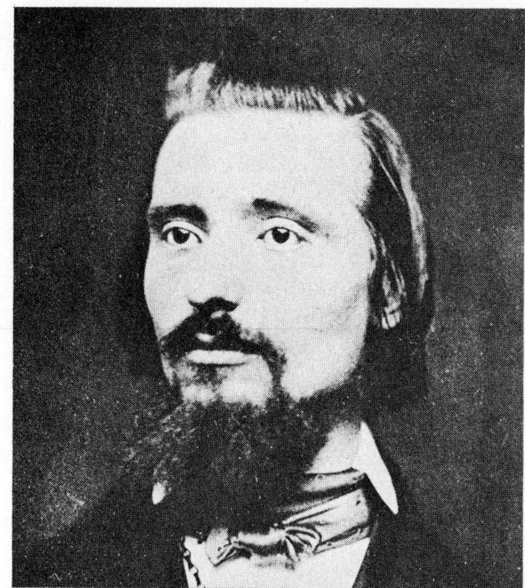

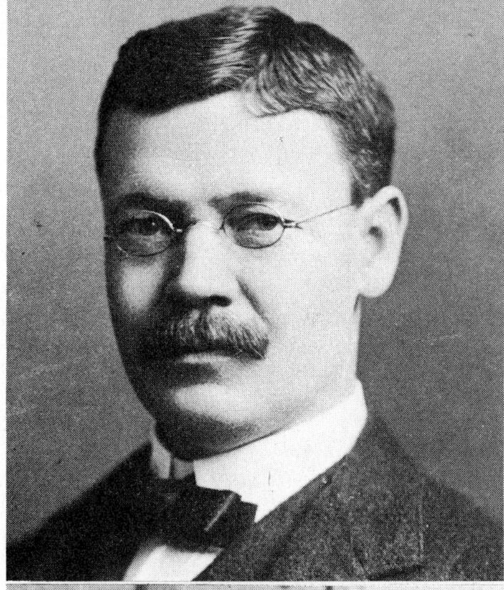

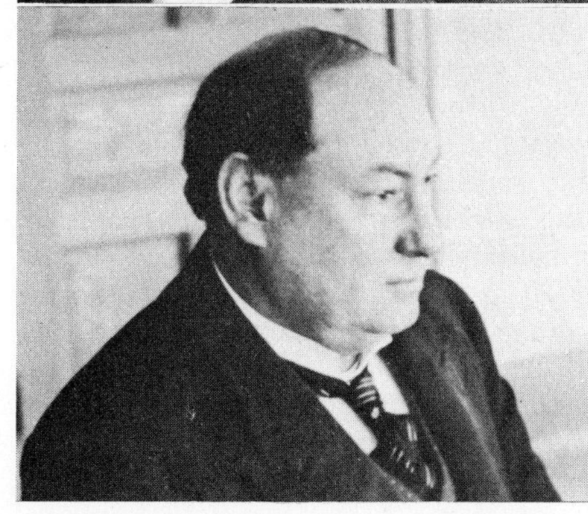

Three men who were instrumental in laying the foundations of modern legislative standards for pharmacy during the three quarters of a century following the American Civil War: Pharmacist John M. Maisch, *top* (1831–1893), as the first permanent Secretary of the American Pharmaceutical Association, reported (1868) the state of pharmaceutical regulation and led the drafting of the first model pharmacy act as a guide for the states. Pharmacist-lawyer James H. Beal, *center* (1861–1945), was largely responsible three decades later for the issuance of a second model state pharmacy act, as he was also for model state statutes on narcotic and poison controls. While Beal was influential in the debate on initiating Federal legislation, the physician-chemist Harvey W. Wiley, *bottom* (1844–1930) was the key figure in both scientific and polemic underpinning for passage of the first Federal Food and Drug Act.

highly desirable. One of these activities is that of supplying the people with genuine and unadulterated foods and drugs.

After enacting a drug-import control in 1848, which placed inspectors in the principal ports of entry, Congress left the field largely to control by the individual states. A model food and drug statute issued by the National Board of Trade (U.S.A.) influenced a number of states to try to deal with the problem of substandard and misrepresented foods and drugs.

A complex of factors placed Federal legislation in this field beyond the possibility of Congressional enactment until the present century. These included: The uneven social development among the states, unwillingness to place Federal power against abuses in the domestic drug market, and inadequate recognition of the states' limitations in such a complex field.

Meanwhile, experience both abroad and in individual states of this country fostered eventual passage of a Federal law. England had attracted attention with its first broad enactment covering both foods and drugs (1875). On returning from Germany, Harvey W. Wiley, who was to be enormously influential, said his experience with the German Imperial Board of Health made him enthusiastic about the possibility of enforcing standards of purity in foods and drugs.[31] He gave this enthusiasm scientific backing and, after 1883, political leverage from his vantage point in the Bureau of Chemistry of the U.S. Department of Agriculture. Wiley's work helped to stimulate the enactment of food and drug provisions in state laws, as it later did the national legislation.

Crude controls aimed at fraudulent or willful adulteration of drugs often entered state statutes through the first modern pharmacy practice acts, discussed previously. The results were disappointing to the American Pharmaceutical Association, which editorialized that "One reason for this is undoubtedly the fact that to carry on such work systematically and continuously requires such expenditures as have never been granted to any state pharmacy board."[32] It was symptomatic of a new line of development when the section on adulteration was omitted from the second model state pharmacy act drafted by the American Pharmaceutical Association.

Yet, more carefully drawn separate statutes did not prove to be adequate to the problem either; and frustration became apparent among those who wanted specific and effective drug standards. In 1895 the journal *Pharmaceutical Era* concluded that "state regulation has been fairly tried, and the discovery made that State lines have little force in maintaining standards for food and drugs. . . ."[33]

Harvey Wiley became the key figure in the campaign for enacting a national food and drug statute because he emerged as a fervent crusader as well as a scientist informed authoritatively about the need for reform. He consolidated scattered discontent into a pressure group effective upon Congress. He and his associates provided much grist for the mill of journalistic muckrackers in national media. Colorful exposés appeared, about shocking conditions in the food-processing industries and, later, about dangerous ingredients and fraudulent advertising of many products of the drug industry. Magazine series, notably in the *Ladies' Home Journal* and *Collier's*, had heavy impact (1890's–1906); and two books that became all-time classics in the field of food and drug abuses were Upton Sinclair's novel, *The Jungle* (meat packers) and Samuel Hopkins Adams' *The Great American Fraud* (a collated series on "patent" medicines). Aroused public opinion greatly strengthened proponents of Federal legislation, while Congressional compromises on some legislative clauses offensive to industry tended to undermine the strength of opponents.[34] Moreover, the Progressives were creating a political fervor pointing toward American social-welfare legislation, of which the Federal Food and Drug Act of 1906 was to become a pioneer example.

To the extent that drugs (as well as foods)

could be considered *inter*state commerce, the Food and Drug Law that was finally passed in 1906 could exact penalties for certain types of misbranding and adulteration. Despite loopholes in the statute, and consequent problems of administration, it had far-reaching influences that in retrospect have been considered beneficial to the pharmaceutical field as well as to the public. To make state legislation mesh with Federal requirements and reach violators engaging only in *intra*state transactions (hence beyond Federal reach), at least two thirds of the states revamped their food and drug statutes in the years immediately following passage of the Federal law.[35]

While professionally conscious pharmacists welcomed new statutes as desirable improvements,[36] the new style of control ended administration of this segment of pharmaceutical law by state boards of pharmacy. Earlier laws had been occasionally administered by a dairy and food commission or by a board of health, but by 1912 the new union of food control with drug control left only 7 boards of pharmacy still retaining primary jurisdiction in this field.[37]

In making food and drug control hinge primarily on Federal enforcement, Congress took a historic step in using its power to regulate interstate commerce as a weapon in the direct furtherance of public health and safety for the first time.[38]

Legal loopholes, weak penalties and changing conditions built up pressure by the 1930's for markedly strengthening food and drug legislation, and this was reinforced by wider governmental concern for social welfare during the administration of President Franklin Roosevelt. The need for such control was dramatized, and previously effective opposition overcome, when a tragic wave of at least 73 deaths in the country was caused by a toxic "Elixir Sulfanilamide" (fall of 1937).[39]

This tragedy shocked the country and gave impetus to the passage of the Food, Drug and Cosmetic Act of 1938. Significantly, a new and demanding section on marketing "new drugs" was added to the proposed bill, a section designed to prevent another pharmaceutical catastrophe analogous to the lethal "Elixir Sulfanilamide." The drastically revised law also gave the Federal government jurisdiction over medical devices (e.g., instruments, apparatus, sickroom accessories) and cosmetics for the first time; and the requirements and the penalties for violation were broadened in many respects. To provide more effective control over false advertising of foods, drugs and cosmetics, and over deceptive or unfair practices, the same 75th Congress passed separate legislation (called the Wheeler Lea bill), which amended the Federal Trade Commission Act.

Although pharmaceutical opinion once again had been divided, on principle and on details, the American Pharmaceutical Association expressed "its conviction that further delay was against the public interest, and has done what it could toward the successful outcome."[40]

A separate law helps to assure the reliable potency and safety of pharmaceutical products of biological origin (e.g., vaccines and antitoxins), through a system of product licensure and inspection of producers. This special class of products had been controlled through the U.S. Public Health Service (Division of Biologics Standards), until 1972 when both the regulatory and research functions were transferred to a new bureau within the Food and Drug Administration. The "biologics law" itself had been strengthened in 1944, although claimed by critics still not to be as stringent in effect as the controls applied under FDA jurisdiction to the other categories of prescription drugs. The first such law was passed in 1902 because of special control problems arising from immunologic agents then available for the first time (initially, the diphtheria antitoxin developed in Germany). Trivalent organic arsenicals, used as injectable drugs, were brought under the same law when World War I cut off imports of early chemotherapeutic drugs from Germany (notably Ehrlich's arsphenamine compounds), thus making home production imperative. The biologics law helps to assure reliable potency and safety of products in its special field through a system of product licensure and inspection of producers.[41]

An important, and debatable, pharmaceutical amendment to the Federal Food, Drug, and Cosmetic Act (Section 503b; effective 1952) holds particular import for practicing pharmacists with respect to dividing drugs more definitely into prescription-only drugs and those that must be labeled with adequate directions for non-prescription use, the handling of oral prescriptions, and the requiring of authorization by the physician for prescription refills.[42]

More far-reaching, although not so directly involving the community practice of pharmacy, were the Drug Amendments of 1962 (Public Law 87-781). These resulted from nearly 3 years of Congressional investigation and hearings, concerning hazardous laxity in many instances of the testing and marketing of new drug products. During these investigations led by Senator Kefauver, a sense of persecution pervaded the pharmaceutical industry because of what most industrial leaders considered to be unfair methods and unwarranted sensationalism on the part of the investigating subcommittee in seeking public attention and support for tighter legislative control.[43]

The complexity of the issues and the circumstances surrounding the proposed major amendments left the outcome deeply in doubt, until there appeared in Europe a pharmacomedical tragedy even more devastating than the poisonous "Elixir Sulfanilamide" of 1937, which had generated the emotional drive behind revision of the Federal law at that time. Now it was discovered that several thousand infants had congenital malformations resulting from the use of a new sedative by the mothers during early pregnancy. Meanwhile, the offending drug (thalidomide) was undergoing widespread and not too tightly controlled clinical trials in the United States. Although the tragic aftermath experienced in Europe was averted here, press photographs of the grotesque limbs and afflicted infants brought home to Americans once again that many drugs are a two-edged sword and reminded them of the extent of their reliance on the competence and the dependability of the pharmaceutical industry.

Spurred by public apprehension, Congress adopted more stringent drug legislation to provide added safeguards. It placed rigid controls over the use of drugs still in the investigational stage; it required that a new drug be proved as effective as claimed, not just safe; it became easier for the government to remove from use a drug found to present some unexpected hazard; it revolutionized advertising practices in promoting prescription drugs to the health professions, among other provisions.

The public clearly benefitted from enforcement of these controls. The public also took unexpected losses, which some industrial economists contend outweigh the gains. For example, the tight network of restrictions forced down the number of new drugs that could be brought each year to the stage of routine use. Even some new drugs introduced must be delayed for experimental check of long-term side effects, perhaps jeopardizing the chance for recovery of certain patients. Yet, the uncertainties of assessing risk-to-benefit ratios in drug therapy, and the public preference toward maximizing safety, prevented repeal of the 1962 amendments from becoming a serious issue.[44]

Moreover, the higher demands for proof of efficacy instituted for *new* drugs led the Food and Drug Administration in 1966 to obtain an expert review of about 3,000 older drugs, (introduced between 1938 and 1962). The results swept into oblivion hundreds of drug products and drug claims that had traditional usage. Yet, with each escalation of legal controls—permitted by each new stage of pharmaceutical and pharmacological knowledge—historical evidence reconfirmed that no law can make even the most valued drugs harmless in all circumstances.

## CONTROL OF ADDICTIVE DRUGS

The unsupervised use of narcotics has such grave consequences and is so difficult to control that early in this century special legislation came to be a common goal among both professional and lay groups, only the approach and the details remaining at issue. During the 1870's the distinctive character of addictive drugs had been made clear by scientific medicine in Germany. This understanding required several decades, however, to displace older notions among American practitioners and citizens. Attempts to obtain a legal ban on nonmedicinal use of narcotics had to counter attitudes that it was largely a private moral concern and that, as a social problem, Eastern peoples were peculiarly more susceptible to addiction than those in Western countries.[45]

Opiates were being dispensed freely and legally without a prescription order; and, perhaps worse still, home remedies of secret composition and high-pressure promotion sometimes contained an opium derivative.

By the early years of this century, what had been of concern only among the best informed became alarming to a larger segment of the population. When a committee of the American Pharmaceutical Association looked into the extent of the problem and the demand in pharmacies for addiction-producing drugs (1901), it brought back data termed "appalling."[46] Tradition, the Association's experience (state pharmacy acts) and the members' preference help explain the decision to develop and promote a model state narcotic bill, rather than to appeal for Federal control.

Although state laws were passed, regulation by individual states alone soon became notorious for inadequate enforcement. An earlier Federal act prohibiting the import of nonmedicinal opium (1877; broadened in 1908) likewise had proved to be quite inadequate.

Meanwhile, the Federal government had been an active participant and signatory to the first international agreement to bring the opium and coca traffic and the addiction problem under control (Hague Treaty, 1911). The United States became one of the first nations to try to meet its obligations under the new international agreement when Congress passed the Harrison Narcotic Act in 1914. During ensuing decades the Federal government, through a Bureau of Narcotics, mounted a massive police action against the underworld network that soon developed to create and feed drug habits. The prices of "street drugs" escalated with each new effort to stamp out illicit supplies; and those with compulsive addictions became notorious for crimes committed to fulfill their daily craving for drugs. International efforts—first through the League of Nations then, after World War II, through the United Nations—tried to untangle the scientific, moral, legal and social issues involved and, with only spotty success, to choke off the sources of supply.

Nationally, the Harrison Narcotic Act was amended and added to several times to achieve better control, with nearly all states passing analogous legislation to reinforce control locally.[47] The law regulated "narcotics" within its scope at every level, whether for licit or illicit use, the established network of pharmacists providing a responsible channel for meeting therapeutic needs. Based on his career experience as U.S. Commissioner of Narcotics, Harry J. Anslinger expressed the view that no evidence exists implicating "pharmacists as being in any way responsible for one case among the 46,000 non-medical addicts [then] known to the authorities." Moreover, it was his opinion that "pharmacists accounted for uncovering more forged prescriptions than Federal, state and city authorities combined."[48]

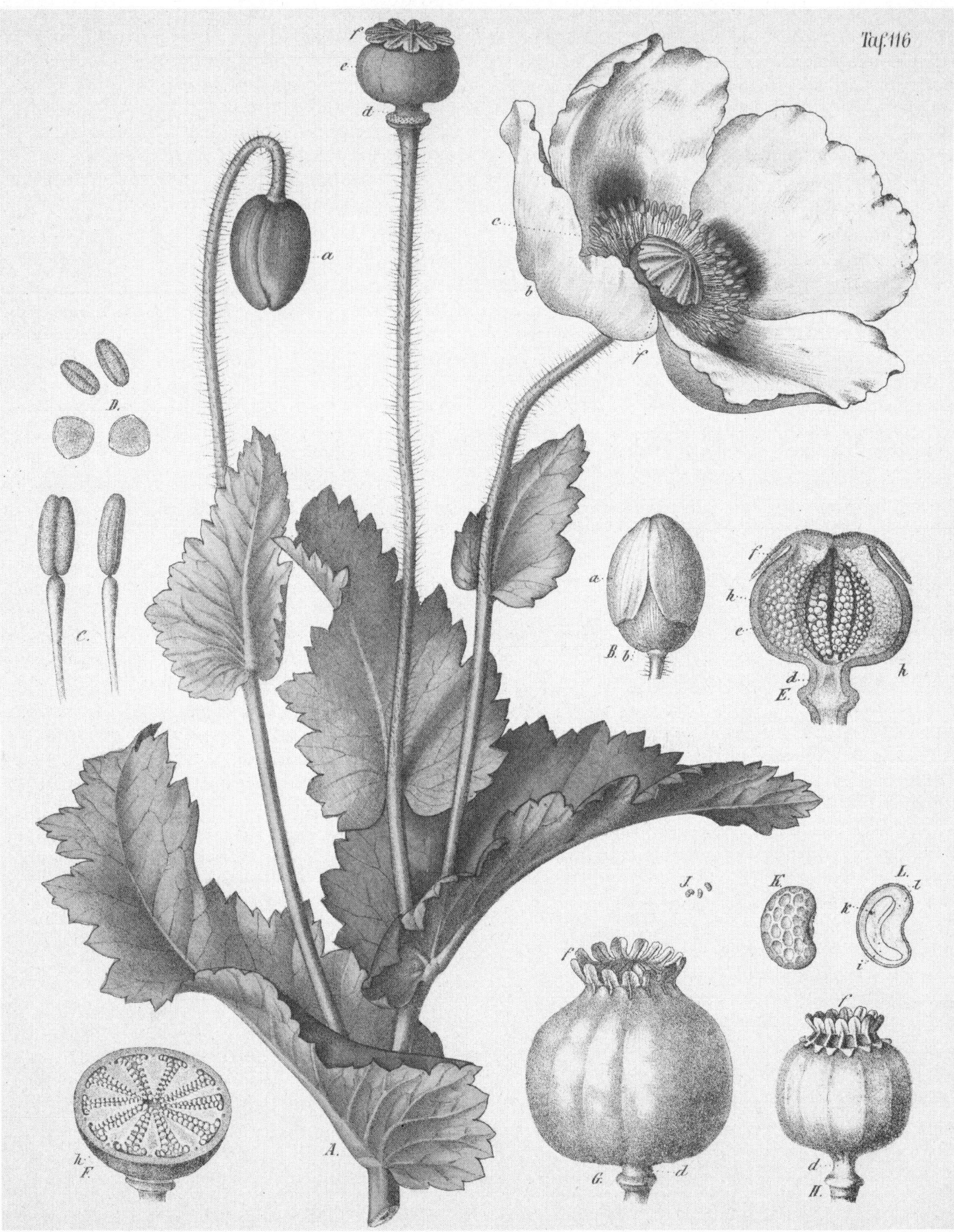
Taf. 116
a
b
c
d
e
f
A.
B.
C.
D.
E.
F.
G.
H.
J.
K.
L.

Yet, the basic problem of misuse and its control remained an enigma. During the 1960's the problem even intensified as new psychoactive drugs were developed for medicinal use, but soon appeared on the black market as "drugs of abuse," whether stimulants, depressants, or hallucinogens. Moreover, dangerous experimentation with psychoactive drugs faddishly spread into middle class segments of American society during the 1960's, especially among youth, whereas earlier drug abuse had seemed most prevalent among the disadvantaged, the alienated and susceptible bohemians in the arts.

Although the medical dimensions of the problem had become more widely recognized since about the 1950's, a public clamor for more effective legal control led the Federal government to set up special offices and commissions. In addition, a series of statutory and regulatory changes during the late 1960's transformed the original Bureau of Narcotics, and in 1970 a new framework was set when Congress adopted the Comprehensive Drug Abuse Prevention and Control Act, and the Controlled Substances Act. The latter provides a new model for parallel state enactments that supersede those based on a model bill of the 1930's. Nationally, all enforcement efforts are coordinated through a Drug Enforcement Administration set up in 1973.[49]

The kaleidoscopic change since the 1960's reflects David Musto's conclusion that "American concern with narcotics is more than a medical or legal problem—it is in the fullest sense a political problem. The energy that has given impetus to drug control and prohibition came from profound tensions among socio-economic groups, ethnic minorities, and generations—as well as the psychological attraction of certain drugs." One consequence has been that "Public demand for action against drug abuse has led to regulative decisions that lack a true regard for the reality of drug use."[50]

Serious public education about the place of all drugs in modern life—in contrast to overreliance upon propaganda techniques and police action has been one approach to such greater "regard for the reality of drug use," in which pharmacists and pharmacy interns have been sharing in an instructional and counseling role.

←

The dried juice from the flower capsule of opium poppies yields an analgesic indispensable since antiquity, but also a drug dependency so enslaving that the special control measure enacted for the USA (1914) found a counterpart in most other countries. No other medicinal plant has exacted such a high social and economic cost world wide. (From Otto K. Berg and C. F. Schmidt: Darstellung . . . offizinellen Gewächse, Tafel 116, III, Leipzig, 1858–63)

## CONCLUSION

Almost every decade of the present century has brought some elaboration of the complex structure of law and regulation over pharmaceutical activities, partly because of the "consumer movement" to maximize protection of citizens in all areas of life, partly because both licit and illicit drugs have become an increasingly significant part of American life. Moreover, the ubiquitous Federal intervention elaborated during the past third of a century—beyond what previously seemed Constitutionally possible—results from new Supreme Court interpretations and from Congressional "declarations" of intent in more recent statutes. All this places added responsibilities upon the pharmacist as the legally mandated custodian of not only the entire range of drug supply but custodian of the expert knowledge that has become crucial to safe and effective use. These specialized duties and recognition would not be possible without the evolving system of professional education that creates "pharmacists."

# 14

# The Development of Education

## PRIVATE SCHOOLS

European civilization was not to be achieved in the New World simply by transferring the European cultural achievements of the late 18th and the early 19th century to the virgin soil of America. Conditions were too different. The exigencies of conquest and settlement, for centuries past only a matter of history in Europe, determined the actual life of people in the United States up to the time of the Civil War. Thus the young republic had to experience the processes of evolution which had characterized the earlier European development—ultimately arriving at a specifically American cultural pattern. Professional education was not a matter of tradition here and still less an effort to impart comprehensive knowledge. Rather, it centered around the kind of people wanting an education and the kind of actual, practical work for which they were to be educated. For some decades, most of the professions that are now replenished by academic graduates depended largely on preceptors who passed their knowledge on to apprentices, academic study being minimal or entirely optional.

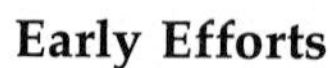

### Early Efforts

Already in 1789 the College of Philadelphia included pharmacy in the title of one of the professors in its medical school (Samuel P. Griffits, professor of materia medica and pharmacy),[1] and the same was true at some

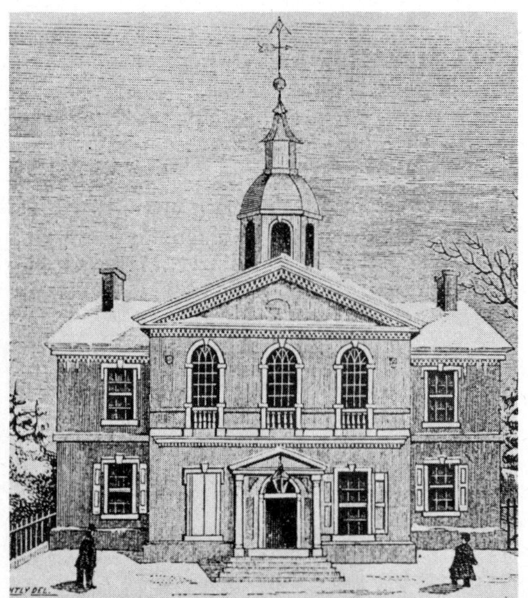

Carpenter's Hall in Philadelphia as it looked when the Philadelphia College of Pharmacy was founded there in 1821. Erected by a guild of master carpenters (1770), the building has served as the cradle for various national institutions and is still preserved as a historic landmark in Independence National Historical Park. The Philadelphia College of Pharmacy operated the first and most influential of the association schools serving 19th-century American pharmacy.

other early medical schools. But this was pharmacy taught by and for physicians. Chemistry also was taught in connection with medicine. At the University of Pennsylvania (about 1810) it was stated that the professorship of chemistry is "almost exclusively" supported by students of medicine, who "are induced to do so in consequence of its application to pharmacy and the different branches of medicine."[2]

Prior to the founding of the Philadelphia College of Pharmacy in 1821, only a few ineffectual attempts to provide instruction in pharmacy for pharmacists are known to have been made.

As early as 1769, a physician (Lewis Mottet) suggested that the colonial commonwealth of South Carolina establish a "botanic garden" and "a chymical Laboratory." He offered himself "for the Direction of the Laboratory, chymical and galenical; and when erected, to collect, analyse and read the General System of Materia Medica." That is, Dr. Mottet was willing to undertake the venture on his own account "if the Public will favour him with the Loan of Six Thousand Pounds Currency." As was to be expected, the proposal was " 'found by the learned Committee, appointed by the Honourable House of Assembly, to be too premature' and the public did not favor Dr. Mottet with six thousand pounds, so the project died aborning."[3] Since he was a native of France, it is not surprising that Mottet's suggestion (of a combination botanic garden and chemical laboratory for the teaching of pharmacy) closely followed the example of the *Jardin du roi* in Paris.

A different attempt 43 years later was more consequential. James Cutbush, a versatile Philadelphia chemist and apothecary, in 1812 advertised "a series of Lectures on the Theory and Practice of Pharmacy, accompanied with the necessary chemical elucidations."[4] He was the first known scientific writer on pharmacy of some importance in America and the first teacher of pharmacy from the point of view of professional pharmacy. For some decades, he was the only one. The other early attempt at theoretic instruction of pharmacists in the sciences of their profession was made in 1816, by a Philadelphia physician, James Mease. Both attempts evidently were unsuccessful and did not receive much attention, "for no further mention was ever made of them."[5]

## Problems of Optional Education

At that time pharmacy in America was considered, by most of those active in this field and by the majority of physicians, as an art that did not require theoretic knowledge; it could best be learned by practice, "by daily handling and preparing the remedies in common use." Had it not been necessary to discourage imminent steps by physicians to bring the dispensing of drugs under medical control, educational pharmaceutical institutions in this country would have remained for a long time only the dream of a few far-seeing pharmacists. Even after their founding, the schools of the early colleges by no means enjoyed continuous prosperity. Thus the Massachusetts College of Pharmacy, founded in 1823, arranged to present occasional lectures but did not provide regular instruction until 1867.

> Some of the institutions, while anxious to educate better the rising generation of pharmacists, found that they were in advance of the time. Even the large cities in which these colleges were situated did not provide a sufficient number of students to pay the professors a moderate lecture fee. Thus after several attempts in New York, Dr. Squibb offered his services free and even dragged his lecture equipment from his Brooklyn factory to the lecture room in New York City. In St. Louis the preceptors appear to have been interested more than were their apprentices.[6]

The number of pharmacists attending lectures in the few American colleges of pharmacy before the Civil War was small, and the number who graduated naturally was still smaller. Most of the schools had to struggle to remain alive, at least until the last third of the century.[7] The whole situation cannot be characterized better than it was in the "address to the pharmacists of the United States," which was composed by a commission under the leadership of Wm. Procter, Jr., and Edward Parrish (accepted by the American Pharmaceutical Association in 1854 and printed "for general distribution").[8] The address complained that there was at that time usually neither a legally indentured apprenticeship nor an honor-bound obligation and therefore, that:

> Our country has been deluged with incompetent drug clerks, whose claim to the important position they hold or apply for is based on a year or two's service in the shop, perhaps under circumstances illy calculated to increase their knowledge. These clerks in turn become principals, and have the direction of others—alas! for the progeny that some of them bring forth, as ignorance multiplied by ignorance will produce neither knowledge nor skill. . . . It has been found that there are three classes of individuals engaged in pharmaceutical pursuits . . . to whom particularly this address is directed: First, those who are imperfectly acquainted with pharmacy and are in business for themselves; secondly, those who have been but half educated as apprentices and who are now assistants receiving salaries, having the responsibility of business entrusted to them; and thirdly, those who are now apprentices or beginners under circumstances and with ideas unfavorable to the acquirement of the thorough knowledge of the drug and apothecary business.

It is significant that the Association did not expect the people to whom it appealed, even the beginners, to study at one of the pharmacy schools. It merely admonished all of these groups to read pharmaceutical literature "regularly and understandingly" and to "assist the reading when necessary by experiment and observation." The graduates of the schools of pharmacy were given the admonition to "act as examples to their less favored brethren." The address states that the American Pharmaceutical Association, recognizing the "vast importance of good schools of pharmacy, where the sciences are regularly taught," will "freely extend its countenance and encouragement to those already existing and to all new efforts."

An important step had been taken with the establishment of a professorship of pharmacy not connected with materia medica, and held not by a physician but by a pharmacist, for the sole purpose of teaching prospective pharmacists. Just 25 years after the founding of the Philadelphia College of Pharmacy (1846) the trustees thus divided the chair of materia medica and pharmacy and unanimously elected to the new chair William Procter, Jr. The report of the committee appointed to consider creating a Professorship of Pharmacy, which was unanimously adopted, said:

> In organizing the school of pharmacy, it was found necessary to seek professors in the ranks of the medical profession—few, if any, of the apothecaries had so accustomed themselves to the systematic study of the several branches connected with the practice of our profession, as to be prepared to assume the office of teachers. Hence it is not surprising that the theory and practice of pharmacy, although held to be of the highest importance to the student, was not allotted to a professor as a separate branch of instruction, but was appended secondarily to the branches of materia medica and chemistry. The question now arises whether, by the lectures in our school, and by other means tending to create a greater taste for scientific attainment among those who practice our profession, so much advancement has been made, as to warrant the appointment of a practical apothecary to teach in a scientific manner, *what has hitherto, in America and England, been the confused and unsystematized art of Pharmacy*. . . . The professor of Pharmacy, if one should be elected, must enter a field of labor scarcely less extensive than that of either of his colleagues in the school, [i.e., the teachers of pharmaceutical chemistry and materia medica] and one which he will have to traverse in the double capacity of teacher and learner. *We look in vain amongst the medical literature of the English language for a single work devoted exclusively and systematically to this branch of knowledge.* To French and German Pharmaciens and books we are indebted for most that is in-

teresting, instructive and original in regard to Pharmacy. The latter are only available to a limited extent in this country, and are not well adapted to our different circumstances. . . . We would suggest, that as Philadelphia was the first city in the Union to organize a College of Pharmacy, and has continued to be regarded as the metropolis of Pharmaceutical as well as Medical Science in America, it is peculiarly appropriate that this measure, *so imperatively demanded by our present circumstances, and so necessary to an advancement of our profession,* corresponding with the progress of science and general intelligence in our country, should be consummated here.[9*]

These two documents supplement each other. Procter's address of 1854 pictures the general situation among members of the calling who needed to become educated; the College report of 1846 shows the difficulties that educators faced in the fulfillment of their task. Conditions in the drug trade for decades afterward made a scientific basis for the whole of American pharmacy a remote objective. The lack of suitable literature in English made each American teacher in pharmacy a pioneer in his field. The ostensible motherland of the American people, England, had neglected pharmacy and could offer neither a pattern to be followed nor the means to be used to build up American professional pharmacy. The standard of the French and the German models and achievements was too high, and their spirit was too different. America could not simply copy them. The trustees of the Philadelphia College of Pharmacy were taking a courageous step in that they were painfully aware of the difficulties involved. How great a need was being filled by them, and how highly esteemed this instruction in pharmacy proper was, is illustrated by the following comparison: "There had been an average number [of Philadelphia graduates] annually for the nineteen years preceding the election of Procter to the new chair of pharmacy in 1846 of only 5½, while in the 19 years which followed the average number receiving the diploma annually was 21."[10]

The establishment of the professorship of pharmacy at the Philadelphia College of Pharmacy had a remarkable prelude. William Procter, Jr., the first man to occupy this chair, as well as Edward Parrish, the secretary of the College, were both graduates of the College. Both had experienced the inadequacy of pharmacy "for physicians taught by physicians" as the basis for professional practice of pharmacy. However, Parrish went a step further. If pharmacy was indeed a special branch of medicine, it must receive acknowledgment of its independence. As a separate art, it had the right to declare its own standards and curriculum. Only those who had mastered its scientific foundations and could demonstrate a complete knowledge of all departments, including its practical applications, could qualify as teachers. Pharmacists, physicians or other persons who wished to practice pharmacy were to be taught by these learned pharmacists. Physicians had lost their foothold in the teaching of pharmacy, in the opinion of Parrish; in fact, if they were to practice pharmacy, they should now be taught by pharmacists. Thus Parrish turned the tables on the medical profession:

> In 1843 he purchased the drugstore . . . adjoining the building of the University of Pennsylvania, which brought him in contact with medical students and their wants. He believed that those who should return to their homes, often in isolated communities, would be without the information that would enable them to compound and dispense medicines for their patients, and that pharmaceutical knowledge was necessary to them, since they would be far removed from prescription drugstores, *still to be found only in the largest towns and cities.** He therefore started a School of Practical Pharmacy in the rear of his building . . . and gave courses of instruction to those who wished to avail themselves of them. Later (1850) . . . the school was removed to a place, where better accommodations were had and instruction was given to both pharmaceutical and medical students.[11]

---

*Italics added.

When appointed "superintendent of the practical department of Parrish's" (1859) the master pharmacist John M. Maisch offered "all manipulations required in a pharmaceutical establishment" and made known the opening of "a laboratory for practical & analytical chemistry, designed in particular for the wants of pharmaceutists." "For students, sufficiently advanced" Maisch even held out the prospect of "a practical course of toxicological analysis."[12]

This School of Practical Pharmacy, existing side by side with the new chair of pharmacy of the College, paralleled the pioneer instruction in pharmaceutical and chemical laboratory work, being given by German pharmacists about 1800. In their capacity as professors of pharmacy and materia medica, or of pharmaceutical chemistry in German universities, they gave the practical instruction in backroom laboratories of their pharmacies to students of medicine and of pharmacy.

The separate professorship of theory and practice of pharmacy at the Philadelphia College of Pharmacy had a precursor two years earlier at the Maryland College of Pharmacy, suggesting the need felt for a more academic approach to pharmacy, at least in urban centers. The Maryland professorship specifically in pharmacy was different and far less consequential from that at Philadelphia. One difference was that the man appointed, David Stewart, was a physician as well as a pharmacist and opened his lectures to students of medicine as well as pharmacy. A more significant difference was Procter's long service and far-reaching influence, while Stewart taught pharmacy only 2 years (1844–1846) and did not long remain prominent in the profession.[13]

Until well after the Civil War, however, physician-teachers were more the rule than the exception. To Edward Parrish it was a point of self-respect to "cut loose from that vassalage to physicians . . ."[14] Yet, American pharmacy—underdeveloped and perhaps partly underambitious—did not itself quickly yield men qualified to staff the schools. Teachers holding the "M.D." were first displaced in pharmaceutical chemistry, and by the end of the 19th century were disappearing from all departments.[15]

The courses and the students during the first period of the Chicago School of Pharmacy (1850–1860) have been described as follows:

> The course continued for twenty weeks. Lectures were given upon three evenings each week, two hours each evening. . . . The students were earnest young fellows, employed in drugstores during the day, and though the course was necessarily presented in the briefest manner, they were encouraged to read, study, and experiment, utilizing the opportunities afforded in the shops. . . . The teachers possessed the equipment necessary for demonstration of the lectures but there were no laboratories.[16]

At Philadelphia in 1868:

> The courses of instruction were still given only in the evening—on Monday, Wednesday and Friday evenings, from about October, until the end of February. The school, as from the first day, was set to answer the needs of apothecaries' apprentices. . . . Diplomas were given only to persons of good moral character of the age of at least 21 years. They must have attended two courses of each of the lectures delivered in the college, or one course in the college and one course in some other reputable college of pharmacy *or medical school* in which the same branches might be taught. They also must have served out at least four years with a person or persons qualified to conduct the drug or apothecary business.[17]

These quotations give a true picture of the scope and the quality of professional education enjoyed by that small minority of American pharmacists who attended one of the pharmacy schools before 1870. The fees did not provide a living for the teachers, whose main activities consequently lay outside the college. Materia medica was one of the most prominent subjects taught in this period, including whatever elementary botany was taught. Physics, if taught at all, was an introductory part of chemistry instruction. The instruction was almost exclusively through lectures. Unsatisfactory financial conditions were largely responsible for the lack of laboratory instruction. Even when the Philadelphia College of Pharmacy erected (1868) a new building, which was remarkable for that period, it did not equip a laboratory immediately. However, by means of funds collected from alumni, "a pharmaceutical and chemical laboratory for individual instruction" was opened in 1870.[18] It was directed by John M. Maisch, the same man who had conducted the first individual laboratory instruction for pharmacists and physicians, about 10 years before, in Parrish's School of Practical Pharmacy.

The era of pioneer pharmacy schools, established by the early pharmaceutical associations, called colleges of pharmacy (see p. 190), ended with the Civil War. Until 1865, when the St. Louis College of Pharmacy opened, there existed five such association schools, and only one other pharmaceutical educational institution, the Course in Pharmacy of the Medical Department of Tulane University, New Orleans (founded in 1838).

From that time on, various pharmacy schools were founded privately by groups of pharmacists organized only for that purpose, or as part of private or denominational universities and colleges, or as divisions of medical colleges.

During this last third of the 19th century, even more frequently in medicine were colleges operated not so much to promote medical knowledge as to turn a profit for the people creating these so-called "proprietary schools."[19]

Whenever these colleges offered courses in pharmacy, as a rapidly increasing number of them did, it was at least questionable whether their departments of pharmacy were created for bona fide pharmaceutical instruction or whether they were mainly "feeders" for the medical courses. However, the opposition of the men representing professional

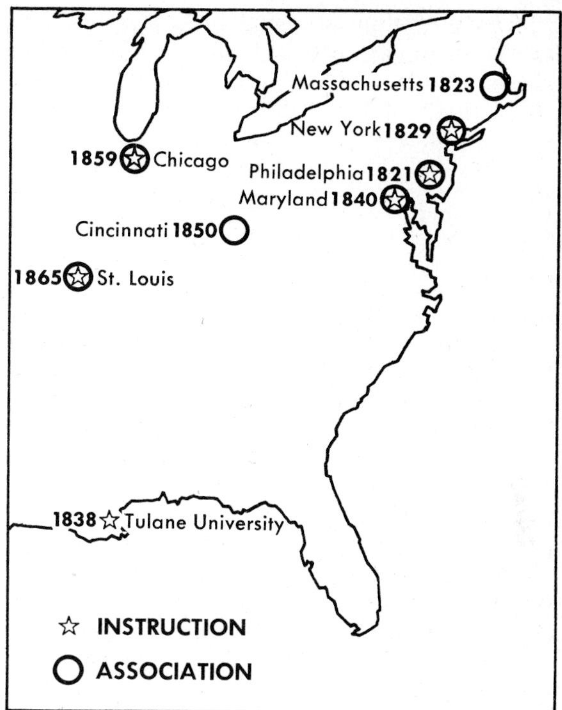


The map illustrates that nearly all organized endeavor and instruction in pharmacy was in the northeastern quarter of the present United States until after the Civil War. An exception was the pharmacy course, in conjunction with medicine, offered in New Orleans. A regular course of instruction was offered by five of the seven local associations of pharmacy founded by 1865. Dates on the map are those of the founding of the associations.

pharmacy was not directed primarily against inadequacies within these schools; it was based on principle. Such men had created and fostered the old colleges of pharmacy to make American pharmacy an independent profession and to secure a special education for the pharmacist in the United States. While they were ready to recognize a period of study at a medical college as an equivalent of study at a college of pharmacy, they could not sanction any step that might surrender pharmaceutical education to medical domi-

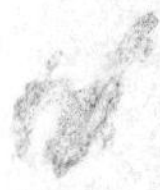

nation, and thus lead the profession back to the situation from which it had scarcely escaped. A.Ph.A.'s astute secretary, John M. Maisch of Philadelphia, looked upon the medical-college intrusion

> . . . with the same favor with which we should regard the attempt of a college of pharmacy to confer the degree of Doctor of Medicine, honoris causa or otherwise. . . .[20]
>
> We are earnestly advocating the proper education of the pharmacist, and are in favor of the multiplication of colleges of pharmacy, but not to an indefinite number, which would be fraught with results similar to those which the medical profession throughout the country is endeavoring to correct.[21]

The private schools, depending partly on the approval of the practicing pharmacists who functioned as their trustees and financial supporters, and depending always on the fees of their students, developed pharmaceutical education along the same lines as did the old-line colleges (associations). Serviceable in its time, this mold for pharmaceutical education became increasingly cramped and limiting. It was to be broken by a strikingly different educational program, thrusting out of a different environment, the state university.

## STATE UNIVERSITIES

As early as 1847, William Procter, Jr., noted the necessity of state-controlled practice of medicine and pharmacy, when he said:

> It is a characteristic of our national and state governments to interfere as little as possible with the working of private interests, and competition is left unimpeded to control the business affairs of society. This liberty of action, so advantageous in the common intercourse of men, is unfortunate in reference to medicine, which, as no guarantee of qualification is required by law of its practitioners, is thrown open to any individual who chooses to adopt the title of doctor or apothecary, be he ever so ignorant.[22]

Yet, Procter, and also Maisch, the influential proponent of state pharmacy laws (see p. 216), opposed the advancement of pharmaceutical education through an agency of the state. This seems scarcely comprehensible unless we understand their commitment to an educational ideology of the old-line colleges that was based on an apprenticeship system. Formal study was intended merely to round off a prolonged apprenticeship that was prerequisite to graduation.

After pharmacy made connections with general institutions of higher learning, through state universities, old ways and traditions of creating new generations of pharmacists were challenged. Moreover, leaders such as Procter and Maisch knew the effort that many had invested in developing pharmaceutical education independent from the medical profession; hence their reluctance to accord the state university the privilege of intruding into a field that pharmacy had claimed for its own and developed largely on its own is understandable.

At the first state-supported institution to produce graduates in pharmacy (1867), the Medical College of South Carolina, pharmacy instruction had a precarious existence until almost the end of the century.[23]

However, the transformation of pharmaceutical education was to draw its power and pattern from another quarter, the midwestern state universities, first and notably exemplified by the pharmacy curriculum approved at the University of Michigan in 1868. Unlike some states in subsequent years, Michigan embarked on a vigorous and full program of instruction without either the suggestive influence of pharmacy legislation or the support of the profession itself. Instead, the course grew out of pharmacy's earlier connection with medical instruction there, through the intermediary of an outstanding chemical laboratory, backed by an administration noted for its pioneering.

In a bold innovation the University of Michigan introduced extensive laboratory instruction coupled with basic science, made the academic study of pharmacy practically a full-time occupation and refused to accept responsibility for apprenticeship as a prerequisite to graduation.

A key figure in this development was the physician-chemist placed in charge of the new pharmacy curriculum, Albert B. Prescott, "Professor of Organic Chemistry and Pharmacy." In pharmaceutical circles Prescott gained widespread respect for himself but unpopularity for his pharmacy program. Therefore, it was before a rather unwilling audience that Prescott presented his classic address on "Pharmaceutical Education" at the 1871 meeting of the American Pharmaceutical Association.[24]

With brevity and clarity, Prescott explained the advantages of a real scientific education and gave his reasons for believing a preliminary apprenticeship, before graduation, unnecessary. These reasons are met again and again, in the frequent discussions of the same question in almost all European countries within the past century.[25]

Apprehension about the University of Michigan's rejection of the responsibility for the apprenticeship can be understood, however, if we recall that in the 1870's few states had a pharmacy law or an administrative board to which that responsibility could be shifted. The idea that the neophyte needs to learn to apply academic knowledge to pharmaceutical practice has a long tradition. Thus, the A.Ph.A Secretary, John Maisch, could have been writing on similar occasions in other times or countries when he argued:

> We grant that as much knowledge in physical and chemical science, and natural history generally, as a young man may possibly acquire before he enters a drugstore, is extremely desirable; but we believe that with all his knowledge of chemistry, natural history, and natural sciences generally, he will not be a pharmacist until he has gone through a regular system of [practical] training, and that is exactly where the colleges of pharmacy throughout the country differ from the University of Michigan. . . . *The colleges are not discouraging preliminary education before the apprentice enters the apothecary business; but what we insist upon is that it is wrong to give a pharmaceutical degree before the graduate has had pharmaceutical experience.*[26]

The break with tradition was sharp and the results uncertain, and within the old framework one could say that the American Pharmaceutical Association only did its duty when it did not recognize the School of Pharmacy of the University of Michigan as a "college of pharmacy within the proper meaning" of the constitution and by-laws of the American Pharmaceutical Association, "it being neither an organization controlled

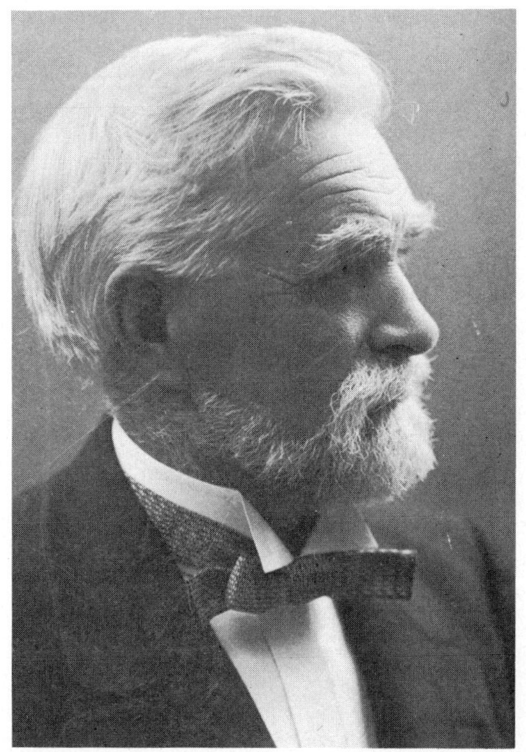

One of the most influential men in the molding of modern pharmaceutical education in America, Albert B. Prescott (1832–1905) was a physician-chemist at the University of Michigan. There he established a school of pharmacy in a pattern radically different from that of schools elsewhere.

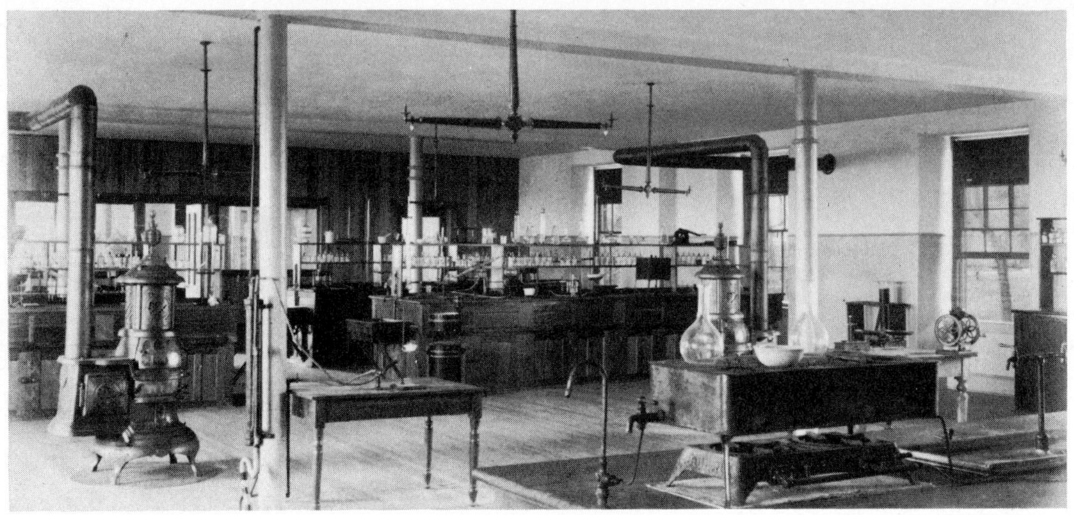

Pharmaceutical laboratory at the University of Wisconsin (1890), just before its school of pharmacy became the first in the country to offer a standard baccalaureate program of four years. Michigan and Wisconsin, like other state schools that followed their pattern, gave a wholly new emphasis to the sciences underlying pharmacy and to laboratory instruction in particular. (Photo: University of Wisconsin)

by pharmacists nor an institution of learning which, by its rules and requirements, insures to its graduates the proper practical training to place them on a par with the graduates of the several colleges of pharmacy represented in this association."[27]

A report on the first graduates of the University of Michigan School of Pharmacy shows that non-pharmacists indeed availed themselves of the opportunity to enter the course without practical pharmaceutical experience.[28]

The second state-university school of pharmacy, founded 15 years later (1883) at the University of Wisconsin, competed with Michigan in its scientific emphasis, yet remained within the old lines in its relationship to the practice of pharmacy. The reason lies in the different circumstances under which the first two schools of pharmacy in American state universities were founded. The design of the older one was a bold revolutionary attempt at the beginning of reconstruction after the Civil War, while the younger one was a product of evolution within this period.

The Michigan school was the outgrowth of a course of pharmacy, which "when first established was by no means mainly designed for students looking forward to the practice of pharmacy. . . . In 1860 the design was more for students of medicine, to give them help in handling medicines when they should come into practice, but it was quite as much intended as general practical training in applied science."[29] The school was started without the cooperation of the pharmaceutical practitioners, who in fact were opposed to the idea. This took place 6 years before the founding of a state pharmaceutical association in Michigan and 17 years before enactment of a state pharmacy law.

The department of pharmacy at the University of Wisconsin, in contrast, was established by legislative act on special request of the pharmacists of the state, assembled in an annual meeting of their state association, 3 years after the founding of this association and 1 year after the enactment of a Wisconsin pharmacy law. As a result, Frederick B. Power, the first leader of the University of Wisconsin School of Pharmacy, had to take into consideration the established pharmaceutical forces and evolution to which his school owed its existence. Unlike Prescott of Michigan (a physician), Power himself came from the ranks of practical pharmacy and was a graduate of the Philadelphia College of Pharmacy. He recognized the desire of community pharmacists not to risk losing the identity of the concept of "pharmacy" with that of "drugstore," by awarding a pharmaceutical degree to persons without practical experience. Wisconsin therefore made this experience a requirement for a diploma, although not a prerequisite for admission to the course.

The problem of dealing in a balanced way with the science and the practice of pharmacy eventually was solved through the development of licensure examinations in the various states (see p. 215). By this means the pharmaceutical practitioners took on themselves the responsibility for appraising the practical experience and the knowledge of the candidate. The requirement that a candidate for a license have experience before taking the state-board examination made it unnecessary for the schools to require this experience for graduation.

## CONSOLIDATION OF THE SCHOOL SYSTEM

New concepts of American pharmaceutical education, both graduate and undergraduate, flourished in the environment of state universities and land-grant colleges. Unlike the old-line universities on the Eastern seaboard, they did not hesitate to harness intellect for a wide spectrum of the world's work, helping to staff an expanding group of university-educated professions and avidly cultivating applied science. Unlike many of the private and association schools in pharmacy, they had the resources to place the student's instruction in pharmacy on a foundation of basic laboratory sciences and to widen his intellectual horizons beyond purely vocational limits.

In the end, only the strongest of the old independent schools could compete effectively for students without soiling academic robes with the appeal of cheaper degrees and lower standards. Many did not survive; many others affiliated and merged with general institutions of higher learning. In less than a half century United States pharmacy moved from a handful of hard-pressed night schools in rented rooms to a plethora of schools of disparate standards and types by the turn of the century, and then, after the first World War, into a period of consolidation and strengthening.

In the chronologic table prepared as Appendix 4 (p. 383) can be seen the spread of different types of schools across the country. It has been noted that four of the five schools regularly teaching before the Civil War were operated by local associations of pharmacists, the fifth by a medical college. The Civil War dealt the adolescent educational system a heavy blow; but after the war each passing decade put formal education within easier reach of prospective students. While each of the four preceding decades had seen one school or at most two begin pharmaceutical instruction, there were ten new schools in each of two postwar decades, a figure doubled in the 1880's and tripled in the 1890's.

From the 1880's onward a majority of the new schools were associated with general institutions of higher education; few any longer were born under association auspices. Proprietary schools, which often smacked of being business ventures, helped to swell the total late in the century, although pharmacy was not plagued with them as medicine was.[30]

Shortly after the turn of the century, however, there apparently were more pharmacy schools than there have been at any time since. All evidence suggests there were too many schools, pressed too hard for sufficient students to remain solvent, to permit steady or uniform progress. Among 80 schools teaching pharmacy (surveyed in 1905), 32 were affiliated with a university or a general college, where there were none a half century earlier. It was to be a persistent trend. Seventy years later (1975) there were fewer schools; and all but 4 of the 73 were affiliated with a university or general college. Meanwhile, the distribution of the schools geographically had improved somewhat, with at least one in all but 7 of the states.[31]

A well organized system of pharmaceutical education had matured by mid-20th century, more than adequate to educate the number of pharmacists needed for pharmaceutical services nationally. In relation to the population served, the number of schools of pharmacy was roughly the same as in some other countries during the 1960's (e.g., Canada, France and Italy), but more schools than in certain other countries (e.g., United Kingdom, West Germany, Sweden and Spain).[32]

## PRELIMINARY EDUCATION

In a first, ill-fated associational effort among schools of pharmacy (1870) the hope had been expressed that pharmacists would insist on better educational background in selecting apprentices for their shops. Here was where the screening took place, it was traditionally assumed, and the schools had not ventured to interpose any actual requirement themselves in regard to preliminary education.

If a youth of the 1870's had asked how much "book learning" he needed to enter pharmacy, Pharmacist A would have replied, ". . . Any boy of 12 to 15 years, who can read, write or cypher a little, is well enough educated to be placed in any store." If the boy turned to Pharmacist B, he would have been told that to be a real pharmacist he first needed the education "which the common schools supply, supplemented by systematic instruction in natural and physical science where attainable, and by the elements of Latin and Greek, and one or more of the modern languages of Europe."[33] If pressed, this pharmacist might have conceded: "At least that's what we hope to find in coming generations of American pharmacy; but we need sincere lads like you. If you know your arithmetic, grammar and can write a good hand, I'll take you on at my shop."

Whether a preceptor even that demanding of preliminary education was the exception or the rule is no longer easy to discern. It does seem clear that the schools generally found it expedient to accept the apprentices sent to them by members of their association-sponsor, rather than see such youths proceed headlong into the practice of pharmacy without any formal pharmaceutical education at all.

The first serious attempt to require of matriculants some definite preparation arose in the state schools of pharmacy. In this the schools were encouraged by the public support that largely freed them from worrisome dependence on student fees to remain solvent, and by the strong though sometimes hidden forces that hold individual departments to some semblance of a general university standard.

State universities in the old Northwest (i.e., Middle West) were better able to withstand pressure against admission standards. Their requirements around 1885 varied from a common school education as at Purdue, to high school graduation (or, alternatively, scores on an admission examination that probably lay between common-school and high-school attainment) as at Michigan and Wisconsin.[34] Yet, in the country as a whole at this time, Professor E. S. Bastin maintained, "it is the rarest occurrence that an applicant is rejected on the ground of lack of preliminary education."[35]

By the turn of the century, pharmacy seems to have been pretty well abreast of medicine and law in the proportion of schools requiring the equivalent of a high-school education for entrance. Below this layer of the most demanding schools of pharmacy—mostly in state universities—requirements fell off sharply, in comparison with medicine and law.[36]

Agitators for better preliminary preparation of students met a sluggish, apathetic response in the profession. A Section of the American Pharmaceutical Association, considering the ignorance of matriculants a pressing problem, attempted for a second time (1898) to sound out opinion among the state boards and state associations. James H. Beal, who conducted the survey, reported back that "Only two state associations seem to have given the matter any consideration . . . No report was received from any Board of Pharmacy."[37]

An organized stand by the schools themselves became possible after they joined together in what is now called the American Association of Colleges of Pharmacy. In a move made effective for the school year 1908–1909 "satisfactory completion of at least one year of work in an accredited high school or its equivalent" became an obligatory minimum for member schools (excepting, for a few years, matriculants from 13 Western states and Indian Territory).[38] This standard was soon advanced to a prerequisite of 2 years of high school or the equivalent (effective 1917–1918). Finally, in the fall of 1923 a 4-year high school requirement became binding on the 42 schools in the association (of which more than half already were meeting such a standard voluntarily).

The hesitant advance of the schools was conditioned at least partially by a still greater reluctance on the part of the members of the state pharmaceutical associations. The lack of professional recognition (hinging on inadequate educational standards) in the armed forces during World War I led to an awareness, as Blauch and Webster phrase it, "that the profession had suffered from a too-conservative educational philosophy."[39]

Yet in a little more than one decade, between 1920 and 1932, American pharmacy finally caught up with European standards, by adding to the preliminary requirement of graduation from a secondary school the requirement that a pharmacy curriculum lead to a standard baccalaureate college degree. Within this short time, the united endeavor of the American Pharmaceutical Association, the American Association of Colleges of Pharmacy and the National Association of Boards of Pharmacy gave American pharmacy a recognized academic basis. However, before this progress could become effective for the whole of American pharmacy, meeting the college standard had to be made a prerequisite to taking a state examination to qualify for a license to practice. It was only through legal requirement that better and more uniformly educated pharmacists could be guaranteed.

New York became the first state (1905) to require college graduation in pharmacy of all candidates appearing before the State Board of Pharmacy[40] and was followed the next year by Pennsylvania. After another decade 17 other states had passed similar laws.[41] By 1949 only Vermont and the Territory of Alaska were holding out against a mandatory college diploma.

## INTERNSHIP

Whatever the academic requirements, apprenticeship had always been at least part of the education of a pharmacist in Europe and later in America. Until pharmacy laws swept through state legislatures in the late 19th century, an apprenticeship of variable length constituted pharmaceutical education for most American-trained practitioners, and in some states long after that. It was a watered-down version of the old apprenticeship system of Europe, lacking clear standards.

The preceptors of apprentices often had been prominent in founding and controlling the independent schools of pharmacy, because they saw the need for some academic supplement to their on-the-job training. The university schools, in contrast, tended to see on-the-job training as a supplement to academic instruction. In any event, apprenticeship was not to be considered a proper university subject, hence it was separate from university programs and outside their responsibility.

As academic requirements among the states advanced, the length of apprenticeship dwindled stepwise to a single year after 1932, in the period when most states agreed that their pharmacists should be graduates of a 4-year academic program. Few questioned the basic assumption, however, that a novice pharmacist, even after college graduation, is not yet fully competent, and that apprenticeship permits a maturing of skill in actual practice and a kind of learning that does not, and probably should not, take place in an academic institution.

The National Association of Boards of Pharmacy had become interested in encouraging more uniformity among the states in the supervised practical experience required for licensure, partly to make it easier for a pharmacist to transfer his license from one state to another. Probably the first systematic move toward uniformity and standards came in 1936 when the N.A.B.P. set up the Committee to Study and Correlate Practical Experience Requirements. This committee promptly became productive under the chairmanship of Robert P. Fischelis, Secretary of the New Jersey Board of Pharmacy, which in 1936 had adopted minimum standards far in advance of those typical of the period. By 1940 the committee had generated national guidelines for the period of practical experience in a pharmacy required of graduates; but the N.A.B.P. did not make these standards effective for another 6 years because of divergent opinions and the distraction of World War II, and still later it weakened them by amendments. As late as 1951 only about half the states had adopted the N.A.B.P.'s minimum standards.

Scrutinizing the wide gap between aspirations and performance in making the average apprenticeship a learning experience, the Pharmaceutical Survey in 1950 admonished the state boards of pharmacy that either experience "as a prerequisite for licensure be modified to be of more practical value or else abolished."[42] Few practitioners or educators believed that the requirement should be abolished. More debatable was the question of proper content and how to assure it in the pharmacies where students experienced what came to be called, during the 1950's, their "internship."* Some states tightened reporting requirements placed upon preceptors and interns. The N.A.B.P. generated its valuable *Preceptor's Guide,* which was first distributed in 1962. Also in 1962, a conference of 8 interested societies called by the American Society of Hospital Pharmacists culminated in the first "Statement on Accreditation of Hospital Pharmacy Internship Training Programs"; and on this basis the ASHP has had a consistently constructive influence on internships and residencies in hospital pharmacy. Still more promising was a prototype created by Wisconsin in 1966 when the state employed a full-time Director of Pharmaceutical Internship to administer a structured 1-year program conducted by preceptors in specially selected training pharmacies. This internship program was placed under the control of a tripartite commission (representing the state board, organized pharmacy, and education). The mechanism of tripartite sponsorship was in place or in process in 40 states three years later, with N.A.B.P. encouragement, although few states were yet ready to adopt the rather carefully structured and controlled content of the Wisconsin internship.[43] Moreover, the changing character of academic education for pharmacy was generating pressure upon the N.A.B.P. to modify its 1-year standard for

*Various terms used to designate supervised experience—"apprenticeship," "internship," "externship," "clerkship," "practical training"—often have distinctive differences in meaning; but usage has not been well stabilized between decades and between states, so for present purposes the question has been ignored.

the internship component of education. This changing attitude was rationalized partly on grounds that "in light of the increased emphasis on programs of this type [that require "patient-orientation" and patient contact] that less time might be required for the total period of internship." The Association therefore adopted in 1971 a much more flexible policy (expressed as a 1500-hour minimum after two years of college, which could include 400 hours concurrently with college in an approved program).

In the 1970's a variety of experimental approaches were being tried, and the experience requirement again appeared to be in transition, tending to reintegrate with academic education under the impact of extended programs infused with the concept of "clinical pharmacy"; diversity rather than uniformity became in this period the keynote; and a growing mood of mutual responsibility for the practical-experience requirement emerged between the colleges and the state boards. Although the N.A.B.P. had never seriously considered "that internship should be abandoned," the accrediting body (A.C.P.E.) recognized since 1974 a prospect (if not yet the fact) that "the experiences students gain in the clinical courses (including clerkships and externships) should be of such caliber so as to serve in lieu of the internship requirement for licensure."[44]

The old dividing line between academic and practical learning experience was blurring. In the course of a century the relationship of the supervised experience to formal academic study, in one sense, had come full circle.

## CURRICULUM

What should the schools teach students who come to them? Before the present century there had been no detailed agreement, either among schools or between the schools and the state boards of pharmacy. The question of what qualifications a pharmacist ideally should have came into sharper focus as states began to require a college diploma as a prerequisite to licensure.

When the first state to require a diploma (New York) tried to decide what training the diploma should represent, it became apparent that the problem was of national scope. Efforts to solve it led to the formation of a National Syllabus Committee (1906), which outlined a curriculum and recommended the proportion and the character of constituent subjects. To continue such work permanently, the Committee was organized formally to represent the American Conference of Pharmaceutical Faculties, the National Association of Boards of Pharmacy and the American Pharmaceutical Association.

In successive editions of its manual, *The Pharmaceutical Syllabus*, the joint Committee endeavored to leave the schools freedom in their methods and curricular decisions and yet provide "suggestions and outlines that may serve as a rational basis for instruction and that will afford scientific tests to determine the fitness of applicants seeking license as pharmacists." However, apprehension about possible regimentation grew, and disagreements became intensified in the 1940's about the direction and the influence of the work of the joint Syllabus Committee. This culminated in the dissolution of the Committee (1946), and a fifth edition of the *Syllabus* never got beyond a tentative mimeographed version.

The American Council on Pharmaceutical Education, which had become active (1932) as the agency to maintain standards in pharmaceutical education, has persistently avoided charges of putting education in a straitjacket by dictating specifics, which had brought about the demise of the Syllabus Committee. Instead, it has emphasized more general requirements for admission and graduation (e.g., years, clock hours of instruction, proportion of laboratory work). The detailed curricular guides that the Syllabus Committee had provided dropped out of sight, but in an advisory capacity, the Curriculum Committee of the American Association of Colleges of Pharmacy has continued to analyze specific issues and segments of the instructional programs.[45]

Part of the problem of deciding curriculum content lay in breaking up the hardened traditions of classical pharmaceutical education, which pre-dated the rise of organic chemistry, bacteriology and pharmacology during the late 19th century. Another part of the problem lay in the tendency of state-university schools to provide for the practical needs of community pharmacy without feeling limited by them. The educational needs of the pharmaceutical field in its totality and at all levels more nearly expressed their eventual aim. Other schools spoke more modestly on behalf of education conceived for the corner druggist of America's main streets.

This major difference of view tended to polarize and perplex those who were shaping pharmaceutical education during the late 19th and early 20th centuries. The University of Michigan took the first steps already at the end of the 1860's toward setting a new direction. It raised academic instruction in pharmacy to the level of a systematic approach to the underlying sciences. It substituted full-time day instruction for the old-time evening courses, besides making intensive laboratory work obligatory. Gradually, other schools followed suit.

The announcement of the new curriculum at Michigan said that the course was to be comprised of "lectures in inorganic and organic chemistry, materia medica and principles of pharmacy; with laboratory courses in qualitative analysis, toxicology, analysis of urine, volumetric analysis, and a somewhat extended course in pharmaceutical operations. Also class exercise in botany."[46] Quantitative analysis, organic analysis, botany and microscopic botany were optional at first but within a few years were required. This was a comprehensive program and for that time an exemplary one. The course was covered in 2 years, each consisting of 2 terms of 3 months each (soon extended to 2 full semesters of about 4½ months each).

The University of Wisconsin started with a similar program, then, in 1892, made a bold innovation. In addition to the 2-year minimum course, it offered the first 4-year course in pharmacy in America, thus placing pharmaceutical instruction on a par with other academic courses. This innovation by its new head, Dr. Edward Kremers, was not achieved without opposition. Like all ideas that are ahead of the times, it had to run the gauntlet of ridicule before recognition could come. Reluctantly, here and there, the 4-year course was imitated; finally, it was generally adopted.

The first school to respond enthusiastically was Ohio State University, where the freshman class entering in 1925 faced 4 years of study, before they could receive their pharmacy degrees. Only the Universities of Georgia, Nebraska and Minnesota had the courage to follow Ohio State's bold lead in requiring a 4-year curriculum before it was made a uniform requirement for all accredited schools.[47]

All schools in good standing with what is now the American Association of Colleges of Pharmacy had adopted a 2-year curriculum (at least 50 weeks) as the minimum requirement in 1907, then a 3-year course in 1925, and the 4-year course in 1932.[48]

After adoption of a 4-year, science-based, university education, it seemed that the pharmacist had clarified his place as a professional in modern medical care, rather than as a technician. Less clear was the constellation of functions that society would expect of him after industrialization of the preparation of drugs had run its course. Even the analysis in the late 1940's by the Pharmaceutical Survey did not entirely come to grips with this question. In calling for establishment of an alternate curriculum of 6 years, as an advanced option, the Survey stressed that in building an educational program "one must know what are the duties and responsibilities of the pharmacist, in other words, what are his functions. One must also know what are the aims and ideals of the profession. And, lastly, one must know what kind of a person the pharmacist is to be."

The Survey did not itself answer this question of knowledge explicitly enough to win the profession over to what then seemed a radical concept for pharmaceutical education, a 6-year program for a professional doctorate. Nor did the American Association of Colleges of Pharmacy approve a proposal in 1950 to embark upon such a program nationally.[49] The opportunity to set up a framework within which education for the pharmacist could develop on a new basis nationally, while not destroyed, was kept pending for another quarter century. The continuation of the 4-year curriculum, a vote for the status quo, had seemed too conservative to some; the alternative posed by the Survey, a 6-year curriculum, had seemed too progressive to others in pharmacy. The pattern for a compromise "solution" was already available at Ohio State University, where Dean B. V. Christensen had inaugurated a required 5-year curriculum beginning with students entering in the fall of 1948, while the Survey still was in progress. Eventually this compromise position became the minimum requirement in all accredited schools, beginning with students entering college after the spring of 1960.

The 6-year professional doctorate had been a program ahead of its time although the University of Southern California pushed ahead to inaugurate it as the required curriculum beginning with the class entering in 1950. The University thereafter has awarded a Doctor of Pharmacy degree for 2 preprofessional years in addition to a 4-year pharmacy program.[50] A few additional schools were offering the same type of program by the 1960's. A dual system of pharmaceutical education was emerging, reflecting, as Prof. Donald C. Brodie of California observed, "two concepts of practice, two philosophies of pharmaceutical education and two levels of educational preparation for practice." The professional climate was changing among practitioners; so was the curriculum emphasis in the schools (especially toward biological sciences), and debate grew.

Dean Linwood F. Tice of Philadelphia, born to the old tradition of practice and education, probably spoke for many by 1966 when he observed:

"While the pharmaceutical curriculum must continue to provide sound training in the pharmaceutical sciences, there is a need for changing the emphasis given certain courses and for the introduction of others. For practicing pharmacists, it is pharmacology which is the most important and, indeed the keystone course in the curriculum. In any school of pharmacy where it is taught at a lower level than to medical students, it is a disservice to the profession and a betrayal of the students' trust," Dean Tice maintained. "The practicing pharmacist must be an expert on drugs, and pharmacology is the bulwark of this expertise." This pharmacist he foresaw would master therapeutic incompatibilities, understand adverse drug reactions, involve himself in the control of drug use (not be only "a custodian of drugs"), and be able to evaluate the best drug for a given purpose from among a series of analogs—whether counseling with other health professionals on prescription medication or with laymen on non-prescription medication.

Speaking as President of the American Pharmaceutical Association, Dean Tice concluded, "I predict that the counting and pouring now often alleged to be the pharmacist's chief occupation will in time be done by technicians and eventually by automation. The pharmacist of tomorrow will function by reason of what he knows—increasing the efficiency and safety of drug therapy and working as a specialist in his own right. It is in this direction that pharmaceutical education must move without delay."[51]

An outside influence for change in just that direction came 3 years later from a Task Force on Prescription Drugs in the federal Department of Health, Education and Welfare. It recommended the development of curricula "for training pharmacists to serve as drug information specialists on the health team," to be backed up by the education of a class of "pharmacist aides" (technicians) to take care of routine functions under pharmacist-supervision.[52]

By the early 1970's a nationwide shift in the character of the pharmacy curricula was under way, in the direction for which Tice had argued. Forty-eight of 69 schools reporting required at least some "clinical pharmacy" (a term not then clearly defined). About 1 in 7 required some experience in a clinical clerkship or externship for academic credit (1972); and the accrediting agency had concluded that every school should develop such a program. Although a component of clinical pharmacy was being fit into the standard 5-year program, at least an optional Doctor of Pharmacy program was being offered in 19 schools by 1975.[53]

In the mid-1970's the question of a duality of professional thought and of education had come to seem more pressing, one orientation in terms of a "drug therapy specialist" (or clinical pharmacist), the other in terms of a "drug delivery specialist" (dispenser). The profession seemed to be moving in the direction of certified specialties, which could have a profound effect on education.[54]

### Which Professional Degree?

The question of what degree, if any, should be awarded to graduates of schools of pharmacy has generated many divergent opinions. The Philadelphia College of Pharmacy, having started partly in protest against the Master of Pharmacy offered by the University of Pennsylvania, was at first somewhat shy of titles.[55]

Thus the diplomas of the college (first issued in 1826) declared the successful student "to be a Graduate in the Philadelphia College of Pharmacy." For more than a century thereafter, "Graduate in Pharmacy" was the modest but significant title of most graduates of American colleges of pharmacy. True, several other degrees were bestowed from time to time, but none was generally accepted. Not infrequently, colleges offered higher degrees to their regular graduates because of competition. Thus the doctor's degree was offered as a "drawing card" by some pharmacy colleges during the 19th century, when several professions swarmed with self-styled "doctors" who lacked respectable academic credentials.

The confused situation becomes evident from Scoville's survey, in 1905, which showed that:

the degree of Graduate in Pharmacy was being given "by one school for 3 months course, 7 schools for 1 year course, 41 schools for 2 years course, 1 school for 3 years course";

the degree of Doctor of Pharmacy, "by 6 schools for 2 years course, 9 schools for 3 years course, 1 school for 4 years course";

the degree of Pharmaceutical Chemist "by 1 school for 1 year course, 16 schools for 2 years course, 8 schools for 3 years course, 1 school for 4 years course, 1 school for 5 years course";

the degree of Master of Pharmacy, "by 1 school for 1 year course, 2 schools for 2 years course, 6 schools for 3 years course, 1 school for 4 years course";

the degree of Bachelor of Pharmacy "by 4 schools for 2 years course, 1 school for 3 years course" and the degree of Bachelor of Science, "by 1 school for 1 year course, 13 schools for 4 years course";

the degree of Master of Science "by 4 schools for 5 years course each."[56]

Such confusion was certain to attract strong bids for reform. Within a few years (1913) the first official statement of the American Conference of Pharmaceutical Faculties as to degrees was adopted, requiring "for the degree of Graduate in Pharmacy a minimum course of 1200 hours." This was followed by a recommended standard that the degree of Pharmaceutical Chemist (Ph.C.) be a 3-year course in pharmacy, based on 4 years of high school (1914). The by-laws refer to the Doctor in Pharmacy for the first time in 1924 by asking for "at least a four-year college of pharmacy course" as "the minimum requirement." In 1937, the Graduate in Pharmacy diploma disappeared from the by-laws, followed in 1938 also by the degree of Doctor of Pharmacy.

The accredited colleges of pharmacy thereafter uniformly awarded the following degrees: Bachelor of Science (B.S.) or Bachelor of Science in Pharmacy (B.S. in Pharm.), for the completion of the 4-year course and later for the 5-year course. Although some wanted a more distinguishing degree, to acknowledge the longer curriculum, no accepted designation was at hand.

Since the 1950's, however, the old Doctor of Pharmacy degree (Pharm. D.) has been resurrected, with new significance, to designate the professional doctorate that could be earned at an increasing minority of American schools in a 6-year curriculum (first offered in 1950 at the University of Southern California). Both the character and stature of the "Pharm. D." were still being resolved during the 1970's, as pressures developed to compress the study into a shorter program and to award the degree for specializations in addition to the original one of "clinical pharmacy."

### Research Degrees in Pharmacy

The professional degrees, even at the level of a doctorate, did not necessarily imply research. This ordinarily was implied, however, by the advanced study designed to supply the creative force in fields of pharmaceutical science. For such work, degrees have been awarded in accordance with the general requirements of graduate schools—which were getting a foothold in American universities during the last third of the 19th century. Such study leads to the degrees of Master of Science (M.S.) or Master of Science in Pharmacy (M.S. in Pharm.) and the Doctor of Philosophy (Ph.D.) or, in earlier decades, the Doctor of Science (D.Sc.)

Before these degrees could be earned on the basis of graduation in pharmacy, it was necessary to elevate pharmaceutical education to the level of a baccalaureate undergraduate degree as a foundation for such advanced study. Edward Kremers was well aware of this when he introduced the 4-year course at the University of Wisconsin. Imbued as he was with scientific standards for pharmacy and a spirit for research brought back from Ph.D. studies in Germany, Kremers superimposed on this foundation the first Doctor of Philosophy programs in pharmaceutical specialties to be based on the regular postgraduate requirements of a recognized American university. The first such Ph.D. was awarded at Wisconsin in 1902.[57]

To give scope to this pioneering program and to reinforce its then meager resources, the University of Wisconsin established the first "Pharmaceutical Experiment Station" in the United States (1913). No person or firm had a claim on the Station's research findings, for in cooperation with the Federal government (Bureau of Plant Industry) it stood under statutory obligation to serve the public. This first American institution of its particular type found endorsement and promotion through the Wisconsin legislature; but the great depression finally choked off its legislative appropriation (1933), and this unique part of the research program by the School of Pharmacy had to be discontinued.

Wisconsin's graduate program was gradually emulated in other strong schools, although at midcentury still only 19 schools offered both master's and doctor's degrees in pharmaceutical research fields. Graduate pharmaceutical students of all types then totalled 357 in American schools representing a 4-fold increase during the preceding 17 years. After World War II, schools in general were strengthened, and research funds became more readily available, bringing a more vigorous response in American pharmaceutical education to the demand for research personnel. Between 1955 and 1975 the number of graduate students rose from 612 to 2,287; and the number of colleges offering graduate degrees rose from 49 to 54 (out of 73 A.A.C.P. full members).[58] Changes in the structure and the dynamics of the pharmaceutical field itself thus have accelerated a trend toward making such advanced work an increasingly important segment of pharmaceutical education.

## HOME-STUDY AND SHORT-COURSE: SUBSTITUTE OR SUPPLEMENT?

Before pharmacy laws requiring an examination for a pharmacy license, the student's belief in the value of systematic instruction under qualified teachers ordinarily would be the decisive factor inducing college attendance. With attendance hinging on such a far-sighted view and so few schools operating, scarcely more than 500 pharmacists had earned an American diploma before the Civil War. The new state laws required that pharmacists have some knowledge but did not state how and where this knowledge was to be obtained. This requirement and the opening of new schools help to account for a sharp increase in the number of graduates by the 1870's, a decade that marked a kind of turning point in education as it did in other areas of pharmaceutical activity. Still, near the end of the century, only about 12 per cent of the pharmacists in American practice apparently had any technical education aside from apprenticeship.[59] If the passing of the state board examination was all that the applicant wanted, there was an easier way than the toilsome one offered by the colleges of pharmacy.

The new pharmacy laws were not retroactive. They recognized and registered the pharmacists in practice at that time, without an examination, just as the boards of medical examiners had recognized the old medical practitioners as physicians. Consequences sometimes ensuing from this practice are illustrated by a report out of Michigan as late as 1896 about

> . . . a practicing physician by the name of O. Barber, who is also a retail druggist. Recently, Dr. Barber had a case of diphtheria which he failed to report. For this oversight he was overhauled by the Health Board and the matter was brought into court. To the amazement of that body and probably to the horror of his patients he gave testimony that he could neither read nor write.[60]

This was an extreme case. Nevertheless, well-educated pharmacists were rare, and at times it was even difficult to find competent examiners within the ranks. For example, when the first West Virginia Pharmacy Act was passed (1881), the legislators did not dare to require a college education of the examiners. "Five years experience in a drugstore was the only requirement." Of 326 pharmacists registered during 2 years after passage of the act, only 2 were college graduates.[61]

To pass an examination under such conditions did not require lengthy academic study. Another kind of preparation, restricted to a knowledge of questions commonly asked in the state board examinations, promised as good or even better success. Therefore, it is not surprising that different ways of preparing for these examinations were offered to all who wanted them, (1) by correspondence courses, (2) by home study of books especially written for this purpose, and (3) by so-called "cramming schools."

### Instruction by Correspondence

The widespread lack of even minimal technical education and the modest legal demands in 19th-century American pharmacy made even home study, at its best, seem to be a constructive effort. Therefore some pharmaceutical journals and educators offered collaboration, as reflected in the two best-known attempts of education in pharmacy by correspondence.

The first operated out of Chicago as the "National Institute of Pharmacy," managed commercially by the publisher of the *Western Druggist*. In a series of 24 "lectures," covering a period of 1 year, a complete course in pharmacy, chemistry and materia medica was given. The main purpose, as explained in the announcement, was to enable clerks, assistants and druggists engaged in business and contemplating a removal "to another state having a pharmacy law . . . to cover the most ground in the least possible time (an important advantage when preparing for a Board of Pharmacy examination)." Upon passing an examination by mail, the student received "a certificate of graduation in the institute." The announcement denied intention of giving this certificate "any legal force whatever under pharmacy laws, the great advantage in this respect to be derived from the lectures being to qualify members for passing Board of Pharmacy examinations."

The other popular venture that exemplifies pharmaceutical instruction by correspondence was launched (1897) by the journal *Pharmaceutical Era*. This course mirrors progress during the decade that had passed since the first announcement of a correspondence course by the National Institute of Pharmacy in Chicago. The course was to cover "a period of two years, to be known respectively as junior and senior. Both years will include two series of lectures of twenty weeks length each." For a number of years, the lectures were printed in the weekly issues of the journal, while the quizzes and examinations were conducted by mail with individual students.[62] The director of this "Course of Home Study in Pharmacy" was no less a person than James H. Beal; among the contributors were men of similar standing in American pharmacy (for instance, Virgil Coblentz, Henry Kraemer, Edward Kremers, John Uri Lloyd and Oscar Oldberg). Their lectures were read by thousands.

There were other less ambitious correspondence schools. J. H. Beal probably spoke for most representatives of scientific and professional American pharmacy when he said,

> In so far as these agencies have honestly striven to raise the standard of education among drugclerks and to promote habits of study and self-help, they should have our commendation; but any proposition or suggestion to the effect that any course of instruction by mail, is or can be made to be the equivalent of a residence course of instruction at a respectable college of pharmacy is false absolutely, and stamps those who make such claims as guilty of misrepresentation and attempted fraud.[63]

More than a few schools were not above using "bait advertising." For example, a Chicago enterprise, named not so modestly the "Lincoln-Jefferson University," offered "ten large lessons forwarded by mail" for $65 "cash in advance" (marked down from $100). Prospective students were told glowingly that "the diplomas are large and beautiful, bearing no statement that the work was done by correspondence."

This course was not discontinued until 1926, and others survived still longer in states lacking legal restrictions.[64] The deathknell sounded for correspondence courses as a substitute for undergraduate academic education when one state followed another, led by New York (1905), in requiring graduation from a recognized school as a prerequisite to licensure.

## Books Especially Written for Home-Study

A demand for cheap and painless learning spawned a modified form of correspondence work, the home-study books. The best known was Oscar Oldberg's *A Course of Home Study for Pharmacists* (1891). This aid to preparing to meet the state board requirements originated in Chicago with the Dean of the College of Pharmacy affiliated with Northwestern University, who worded his preface carefully. He emphasized that "no course of study at home takes the place of a good college with its experienced teachers and its invaluable laboratory practice." At the same time he pointed out that of 75,000 persons employed in the drugstores of the United States "only a few thousand have enjoyed the advantages of a college of pharmacy education." He therefore recommended "home study" as being "of the highest importance to those who are prevented by circumstances from entering college. . . . The pharmacy laws, too, oblige many thousands to study at least enough to pass the State Board examinations." In the same year that Oldberg published his *Course of Home Study for Pharmacists* his College took up "the work of applying the principles of University Extension by conducting an elementary or preparatory course of home reading in physics, chemistry, materia medica, and pharmacy,"[65] in which Oldberg's book of course played a key role. The material was supplied in installments with questions, by mail, "primarily as a preliminary course for prospective college students," which required three to ten months depending upon the time available to a student.

### Cramming Schools

If the prime intention of the correspondence courses and of the home study books and similar attempts was narrowly aimed at preparing for the state board examination, some of them (especially the above-mentioned courses of the National Institute of Pharmacy and *Pharmaceutical Era*) also endeavored to impart a better understanding of the subject matter. However, this can scarcely be claimed for any of the so-called cramming schools. Their objective was the preparation of their students for state board examinations by cramming their brains in the least possible time with answers to commonly asked questions. As late as 1947, an establishment with the high-sounding name "Bay State Institute of Pharmacy, Inc.," located at Boston, sent out circulars "to the unregistered drug clerks of U.S.A." offering "preparation for the Board of Pharmacy license in the states of Massachusetts, Nevada and Vermont," where graduation from a school of pharmacy still was not a legal requirement for the board examination. The fee for a "Six-Week Resident Course in Pharmacy" or a "Fifteen-Week Correspondence Course in Pharmacy" was $300. Said the circulars, "This is the last chance offered to drug clerks. . ."

However, a few cramming schools survived even the laws requiring college graduation. They were given a new lease on life because of the continuation of examinations for a kind of second-class licentiate, usually classed legally as "assistant pharmacists." A strong movement to abolish these second-class certificates arose from abuses and arguments concerning the pharmacy assistant's proper role in a pharmacy. Efforts to solve the problem by abolishing legal provision for licensing any new "assistants" had succeeded by 1947 in all but 8 states. To hasten this solution, a number of states permitted experienced pharmacy assistants of limited education to attempt an examination, during a limited period, to qualify fully as pharmacists. In this situation the surviving "cram" schools found a further market for their brand of instruction.[66]

### In-Service "Continuing Education"

The development of "extension work" in higher education—beginning in the 1890's, under British influence—offered some encouragement or at least surface justification to home-study endeavors which coincided with a particular need and stage in the development of American pharmacy.[67] However, the most that can be said for these study endeavors, is that they simplified and systematized the self-education of perhaps thousands of youths in pharmacy who never would enter the doors of a school of pharmacy. In contrast, extension work characteristic of the present century has been primarily to simplify and systematize a continuing education for practitioners who already have a sound academic education.

The first university extension divisions were being organized during the early 1890's in midwestern universities, and striking some sparks in pharmacy. For example, the abovementioned correspondence course conducted by Oldberg was associated with a general pioneering effort in this field by Northwestern University and could be considered one of the earliest responses in academic pharmacy to the concept of extension study. At about the same time, Buerki's study found, members of the pharmacy faculty at the University of Wisconsin had "presented four of the first six-lecture courses offered as true extension work" at that University, although in basic sciences rather than pharmaceutical subjects.

Beginning in 1909, as part of a general resurgence of extension work at the University of Wisconsin, the pharmacy department featured several series of extension lectures and no less than 13 correspondence courses on a variety of pharmaceutical subjects (40 weekly lessons each), mainly designed for students preparing to enter the University—the same rationale used by Oldberg at Northwestern University.

With federal funding generated during the great depression, extension work in universities flourished; and in 1935 Robert P. Fischelis, as President of the American Pharmaceutical Association, focussed American pharmacy's attention on the need for more systematic use of continuing education. During the next several years, as Chairman of an A.Ph.A. Committee on the Study of Pharmacy, Fischelis continued to press for expanded programs. His efforts were reinforced by the attention and resources generated by the George-Deen Act of 1936. Although designed primarily for nonprofessional employees of distributive occupations, the authorized resources could be drawn upon under a "Wisconsin Plan . . ." devised under the leadership of Sylvester H. Dretzka of the State Board of Pharmacy. This "became the model upon which many subsequent state programs were based after 1938," Buerki concludes, although apparently other states did not draw substantial funds from the George-Deen Act. Buerki estimates that by 1940 at least 35 of the schools of pharmacy nationally had initiated some activity in continuing education, but not more than half of these were on a regular basis. At the end of the 1940's the Pharmaceutical Survey found that 43 of 50 schools reporting had no "in-service" or "off-campus" training program for practicing pharmacists, and urged each school to accept responsibility in this field. In response a number of schools resumed activity, especially weekend "refresher courses."

Then, in 1950, the University of Wisconsin and Rutgers University instituted what Buerki terms "the first modern pharmaceutical extension services."[68] A further stimulus came from a Committee on Continuation Studies created by the A.A.C.P. (1955). Another proposal in 1965 called for "a redefinition of in-service education in terms of serious postgraduate academic endeavor" for practicing pharmacists, and for "pilot studies to devise methods and patterns" for putting continuing education programs on a regional or national basis (rather than state basis.[69]) The possibility of realizing such potential was enhanced in 1966 when the University of Wisconsin announced the first graduate program to prepare specialists for research and administration in the field of continuing education.

Implementation remained spotty nationally until a trend toward massive in-service education emerged during the 1970's, partly motivated by "declarations at the federal level that professionals in the health-care field should be responsible for continually gaining knowledge of developments in their respective areas."[70] A number of states (beginning with Florida and Kansas in 1967) established by law or regulation a minimum of continuing education as a condition for renewal of a pharmacist's license. This stimulated the production of new resources for fulfilling such requirements, and concern in organized pharmacy to develop appropriate standards for assessing instructional units and the results achieved.[71] Whatever temporary problems stood in the way, the long-term shift toward formal assurance of continuing competence in pharmacy and other health professions augured well for the patient.

## ASSOCIATIONS OF SCHOOLS

### The Conference of Teaching Colleges

The first organization for pharmaceutical education, the Conference of the Schools of Pharmacy, followed a meeting of delegates from 5 "teaching colleges of pharmacy" (Chicago, Maryland, Massachusetts, New York, and Philadelphia) and from the New Jersey Pharmaceutical Association in 1870 (at the A.Ph.A. meeting). By constitutional definition, the Conference consisted of schools requiring apprenticeship before graduation. This explicit exclusion of the University of Michigan confirms other evidence that the threat of change and challenge represented by the state university helped to spark the impulse to form a special organization. In addition, the first association of medical colleges, formed just 4 years earlier, set an example that scarcely could have passed unnoticed among pharmaceutical educators.

Both the nature and the fate of this earliest associative attempt of the medical colleges found a remarkable parallel in the procrastination and the ineffectual short life of the Conference of the Schools of Pharmacy. The Conference was ineffectual largely because, among other reasons, the delegates were without real policy-making powers; they "recommended to the Colleges," which in turn might "urge their members" (practitioners) to take action. For example, recognizing a key limitation in the lack of a uniform requirement of preliminary education, the Conference considered the question at four annual meetings—and four times did nothing—recognizing that in effect the selection of future students rested with the preceptors, because it was they who selected youths for the preliminary apprenticeship. The effects of this basic idea pervade all aspects of the association schools during the 19th century.

One case in which there was action as well as theoretical agreement can be found in the refusal by the Conference (1874 and 1875) to recognize the "Doctor of Pharmacy" degrees offered by two recently established schools (National College of Pharmacy at Washington, D.C., and Tennessee College of Pharmacy, Nashville, Tenn.) for ordinary course work, and partly even to students who did not attend the courses but merely took the examination and paid the fees. Apart from such common defense against unfair competition, there could hardly be united action of the American schools of pharmacy at this time. There were still no definite educational requirements asked for by the licensing boards (and often no such boards!), such as would make systematic schooling a prerequisite for the pharmacist-to-be. The necessity of using all possible means to attract students to keep up the mere existence of most schools was stronger than the desire of some professors to elevate the educational standards.

After 13 frustrating years the Conference of Schools of Pharmacy dissolved. The last yellowed page of the minute book reports in the scrawl of an acting secretary that in 1884 only 3 college representatives carried credentials as delegates; so no meeting could be held for lack of quorum.

Bitter disappointment with lack of results may have colored the judgment of the Secretary of the American Pharmaceutical Association, John M. Maisch, when he wryly reflected that "there was very little talked about that can be considered of any importance for pharmaceutical education." Actually much of importance was discussed; delegates saw the problems, grappled with them and failed to solve them. Yet it is difficult to believe that pharmaceutical education did not benefit eventually by the exchange of views and experiences during the years of the Conference.[72]

### The American Association of Colleges of Pharmacy

Shortly after the dissolution of the ill-fated Conference, a section on Education and

Legislation was established (1887) in the American Pharmaceutical Association, which provided a forum *pro tem* for educational affairs. But when a new Association of American Medical Colleges was founded (1890), Professor William Simon of Baltimore told the Section, "this is what we have to do, and what we ought to have done long ago."[73] Another decade passed before a new association was founded, but this time it would be successful.

James H. Beal, a pharmacist-lawyer who consistently helped to usher in modern American pharmacy, describes in his memoirs the founding of the new college association:

> I conceived the idea that if representatives of the various colleges could be brought together where they could speak face to face, their jealousies would subside, and prior to one of the American Pharmaceutical Association meetings I sent a circular letter to the various colleges suggesting that we have a meeting to see if some of these conflicting views could not be harmonized. Only two [individuals] responded favorably, Dr. [William] Simon of the Maryland College of Pharmacy and Henry P. Hynson of Hynson, Westcott and Dunning of Baltimore [likewise professor at the Maryland College of Pharmacy]. When the association [A.Ph.A.] met at Richmond, Virginia (1900), I made the motion to call for a meeting of Pharmaceutical Faculties. A committee was appointed to consider the question, of which Professor Remington of the Philadelphia College of Pharmacy was made Chairman. Remington was very skeptical of the idea but turned it over to me to work out a report, and knowing of the magic in the word "conference," I used it in recommending a meeting. Since there seemed nothing dangerous in the coming together in the same room, the other members of the Committee agreed to the report. When the members found that no compulsion was intended, they discovered they could discuss these questions in good temper and this was the origin of what was known for many years as the American Conference of Pharmaceutical Faculties but is now known [since 1925] as the American Association of Colleges of Pharmacy.[74]

This new organization, founded by the representatives of 21 American pharmacy schools, originated under circumstances quite different from those of the Conference from 1870 to 1885. In the meantime, the idea of education as a duty of organized society (i.e., of the state) had finally been given recognition by the people of the United States, and farseeing men in American pharmacy, educators and practitioners as well, had taken advantage of this fact. A large proportion of the pharmacy schools founded in this country between 1883 and 1900 were an integral part of the educational systems of individual states, as departments of state universities or of state colleges. In this general and officially approved trend toward higher education, the educational reformers in American pharmacy were given their opportunity.

True, private schools with no university affiliation were still in the majority. A representative of the then-still-private Maryland College of Pharmacy, Professor Henry P. Hynson, was the temporary President of the meeting to organize "The American Conference of Pharmaceutical Faculties." The dean of the time-honored Philadelphia College of Pharmacy, Joseph P. Remington, acted as the chairman of the Committee on Organization. However, the man who was elected the first president of the Conference was Albert B. Prescott, dean of the first university pharmacy school of consequence in the United States, that of Michigan. There could not be more convincing proof of the change of mind in the field of pharmaceutical education than the selection of this man. Thirty years before he had been condemned and ostracized by his fellow teachers for introducing and advocating academic pharmaceutical instruction based on scientific considerations only, instead of instruction intended merely as a supplement to the knowledge acquired in "the store."

Joseph P. Remington, president of the Conference in 1902, although emphasizing in his presidential address that drugstore experience should go hand in hand with college work to achieve the best results, did not hesitate to say,[75]

A student who carefully follows the instruction will certainly acquire more sound knowledge of the essential facts which lie at the foundation of pharmacy, in three years at college, than one who has spent his time exclusively in the store for twenty years, gathering knowledge on the installment plan.

Moreover, what had once seemed remote, now became a common goal—hence brought within reach—as this distinguished spokesman of the old-line schools emphasized the necessity "to secure from the legislature of our various states the recognition of the possession of the college diploma before a candidate is permitted to take the state examination." A cornerstone of adequate professional standards thus was recognized, never to be lost sight of again.

Besides its successful endeavor in placing pharmaceutical education in this country on a full academic basis, in improving curricula and faculties, and in promoting research, the American Association of Colleges of Pharmacy created a spirit of collegiate solidarity and friendly emulation among the schools and the teachers of pharmacy which guarantees an orderly development. It would be hard to overestimate the role in this development served by the *American Journal of Pharmaceutical Education*, founded in 1937 by the A.A.C.P. and apparently the first periodical of its scope internationally.

Until the A.A.C.P. helped to set up a separate accrediting agency in 1932 (see below), much of its effort centered about setting and fostering compliance with group standards for pharmaceutical education in America. Having matured within this concept, the Association continued to emphasize the aims and policies of administering the individual schools, of creating a system of pharmaceutical education and of representing this system at the interface with other educational agencies, government, and the pharmaceutical field at large. These matters traditionally were dominated by the deans.

An increasing number of faculty members, lacking an organized endeavor of their own, became dissatisfied with an Association that they saw partly in terms of a somewhat conservative "deans' club." During the early 1970's thousands of man-hours were spent by a coalition of deans and faculty members to hammer out plans for a thorough reorganization, which received final adoption at the 1973 meeting. Responding to the more egalitarian views of American university life in the 1960's, the A.A.C.P. became a more balanced and broadly democratic organization, if a more complicated one (having four Councils, which linked together through a policymaking House of Delegates). Reinforcing this move, there has been since the 1960's an increase in the staff and activities of the year-round headquarters office of the Association, including establishment of an office of educational research and development.

Dean L. C. Weaver of the University of Minnesota, who had led the reorganization committee, pointed to two of the main purposes when he said, "The functional reorganization . . . will guarantee fair representation of the faculty, students, and administrators of colleges. Another feature is that the objectives are being expanded into areas which will require us to take positions on the many prickly problems facing pharmacy today."[76]

## AMERICAN COUNCIL ON PHARMACEUTICAL EDUCATION

As the American Association of Colleges of Pharmacy gradually increased educational standards, their acceptance served as criteria for admission to the Association and for maintenance of a school's membership. In effect, this provided a kind of accreditation system for American schools until the American Council on Pharmaceutical Education was established (1932).

Through the Council, the Pharmaceutical Survey observed, "the upgrading and the systematization of the training institutions were promoted and the reciprocal recognition of licenses among the several states greatly extended."

These purposes served the interests of both the citizen and pharmacist; and in setting up an accreditation agency to pursue them systematically, pharmacy followed an established American tradition. Such an agency operates under the aegis of a federation of institutions of learning (within a specified scope) or of organized societies of a profession. Although accrediting agencies are private (i.e., extra-legal) bodies, their affairs are conducted so that legal authorities may accept their results and evaluations as a rough guide to the adequacy of professional education offered by applicants for licensure.

Thus it was that the National Association of Boards of Pharmacy (i.e., federated state licensing bodies) took the lead in organizing the American Council on Pharmaceutical Education. Joined with the N.A.B.P. ever since as co-sponsors have been the American Pharmaceutical Association and the American Association of Colleges of Pharmacy (each with three representatives on the Council) and the American Council on Education (one non-pharmacy representative). The Council is responsible for drafting standards and periodically it sends inspection teams for a searching examination of each school—its staff, program, standards, facilities, administration and finances—to evaluate compliance with published accreditation standards. Until 1974 these standards spoke primarily to the quality of the institution. Thereafter, revised standards have shifted the focus more toward accrediting specific programs (based on evaluation of goal accomplishment) within an institution. Moreover, clinical training (including clerkship or externship) had come to seem so much a condition of adequate pharmaceutical education that for the first time it was placed as an expectation upon every accredited school (with the expressed hope of eventually superseding the traditional internship separate from formal education).

Through its reports to the respective universities and schools, its counsel, and its published list of accredited schools, the Council has had a unifying and elevating influence, has provided one basis for helping prospective students to select schools, enhanced interschool relationships and helped schools to recognize more clearly their potentialities and deficiencies.

The Pharmaceutical Survey gave strong support to the functioning of the Council, and in response to its recommendation a central office with a full-time administrative head (Director of Educational Relations) was set up in association with offices of the National Association of Boards of Pharmacy.[77] The Council's services, like much else of educational value, would have been greatly hampered without the help of the American Foundation for Pharmaceutical Education.

## THE AMERICAN FOUNDATION FOR PHARMACEUTICAL EDUCATION

Some of the schools of pharmacy were in straitened financial circumstances on the eve of World War II (often those not well integrated with a strong university); and in wartime conditions worsened. Moreover, financial pressures upon individual students were squeezing some of the most capable of them out of pharmacy, which had no centralized funding agency, no pooled funds. These needs have been alleviated since 1942 when the American Foundation for Pharmaceutical Education was established.

Within the National Drug Trade Conference, the Chairman of a Committee on Endowments, Dean Earnest Little of Rutgers University, had strongly urged a systematic effort in this direction; but the Conference was not well designed to supply more than a sympathetic ear. One who heard was a man with the unusual combination of insight, energy and authority to get things done. This man was E. L. Newcomb of the National Wholesale Druggists' Association. Taking independent initiative, the Association (through Newcomb) invited 50 leading pharmaceutical and chemical manufacturers and chain-store executives to discuss "facts relative to the future functioning and financial status of colleges of pharmacy, particularly those which did not receive state aid." This conference directed "the group which called the meeting to organize an all-industry committee" for assembling information and to assist in solving the serious financial problems confronting pharmaceutical education.[78] Subsequently the National Drug Trade Conference resolved "to advocate the formation of an *American Foundation for Pharmaceutical Education.*" But it was left for the National Association of Wholesale Druggists, especially as represented by E. L. Newcomb, with the support of George V. Doerr, to take the practical steps that led to assurance of the necessary philanthropies and, in 1942, the organization of the Foundation as a permanent institution. It was sponsored by all national pharmaceutical organizations holding membership in the National Drug Trade Conference, which meant by organized pharmacy as a whole, manufacturers and wholesalers as well as practicing pharmacists and educators. Among its stated purposes, the Foundation endeavors—

- To uphold and improve pharmaceutical education by aiding . . . colleges of pharmacy and students therein;
- To aid in the creation of sources of unbiased and authoritative investigation and experimentation on pharmaceutical problems;
- To assist in the selection of important research problems and to provide that the investigations be adequately financed, and to insure as far as possible that they be carried out by competent investigators under the supervision of recognized scientific authorities.

After helping to rescue some needy schools during the World War II period, the Foundation increasingly turned its resources to undergraduate scholarships and, of more recent emphasis, to graduate and postdoctorate fellowships (totalling, in A.F.P.E.'s first quarter century, 3,015 undergraduates and 685 graduate students aided). Among other long-term projects most productively underwritten by the Foundation, wholly or partly, have been the influential Pharmaceutical Survey of 1946–49, the American Council of Pharmaceutical Education, the *American Journal of Pharmaceutical Education,* and the annual national seminars to improve pharmaceutical instruction in the schools.[79]

There scarcely could be a better demonstration of the willingness of the pharmaceutical industry to accept its share of responsibility to society in matters pertaining to pharmacy.

## PHARMACEUTICAL SURVEYS

Because education is basic to renewal and progress in any profession, periodic inquiries into the status of American pharmacy often have been focused sharply on its educational facilities.

Perhaps the first pharmaceutical "survey" was that launched by the American Pharmaceutical Association soon after its founding, to secure statistical data about pharmacy throughout the country (see p. 290). However, not until the 1920's was an attempt made to obtain a comprehensive picture offering, in addition to statistics, the basis for evaluating the degree to which the needs of society were being served by contemporary pharmacy.

As a result of studies "made possible by a subvention granted by the Commonwealth Fund . . . and by the co-operation of the American Association of Colleges of Pharmacy . . . the National Association of Retail Druggists, and the National Association of Boards of Pharmacy,"[80] a book appeared entitled *Basic Material for a Pharmaceutical Curriculum* (1927). It was prepared by the director of the investigation, W. W. Charters, then professor at the University of Pittsburgh, and A. B. Lemon and Leon M. Monell, professors at the University of Buffalo School of Pharmacy, with collaboration by Dr. Robert P. Fischelis,[81] then of New Jersey.

The reception of this report was enthusiastic and of great consequence. "A careful study of the Dr. Charters report," said Dean D. B. R. Johnson of the University of Oklahoma, in his address as President of the American Association of Colleges of Pharmacy in 1927, ". . . has convinced me that we must sooner or later come to a four-year course for a degree in pharmacy. I therefore recommend that, as soon as possible, the four-year course be adopted."[82] In the same year, H. C. Christensen, Secretary of the National Association of Boards of Pharmacy, called the book "a classic . . . so far-reaching in its possibilities for pharmacy . . ." that everyone, in whatever branch of the profession, should read it. He also put a significant question: "Why not have a survey made every ten years . . . ?" In conclusion, Christensen stated, "We now need a survey to show the requirements of the commercial and administrative side of pharmacy. Well, we have opened up a big field."[83]

The National Association of Boards of Pharmacy, indeed, took steps to initiate a survey on a broader scale, joined by other associations; but the United States had entered the great depression. Funds were not forthcoming, and in 1932 the proposal had to be dropped.

The general idea remained alive. Its first fruit was the so-called Bernays Drug and Pharmaceutical Survey, paid for by "a group from the pharmaceutical profession and the drug trades" and conducted by a public relations agency. This study was concerned mainly with "a better relationship between the drug trades and the pharmaceutical profession, and the public." The conglomerate of data collected and the conclusions drawn, (covering 1,200 typewritten pages) remained unpublished. A report, presented to the American Pharmaceutical Association (1943)[84] by Edward L. Bernays, the head of the public relations agency conducting the survey, did not find the favorable reception given to the Charters survey.[85]

It was symptomatic when, on the same day that Bernays spoke, the American Association of Colleges of Pharmacy adopted a resolution recommending a study of "the possibility of supplementing the Charters, Lemon, and Monell Study." An urgent request was submitted to the American Foundation for Pharmaceutical Education, with the endorsement of four national organizations, asking the Foundation to "underwrite a comprehensive study of pharmacy, pharmaceutical practices, and new areas of pharmaceutical specialization . . ."

The Foundation reacted favorably, and the study called The Pharmaceutical Survey was inaugurated (April 15, 1946), to be conducted by the American Council on Education and directed by Edward C. Elliott, a nationally known educator, a nonpharmacist, and, as an investigator and analyst, bold and searching.[86]

This survey produced the broad-ranging evaluation expected of it, placing the needs of pharmaceutical education in relation to the status of other segments of American pharmacy at mid-century. If not revolutionary, the findings were incisive in exposing the evidence for needed change. One major flaw—no fault of the Survey staff—was the lack of a well planned and sustained implementation of these findings. Nevertheless their influence has been persistent, although never systematically assessed. Certainly, *The General Report of the Pharmaceutical Survey 1946–1949* represents a unique milestone in the history of pharmacy, and repays study even today.

There have been various specialized studies, meanwhile, but none more probing and provocative than the Audit of Pharmaceutical Service in Hospitals led by Dr. Don E. Francke and his associates in the early 1960's. It went beyond reporting comprehensively on the professional and administrative services then being offered by American hospital pharmacists. It also set a philosophical framework and raised questions that called for further study. When published, the "Audit" by Dr. Francke and his co-authors offered insights that related to the needs and goals of professional pharmacy at large; yet, the influence undoubtedly has been largely restricted by its specialized scope and audience.[87]

About the same time there were calls for a more broadly based analysis that might set some guideposts for the future direction of American community pharmacists, especially since new conditions had begun to make the old Pharmaceutical Survey of the 1940's seem dated and doubtful as a continuing guide. One response was an exploratory probe commissioned by the American Pharmaceutical Association, which blueprinted problem areas for selective analysis and problem-solving by applying the tools of social science, and was approved in principle.[88]

When neither this nor any other study had materialized after another 7 years, however—perhaps because of problems of unifying the expected multi-sponsorship—the American Association of Colleges of Pharmacy decided the time had come to grasp the initiative. Said President Arthur Schwarting, "There is no single agency, organization or governing instrument within the health professions which has the capacity or the leadership to accomplish this study. . . . We must therefore separately undertake an analysis of ourselves to determine the rightful place of pharmacy in the system." He proceeded to call for the prompt appointment of a Commission on Pharmacy, which would "determine the scope of pharmacy services in health care and project the educational processes necessary to insure that these services are obtained."[89]

By that fall the distinguished John S. Millis had been chosen to lead what came to be known as the "Millis Commission." Dr. Millis brought to the difficult analysis and conclusions an exceptional combination of abilities and education as it articulates with the needs of society, as had Edward C. Elliott before him, who headed the rather different national survey three decades earlier. How the profession as a whole and pharmaceutical education in particular reacted to *Pharmacists for the Future; The Report of The Study Commission on Pharmacy* (Ann Arbor, c. 1975) would help determine the direction of American pharmacy's efforts during the rest of the century.

While such surveys assume that new analysis and insight were to be a prelude to progress, by no means everyone welcomes the change and the uncertainty and perhaps sacrifice that this might imply. In education for pharmacy, as in other fields, advances in requirements often have been a response, not to the active demand of a majority, but to that of a minority who aspire to leave their profession a step beyond where they found it. Rufus A. Lyman of Nebraska, founding editor of the *American Journal of Pharmaceutical Education*, looked back on efforts to advance pharmaceutical education as he had experienced them over four decades, and concluded:

> Some were violently opposed, the majority were indifferent. Support did come from a few farseeing laymen who recognized the importance of the pharmacist and the drugstore in the public health service. It also came from a handful of practicing druggists who were readers of pharmacy's history and who had learned the part the pharmacist has played in the past in science, in industry, in research, in education, and in the art of living, and who had a vision of greater things for the future.[90]

# 15

# The Establishment of a Literature

## BOOKS IMPORTED FROM EUROPE

Before America had a pharmaceutical literature of its own, practitioners of medicine and pharmacy generally used the European books with which they felt most at home, whether by tradition or language or training. Most American-born physicians who had an academic education in this early period received their training at medical schools in Edinburgh or London. Naturally, on returning to their native country they used and taught to American students or apprentices the medicine taught in the British Isles and the literature used there.

The literature that seemed important on American soil early in the 19th century may be inferred from resolutions on a proposed American pharmacopeia (New York State Medical Society, 1818) which point out that various pharmacopeias then were used "in the different sections and States of the Union such as: the Edinburgh Dispensatory, the London Dispensatory, the London Pharmacopoeia, the Dublin Pharmacopoeia, the Parisian Pharmacopoeia,"[1] and also mention the few formularies issued in America between 1806 and 1818. This list makes no pretense at completeness, and the omission of the Edinburgh Pharmacopoeia was surely not deliberate. However, the fact that the Edinburgh Dispensatory was mentioned, and not the pharmacopeia on which the dispensatory was based, tends to confirm that in America the dispensatories (which combined the pharmacopeial text, explanatory comments and additional material) were much more in practical use than the pharmacopeias themselves.

Practitioners who had immigrated from various countries tended to make some use of pharmaceutical literature from their country of origin, despite the already confusing number of formularies; but it did not negate the dominance of English pharmaceutical literature.

## ATTEMPTS TO ESTABLISH AN AMERICAN PHARMACOPEIA

### Philadelphia

The first known step toward an American pharmacopeia was taken by the physician John Morgan, who already had distinguished himself by establishing the first medical school. American pharmacy was indebted to him for his efforts in the movement to separate pharmacy and medicine in this country. Then, in 1787, Morgan "proposed to the College of Physicians of Philadelphia the compilation and publication of a pharmacopoeia for Pennsylvania."[2] Since the Federal Constitution had not yet been ratified by all of the 13 states, national standards apparently were not considered. But when the United States of America had become a reality a year later, the plan of the

College of Physicians of Philadelphia was expanded.

A circular (ordered 1789) went to 100 "proper persons," stating that "one of the objects of the college has been that of forming a pharmacopoeia adapted to the present state of medicine in America; for which purpose a committee of their members has been some time since appointed, who have made some progress in their work." Furthermore, the circular pointed out "the absolute necessity of some standard amongst ourselves to prevent that uncertainty and irregularity which in our present situation must infallibly attend on the compositions of the apothecary and the prescription of the physician." It asked that the addressee "particularly inform us what native American remedies have been discovered amongst you."[3]

There was little response, although encouraging replies were received from medical societies of Delaware and New Haven, Connecticut. Not daunted, the College named a committee on pharmacopeia to compile material on pharmaceutical substances and processes, but apparently a completed study was never presented.

A new appreciation of native resources and pride in young nationhood after the Revolution reinforced interest in indigenous drugs and in an American pharmacopeia. For example, one member of the Philadelphia committee, the botanist Benjamin Smith Barton, stressed (1798) the desirability of giving American drugs "a place in the Pharmacopoeia of this country," that is, "when such a desideratum shall be supplied."[4]

### South Carolina and Connecticut

The idea of "the establishment of an independent American Materia Medica" was mentioned also in a letter published by the Medical Society of South Carolina (1798). Later on, the society touched on the objective again in a letter to the Massachusetts Medical Society (1808), refusing to adopt the *Pharmacopoeia of the Massachusetts Medical Society*.

The Connecticut Medical Society had voted "that the professors of the Medical College be requested to communicate to the next convention [1816] the best mode of producing a general and uniform pharmacopoeia; there it was voted "to accept the report of the committee . . . to compile a pharmacopoeia and to submit it to the next convention."[5] Whether the committee appointed for that purpose ever did preparatory work is unknown.

## THE MASSACHUSETTS PRECURSOR

The unfulfilled plans of the physicians in Philadelphia, South Carolina and Connecticut were fully attained by their Massachusetts colleagues. The Massachusetts Medical Society had shown its concern for genuine and adequate medicines as early as 1786, when it petitioned the legislature to prevent the sale of bad or adulterated drugs. The compilation and the publication of a "pharmacopoeia" was another step in the same direction.

> At different periods, the Society has expended no small amount of labor to secure a uniform mode of compounding medicines, and to protect the community against the dangers incurred by the use of such as are spurious. At a meeting of the Counsellors, October 3, 1805, a committee was appointed to draw up and lay before them a pharmacopoeia or formulary, for the preparation of compound medicines, with names affixed to the same, to be called the Massachusetts Pharmacopoeia.[6]

In 1807 "the committee . . . presented the manuscript of a pharmacopoeia" at a meeting of the Counsellors of the Society, and it was voted "that the said pharmacopoeia be printed for the use of the Society."[7] The book, a volume of 272 pages listing 536 drugs and preparations, appeared early in 1808. An illuminating preface revealed that the Society resolved to adopt the pharmacopoeia of the Edinburgh College as the basis of their own; but to permit such omissions, alterations, and additions as, upon minute examination, should be found necessary. It was not desirable however, to give to this the appearance of originality; on the contrary, trifling considerations have not induced any variation from that excellent work.

The most important of the additions mentioned were indigenous American drugs not included in the Edinburgh pharmacopoeia.[8]

The authors of the Massachusetts pharmacopoeia were in advance of their time in another innovation. Their model, the Edinburgh pharmacopoeia, like most similar books of that period, was written in Latin. The text of the Massachusetts book was in English, except for drug titles in Latin as well as English. The preface justified the bold innovation with the statement that a Latin book "is not adapted in this country, where the apothecaries are not necessarily instructed in that language." The same statement held true for most of the American physicians.

The apothecaries are mentioned several times in the preface, such as in the statement that "it is the business of the physician to prescribe, and of the apothecary to prepare medicines."[9] This unreserved recognition of the separation of medicine and pharmacy, as early as 1808, implied an advanced position. It was the first known official declaration of this kind to be made, not by an individual physician (like John Morgan; see p. 160), but by an organized group of American medical practitioners. However, the preface implied recognition that this desirable separation was of necessity restricted to the larger cities:

In them, the professions of physician and apothecary are most distinct; and between those, whose relation to each other is so important, a perfect understanding should exist. As this cannot be established between them as individuals, it is necessary that there should be uniformity, both in the pharmaceutical preparations and language.

The authors chose an excellent way to induce pharmacists to adopt their work. They appealed to self-interest and professional responsibility. "The Medical Society indeed is not empowered to require of apothecaries a compliance with the directions of this pharmacopoeia; nor does such power seem requisite. It has a sufficient substitute in the apothecary's regard to his own interest, and to his duty to the public."[10] This appeal found the expected response within the state of Massachusetts.

Was this local success all the authors of the Massachusetts pharmacopoeia had hoped for? The sentences with which they closed the preface of their work reveal a higher and more comprehensive aim. The authors

cannot hesitate to solicit the aid of all scientific men in effecting a revolution, so very desirable for the correct practice of medicine; a revolution, which concerns the reputation and success of every medical practitioner, and the health and safety of every individual.

"Revolution" is too strong a word to have been used by men so deliberate as Jackson and Warren with reference only to Massachusetts. They must have had in mind all of the United States. Indeed, attempts were made to secure general recognition for the book. Copies and a circular letter, emphasizing the advantages of "a pharmacopoeia calculated for the practice of the United States"[11] were sent to the medical societies of other states. The New Hampshire Medical Society was the only one to adopt the book.[12] One other response, the letter from the Medical Society of South Carolina mentioned previously, expressed the opinion that a "perfect pharmacopoeia" can be obtained only by "the concurrence of different States," by requesting "the different Medical Societies, at a future date . . . to refer such a compilation to someone of the learned Medical Association."[13]

It was exactly this idea, the recognition of all medical organizations in the compilation of such a standard, that the physician Lyman

Spalding of New York made the basis of his attempt at a national pharmacopeia. The Massachusetts Medical Society had appointed a committee to revise its pharmacopeia, but after receiving the request of the New York State Medical Society for cooperation in preparing a national pharmacopeia according to the plan of Spalding, the Massachusetts Society concurred (1818). Through this collaboration "more than ninety per cent of the articles in the Massachusetts book were included in the later publication."[14] In this way the book which had been refused general recognition constituted 12 years later the greatest part of the first generally recognized pharmaceutical standard in the United States of America. While the Massachusetts pharmacopoeia had no legal force such as we have come to expect of a pharmacopeia, it did have the authority of the state medical society behind it and the intent to bring about more uniformity of drugs and more precision of physician-pharmacist communication in the community.

## HOSPITAL FORMULARIES

Differing from the Boston book of 1808, the New York booklet appearing 3 years later was more modest in both appearance and purpose. Although called a "pharmacopeia" it was so-titled only in the old etymological sense of a book on how to make drugs. It was a compilation of written formulas for medications to be used within a specific hospital, the second such institution founded in the United States. *The Pharmacoepia Chirurgica in usum Nosocomii Novi Eboracencis* . . . [sic] of 1811, by Valentine Seaman, M.D., thus may be the earliest known example, for an American civilian hospital, of a category of pharmaceutical literature that has a long tradition. Such hospital formularies in manuscript form are known from medieval Islam and Europe, and printed hospital formularies go back at least to the 17th century.

The 1811 edition of the formulary of the New York Hospital had almost dropped from sight for more than 60 years, partly because of its rarity, but perhaps also partly because it was so limited in scope, defectively organized, and poorly edited. The hapless author, although outstanding medically, allowed two misspellings even in the aforementioned title of the booklet! Because of still other deficiencies, this early formulary was castigated or at best received with faint praise by important medical journals. Probably for this reason, it was only 4 years after publication that Dr. Seaman, compiler of the formulary and attending surgeon at the New York Hospital, began a collaboration with Samuel Latham Mitchill, a prominent attending physician at the Hospital, which culminated in the much better known and respected *Pharmacopoeia Nosocomii Neo-Eboracensis* of 1816.

It was a new and quite different formulary, almost four times larger than was the ill-starred venture of 1811; the number of dosage forms was tripled, the number of drugs increased to 430 (if we include the list of materia medica), nomenclature modernized, and compounding procedures more uniformly included. Unlike its predecessor, the *Pharmacopoeia of the New-York Hospital* proclaimed that it carried "the Authority of the Physicians and Surgeons of that Institution." Yet, the suggestion that the Hospital's pharmacopeia "be considered as directions for our Physicians and Surgeons in the manner they may think fit to prescribe" was not accepted—an early instance of the continuing debate over the limits of authority of a hospital formulary.[15] In this and other respects the formulary set a pattern for innumerable American hospital formularies that have since been prepared, both printed and unprinted, designed for local use and instruction within particular institutions. The formulary of 1816 was already seen by its authors as somewhat of a model, which not only was to serve the medical staff and students of the New York Hospital, but also as "a manual of prescription and selection of official preparations" for those "Apothecaries, who reside in parts of the United States where no regular pharmacopoeia has been established."[16] The potential geographic scope was considerable, since the Massachusetts pharmacopoeia was the only "regular" one previously issued in the United States. In fact, little distribution of the formulary of the New York Hospital apparently was achieved beyond New York. However, it stimulated the interests of the senior author, Samuel Latham Mitchill, concerning the need for drug standards; and a few years later we find him playing a key role in the movement that led to the issuance of the first *Pharmacopeia of the United States.*

In subsequent decades an occasional local hospital formulary followed the precedent of the New York Hospital, collecting on the printed page the favorite drug formulas of the medical staff, for convenience and instruction in prescribing. Then, in the late 1920's, a reassessment of the centuries-old function of the hospital formulary was undertaken, in which the New York Hospital again helped to provide the prototype. However, it was at Syracuse University Hospital that "probably the earliest effort to establish a scientific basis of drug control and standardization in an American hospital occurred in 1925" when 45 physicians and a pharmacist "embarked upon a program of rationalization of hospital drug therapy. . . . " The New York Hospital project came to similar results in 1932. The consequence has been adjudged by the historian Alex Berman this way:

> These two pioneer efforts were prototypes of formulary systems subsequently adopted by many hospitals in the United States. The hospital formulary had now become the focal point for the control and standardization of therapeutic agents; it reflected the policies of pharmacy and therapeutics committees; it prevented product duplication; it was a teaching aid; it helped set realistic drug inventories; and it was the product of progressive pharmacological knowledge. In this new world of the formulary system, the pharmacist had become a key individual acting as Secretary to the Pharmacy Committee, consultant to the medical staff, and compiler of the formulary itself.[17]

By mid-century the use of hospital formularies in this sense had become widespread. With all but a remnant of drug making removed from hospitals into the large-scale scientific and production facilities of drug manufacturing firms, the actual instructions for formulating each medication—the hallmark of earlier hospital formularies—were rapidly being displaced by pharmacologic and therapeutic information, as well as pharmaceutical specifications, for representatives of each category of medication. When the University of Michigan Hospital published its *Hospital Formulary of Selected Drugs* (Ann Arbor, 1954), under the editorship of chief pharmacist Don E. Francke, it set a new American standard of its kind and generated a national influence and usage. From this editorial burden, Dr. Francke "was struck by the great amount of time and effort required to prepare a formulary. I realized that the work I was doing was being duplicated by numerous other hospital pharmacists throughout the country." So, "about the time the *Hospital Formulary of Selected Drugs* was being printed," he recalls, "I presented the proposal for the development of a National Hospital Formulary Service" in 1954. The American Society of Hospital Pharmacists implemented the proposal the following year and began publication of the *American Hospital Formulary Service* in 1959.[18] Significantly, the Society stressed that it was establishing, as Donald E. Francke had recommended, a loose-leaf "service," which institutions could utilize selectively, not an inflexible national hospital formulary. It passed the 10,000-mark in its list of subscribers within 8 years, and continues to grow in influence.

## THE U. S. PHARMACOPEIA

The founding of the present United States Pharmacopeia was a signal event in the development of American medical care, which depended heavily upon the initiative of two men. Which of them deserves more credit as "father" of the *Pharmacopeia* has been open to discussion.[19]

In comparison with Lyman Spalding, Samuel Latham Mitchill was unquestionably the greater and more brilliant personality. A graduate of the University of Edinburgh, Mitchill was older and much more versatile and experienced; his reputation as a physician was of the best. He was one of the founders (1797), and for 16 years the principal editor, of the earliest medical journal in the United States. He had served as teacher and chemist. Once he had been a senator and twice a representative. Yet, all of this could not guarantee success in a venture which in the previous decades had several times been tried in vain.

The statement, coined by Barton in 1798, that a national pharmacopeia was a "desideratum" of American medicine and pharmacy had been quoted in the medical literature again and again. No one in the country knew this better than Mitchill. He was exactly informed in regard to the different attempts to create such a book. He knew why they had failed. To have tried under the circumstances would have been hazardous for him. True, all scientific and practical sources and resources were at his command; nevertheless, instead of issuing the first *United States Pharmacopeia,* the cautious Mitchill launched a hospital formulary.

To make the dream of an American pharmacopeia a reality required a man who had less to lose and more to gain; a man willing to devote himself entirely to the difficult task. This man was Lyman Spalding. Although Mitchill was not willing to take the risk, he still wished to manage the undertaking. Spalding had gained his friendship through correspondence, and Mitchill helped the young physician to settle in New York. Later he encouraged Spalding in the plan of initiating a *United States Pharmacopeia,* to be prepared as a cooperative task by the medical associations of the entire country. Although Mitchill gave sanction to this plan and assisted in its execution, he left both the responsibility and the glory to Spalding.

The real start of the new and finally successful enterprise was made by Lyman Spalding on January 6, 1817, when he submitted

> to the New York County Medical Society, a project for the formation of a National Pharmacopoeia, by the authority of all the medical societies and medical schools in the United States. The plan proposed was, (1) That a convention should be called in each of the four grand divisions of the United States, to be composed from all the medical societies and schools; (2) That each district convention should form a pharmacopoeia, and elect delegates to meet in general convention in the city of Washington, on the first of January, 1820: (3) That the general convention should, from the district pharmacopoeia, form the national work.[20]

The development of the project now proceeded rapidly. Only one month after Spalding submitted his project to the New York County Medical Society, the New York State Medical Society, at the suggestion of Mitchill, approved "the formation of an American Pharmacopoeia of delegates from the several State Medical Societies."[21] A committee with Lyman Spalding as secretary was appointed to "correspond with all the incorporated state medical societies, etc., in the Union and such influential medical men as they may deem proper." On March 4, 1818, the committee issued the first circular. The response received made it clear "that the design of forming a National Pharmacopoeia had met the approbation of a majority of the medical associations in the U.S." A second circular in-

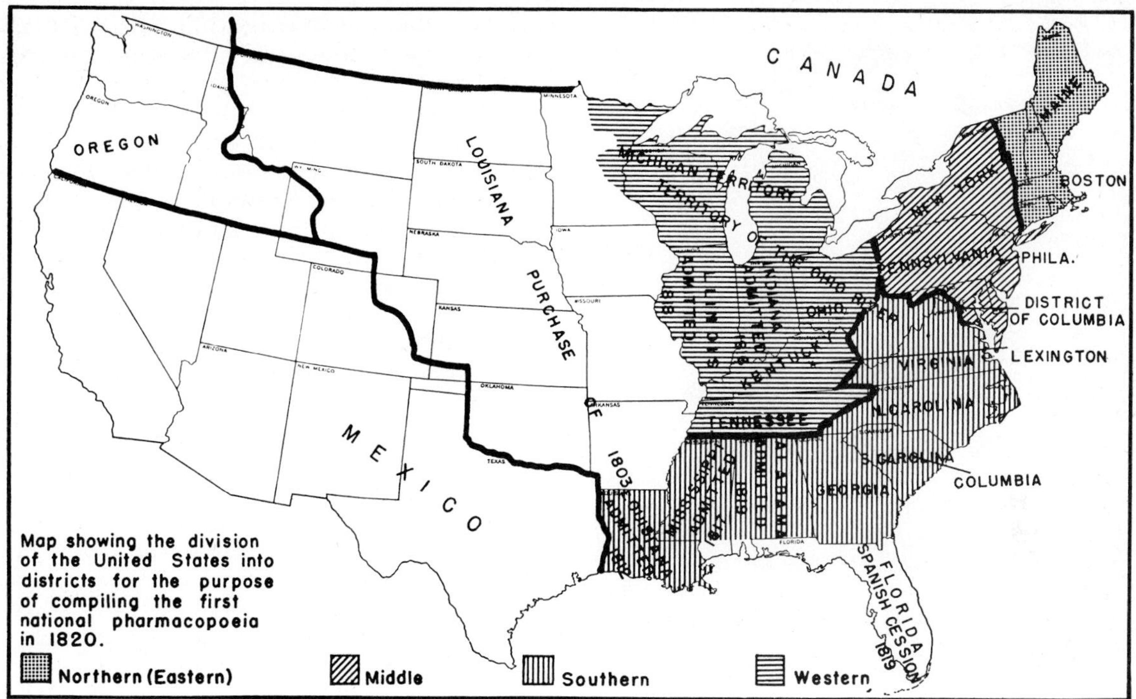


Map showing the division of the United States into districts for the purpose of compiling the first national pharmacopoeia in 1820.

vited "the said associations to designate a time and a place for the meeting of each of the district conventions: and in conformity therewith the following places were designated, viz., Boston, Philadelphia, Columbia, South Carolina, and Lexington, Kentucky."[22]

Most of the work was accomplished within the Northern (Eastern) and the Middle districts, more particularly by the delegates of Massachusetts, New York and Pennsylvania. "There were no conventions held in the Southern and Western districts, but measures were taken by those concerned, to secure a representation of the Southern district in the General Convention at Washington."[23]

Only a scattering of men took seats when the General Convention convened on the first day of January, 1820, in the Senate Chamber of the Capitol in Washington, D.C. They had no power to legislate or even to make the proposed pharmacopeia "official." Yet they formally represented their constituencies and would bring into being the first Pharmacopeia of the United States in a typically American way.

On that first day, we are told, only a half dozen delegates participated; on the second day five more delegates appeared. All were physicians, the majority coming from the pharmacopeial Middle District lying just North of the Capital. At that time no society or school of pharmacy existed in the United States, to offer the possibility of organized pharmaceutical representation. (By the time of the second revision of the U.S.P., representatives of American pharmacy assumed a working partnership and in subsequent revisions were officially recognized and increasingly important.)

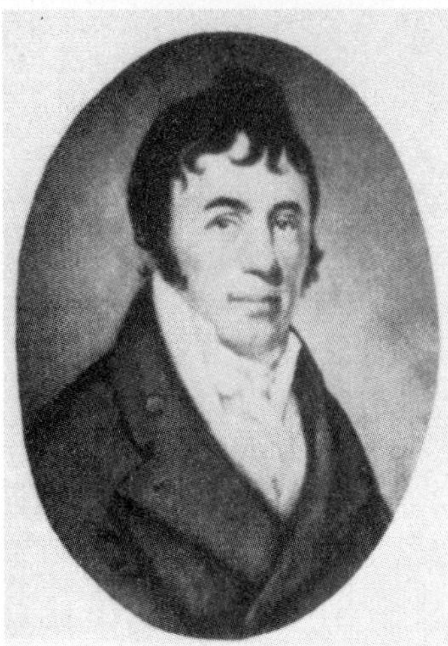

The physician Lyman Spalding *(above)* was more responsible than anyone else for the successful planning and work that produced the first *Pharmacopeia of the United States* in 1820. It is said that he was urging the idea of a national pharmacopeia on his friends as early as 1815.

It was a relatively young group that assembled at the founding Convention, 9 of the 11 being under 48 years of age. Their professional stature varied considerably. The dominance of the College of Philadelphia (later called the University of Pennsylvania) in early medical education shows up in the background of at least half the delegates, who either graduated from its medical department or at least studied there. Two others had studied medicine at the University of Edinburgh, whose famous medical department had been the model for American beginnings at the College of Philadelphia. This educational background suggests an informed awareness of European pharmacopeial experience among the delegates and helps to explain the influence of the respected Edinburgh Pharmacopeia on American developments.[24]

At the close of the founding assembly, Lyman Spalding wrote to his daughter. "We have completed the objects [of] our mission in the most amicable and harmonious manner possible to the perfect satisfaction of ourselves and every body else. The Government has agreed to adopt the Pharmacopoeia for the use of the Navy and Army . . . The great national work is spoken of by the President [James Monroe] as an undertaking which will assist in giving us a National character."[25]

When the first *U.S. Pharmacopeia* was published, the preface mentioned the "Pharmacopoeia of the Massachusetts Medical Society," but an intent to minimize its importance seems evident. The evidence shows, however, that a revised Massachusetts pharmacopeia recommended by the Eastern district was consolidated with a prospectus recommended by the Middle district and revised for publication as the first U.S.P.[26]

The report of the Philadelphia delegate states that "in the arrangement of the materia medica the plan proposed in the Middle district [virtually, New York and Philadelphia] has been departed from," but "the list of preparations and compounds is pretty nearly what was agreed on in the convention of the Middle district."[27] Since "more than 90 p.c. of the articles in the Massachusetts Pharmacopoeia were included" in the *Pharmacopoeia*, either the draft of the Middle District was itself based on the Massachusetts book or its authors came independently to similar conclusions.

The entire editorial work had to be done by the committee of publication under the active chairmanship of Lyman Spalding. How thoroughly the original draft was revised and corrected becomes apparent from a printed copy of items of the materia medica as well as of the *medicamenta praeparata* that the chairman sent to his committee members.[28] Finally, the book was printed in Boston and appeared on December 15, 1820, bearing the title *The Pharmacopoeia of the United States of America*, published "By the Authority of the Medical Societies and Colleges."

The national successor to the *Massachusetts Pharmacopoeia* differed strikingly in that it did not confine itself to the use of the English language—the text on facing pages being both in Latin and in English. In contrast with the authors of the *Massachusetts Pharmacopoeia* the majority of the delegates responsible for the national standard was of the opinion that "no well-educated physician or apothecary is unacquainted" with Latin.[29] Another significant remark in the preface, one of the earliest official American statements concerning pharmaceutical manufacturing on a large scale, reads: "Those compound substances which are prepared in the large way at manufactories, and which are to be kept by the apothecary, *though not necessarily prepared by him,** are inserted on the materia medica list. Those which are to be made by the apothecary alone, are placed among the preparations and compositions."[30]

The uncertainty of the authors in selecting drugs is illustrated by the fact that they divided the materia medica list into two parts, one containing "articles of decided reputation or general use" and another containing "those the claims of which are of a more uncertain kind." This dual list was continued until radical changes were effected in 1882 (6th revision).

This procedure had a European pattern. However, there is one difference. In European countries the discrimination had a very practical meaning. There the articles of the first list *(series medicaminum)* had to be kept in stock in even the smallest pharmacy. Thus the availability of these drugs to prescribing physicians was guaranteed.

In general, the new book met with a kind reception, although there were some disapproving voices. In a Philadelphia medical journal, an anonymous reviewer, after a long and detailed criticism, concluded that the work "will probably require immediate revision."[31] The senior surgeon of the Navy, Dr. Edward Cutbush, stated to the Secretary of the Navy that he was not able to give his "unqualified approbation of the work for the use of our naval surgeons."[32] The members of the medical and pharmaceutical professions accepted the book, so far as they were interested, and in 1828 a somewhat modified second issue of the first U.S.P. appeared.[33]

The importance of first publications such as this lies not so much in their perfection and immediate results as in the simple fact that a beginning has been made. At the close of a 12-page review, the *Medical Repository* stated:

> This work forms an era in the history of the profession. It is the first one ever compiled by the authority of the profession throughout a nation. Collections of this sort have been made in other countries, but none, so far, under the impressive sanction which distinguishes this. Many of the authorities of the Past compiled similar works, later still, the Colleges of Great Britain have followed their examples. France by command of her Monarch has furnished her "Codex," but it has remained for American Physicians to frame a work which emanates from the profession itself, and is founded on the principles of Representation. It embodies a Codex Medicum of the free and independent United States.[34]

## REVISING THE PHARMACOPEIA

While the first revision was underway a dangerous schism developed among those most interested in developing effective drug standards for America through the new *Pharmacopeia*. Misunderstandings arose largely because of crude procedures for administering the U.S.P., intensified by an old rivalry between New York and Philadelphia factions. Under the leadership of the eminent New York physician Samuel L. Mitchill, then U.S.P. president, a second General Convention was held in New York, and a FIRST REVISION was published on schedule, at New York in 1830.

A bizarre sequel was the appearance of another and different First Revision, imprinted Philadelphia, 1831![35] This edition

*Italics added.

gained more recognition than did the competing New York edition. And the New York book had no successors. Before the time for a third General Convention, two key figures in the founding period of the *Pharmacopeia,* the New Yorkers Mitchill and Spalding, both had died. No one comparable came forward in the New York area to do the work and to fight for it.

However, in the Philadelphia contingent were two physicians whose competent work and influential personalities would be decisive for the future of the *Pharmacopeia of the United States:* George B. Wood and Franklin Bache. Among medical practitioners in general, now that the *Pharmacopeia* seemed to be well established, interest in it waned. So much so that it is doubtful that pharmacopeial work would have persisted except for the sustaining prosperity of the *United States Dispensatory* prepared by Wood and Bache (see p. 279), who were now the key figures in carrying forward the further revision of the *Pharmacopeia.*

These physicians were both on the faculty of the Philadelphia College of Pharmacy, and thus arose a collaboration on the *Pharmacopeia* between physicians and pharmacists of scientific attainment that had been lacking.

To conduct experiments for use by the Committee on the Pharmacopeia, an eminent Philadelphia pharmacist, Daniel B. Smith, was employed. When the Philadelphia edition (1831) appeared, the preface alluded to this work, to improvements due to the "zeal of pharmacists as well in this country as in Europe," and to the entire *Pharmacopeia* having "passed the examination of pharmacists of acknowledged eminence in their profession."[36]

The pharmacopeial revision work now developed into a definite routine, which persisted through the Fifth Revision (6th edition, 1873). The decennial revisions were carried out by a Committee of Revision authorized and appointed by each subsequent Washington Convention. George B. Wood and Franklin Bache of Philadelphia continued to be the most active members of the Committee.

In the First Revision cooperating pharmacists included only members of the Philadelphia College of Pharmacy. The SECOND REVISION (published 1842) took advantage of the advice of still other pharmacy colleges then operating. Helpful response came from both Boston and New York, but the most important pharmaceutical collaboration again came from Philadelphia, consisting of "amendment of the whole Pharmacopoeia, by a special committee. . . ."[37] Among the collaborators was that remarkable pharmacist, William Procter, Jr.

This Second Revision appeared only in English. A notable technical innovation was the approval of percolation as an optional method of extraction, a progressive step taken earlier only by the French and the Scottish (Edinburgh) pharmacopeias. Brief notes on purity tests for some U.S.P. drugs were introduced, following the example of the London and the Edinburgh pharmacopeias.

Participation of pharmacists in this 1842 edition was more extensive but still only semi-official. With the THIRD REVISION (1851 edition) pharmacy was accorded official representation in the General Convention. A new period dawned. The period of the pharmacopeial convention as a purely medical organization had come to an end.

By including pharmacy, the representatives of medicine publicly recognized two factors: (1) the existence of American professional pharmacy and its representation by the colleges (i.e., local associations), and (2) the necessity of having pharmacy share not only the work but also the responsibility.

At the 1850 Convention two of the five pharmacists participating were made members of the Committee of Revision: William Procter, Jr., of Philadelphia, and John Milhau of New York City.

When the 1851 edition appeared, fluid extracts were a notable innovation among the dosage forms.

At the U.S.P. General Convention of 1860, 11 pharmacists participated (from four colleges along the Eastern seaboard); pharmacists comprised half the new Committee of Revision; and the American Pharmaceutical Association (founded just 8 years before) transmitted new technical material as published in its *Proceedings,* for use in the work of revision. This convention also was noteworthy for a contribution from the New York medical profession, read by Dr. E. R. Squibb, which was the first proferred from New York in the three decades since the severe schism of 1830.

This FOURTH REVISION appeared as the 5th edition in 1863 (reprinted 1864, 1866, 1868). Its lateness probably can be attributed partly to the numerous changes (requiring some 119 meetings and 138 written reports of subcommittees), partly to a wish to take into account innovations in a forthcoming edition of the *British Pharmacopoeia,* with which there was growing American cooperation. One significant change was the grading of powder fineness according to five different sieve meshes. The use of apothecaries' weights was de-emphasized.

Work on the *Pharmacopeia* now had entered a period of transition. When the FIFTH REVISION of the *Pharmacopeia* appeared (1873), Franklin Bache had died and George B. Wood was diligent but old. His energy and authority, after four decades of pharmacopeial work, were strong enough to hold the new edition within old lines; but there were new men among the 60 delegates at the General Convention (1870), men with new ideas, and their presence implied change.

The old guard, as symbolized by Wood, must have realized that they were on the defensive, since they emphasized the "conservative character necessarily pertaining to a National Pharmacopoeia" and rejected any thought of a "mission to lead in the paths of discovery." They spoke disdainfully of "pandering to fashion or to doubtful novelties in Pharmaceutical Science," and complained of the "meagreness of details" in reports submitted for use by the Committee of Revision.[38]

Although the medical colleges represented at the Convention of 1870 had still outnumbered pharmacy colleges 3 to 1, 4 of the 6 technical contributions presented to the Convention for the next revision came from pharmacists. Without doubt, pharmaceutical interest in the *Pharmacopeia* had increased gradually, while that of the medical profession had decreased.

Dr. E. R. Squibb was among those who felt that the pharmacopeial work had not kept pace with the times; and he was dissatisfied with the dependence of the *Pharmacopeia* on the private success of Dr. Wood's *Dispensatory of the United States.* Some of the proposals Squibb now put forward were a paid full-time director of revision, revision every 5 years (instead of 10), a pharmacopeia embracing so much commentary that it need not be supplemented by a dispensatory, plus publication of an inexpensive annual that would provide a semi-official progress report on innovations in drugs, processes and equipment.[39] Dr. Squibb thought that such a program should be administered by cooperative action of the American Medical Association and the American Pharmaceutical Association, medicine taking the lead and the responsibilities, with pharmacy assisting, as a special branch of medicine.

In pharmaceutical circles this plan was treated with reserve, for rather obvious reasons. At the American Pharmaceutical Association it was clearly recognized that physicians "certainly have a right to direct what substances shall enter into the Pharmacopoeia, their general character, and the preparations, but the details of the work devolve certainly upon pharmacists and pharmaceutical chemists. . . ." The pharmacists' Association seemed ready to cooperate with the American Medical Association—but on a basis of equality.[40]

In medical circles the plan perhaps met more indifference than active opposition. The American Medical Association not only

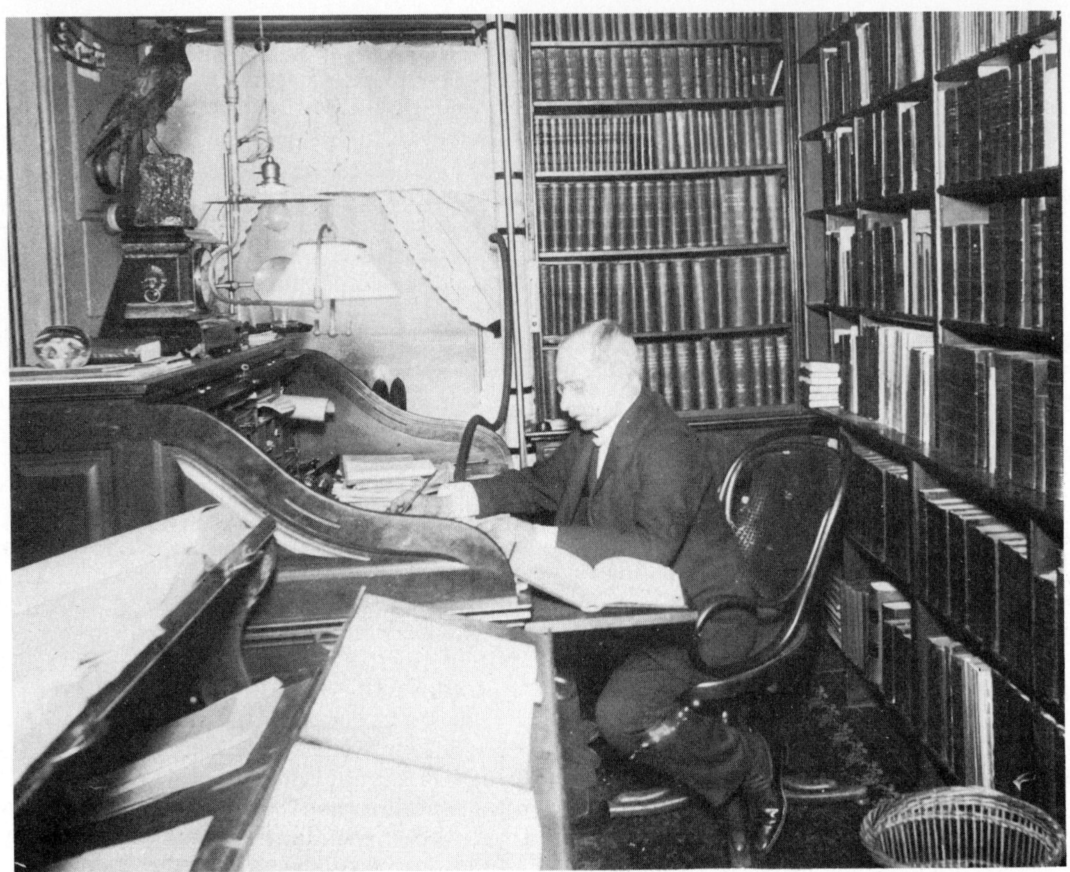

Charles Rice (1841–1901), one of the most remarkable American pharmacists, did most of his work at his desk in Bellevue Hospital *(above)*, where he served as superintendent of the General Drug Department. At the lower left can be seen part of the revolving dictionary rack that he used in reading 18 languages of East and West. He was the key figure in giving the U. S. Pharmacopeia (1882) its modern outlook and format; he was chairman of the committee to develop the first National Formulary and he contributed brilliantly to other pharmaceutical publications.

failed to adopt the proposal but called any arrangement for pharmaceutical responsibility "inappropriate" to the Association.[41]

This circumstance created an opportune hour for American pharmacy. Fortunately, members of the American Pharmaceutical Association had the ability and the farsightedness to comprehend the great task confronting them and to grapple with it. At the 1877 meeting, high level discussions were held, with initiative particularly in the hands of Frederick Hoffmann of New York. In a resolution adopted by the assembly, he pointed to the necessity for a more frequent, comprehensive and generally satisfactory revision on a new basis, and placed that task in the hands of the American Pharmaceutical Association.[42]

In place of its old Committee on the Pharmacopeia, which had no authoritative influence, the American Pharmaceutical Association named a new 15-man committee with a great task: not only to draft a new edition of the *Pharmacopeia of the United States*, but actually a new type of pharmacopeia.[43]

There remained a question: What trouble might ensue with distinguished oldsters still in pharmacopeial positions, who felt themselves challenged and their prerogatives put in question? To forestall dissension, the old Convention was left externally untouched. The presidency was filled by a physician, as from the beginning in 1820. Yet, the internal workings definitely changed.

Previously, the Committee of Revision had played the role of an executive body, largely through the authoritarian dominance of one man, George B. Wood. The Committee was now made the official executive, with the backing of the American Pharmaceutical Association. It was given authority to "report a complete plan for the revision of the Pharmacopoeia at the next Decennial Convention," instead of the traditional procedure of revising and amalgamating various drafts and contributions first brought before the Convention by constituent groups.

Pharmacists now held a majority in the Committee of Revision (14 of 25). At its head was the learned and versatile hospital pharmacist, Charles Rice of New York, who was also chairman of the American Pharmaceutical Association's committee, which published a remarkable comprehensive report in 1880. When the Association placed the Committee's proposals on the Pharmacopeia before the General Convention, they became the foundation for the renowned SIXTH REVISION, the 1882 edition.

Any pharmacist who holds this book in his hands and compares it with its predecessor will recognize the advent of the modern *Pharmacopeia of the United States* and will appreciate why this edition signaled a fundamental advance in drug standards for the American health professions and the public.

The new *Pharmacopeia* turned more sharply away from the outworn concept of the community pharmacy as the place of manufacture of most of the pharmaceutical preparations. Instead it tried to establish in the pharmacy another kind of responsibility: examination of medicinal substances by the pharmacist as a check on quality. Casual mention of a few tests was replaced with detailed tests for identifying and determining the purity of many of the drugs. Detailed processes for assaying the alkaloids appeared for the first time. Drugs from the vegetable and the mineral kingdoms were more meaningfully described as to physical characteristics and, where possible, chemical properties. Symbolic formulas and molecular weights were introduced.

The old division of the *Pharmacopeia* into primary and secondary lists of basic drugs and a section of preparations was abandoned. A single alphabetic arrangement of all drugs in the new edition was similar to that in the *British Pharmacopoeia*.[44]

The fullness of description and explanation in the Sixth Revision especially impressed the pharmaceutical and medical world. Nomenclature was revised and one class of preparations appeared for the first time: abstracts (dilutions of powdered extracts). Still other innovations reinforce the special place that the 1882 edition holds in the history of the *United States Pharmacopeia*.

With authority for drafting subsequent editions now centering in a single executive body, the preparatory work went forward in a more systematic way. One offshoot of work on the SEVENTH REVISION was the serial *Digest of Comments* on the *United States Pharmacopeia*, which would find a useful place in pharmaceutical literature for several decades (after 1905 appearing as *Bulletins* of the Hygienic Laboratory of the U. S. Public Health Service; from 1926 to 1948 as part of the *Abstracts* of the American Pharmaceutical Association).

With the Seventh Revision (8th edition) there was established the present policy that requires announcement of "a definite date, reasonably distant from the actual date of publication, when the new Pharmacopoeia is intended to go into effect and to supersede the preceding one." Thus the new book was made effective on January 1, 1894 (although it had been published in September, 1893). Such evidences of increasing formality in procedure and precision in content reflected increasing legal implications, for although the Federal Food and Drug Act had not yet been passed, the *Pharmacopeia* had already been made "official" under a number of state laws, a fact recognized by the change in this edition from the old term "officinal" to "official."[45]

The *Pharmacopeia* effective from 1894 contained other evidences of a new time. Assays for active principles of both drugs and preparations were added wherever possible. Standards of purity were made "as high as practicable for legal enforcement, but not beyond a point reasonably attainable by the manufacturer." Chemical formulas were modernized. Use of the metric system was encouraged, "solids to be weighed and liquids to be measured." Substances were excluded that could be produced only by a patented process or that were otherwise protected by proprietary rights.

The General Convention of 1900 remains memorable particularly because it took action to incorporate as "The United States Pharmacopoeial Convention" (June 11, 1900), with the purpose of "establishing one uniform standard and guide for the use of those engaged in the practice of medicine and pharmacy in the United States, whereby the identity, strength and purity of all medicines and drugs may be accurately determined and for other like and similar purposes."[46] Some of the organizational changes introduced at this time remain functional today. A Board of Trustees was established to handle business affairs. Additional delegates to the Convention were authorized, including representatives from the American Chemical Society and branches of the United States government (such as the Army, the Navy and the U. S. Marine Hospital Service). With the establishment of this newly chartered organization, the American Pharmaceutical Association had fulfilled its diplomatically pursued goal of giving the *Pharmacopeia* and its revisions a solid and lasting foundation.

Shortly after his re-election as chairman of the Committee of Revision, Charles Rice died (1901). From among the 18 pharmacists and 7 physicians on the Committee there was chosen as Rice's successor Joseph P. Remington of Philadelphia, one of the master pharmacists of his generation.

While the collaboration of physicians was eagerly sought, the preponderance of pharmacists on the Committee of Revision reflects the fact that the entire painstaking and detailed technical work was pharmaceutical in nature and hence devolved on pharmacists, "while the field of the physician in connection with the revision of the Pharmacopoeia is restricted mainly to deciding upon the admission or exclusion of articles."[47]

The General Convention of 1900, faced with the economic realities of modern research and development, modified its policy that had excluded indiscriminately the patented and other proprietary drugs. The Committee of Revision was now permitted to consider any "product of definite composition which is in common use by the medical profession, the identity, purity or strength of which can be determined. No compound or mixture shall be introduced if the composition or mode of manufacture thereof be kept secret, or if it be controlled by unlimited proprietary or patent rights."[48] The Committee also was instructed to introduce average approximate doses (but not to give a minimum or maximum). The general advice that as many assays and tests of identity and purity as possible should be introduced led to a remarkable increase of U.S.P. assays.[49] A purity rubric was to be given for each chemical substance "used solely for medicinal purposes. . . . " With the prospect of Federally enforced drug standards pending, these changes involved new considerations and import.

Under the new chairman, Joseph Remington, revision was carried forward with great care. The United States honored the recommendations of the International Conference on the Unification of Potent Medicaments (1902) in this edition, with one or two exceptions. For example, a strength of about 10 per cent for potent tinctures became a uniform rule. Inauguration of a new class of drugs, the biologicals, was signaled by admission of antidiphtheria serum to the *Pharmacopeia.*

With this EIGHTH REVISION, which did not appear until 1905, began the practice of dating the *Pharmacopeia* according to the year when each edition took effect (rather than emphasizing the year of the respective General Convention). The U.S.P. VIII* was the first edition to have full legal recognition of the United States government, which was granted by the first Food and Drug Act (1906). Both this enactment and its successor, the Food, Drug, and Cosmetic Act of 1938, made official the *National Formulary*, then published by the American Pharmaceutical Association (see p. 275), as well as the *Pharmacopeia* published by the independent and newly incorporated United States Pharmacopeial Convention. These books now spoke with the force of law; all they said and did not say took on additional meaning and ramifications. Hence it is not surprising that a modified printing of the U.S.P. became necessary after passage of the Act.

Henceforth the *Pharmacopeia* became nearly indispensable for the entire American trade in drugs, not in pharmacies alone; yet, it is noteworthy that the book could not become "official" in the strict sense of the term "pharmacopeia" traditional elsewhere. That is, under the United States Constitution, the national law could not require possession of a copy nor make observance of the rules and the standards of the *United States Pharmacopeia* compulsory for every licensed pharmacist or pharmacy. Such requirements had to be made effective through laws of the individual states.

When the General Convention (1910) called the general principles that it adopted "recommendations" instead of "instructions," it undoubtedly signaled a trend toward greater authority for the Committee of Revision, with the Convention and its Board of Trustees restricting themselves more to administration and broad policy. With this NINTH REVISION the Committee of Revision was increased to 50 members besides the president of the Convention ex officio. Fifteen subcommittees were appointed, "of which the chairman, elected by the members of the respective subcommittees, constituted an executive committee . . . ."[50]

The subject areas dealt with by these subcommittees may be taken as evidence of the need for a pharmaceutical majority in the practical work of pharmacopeial revision.[51] Only three subcommittees were devoted to medical subjects, namely those on the scope of the *Pharmacopeia*; on therapeutics, pharmacodynamics and posology; and on biologic products and diagnostic tests. The other 12 subcommittees dealt exclusively with pharmaceutical, pharmacognostic and pharmacochemical problems and hence consisted of pharmacists and other pharmaceutical specialists.

It recognized technical advance in a difficult field when this edition admitted "biological tests or assays" as a matter of principle, whereas in the preceding edition they had been expressly barred.

Indicative of the Convention's reaction to a pharmaceutical trend in formulation and marketing was a paragraph discouraging the introduction of new compound preparations, "as far as possible."

The ninth decennial revision, published in

---

*Pharmacopeial numbering is according to the *Revision*—not the edition.

1916, was translated not only into Spanish,[52] as were predecessors, but also into Chinese.

Remington died 2 years before the Pharmacopieal Convention of 1920,[53] which elected as his successor another pharmacist, E. Fullerton Cook of Philadelphia. Like Remington, he was associated with the Philadelphia College of Pharmacy.

Reflecting the difficulty of the task assigned to the medical subcommittee on scope, a further "Referee Committee on Scope" was now established, consisting of 21 physicians of the General Committee, to take the responsibility of deciding disputed questions concerning the admission and the deletion of therapeutic substances.[54]

No matter how wisely such decisions were made, it became increasingly difficult to keep the *Pharmacopeia* abreast of scientific and therapeutic developments; hence interim supplements became more common. A corollary need was for greater specialization and more participating experts. This was reflected in the number of auxiliary advisors who worked on the TENTH REVISION, which appeared in 1926, including the government "Bureaus and Departments responsible for enforcing drug standards, the various medical associations, numerous national pharmaceutical bodies and hundreds of individuals, all working with the appropriate organized subcommittee."[55]

The demands of pharmacopeial work found formal expression when the Convention revised its Constitution and By-laws (1930). The circle of groups entitled to representation in the Pharmacopeial Convention was enlarged greatly, and the number of individuals participating in revision work greatly increased.

The ELEVENTH REVISION (published 1936) would have been financially prohibitive, it was reported, except for the collaboration without charge by many of these specialized agencies and individuals, including "colleges, universities, industrial organizations, private laboratories and the Government," and "voluntary service . . . by outstanding physicians, pharmacists, and other scientists of this country."[56] Sources of some of the important contributions were acknowledged when the new edition stated,

> Portions of monographs, prepared by the American Medical Association and published in "New and Non-official Remedies" have been used to form the basis of a number of new tests. Extensive data published by the American Chemical Society have been utilized in preparing the new reagent standards. The joint "Contact Committee" of the American Drug Manufacturers' Association and the American Pharmaceutical Manufacturers' Association has assisted in developing biological and vitamin assays and in many other problems of the revision.[57]

This Eleventh Revision introduced reference standards for certain drugs and provided for their distribution.[58] It also marked still closer cooperation with the British Pharmacopoeia Convention and, beyond that, increasing adoption of international standards. In this supranational endeavor, which was to culminate in the *Pharmacopoeia Internationalis*, the American U.S.P. chairman, E. Fullerton Cook, played a prominent role.

The TWELFTH REVISION (13th edition, 1942) marked the start of a full-scale program of "continuous revision," under which a new *Pharmacopeia* appears "every five years, a bound 'Supplement' halfway between, and, to meet the frequently occurring situations which require immediate attention, 'Interim Revision Announcements' or sheet 'Supplements' whenever these are required."[59]

This far-reaching decision influenced, and, indeed, even necessitated, another decision that made the chairman of the General Committee of Revision a full-time permanent "Director of Pharmacopoeial Revision" with broad administrative powers. This position is filled through election by each outgoing Board of Trustees.[60]

To house the Director and the Pharmacopeial staff and facilities, the U.S.P. purchased a permanent headquarters building in New York City (converting an elegant town house at 46 Park Avenue), which was occupied in 1950.[61]

The twin innovations of permanent Director and permanent headquarters constituted one of the most important steps to assure the continuity and the fruitfulness of revision work since the establishment of the United States Pharmacopeial Convention in its modern form (1900). To a large extent this step fulfilled efforts of the pharmacist E. Fullerton Cook, who had been connected with the revision work for about four decades.

His tasks were taken over in 1950 by the first Director of Pharmacopeial Revision elected by the Board of Trustees, Lloyd C. Miller. His selection may be construed to symbolize a transformation that had been taking place in the character of the men and the work of pharmacopeial revision, a shift in emphasis from the high art of professional practice to highly specialized scientific research. Before 1880 the pharmacopeial revision work had been headed by physicians; since then it had been headed by pharmacists; and after 1950 by neither a pharmacist nor a physician, but by a biochemist and pharmacologist.

In overhauling its Constitution and By-Laws in the 1940's the Convention made other important changes. Formally adopted was the custom of having the General Committee of Revision consist of 60 persons, one third qualified in medical sciences and two thirds in pharmaceutical and allied sciences (plus the President of the Convention and the Director of Revision ex officio). At the same time the composition of the Board of Trustees was defined to consist of nine persons, including the President of the Convention ex officio. Six are elected from the accredited delegates to the Convention: of these, two are from the pharmaceutical colleges and organizations represented and two from the medical colleges and organizations; the other two are the Treasurer and the Director of Revision ex officio (the last two without voting privileges).

At this time the number of agencies entitled to representation in the Pharmacopeial Convention was expanded considerably in recognition of the fact that the work must be increasingly a collaboration among the professions, the pure and the applied sciences, the governmental branches, and the trade organizations—all directly involved and particularly knowledgeable in the complex ramifications of drug standards and standardization. One stimulus toward maintaining this work at a uniformly high level of expertness stems from the Federal Food, Drug, and Cosmetic Act, which obligates the Food and Drug Administration to draft standards of its own in the event that standards set by legally designated compendia are deemed inadequate. "Thus far," said the U.S.P. Director, Dr. Miller, "this has not proved necessary and it is our aim to be alert to the point that recourse to such action will never be necessary."[62]

Although the "continuous revision" concept had led to the scheduling of a completely new edition approximately every 5 years, the General Convention continued to meet decennially, which had been traditional since the founding.

The Thirteenth Revision became effective (April 1947) less than 5 years after the Twelfth Revision was published. The most striking innovation of this edition placed English drug names ahead of Latin names for the first time, the latter being only vestiges of earlier centuries when Latin had been in common use by physicians and pharmacists.[63]

With English names in first place, the alphabetic arrangement of the Pharmacopeia henceforth gave a quite different sequence to the monographs covering the individual drugs. Moreover, immediately following the material on each basic drug appeared the monographs for its various dosage forms, which heretofore had been grouped by classes (all fluid extracts together, etc.).

After the fundamental changes in the administration, the content and the style of the Pharmacopeia during the 1940's, it is not surprising that the FOURTEENTH REVISION showed little change beyond the routine admissions and deletions of drugs, especially since it became effective only 3 years after the issuance of the previous edition, an unprecedentedly brief period. This edition inaugurated the useful practice of designating with an asterisk each drug known to be protected by a patent.

To illustrate the reciprocal functioning of the *National Formulary*, which has been a companion book of comparable officiality since 1906, it may be mentioned that about 90 per cent of the drugs deleted by the U.S.P. continued to have standards in legal force by transfer into the N.F. Conversely, almost 18 per cent of the drugs newly admitted to the U.S.P. were taken over from the N.F.

In preparing the FIFTEENTH REVISION (effective 1955), it was necessary to deal with an unusual number of new drugs vying for admission (the result of a postwar boom in research) and with advances in analytical procedures affecting assays. Administratively, the Revision Committee had been enlarged and diversified, while the subcommittee structure had been pared down by a third and given more autonomy. The revamped working plan respected tradition in that "scope and posology remained the concern of the physicians on the Committee, whereas the pharmaceutical aspects of revision fell to those trained in pharmacy, chemistry, bacteriology, etc."[64]

Making the U.S.P. a therapeutic guide to the drugs of medical choice at the time of revision remained a central concept. Already in the first *Pharmacopeia* the scope had hinged on the idea of admitting drugs "the utility of which is most fully established and best understood."

With this edition, Latin names—which had been dropped from primary to secondary position in U.S.P. XII—were now "dropped practically entirely, both because of disuse and because they generally differ so little from the English titles." In instances where the Latin stem did differ markedly, the Latin name was placed among the synonyms. Here, too, began the practice of stating the general therapeutic or pharmaceutic "category" of the substance covered in each monograph. The demise of apothecary weights and measures was either hastened or confirmed by their banishment from statements of dosage and sizes available.

The SIXTEENTH REVISION (effective 1960) stated,

> The feature that distinguishes this revision most from all of its recent predecessors is the progress made in adopting new analytical techniques. Thus either much more extensively, or for the first time, use has been made of nonaqueous titrimetry, complexometry, ultraviolet and infrared spectrophotometry, column and paper chromatography, and (in one instance) a phase solubility determination for assay purposes.

Indeed, in the decade that the appearance of U.S.P. XVI brought to a close

> the technology of drug standardization underwent a remarkable transition. . . . Chemical analysis attained a new plane in respect to precision and sensitivity, albeit at a decided loss of simplicity. Thus vastly improved techniques of isolation, coupled with refinements in quantitative instrumental measurement provided means of analyzing drug principles for the first time or served to replace more costly and time-consuming biologic assays. During this decade [1950's], the need first arose for standardizing radioactive drugs, and the use of radioactive tracers was introduced into drug analysis.[65]

A continuing trend toward more and longer monographs now called forth a number of editorial stratagems to keep the *Pharmacopeia* within a manageable size. For example, a single monograph sometimes covered two or more closely related substances, which in the traditional style of previous editions would each be covered in a separate monograph. For the first time the *Pharmacopeia* published a list of the articles that had been approved for admission but for which satisfactory monographs could not yet be completed (81 such titles, as compared with 908 titles for which monographs were actually published in U.S.P. XVI).

The SEVENTEENTH REVISION (effective 1965) reflected a still more conservative approach to selecting drugs admitted to the U.S.P., in view of the heavy emphasis upon safety and efficacy under the 1962 amendments to the Federal Food, Drug and Cosmetic Act. Besides the question of drug products to be admitted, the 1960 Convention had asked that the scope be broadened to include standards for additional *types* of medical products, such as devices for administering drugs, substances for vascular repair and internal splinting, agents for diagnostic tests not conducted on the person of the patient, and so on. The regulations as well as newer scientific capabilities in pharmaceutical laboratories raised in new terms the old question: What constitutes an adequate drug standard? The complex difficulty of getting a definitive answer partly lay with an old problem: the influence on a test result of some substance used in formulating the drug product in addition to the influence of the therapeutic ingredient being measured. Rather than circumventing it, the advent of modern spectrophotometry in applying analytical standards presented this "inadequacy" in a new guise. In moving against the problem, the Revision Committee specified that, wherever possible, the specific ingredient being tested first be isolated from substances that might distort test results and, second, that the extracted substance be tested in comparison with a sample of U.S.P. Reference Standard, under rigidly specified conditions. Standards were tightened further by applying formal test assays more widely to basic drug entities and trying for greater specificity—for example, by utilizing polarography more often. In the field of drug names, a long-term trend had been away from multiple synonyms for medicines. Henceforth, only a single official name could be listed and used for each drug, under Federal law. To propose such United States Adopted Names ("U.S.A.N.") a cooperative program was initiated in 1961 by the U.S.P.C. and the A.M.A., later joined by the A.Ph.A. (1964) and the F.D.A. (1967). Possible differences between "proper" physicochemical constitution and physiological availability of a drug faced the Committee of Revision with a serious challenge; but the scientific means proved to be not yet at hand to resolve the question it posed. Beginning in 1961, the Drug Standards Laboratory (in the A.Ph.A. building) had come under the tripartite sponsorship of the A.Ph.A., U.S.P., and A.M.A., which proved to be "a source of great strength" to the standard-setting agencies.

The EIGHTEENTH REVISION (effective 1970) generated standards in the new perspective of the Food and Drug Administration's heavy emphasis on "good manufacturing practices" in the regulation of pharmaceutical manufacturing laboratories. Although such practices rarely could be quantified sufficiently to set standards in the usual sense, the "procedures by which good manufacturing practice is implemented are decidedly related to drug standards, and consequently much of the revision . . . serves to necessitate and/or demonstrate compliance with what are regarded as the best practices. . . ." (p. xiii) One consequence was far greater attention to a drug's uniformity of content from dose to dose (first introduced in U.S.P. XVII), microbial limits and dissolution rate. The quest to clarify the dimensions of the issue about correlation between physiological availability and compliance with official standards was pursued further though a U.S.P.-N.F. Joint Panel on Physiological Availability. The result was limited progress, and since what had come to be called "bioavailability" depended on the manufacturer's production control as well as on the product formulation, the goal remained elusive.

The NINETEENTH REVISION (effective 1975), reflected the accelerating change in the science and technology underlying drug standards and in the U.S.P.C. attitude toward its public mandate. Although the U.S.P. itself had been revised on a 5-year cycle since 1940, the administrative phase had remained on a decennial basis since the founding. From the 1970 Convention onward, all U.S.P. activities and appointments were placed on a 5-year cycle and provision made (e.g., increased staff) for an increased tempo and scope of activities, including a more continuous representation and communication between the national membership of the U.S.P. Convention and its elected officials. With the retirement of Lloyd C. Miller, a new post of Executive Director was created, with the pharmacist William M. Heller, Ph.D., as the first incumbent. The old post of Director of Revision permitted an inference of divided authority, which, after two stressful years, was continued as the post of Director, Drug Standards Division, in a modified headquarters structure. Pressure for ever more refined standards of quality assurance pushed aside any remaining consideration of the limited resources of small manufacturing laboratories. Thus, for the first time, test procedures included high-pressure liquid chromatography, X-ray diffraction spectrophotometry, and atomic absorption spectrophotometry, as well as far more frequent use of gas-liquid and thin-layer chromatography. U.S.P. XIX maintained its allegiance to the long tradition of recognizing "only the best, established drugs," despite the complexities of reaching an expert consensus. An alternative concept to selectivity, the monumental undertaking to set standards for all drugs, no longer seemed beyond discussion within the Convention, as the prospect of merging the *National Formulary* program (see p. 275) with that of the U.S.P. emerged and as the federal government pushed toward an ultimate goal of permitting on the market only drugs of assured efficacy as well as safety. Already in U.S.P. XIX, because of a decision to recognize all drugs of "equivalent medical merit," 1284 articles were admitted and characterized, more "than have appeared in any USP for 75 years" (p. xiii). This Revision also initiated a policy of "continuous admission," whereby U.S.P. selection and standard setting will keep pace with the introduction of new drugs. Such interim admissions will appear in a companion volume, *The USP Guide to Select Drugs.* To open the standard-setting process to wider scientific review another publication has been established (1975), the bimonthly *Pharmacopeial Forum, with USP-NF Comment Proof.* U.S.P. XIX recognition of automated methods of analysis for the first time signalled an advancing revolution in drug-standardization techniques. These advances did not yet resolve the agitated issue of bioavailability, but did embolden a declaration that "It is the ultimate objective of the Pharmacopeia to provide standards ensuring that all specimens of a given dosage form are bioequivalent" (p. xvi). One significant change to help assure the equivalence of U.S.P.-recognized drugs was the requirement that each product must bear an expiration date on the label. Although the U.S.P.C. remained far from its potential as an information-generating agency for an audience of practitioners (as envisioned under the leadership of Executive Director Heller), the U.S.P. XIX notably included more information unrelated to technical drug standards than before. Such informational portions of the text (often general dispensing guidelines for the pharmacist) have been visually separated from the legally required drug specifications—as part of a varied improvement of U.S.P. format.

As the *National Formulary* (see p. 277)—which always had been parallel with the *U. S. Pharmacopeia* in legal standing—moved ever more parallel to the U.S.P. in policies, criteria, and format, the need and logic of having two standard-setting agencies came into question during the 1960's. This circumstance led the 1970 U.S.P. Convention to recommend not only that the Committee of Revision "intensify efforts to coordinate the activities" of the U.S.P. and N.F., but to "explore the advantages and feasibility of unification . . . producing a single compendium of standards and tests for official drugs and dosage forms" (p. xxxii). A long and thorny negotiation followed, which helped to precipitate the unusual special Convention of 1973, followed by a renewed impetus toward merger that culminated in the U. S. Pharmacopeial Convention acquiring both the *National Formulary* and the Drug Standards Laboratory from the American Pharmaceutical Association (effective 1975).[66] With this move, all standard-setting functions of the official compendia were consolidated in a headquarters building that the U.S.P. had purchased in 1971 in Rockville, Maryland, near the principal standard-enforcing body, the Federal Food and Drug Administration.

The *National Formulary* dovetailed comfortably with the ongoing program of the *U. S. Pharmacopeia*. It had come into being within a quite different concept, however; and during most of its 86-year history the "N.F." had made a distinctive contribution of its own.

## THE NATIONAL FORMULARY

Inherent in the traditional work of the practicing pharmacist, the making of drugs, was a need for collections of formulas, whether scribbled into a notebook or elegantly printed. The *National Formulary* can be considered a culmination of the American expression of this universal need of the preindustrialized period of pharmacy.

Only 3 years after the founding of the first local association of pharmacists (Philadelphia) its members published a small formulary.[67] Only 5 years after the founding of the national association of pharmacists (A.Ph.A.), its members set about to "collect and arrange . . . local unofficial formulae."[68] The trend outran the enthusiasm of many leading pharmacists of the late 19th century, who preferred the formulas of the U. S. Pharmacopeia to the unofficial formulas, "which, however necessary, tend to complicate the labors of the pharmaceutist."[69]

This need for unofficial formulas found other expressions by the 1880's through a number of local formularies, of which the New York and Brooklyn Formulary had the largest circulation. Other local formularies, prepared for similar purposes, were published by the Kentucky and the Pennsylvania Pharmaceutical Associations. Another was published by a joint committee of physicians and pharmacists in Washington, and still others elsewhere. In addition, there were the formularies published by individual authors.[70]

When the idea of a formulary under the authority of the American Pharmaceutical Association was revived (1885) conditions were more favorable to such an undertaking than they had been about 1860. Under the influence of pharmacists, the *Pharmacopeia* (1883) had been radically purified, so far as "obsolete and unused drugs" were concerned.[71] No fewer than 121 preparations had been deleted. No doubt among them were some which conservative physicians in various parts of the country were in the habit of prescribing. Furthermore, preparations representative of so-called "elegant" pharmacy were now being mass-produced under "brands" and prescribed as such by physicians, even though the formulas could be prepared readily in the prescription room of any pharmacy. Practicing pharmacists naturally viewed with concern the growing loss of one of their principal professional functions.

As a countermeasure, support crystallized around the idea of promoting to physicians a variety of formulas improving on or widening the range of drugs recognized by the *Pharmacopeia* and stressing a flexible custom service to fit the needs of the individual patient. It is significant that the father of the modern *Pharmacopoeia* of 1882, Charles Rice, was chairman of the American Pharmaceutical Association committee on unofficial formulas and their ardent advocate. In his report in 1886, Rice explained the origin and the purpose of the proposed formulary:

> Acting on the suggestion of Mr. S. J. Bendiner of New York, the College of Pharmacy of the City of New York, the German Apothecaries Society of New York and the Kings County Pharmaceutical Society, about two years ago, appointed a joint committee to prepare a Formulary of unofficial preparations which was to be brought to the notice of the medical profession, with the request to accept the formulae therein contained—after examination and approval—and thereafter to abstain from specifying on their prescriptions the products of special manufacturers, whenever ordering any preparation for which a formula was given in the book.[72]

The book on elixirs published by John Uri Lloyd (1883) as well as the *New York and Brooklyn Formulary* (1884) "acted as a decided stimulus" in giving a national scope and reality to the ambitions of pharmacists that here and there had found expression through local formularies. The state pharmaceutical associations participated in the Committee's work; and in 1888 a manuscript was presented to the American Pharmaceutical Association and was published in the same year both as an appendix to the *Proceedings* and as a separate book "by authority of the American Pharmaceutical Association."

Taking the title of the *National Formulary of Unofficinal Preparations* at face value, framers of early food and drug bills did not propose to make the American Pharmaceutical Association's book "official" as they did the *U.S. Pharmacopeia*. However, the 1906 Federal law elevated the *National Formulary* to the same legal standing as the *Pharmacopeia*.[73]

At the first opportunity (4th ed., 1916)* the now incongruous part of the title, ". . . of Unofficinal Preparations," was dropped. Moreover, the *National Formulary* developed its monographs on drug standards in a way analogous with the development of monographs in the *Pharmacopeia*; and in 1938 the American Pharmaceutical Association established a laboratory devoted primarily to determining drug standards (which in 1975 was acquired by the U.S. Pharmacopeia). The "N.F." has designated standards for numerous drugs and drug preparations that are used by physicians or laymen but do not qualify for inclusion in the "U.S.P." as the current drugs of choice in their therapeutic class.

A new epoch in the development of the *National Formulary* was initiated in 1938 with a plan for more frequent revisions, approximately every 5 years; and in 1939 the by-laws of the Association were changed to provide for a "Committee on National Formulary" with a full-time Chairman and 10 instead of 15 members. A man of proved capacity thus was given enhanced range of action: Justin L. Powers, Director of the Laboratory of the American Pharmaceutical Association, who continued to head the National Formulary as Chairman until his retirement (1960).[74] Powers' successor, the chemist Edward G. Feldmann, served as Director of Revision of ths N.F. as a major part of his responsibility as Director of the Scientific Division of the American Pharmaceutical Association, until succeeded on the N.F. by the pharmacist-chemist, John V. Bergen, Ph.D. (1970–1974).

By 1942 the book (N.F. VII) showed remarkable changes, testifying that the men responsible no longer regarded this volume as merely a stepping-stone from and to the *United States Pharmacopeia*, supplementary to the latter, but rather as a book of comparable character, differing mainly in point of view as to the kind and the scope of material to be admitted.[75]

Coordination between the two standard-setting agencies increased, sharing in ideas and in developmental work on monographs for specific drugs, according to final decisions as to whether a particular drug should

---

*The roman numbering of the *National Formulary* refers to the successive *editions* (in contrast with the U.S.P. numbering of revisions).

be recognized by the N.F. or by the U.S.P. Mutual accord was maintained in such changes as the format of presenting specifications for recognized drugs, the shift from a 10-year to a 5-year revision cycle, then to continuous interim revision, the setting of effective dates for new sets of standards, basic changes in test methods authorized, and so on. An A.Ph.A. periodical, *Bulletin of the National Formulary Committee* (f. 1930; retitled *Drug Standards*, 1951) provided a medium for mutual exchange of ideas, findings, and work-in-progress among all those interested in the perplexing questions that revolve about "adequate standards" for the nation's drug supply, whether recognized by the N.F. or the U.S.P.

A historic and consequential change in the Twelfth Edition (effective 1965) eliminated *extent of use* of drugs as a central criterion for N.F. recognition. This traditional criterion had helped to maintain a distinctive character in the N.F., since the U.S.P. traditionally emphasized the criterion of selectivity (consensus of relative merit among drugs of the same class). At the time, this policy change "served to elevate the importance of this [N.F.] compendium as a guide to rational medical practice." In retrospect it seems also to have opened the door to questions about the need for two separate standard-setting organizations so analogous in function as the N.F. and U.S.P. were becoming by the 1960's. It was during this same revision period that the Drug Standards Laboratory in the A.Ph.A. headquarters was revitalized through joint support contributed by the U.S.P. and by the American Medical Association (the latter having earlier discontinued its own drug-testing laboratory).

Drastic changes in methods of drug manufacture and in methods of drug standardization and testing had placed the majority of procedures beyond the range of even the largest and best-equipped pharmacies by the 1960's. Moreover, the standard-setting mechanism itself grew vastly more complex and demanding under the impact of both legal and scientific changes. "With ingenuity which rivals that seen in any field of science or technology," the N.F. XIII (1970) pointed out, "pharmaceutical scientists—particularly during the past ten years—have utilized the recent developments in analytical methodology in the testing of pharmaceuticals. The net result permits inspection of infinitely smaller samples, enormously greater selectivity, and drastically improved precision and accuracy." One result of official application of advanced analytical techniques has been a mushrooming growth during the past decade or two of both N.F. and U.S.P. Reference Standard services, which supply samples of prototype drugs for comparative testing purposes to laboratories of the United States (and to some extent abroad).

The National Formulary XIV (effective 1975) was the last edition to appear under the auspices of the American Pharmaceutical Association, which had brought a quite different book into being in 1888. After 4 years of sporadic negotiations, the responsibility for continuing to generate standards for N.F. drugs was transferred to the U. S. Pharmacopeial Convention as of 1975. Observed the Director of the Scientific Division of the American Pharmaceutical Association, Dr. Edward G. Feldmann,

> A major consideration which swayed the A.Ph.A. in reaching its decision on this matter was its conclusion that survival of the drug standard setting function within the private sector —and divorced from direct control from either industry or government—is even more important than having A.Ph.A. continue direct authority over one phase within such a program (i.e., the National Formulary).
>
> Now that this dream is to become reality, it is our opinion that unification of the official compendia will be of enormous benefit in strengthening the so-called independent 'third force'—as distinguished from government and industry—in our three-sided system of responsibility for drug quality.[76]

This system appears unique among the pharmacopeial programs of the world, in that the standards for an entire country were originally devised, and have been generated ever since, by voluntary collaboration of the health professions and supporting sciences—untainted by malfeasance throughout the long history of the U. S. Pharmacopeia and National Formulary and recognized by Federal law since the beginning of this century in the public interest.

What we mean by adequacy of drug standards will change as the sophistication of science and technology change. The need remains unchanged for adequate drug standards as a prerequisite for the safe practice of pharmacy. The American pharmacist of recent history has used the U.S.P. and N.F. only as a source of information for reference, rather than as a guide to drug making. Still continuing, however, is his historic service in supporting the standard-setting agencies (through personal purchase of official compendia and through his professional organizations), thus helping to assure the public security in pharmaceutical services.

## DISPENSATORIES

In the 16th century, the word *dispensatorium* came into general use as a book title having the same meaning as "pharmacopeia." It was in England that "dispensatory" came to designate a kind of commentary which embraced the text of the pharmacopeia or pharmacopeias, and during the 18th and the 19th centuries such dispensatories became an English specialty.

### Coxe's American Dispensatory

Some English dispensatories were commonly used in America, before the creation of an American pharmacopeia, because they were based on pharmacopeias recognized in America almost as much as in England. However, it may seem strange that America had a dispensatory of its own before it had its own pharmacopeia.

The physician John Redman Coxe, who later on indirectly caused the organization of the first American college of pharmacy (see p. 189), edited the first edition of his *American Dispensatory* in 1806. He used Duncan's *Edinburgh New Dispensatory* to such an extent that it was almost a reprint and was considered as such by Duncan. The book was so successful that it went through nine editions.[77]

In 1810 the first edition of Thacher's *New Dispensatory* appeared, and Coxe did not scruple to profit from the work of this competitor. In his third edition he stated that "he has not failed to introduce a considerable addition to the materia medica, for which he is chiefly indebted to Dr. Thacher's very excellent dispensatory."

In his last edition Thacher complained that 40 pages of his were transferred "literally from the last two editions" into Coxe's own dispensatory. He adds that these transfers "are not designated by the customary marks of quotation"!

After publication of the *United States Pharmacopeia* (1820) the volume of Coxe of necessity became, with some reservations, a commentary on this work.

### Thacher's American New Dispensatory

The *American New Dispensatory* of James Thacher, a Boston physician, was the first such work based on an American pharmacopeia and which the author pointedly sought to imbue with an American spirit. The *Pharmacopoeia of the Massachusetts Medical Society* (1808; see p. 256), served as the basis for Thacher's *Dispensatory*. "This Pharmacopoeia," he wrote in the preface of his book, "is not inferior in point of merit to any other and its nomenclature and order of arrangement are strictly followed throughout." Thacher's cooperation with the authors of the *Massachusetts Pharmacopoeia* went so far that he submitted his manuscript to the Massachusetts Medical Society for criticism.

"After having been revised by a committee of the counsellors," the *Dispensatory* was published in 1810 and in three further editions.[78] Its particular merit was that it paid "proper attention to several indigenous substances, not to be found in any other Dispensatory," quoted the American botanists Barton and Cutler (see p. 173) and "that excellent publication, the Domestic Encyclopedia, edited by Dr. Mease," along with earlier British works. Thus Thacher's *Dispensatory* was the first distinctly American publication of its kind.

### The United States Dispensatory

Significantly, neither Coxe's nor Thacher's book survived the appearance in 1833 of the *United States Dispensatory*, edited by George B. Wood and Franklin Bache. For several decades the only book of its kind in America, the *United States Dispensatory* has remained a pharmaceutical book of reference used throughout the country and to some extent internationally.

The secret of its initial success lay in the personalities of its authors, especially George B. Wood. Both men were principal authors of the *Pharmacopeia* (Philadelphia, 1831), and participated decisively in revising all later editions during their lifetimes. They thus gained intimate knowledge of what required exposition, and they were especially well qualified for their work. Both were physicians and professors. For several years, Wood had been a professor of materia medica, and Bache had been a professor of chemistry, at the Philadelphia College of Pharmacy. The fact that Wood, in his preparation of the *Pharmacopeia* of 1831, insisted on avoiding any explanatory notes "as wholly out of place in a Pharmacopoeia," makes it likely that he was already thinking of issuing some kind of commentary. Doubtless, it was because of the commercial success of the *Dispensatory* that the *Pharmacopeia* could be kept alive. Moreover, the fact that both books were issued by the same publisher made possible the requisite financial balancing. Not until after the death of Wood (1879) were the two books produced and published separately.

In the book of Wood and Bache, the English pharmacopeias were considered as in the earlier American dispensatories, but the "almost untouched . . . pharmacy of continental Europe" was also considered and special attention was paid to the "treatises and dissertations . . . on pharmacy . . . of the French writers, who stand at present at the head of this department of medical science."

All possible literary sources were utilized, and the mass of information was well arranged and presented in a clear style. It seems almost incredible that for more than 30 years the two authors alone did most of the comprehensive and responsible work on no fewer than 11 editions.[79] In the preface to the first edition, the authors thanked "Mr. Daniel B. Smith, president of the Philadelphia College of Pharmacy," for "much important information in relation to the various branches of the apothecary's business," for some "prefatory remarks on pharmacy" and for "several articles." Not until after the death of Bache (1864) was such assistance from outside again acknowledged, this time from Wood's "friends, Mr. William Procter, Jr., Prof. of Pharmacy in the Philadelphia College of Pharmacy, and Dr. Robert Bridges, Prof. of Chemistry in the same institution" (12th ed.).

The 14th edition was again begun by Wood (with the assistance of Bridges) but completed by his nephew and successor in the chair of materia medica at the University of Pennsylvania, Horatio C. Wood. After George Wood died (1879) his nephew invited Joseph P. Remington, at that time a well-known pharmacist of Philadelphia, and Samuel P. Sadtler, Professor of Chemistry at the Philadelphia College of Pharmacy, to share with him the editorial responsibility of the 15th edition.[80]

This 15th edition (1883) may, as the authors stated, "very justly be looked upon as a new book," offering in particular a thorough updating of the pharmaceutical chemistry of the drugs explicated, a task that had been neglected ever since the death of Bache. Through the decades the scope of the "U.S.D." made it a veritable encyclopedia of commentary on drugs old or new, foreign or domestic, obscure drug names and forms, botanical lore, historical asides, bibliographic citations and summary explanations of the official compendia. Then, with the 26th edition (1967) the final break was made with the encyclopedia tradition. The *U. S. Dispensatory* henceforth was to concentrate on "those data of importance in prescribing and dispensing drugs . . . ," (p. vii) meaning for the most part those medicines professionally recognized as specific and effective in their pharmacologic action; it tried to ignore therapeutic vestiges and folk medicine of an earlier time, for which the "U.S.D." had served as a storehouse earlier in the century. Within this modernized concept, the U.S.D. has retained its place as the oldest book of its kind in continuous publication, a book originated in Philadelphia, and edited and published there throughout its long history.[81]

**The National Dispensatory**

Because of obvious deficiencies of the *United States Dispensatory* from the 12th to the reorganized 15th edition, the monopoly of this book was destroyed at least temporarily. In 1879, Alfred Stillé and John Maisch published the *National Dispensatory*, which filled the gap at the time, as becomes evident from the fact that the 1st edition was sold out in a few months.[82]

Because of the inclinations of their authors, two differences can be seen between the *National Dispensatory* and its older rival, the *United States Dispensatory*. Alfred Stillé as a teacher of clinical medicine at a time when the physiologic action of medicines was to become the subject of exact experimentation, included "for the first time in a Dispensatory, a succinct account" of the results of those experiments, "occasionally in the theoretical language of the day." He added "another feature, novel in a Dispensatory": a therapeutic index. "Such an Index," the authors stated in the preface to the first edition, "becomes to some extent a therapeutical classification of medicines, and it is believed must greatly enhance by its suggestiveness the working value of the book to the practitioner."

Such an approach to writing a pharmaceutical reference work may seem to foreshadow clinical pharmacy of a century later; but it must be recognized that the "practitioner" Stillé referred to was the medical practitioner. The *National Dispensatory* thus appealed much more to the special interests of the physician than did the *United States Dispensatory*.[83]

A second difference from the *U. S. Dispensatory* resulted from the predilection of the German-born second author, John M. Maisch, who included in the second edition of the book "nearly the entire German Pharmacopoeia."

When John M. Maisch died (1893), the fifth and last edition of the *National Dispensatory* was edited by Stillé, with the cooperation of Maisch's son, Henry C. Maisch, and Charles Caspari, Jr.

Then in 1905 a book completely written by Caspari and others appeared under the title, *The National Standard Dispensatory* (which was discontinued after the 3rd edition of 1916).

Books of similar character, but less influence, played their part in the evolving pharmaceutical literature of America—then disappeared when they no longer adjusted adequately to needs of new times. The earliest of such books had been an American edition of Nicholas Culpeper's *Pharmàcopoeia Londinensis or the London Dispensatory* (Boston, 1720). But during the 19th century

Americans themselves were publishing a number of books of commentary on drugs, about which reference notes may be found in Appendix 6 (p. 438).

## HOMEOPATHIC PHARMACOPEIA

To the American pharmacist today, the *Homeopathic Pharmacopoeia of the United States* seems a curious rather than a practical book. Yet, the book retains some current as well as historical interest because its drug standards are "official" under the Federal Food, Drug and Cosmetic Act in the same sense as are the *U. S. Pharmacopeia* and the *National Formulary*.

The strange medical doctrines on which homeopathic drug therapy rests have a small and dwindling place in American medicine. Introduced by Samuel Hahnemann, a German, at the end of the 18th century, homeopathy at first was one of a number of medical systems vying with one another. Eventually discredited and disowned by regular medicine, it has survived in some countries as a small medical sect largely dependent on its appeal to a lay following (see p. 47).

The special way of preparing homeopathic remedies[84] makes Hahnemann's system interesting pharmaceutically. Homeopathic pharmacy in the United States, unlike that in some other countries, has never become a special branch of study and practice for the average pharmacist. Hence the *Homeopathic Pharmacopoeia* found its main use among those practicing homeopathic medicine and in governmental agencies that are reponsible for assuring that authorized standards for drugs are met. Seven editions of the *Homeopathic Pharmacopoeia of the United States* have appeared, the first in 1897 and the last in 1964. Even though the American Institute of Homeopathy has "kept abreast of the extensive work being done in other countries," especially on the homeopathic pharmacopeias of France and Germany,[85] it remains to be seen whether traditional homeopathic drugs—and the *Pharmacopoeia* whence they derive—can survive the drug-efficacy requirements of the amended Food, Drug and Cosmetic Act in the United States.

## THE PHARMACEUTICAL RECIPE BOOK

As the *National Formulary* became more self-consciously "official" and scientific, more removed from the homely appeal of the old "unofficinal preparations," the gap that the original *National Formulary* had tried to fill seemed to reappear. As early as 1912 a committee of the American Pharmaceutical Association published a report on 114 such formulas, under the chairmanship of Otto Raubenheimer. This led to a standing Committee on Recipe Book (under his chairmanship) which published groups of formulas serially in the Association's *Journal* over the next 5 years.

Then a new committee headed by the eminent New York pharmacist J. Leon Lascoff presented the Association with an unedited collection of 1,500 formulas. The accumulation was pruned, edited, and brought between book covers in 1929 under the editorial direction of Ivor Griffith of Philadelphia. The *Pharmaceutical Recipe Book*, as the title implies, included "only preparations that can be compounded by the pharmacist" and abjured ambitions to set drug standards.

Here the pharmacist found compound formulas not only for unofficial drugs but also for materials for diverse technical uses—household compounds, cosmetics, photographic materials, flavorings, reagents, and so on.

Such a book appealed to pharmacists' pride of craftsmanship and met a need as well. It went through a second (1936) and then a third (1942) edition. The fact that no further editions were considered worthwhile is one more indication of the changes taking place in pharmacy.[86]

## NEW AND NONOFFICIAL DRUGS

The American Medical Association established in 1905 the Council on Drugs (called the Council on Pharmacy and Chemistry until 1958) primarily as a medical rather than a pharmaceutical institution. Nevertheless, the Council included a number of pharmacists and persons with pharmaceutical as well as medical education in the early decades, then became increasingly medical in its composition. The effects of the Council continued to be equally as constructive for pharmacy as for medicine. When the Council was first organized, commercial abuses in marketing proprietary drugs were still largely unchecked; it would be hard to overestimate the importance of the Council's evaluations and publications, especially in the decades before effective government regulation.

The A.M.A. organized the Council on Drugs "primarily for the purpose of gathering and disseminating such information as would protect the medical profession in the prescribing of proprietary medicinal articles."[87] These articles, their advertising, labeling and naming, and even the general policies of the firms manufacturing them, had to comply "with definite rules" and must "present some real advantage," to be admitted, (i.e., to be described as to their essential features) "in the annual publication of the Council, the 'N.N.R.' [*New and Nonofficial Remedies*]. This description is based in part on investigations made by or under the direction of the Council, but in part also on evidence or information supplied by the manufacturer. . . ."

The Council explicitly stated from the beginning that "the admission of an article does not imply a recommendation. It means only that no conflict with the rules has been found by the Council."[88]

During at least its first half century, the annual *New and Nonofficial Remedies* probably should be considered of pharmaceutical importance second only to the legally enforced compendia (the U.S.P. and N.F.). The selectivity and standards of the Council's program understandably came into conflict with the marketers of proprietary prescription drugs occasionally, which probably partly motivated the abandonment in 1955 of the Council's "seal of approval" policy.[89]

The title of the annual volume changed in 1958 to *New and Nonofficial Drugs*, then was superseded by *New Drugs Evaluated by the A.M.A. Council on Drugs* during the years 1965 through 1967. The latter signalled not only a change of name, however, but a change of A.M.A. attitude. *New Drugs* declared that it "differs from its predecessors in scope [individual drugs introduced within the previous 10 years], organization, and format . . . in no sense a list of 'approved or accepted' drugs." The final step came in 1972 when the American Medical Association abolished the Council on Drugs, in the name of "financial restraint." Not only had the drug market changed during the 67 years of service of the Council on Drugs, but so had the A.M.A.[90]

## TEXT AND REFERENCE BOOKS

When the Philadelphia College of Pharmacy created a professorship of pharmacy and bestowed on William Procter, Jr., the honor and the responsibility of this new charge (1846), the professor looked "in vain amongst the medical literature of the English language for a single work devoted exclusively and systematically to this branch of knowledge." What was the explanation? True, English pharmacy at that time was in a period of transition and reconstruction (see p. 107), and an English textbook of pharmacy, written by an English pharmacist, could scarcely be expected.

There was an abundance of French and German textbooks, and England had never—in literature as elsewhere—hesitated to take the good where she found it. Translations of French and German books into English were not uncommon, so the English reserve in not also taking over one of the continental European textbooks on pharmacy probably lay in the fact that these books were of little use to the average English "chemist and druggist" of that period. The scientific standards and objectives of these treatises were too high, and the need for elementary instruction in practical pharmaceutical technic could not be filled by them.

In continental Europe itself there was an obvious need for a book describing and explaining in detail all the instruments and apparatus invented since the rise of modern chemistry and employed by pharmaceutical scientists, manufacturers and practitioners.

In the 16th century the German physician Andreas Libavius (Libau) had given such a comprehensive description in an annex to his book *Alchimia.* The Italian pharmacist Antonio de Sgobbis described the pharmaceutical technic and apparatus of his time (1662) in his *Nuovo et Universale Theatro Farmaceutico*. The book of the French pharmacist Antoine Baumé, *Elémens de pharmacie théorique et pratique* (1762) met the needs of that generation. Now, in the middle of the 19th century, another man was required to fulfill the same task for his time. This man was the German pharmacist Carl Friedrich Mohr,[91] who not only described the modern pharmaceutical contrivances and apparatus but also invented many of them himself. With his *Lehrbuch der pharmaceutischen Technik*, Mohr gave German and Anglo-Saxon pharmacy what it needed. On the continent it was a very useful and much used book. For England and for America it was to become, for the time being, *the* pharmaceutical textbook.

The first German edition of Mohr's book (1847) was scarcely off the press when the English pharmacist and professor at the school of the Pharmaceutical Society of Great Britain, Theophilus Redwood, translated the book and published it under the title *Practical Pharmacy founded on Mohr's Manual* (preface dated December, 1848).

PRACTICAL PHARMACY:

THE ARRANGEMENTS,

APPARATUS, AND MANIPULATIONS,

OF THE

PHARMACEUTICAL SHOP AND LABORATORY.

BY

FRANCIS MOHR, PH. D.,

ASSESSOR PHARMACIÆ OF THE ROYAL PRUSSIAN COLLEGE OF MEDICINE, COBLENTZ;

AND

THEOPHILUS REDWOOD,

PROFESSOR OF CHEMISTRY AND PHARMACY TO THE PHARMACEUTICAL SOCIETY OF GREAT BRITAIN.

EDITED, WITH EXTENSIVE ADDITIONS,

BY

WILLIAM PROCTER, JR.,

PROFESSOR OF PHARMACY IN THE PHILADELPHIA COLLEGE OF PHARMACY.

ILLUSTRATED BY FIVE HUNDRED ENGRAVINGS ON WOOD.

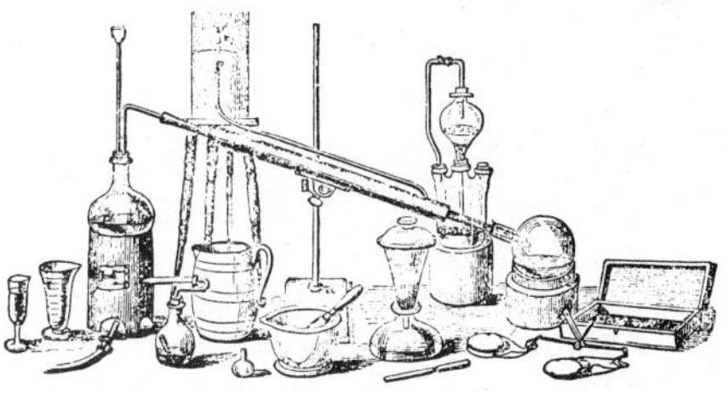

PHILADELPHIA:
LEA AND BLANCHARD.
1849.

Title page of the first pharmaceutical textbook that was adapted to the needs of American students. Significantly, it was based on a British version of a German work (by Carl Friedrich Mohr, whose first name was printed erroneously as "Francis").

As early as March, 1849, William Procter, Jr., edited an American issue of Redwood's enlarged translation "with extensive additions" under the title *"Practical Pharmacy,* with the subtitle *The Arrangements, Apparatus, and Manipulations of the Pharmaceutical Shop and Laboratory*. The earliest reference to the book in the *American Journal of*

*Pharmacy* begins with the significant remark, "The want of a treatise on practical pharmacy, devoted to apparatus and manipulations, has long been a desideratum both in England and the United States."[92] As stated in a later review, the book comprised "the whole of Mohr and Redwood's book, as published in London, rearranged and classified by the American editor, who has added much valuable new matter, which has increased the size of ths book more than one-fourth. . . ."[93]

The book of Mohr-Redwood-Procter "did not go through a second edition by reason of the cost of proper illustrations, which the publishers refused to incur,"[94] and without which Procter apparently did not want to proceed. Thus the way was free for another book of a similar kind, the *Introduction to Practical Pharmacy,* published by Edward Parrish in 1856. It is considered the first truly American textbook on pharmacy. This being granted, the question may well arise whether it was a textbook for pharmacists, designed primarily to meet their needs. A review of the first edition, published in the *American Journal of Pharmacy*, gives the answer. Parrish's book "is not based on the superstructure of any foreign publication, as has usually been the case with books, on similar subjects, issued from the American press, but is original in conception with its author, who, from his experience both as a pharmaceutist and as a lecturer and teacher of practical pharmacy to medical students, has become aware of the want of a textbook in this department, which he has thus endeavored to supply."[95] This corresponds with a statement made by Parrish himself in the preface of his book as well as with its subtitle: "A textbook for the student and a guide to the Physician and Pharmaceutist."

At the time he wrote, Parrish was conducting a private school of practical pharmacy for *students of medicine* (see p. 229). The *American Journal of Pharmacy* stated, "The book . . . was commenced with a view to satisfy this want [of a book for medical students], but in its progress the author determined to enlarge on his original plan, so as, without claiming for it the fullness of a handbook of Pharmacy, to render it very useful to the strictly pharmaceutical students . . . as well as to pharmacists in general. . . ."[96] It is likely that Parrish decided "to enlarge on his original plan" after having learned that no new edition of the book of Mohr-Redwood-Procter was to be expected. Thus the first textbook on pharmacy that could be considered typically American (written by an American pharmacist) was designed primarily to aid physicians in practicing pharmacy and only secondarily to instruct pharmacists. Although the book retained the traditional subtitle, placing the physician as the primary reader, rather than the pharmacist, it became with each new edition more and more a treatise on pharmacy for pharmacists.[97]

Joseph P. Remington published the first edition of his *Practice of Pharmacy* (1885) as "a treatise on the modes of making and dispensing official, unofficial and extemporaneous preparations, with descriptions of medical substances, their properties, uses and doses intended as a handbook for pharmacists and physicians and a textbook for students." The analogy to the title of Parrish's *Introduction to Practical Pharmacy* is evident; but for Remington the pharmacist came first, and the limitation to "practice" was, at least in the early editions, still more definite than in the editions of Parrish's *Introduction* between 1864 and 1884, which became increasingly scientific and theoretical.

With the book of Remington the era of the modern American pharmaceutical textbook started. As Remington himself said, he tried "to frame a system which should embody their [Procter's and Parrish's] valuable features, embrace new subjects, and still retain that harmony of plan and proper sequence which are absolutely essential to the success of any system." The book became very popular.

If *Remington's Pharmaceutical Sciences* now (15th ed., 1975) holds a somewhat different place in the literature, it retains its vitality and remains one of the most encyclopedic and voluminous pharmaceutical books for reference and instructional use.[98]

The development from the introductory treatises on practical pharmacy to voluminous tomes covering the whole of pharmacy created a renewed demand for smaller and more compendious guides. Reinhold Rother published (1887) the first edition of a book of this kind under the significant title *The Beginnings in Pharmacy,* "an introductory treatise on the practical manipulation of drugs and the various processes employed in the preparation of medicines." The book meant an entirely new type of handbook for America, a successful attempt to provide a real apprenticeship through information perfectly adapted to the material and the implements of the ordinary pharmacy.[99]

The idea of a concise treatise on pharmacy also found a realization in the *Handbook of Pharmacy* published by Virgil Coblentz (1894). This book was not restricted to an introduction to practical pharmacy, but also embraced "the theory and practice of pharmacy and the art of dispensing." It began a succession of American textbooks on pharmacy that tried, in a time of simpler pharmaceutical science and technology, "to supply to the student of pharmacy a compendious and yet sufficiently detailed textbook for systematic study, and to those exercising the art a trustworthy guide to be consulted in daily practice" (preface to the first edition). That the book did not live beyond a second edition was most likely due to the appearance of similar book, the *Treatise on Pharmacy for Students and Pharmacists,* by Charles Caspari, Jr. (1895).

Caspari's motive for writing a book was much the same as that of Coblentz. Moreover, he expressed it in almost the same words, adding, however, a direct "dig" at Remington's voluminous book. Caspari's popular book went through eight editions (until 1939).[100]

Of the three American textbooks on pharmacy that were begun in the 19th or the early 20th century, the Remington-Cook-LaWall represents the encyclopedia type, the Caspari-Kelly the systematic-informative type, and Arny's *Principles of Pharmacy,* the common textbook type. In the preface to his first edition (1909), Arny stated that its "frank intention . . . is to explain the Pharmacopoeia from its pharmaceutical standpoint."[101]

While the textbooks mentioned thus far attempted to cover more or less fully the entire field of pharmacy, another type specialized in the art of compounding and dispensing medicines (theory and the practice of filling prescriptions). One of the earliest and best-known examples of this kind was Wilbur L. Scoville's *The Art of Compounding* (first edition, 1895), whose ninth and last edition in 1957 seems symbolic of the dying art of compounding at the "prescription bench."[102] With the first edition of the book of William J. Husa entitled *Pharmaceutical Dispensing* (1937) a systematic scientific treatment replaced the elementary treatment of the subject traditional from an earlier period of pharmaceutical education.

In a series of pharmaceutical textbooks that began in 1945, called *American Pharmacy*, authors belonging for the most part to the younger generation expressed a new idea. Instead of trying to compile all that the pharmacist should know between two covers, each volume of the series presents one phase of the science and the art of pharmacy within the framework of theories and generalizations according to a coordinating plan.

It was symptomatic of a new line of development that special textbooks appeared from the late 1960's onward emphasizing "clinical pharmacy." Texts by Glenn L. Jenkins (1966) and Charles W. Blissitt (1972) and their co-authors—with handbooks by Hugh F. Kabat (1969) and David Angaran (1972)—exemplified a vanguard whose objective was nothing less than to put at the core of the practice of pharmacy a "patient-orientation" dealing with the selection, control and monitoring of drug usage.

By no means do the books mentioned constitute a complete list of textbooks on the technology and the professional services of pharmacy published in America. However, they are representative of the evolution of different types of these books and illustrate the development in the demand for professional pharmaceutical information.

**Pharmaceutical Sciences**

American pharmaceutical education, about 60 years after its first beginnings, had matured sufficiently to begin to provide its own specialized textbooks in the pharmaceutical sciences, which underlie the development of drugs and the dispensing of them with assurance of proper quality and professional judgment. Until the last quarter of the 19th century, besides the subject of pharmacy, American schools ordinarily required scientific instruction only in materia medica and in pharmaceutical chemistry. So it is in these fields that we find the first scientific texts emerging.

*A Conspectus of Organic Materia Medica and Pharmaceutical Botany* was published (1879) by Lucius E. Sayre, a pharmacist then teaching in Kansas. This was followed (1882) by the more popular *Manual of Organic Materia Medica* by the Philadelphia pharmacist and teacher, John M. Maisch. Other textbooks, often still more specialized, soon followed in biologic areas of pharmaceutical work.[103]

Textbooks on pharmaceutical chemistry written by American pharmacists also were comparatively late. For some decades, *Chemistry, Medical and Pharmaceutical*, written by John Attfield, professor of practical chemistry to the Pharmaceutical Society of Great Britain, was the main textbook on chemistry used by American students of pharmacy, as "revised by the author for the followers of medicine and pharmacy in America, the chemistry of the preparations and materia medica of the United States Pharmacopoeia being introduced" (preface). The practical usefulness of Attfield's book carried it through 19 editions (by 1906). By that time a number of competing American textbooks had appeared. The earliest by pharmacists were written by Frederick Hoffmann of New York (1873) and by John Uri Lloyd of Cincinnati (1881).[104]

In the present century, a wide range of textbooks in the pharmaceutical sciences has appeared that not only reflects a trend toward specialization, but adapts to the shifting orientation of pharmaceutical education as a whole. The chemical understanding of drugs could never be ignored in the training of the pharmacist, but the trend begun by Paracelsists more than four centuries ago found new expressions. From the 1880's onward, an emphasis upon organic medicinal chemistry reflected the importance of synthetic organic remedies in therapeutics; and by the 1940's the application of physical chemistry to the understanding of pharmaceutical systems was becoming important in education. The pharmacist's pre-modern orientation toward biological (mainly botanical) sciences no sooner had been thus overthrown, than he was borne back at a different level by two trends: One, the need for scientific understanding of new and important classes of biological products in recent decades (see p. 49) and, two, scientific study supportive of the abovementioned concept of clinical pharmacy. In the 1950's this latter trend was being reflected in the changing textbooks of pharmacognosy and a new depth in clinical pharmacology and, by the 1970's, in a new type of textbook on biopharmaceutics (such as those by James Swarbrick, ed., 1970, John G. Wagner, 1971, and Robert E. Notari, 1971). An important branch of this literature, beginning to be systematized by the early 1970s, concerned the interactions of drugs within the body.[104a]

In such textbooks can be found the cumulated evidence of the scientific progress of pharmacy.

## JOURNALS OF ASSOCIATIONS

Books represent the static aspect and journals the dynamic aspect of pharmaceutical literature. A remarkable number of American journals have appeared, both national and local, reflecting the heterogeneity of the pharmaceutical field. However, they hold collectively the task of conveying information on all phases of pharmacy. In addition, they help to mold opinions and to gain support for new enterprises. Hence, the character of the journals, and of the men who determine their content, has an unusual historic interest and influence.

One way of looking at journals is to see whether they stress information or entertainment, or perhaps reach that highest aim of the ambitious and honest journalist: to achieve educational objectives in the most appealing way. Journals designed for a definite group of readers have to serve their special needs and demands. And needs and demands are by no means always identical. To ascertain the real needs of people and to educate them to the point where they recognize them is a task characteristic of journals with higher ambitions. Following or even creating trivial or incidental demands, without educational aims, characterizes the others.

Accordingly, journals sprang up to serve the two-sided character of pharmacy. One group of publications catered to pharmacy's function in providing professional service to the public based on scientific knowledge. Another group catered to pharmacy as a trade, based on principles and necessities of commercial operation. Hence, some are scientific-professional, and others are commercial. Still others are of a dual nature. Not only the scientific-professional pharmaceutical journals, but also the majority of the more-or-less commercial periodicals, have endeavored to foster professional responsibility.

### Scientific-Professional Journals

Significantly, the first American pharmaceutical journal, which at the same time was the first journal of its kind in the English language, was the child of an association. Its European model was the French *Bulletin* [Journal] *de Pharmacie*, initiated by members of the Société de Pharmacie de Paris. But what a difference in the circumstances creating these publications! In France, pharmacy was an old, dignified and widely recognized profession, whose members had prominently, if not decisively, contributed to the various literatures. Evidence in point is that French natural scientists resented the new journal, fearing that the much appreciated pharmaceutical contributions would be diverted from the general scientific periodicals.

When the Philadelphia College of Pharmacy published the first issue of its journal in 1825, no recognized professional pharmacy existed in the United States of America; and only a few people were able and willing to devote themselves to scientific pharmaceutical work. The French journal was nourished by professional wealth and came as a crowning achievement of pharmaceutical progress; the American journal was a child of need and came at the beginning.

As far as ideologic objectives were concerned, the American journal was amazingly successful. The *Journal of the Philadelphia College of Pharmacy*, as it was called by its founders, soon received nationwide and even international attention. In recognition of this fact the title of the publication was changed (1835) from a local to a national designation. As the *American Journal of Pharmacy*, this oldest American pharmaceutical periodical has served the profession at home and abroad for nearly a century and a half.

However, in spite of its national baptism and international reputation, it has remained the journal of the Philadelphia College of Pharmacy, and all of its editors have been affiliated with the College.

In the early years the *Journal* could be kept alive only by sacrifices on the part of the Publication Committee. "Let it not be said," wrote R. E. Griffith (1832), "that the pharmacists of this country felt too great an apathy and so little zeal in their profession as to permit the only journal devoted to the subjects of their pursuits to languish and die."[105]

The *American Journal of Pharmacy* was indeed the only one of the scientific periodicals, issued by colleges of pharmacy in their capacity as combinations of associations and schools, which survived[106] (although its relative importance diminished as its original uniqueness was increasingly shared among other journals). Distinctively college organs, such as alumni reports, extension bulletins and student journals, represent a later development, with the main objective of serving as a means of internal communication among members of their restricted groups.

The *Journal of the American Pharmaceutical Association*, published since 1912, was born out of a situation quite different from that faced by the *Journal* of the Philadelphia College of Pharmacy. Mainly through the efforts of Philadelphians, and later through the American Pharmaceutical Association, a recognized pharmaceutical profession, interested in pharmaceutical activity of a scientific nature, had been created. Like the *Bulletin de Pharmacie* in France more than a century earlier, the *Journal of the American Pharmaceutical Association* was the crowning of a development. The publication of a monthly journal instead of the annual *Proceedings* was discussed many years before it materialized. There was a widespread aversion to involving the American Pharmaceutical Association in any kind of business or competition.[107] The *Journal* replaced both the annual *Proceedings*, published since the founding (except 1861), and the *Bulletin*, an earlier journal issued since 1906.

True to one of its constitutional purposes, "diffusing scientific knowledge among Apothecaries and Druggists, [and] fostering pharmaceutical literature," the Association has produced a remarkable serial literature through these and other publications which are outlined chronologically in Appendix 6 (p. 433).

Always a means for nurturing American pharmaceutical science, the Association's *Journal* was an indication of a new maturity and stage of specialization when it yielded a separate research journal as an offshoot (Scientific Edition, 1940–1961), which is now called the *Journal of Pharmaceutical Sciences.*

One of the most vigorous and purposeful of the professional journals has been the *American Journal of Hospital Pharmacy*, growing out of modest mimeographed sheets launched (1943–1944) as the *Bulletin of the American Society of Hospital Pharmacists.*[108] In 1964 the Society launched a monumental undertaking, the *International Pharmaceutical Abstracts*, a semimonthly "key to the world's literature of pharmacy"—conceived and initially edited by Donald E. Francke. More recently (1974) the Society founded another remarkable journal, *Drugs in Health Care.*

Another pharmaceutical group of importance, the American Association of Colleges of Pharmacy, journalized its proceedings, thus bringing its work to the knowledge of the profession. In 1937 the Proceedings was absorbed into the Association's new *American Journal of Pharmaceutical Education*, the first specialized periodical of its scope internationally.

## Commercial-Professional Journals

Having secured the passage of the requisite legislation, the main task of the local and the state associations was to see to the proper enforcement of the laws concerning pharmacy and to take care of both the professional and the commercial interests of their members. In the course of decades the commercial interests dominated more and more. As a result, up to about mid-20th century, state associations placed their emphasis on promoting and defending these commercial interests, a situation reflected in their proceedings and in the journals that succeeded them. After World War II some state associations brought professional and commercial concerns more nearly into balance; and the greater professional substance of some state journals may portend a reversal of a trend.

The first state association to journalize its proceedings (the original California Pharmaceutical Society having become inactive after 1895) was the California Pharmaceutical Association. In a new beginning (1907) the *Pacific Pharmacist* was its official publication. Other state associations followed California's lead, especially after World War I.[109] The highly personal interchange possible through local-association journals found early expression and still survives, particularly in urban areas.

The most important association journal stressing the business and management of a pharmacy has been the *N.A.R.D. Journal* (from the beginning in 1902, until 1913, called *N.A.R.D. Notes*), issued by the National Association of Retail Druggists. For its members, the National Association of Chain Drug Stores and American College of Apothecaries both issue newsletters.

These owner-oriented journals had a counterpart for employed pharmacists in the *National Drug Clerk* (f. 1913), which ceased publication with the dissolution of the National Association of Drug Clerks (1934) and had no successors.

Wide areas of the professional, scientific and commercial fields covered by the association-sponsored journals for practicing pharmacists have been covered also by private publishing. Some of these periodicals have been influential, useful media; and a group representative of the late 19th and the 20th centuries are noted in Appendix 6 (p. 434).

Striking features of American pharmaceutical journalism are the almost confusing abundance of the journals—of which only a few illustrative examples have been mentioned here—and the incessant changes they have undergone. The list of American pharmaceutical journals compiled by Minnie Marie Meyer (1933) includes some 350 titles, and even this list is not complete.[110] The ups and downs, the unbalanced mass production, the courage to venture and to experiment have not been restricted to the pharmaceutical periodical literature; they have been characteristic of American life.

# 16

# Economic and Structural Development

## THE COMMUNITY PHARMACY

The community pharmacy has a recognized place in public welfare. This is reflected in legal and educational requirements set by legislatures that reflect, and help to assure the quality of, pharmacy's professional functions. Other functions of a pharmacist's establishment are largely commercial and hence are subject to the general laws and rules affecting commercial ventures.

The situation of the "drugstore"*in colonial times and during the first decades of the young republic has been described in previous chapters. The majority of the few educated pharmacists who then practiced their calling in this country were to be found in Boston, Philadelphia and New York. For the most part they were wholesalers as well as retailers; the first pharmaceutical associations and schools were created through the initiative of these men.[1] These wholesale druggists and the dispensing druggists filled the prescriptions sent to them by the few physicians who did not dispense their own medicines. However, their main professional activity was to provide the rural physicians with drugs, both imported and indigenous, and with compounded medicines that they often produced in their own laboratories.

### Before the Civil War

Until the Civil War, and later, a horde of general stores with drugs as a sideline, and many physicians keeping drug shops, left little career opportunity for the pharmacist as such. A true pharmaceutical profession did not exist before the American Pharmaceutical Association created and developed it. One of the first actions of the Association was to secure reliable statistical information about the condition of pharmacy throughout the country (1851 and 1852). The situation cannot be characterized better than by quoting from some of the reports.[2]

> The State of Maryland contained in the year 1851 about 139 apothecary shops of all grades, about 100 of them in the city of Baltimore, but only 12 were estimated as being owned by real apothecaries.
>
> In the States of Maine, New Hampshire, Rhode Island and Connecticut the number of drugstores kept by physicians surpassed those kept by apothecaries and the stores of general dealers trading also in drugs and medicines far surpassed the number of legitimate drugstores.

---

*The term *pharmacy* is considered preferable, though interchangeable, in relation to the term *drugstore* (modern U.S.A.). In this chapter *drugstore* has been used at times to help imply a pre-professional period (or, for more recent times, an average American pharmacist's establishment), but the usage here carries no fixed degree of distinction. There is merit in the idea that in referring to a variety store or supermarket that includes a pharmacist's practice, only a legally defined pharmacy component should be designated by use of the term *pharmacy* (or *drugstore*).

The situation in Philadelphia was typical of the few large American cities of that period: The sale of medicines by general stores was common and extensive. Fifty-seven drugstores were kept by physicians, who left them much of the time in the hands of medical apprentices or hired assistants. "The competition among pharmacists in Philadelphia is so excessive," the report goes on to say, "as to be a chief obstacle to the attainment of a higher standard of knowledge and skill among them."

Of California it was reported (1852) that "two-thirds of all the drug stores . . . are kept by physicians." In North Carolina, "throughout the State the dispensing and sale of medicines, including nostrums, was in the hands of the physicians." In Georgia "pharmacy was yet in its infancy, and pharmacists and physicians equally ignorant about materia medica in general. The use of nostrums was extensive." The conditions mentioned held true for the early phases of cultural development in most of the southern and western states.

Professional oases could be found where the influence of European continental pharmacy was felt, as in parts of Pennsylvania and above all in New Orleans, St. Louis and New York. Even in these places, "many physicians dispensed and dealt in medicines and kept clerks" (New Orleans); "nostrums are kept and are in general and increasing demand throughout the State" (St. Louis); and in one state (New York) an early "enactment to regulate the preparation and dispensing of medicines . . . had proved unavailing." However, in these parts of the country there was a distinct pharmaceutical calling with professional ambitions and objectives.

It was the concepts and customs of French pharmacy that dominated in New Orleans; German pharmacy in St. Louis, where about half the shops at mid-19th century were conducted by German immigrants; in New York City the first examinations for pharmacists (1872) turned up nearly as many candidates of German origin as of the American-born, and the scientific education that the German applicants brought to pharmacy was shown to be strikingly superior. In other ethnic enclaves, too—such as parts of Wisconsin, Indiana and Ohio—German immigrants who knew the standards of pharmacy in their homeland often had a telling influence as nuclei of professionalism, especially before about 1900.[3] European models tended, however, to take root only locally or else wilt under the conditions of a country so large and relatively uncultivated.

Published reminiscences of old pharmacists, going back as far as the 1840's, show three basic facts: first, that American pharmacy was then considered a simple trade, for the most part, to be changed for another if the expected profit did not materialize; second, that a business frequently had been founded by a physician who later sold it to his clerk; and, third, that because of circumstances the drugstore sometimes became a general store and often a wholesale business, even if it had not been so intended originally.

The occupational fluidity of much of the 19th century is illustrated by J. F. Hancock, who tells of a pharmacy opened in Baltimore (1849) by a physician, "who had but recently graduated in medicine" and had "in his younger days learned the trade of house carpenter." After a few years as physician and pharmacist, this man left his calling and sold the drugstore to another doctor of the same type, who made a partner of the young apprentice whom he found in the drugstore. Shortly afterward, this physician likewise discontinued the drugstore and his practice, to become a lawyer. The young apprentice, who had only 2 years of meager experience, became the sole owner.

Frederick W. Fenn of Delaware reported that "except in a few instances there were no regular pharmacies outside of Wilmington in 1857. The town drugstores were usually combined with hardware, and additional sidelines were stationery and books, wall-

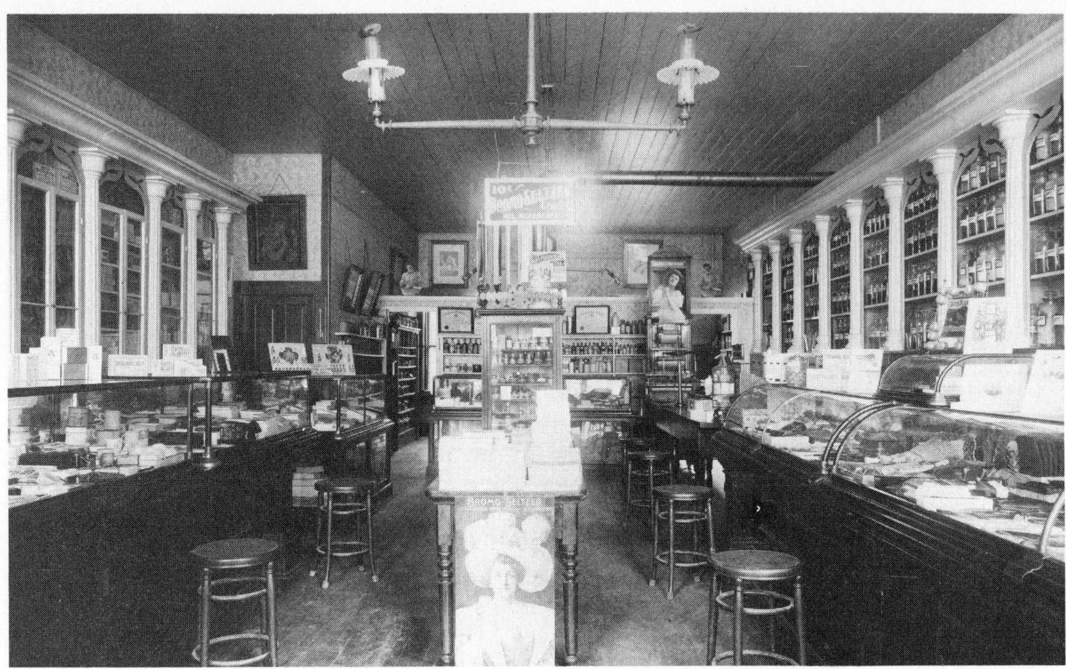

American pharmacies commonly looked like these in the late 19th century *(facing pages)*, and many remained basically unchanged until well into the present century. A typical prescription case can be seen in the rear. Most stock is behind glass or in wooden wall cabinets. Shelves hold typical sets of matched salt-mouth and tincture bottles. Handsome cut-glass urns of various shapes, atop display cases, often held toiletries or confections. (Photograph from The White Drug Store, Pullman, Wash., and from the Frank and Robert Bergmann Pharmacy, Watertown, Wis.)

paper, paints, and oils. Some druggists sent out wagons filled with all sorts of domestic medicines to supply country general stores."[4]

Two early representatives of Wilmington pharmacy grew into general as well as pharmaceutical importance: Joseph Bringhurst, Sr., and Joseph Bringhurst, Jr.[5] The former (1767–1834), born in Philadelphia, obtained his degree of Doctor of Medicine at the University there. Then he went to Delaware (1793) where he established a drugstore in connection with his medical practice. He was intimately acquainted with political and industrial figures in England as well as in the United States and was a partner in the first cotton factory erected in Delaware. Joseph Bringhurst, Jr. (1807–1880), succeeded to his father's pharmacy, from which he retired (1852) to become one of the Delaware pioneers in a number of social and financial ventures.[6]

These pioneers had to be men of courage and industry, and it was with the usual pioneer discomforts that early pharmacists were obliged to study and practice their calling. They did as well as could be expected under the circumstances. By the way of illustration, it was not easy to conduct a business in the town of Helena, Montana, where

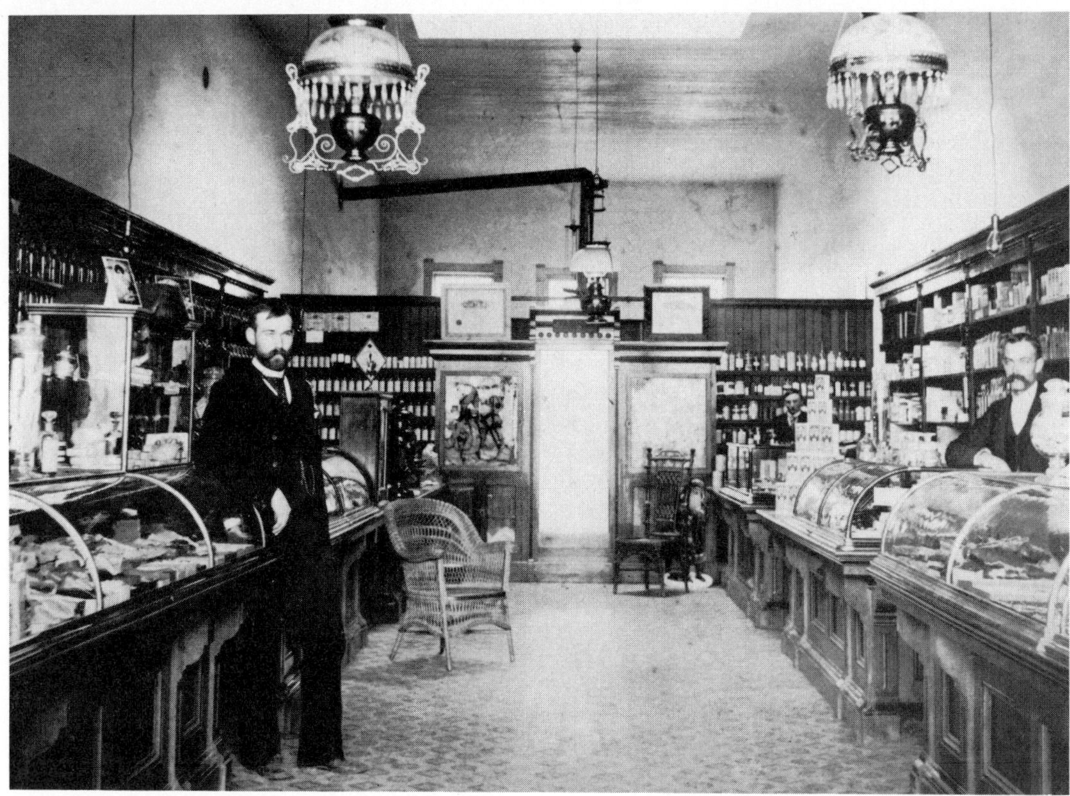

for three months of the year supplies could be brought only by way of the Missouri River and for the remaining months had to be carried overland a distance of 1,500 miles, subject to the constant danger of robbery. "During the winter of 1863 and 1864 a vigilance committee was organized which hung all the 'roadagents' who did not escape, and restored law and order." On the other hand, it suggests that business was profitable, when a druggist in Helena testifies: "With a capital of $3,500 we sold $99,600 worth of goods the first 15 months we were in business and made a profit of over $18,000."[7]

Chicago's first druggist (1832), Philo Carpenter, wanted to run an exclusively professional pharmacy but was unable to do so, for "owing to the scarcity of currency a large part of the business done was by a system of barter, called 'store pay.' Farmers and others who needed goods took what they had to sell and traded it at the stores for what they needed. The storekeeper then had to dispose of the goods so left in whatever way might be most advantageous."[8] In Detroit the hunters brought buck, beaver and fox skins in exchange for the goods they needed.

Such conditions paved the way to the combination drugstore, general store and wholesale establishment. A large portion of the drugstore business in the country consisted of all kinds of dyestuffs and oils and paints, for houses were built which had to be painted, and homespun textiles were made which had to be dyed. The need for these articles was greater than for medicines and drugs, and the latter very often became a sideline, at least in terms of the volume of business transacted.

## After the Civil War

All this changed with the Civil War, a decisive turning point in the development of the North American continent. Pioneer society had been self-sufficient as well as primitive. It was scarcely touched, and by no means penetrated, by the intellectual spirit that radiated from individuals and the few centers of learning and culture along the eastern seaboard. At this time society was confronted with a rapidly developing industry that demanded the highest technical achievements. The drugstore business in dyestuffs for home-dyed cloth and similar goods vanished with the rise of the American textile industry, which became one of the largest in the world. A similar dismemberment occurred when the growth of the building industry took away the drugstore's paint and oil business. With these changes, American pharmacy had opportunity to develop its professional character. Had full advantage been taken of this, the "pharmacy" might have replaced the "drugstore," permanently.

In some districts, professionalized pharmacy was achieved, as a full-time scientifically based service, but could not sustain itself and never became the norm. The rise of a large and powerful pharmaceutical industry partly accounted for this, taking over the manufacturing previously carried on, to a large extent, in the drugstore laboratories. Another reason for the stunted growth of pharmacy as a full-time occupation was the fact that, on the one hand, there were too many drugstores in proportion to the demand for pharmaceutical service; and, on the other hand, the number of educated pharmacists available was comparatively small.

## Comparison With Europe

A comparison with the development in Europe helps to support this statement. There also, the rise of a powerful pharmaceutical industry during the second half of the 19th century diminished the manufacturing previously carried on within the pharmacies. However, only the face and not the character of continental European pharmaceutical practice changed. It was controlled by high educational requirements limiting the number of those entitled to ownership of a pharmacy.[9] In addition, the number of pharmacies often was restricted to the proportion needed to handle the demand for pharmaceutical service.

The scientific training and the economic security of the pharmacists enabled them to concentrate profitably on their function as the responsible distributors of medicinal products. The standardization of the strength of pharmaceutical products, which began in the late 1870's, was no challenge to them; and the manufacture of galenics in the laboratories of the pharmacies was inspired by long tradition and professional ambition.

In America the development of pharmaceutical industry encountered conditions very different from those in continental Europe, as previously shown. On the one hand, the dispensing of proprietary medicines for self-medication was of great importance to the American pharmacist at a time when it meant little to European continental pharmacy. On the other hand, the increasing medical tendency to prescribe prefabricated proprietaries instead of writing individualized prescriptions, which was so threatening to the continental European pharmacist accustomed to extensive compounding in a large prescription practice, seemed much less important to the average American pharmacist. He had less to lose from the shift to factory-made medicaments, since most American physicians dispensed their own medicines, even if they did not have public drugstores, and thus the average American pharmacist had never enjoyed a large prescription practice. As late as 1904, for example, an inquiry answered by 41 Illinois pharmacists showed that "in 7 cases the physicians write prescriptions, in sixteen they dispense their own medicines, and in eighteen they do both."[10] Not only were American conditions less conducive to voluntary professional development, as compared with Europe, but there was more reluctance to use state authority to separate and nurture particular professions even in the name of a higher level of service to the public.

While the impact of industrial output on the back-room laboratory of community pharmacies could not be gainsaid, there was prospect by the 1930's of a "tendency for a greater amount of prescribing and a lesser amount of dispensing from the doctor's office."[11]

Another quite different factor, rising out of sharp competition between too-numerous drugstores, had a remarkable influence on the way the American pharmacist's establishment evolved and on the economic structure of the entire calling. This factor was price cutting.

## Price Cutting versus "Fair Trade"

Competition in prices is an integral part of trade and as old as commerce itself. Its advantage to society has its limitations at that point where it becomes profitable only for a certain group of individuals and threatens the general economic order on which society is built. It is from this concept that the terms "fair" and "unfair" trade practices are derived.

As early as the first decades of the 19th century, price cutting was a striking feature of American pharmacy. For a long period after the founding of the Massachusetts College of Pharmacy (1823), "almost all the business [it] transacted was in reference to prices." T. W. Dyott, perhaps America's first price-cutter, not only sold drugs and proprietaries more cheaply than his competitors, but the example of his own success helped to establish price-cutting and its continuous advertising as a common practice. Dyott had come to Philadelphia from England (1806) and opened a patent-medicine warehouse.[12] Until its demise during a financial crisis, this venture enjoyed many years of success. The pharmacist-founder of the George A. Kelly Company of Pittsburgh, who practiced price-cutting, used methods that foreshadow the chain-store system. Under the firm name of Beckham and Kelly, his four drugstores in Pittsburgh (around 1860) bore signs that read, "Cut-rate Drugstore."

The demoralizing expansion of price-cutting followed the expansion of the American pharmaceutical industry during the late 19th century, which glutted the market with proprietary remedies for self-medication. This was partly because proprietaries could be bought in department stores, which advertised them at a price lower than that marked by the manufacturer on the package, and partly because of the business methods of drug manufacturers and wholesalers. To induce pharmacists to purchase large amounts of their products the manufacturers as well as the wholesalers rewarded such purchases with special discounts and bonuses, thus enabling pharmacists to sell the products for less than the usual resale price.

Among American drugstores of the early 1880's, "the pioneer price-cutting of the 'big four'—Evans of Philadelphia, Robinson of Memphis, Dow of Cincinnati, and Jacobs of Atlanta—aroused national attention. . . . Price cutting became, in a few years, practically universal. . . . The first cut-rate drugstore in New York City was established by George Ramsay, of the Hegeman Company."[13]

Significantly, some of the most successsful cut-rate drugstores were established not by educated pharmacists but by enterprising businessmen. Impressed by the success of Hegeman in New York, one man founded the "Economical Drug Store" in Chicago with borrowed money (1892), after he had made and lost a "fortune in the show business."[14] The Chicagoan who established "The Public Drug Company . . . a large drugstore organized and conducted on the Department Store Plan" (1900) was not "a pharmacist by training or education, but on the contrary a shrewd and resourceful commercial man."[15]

To combat this trend, a "Campion plan" first was attempted. It depended upon a manufacturers' rebate system applying only to pharmacists selling at regular prices. Concerns which did not employ the rebate system were supposed to be under obligation not to sell to "cutters" at all.[16] The plan proved to be a failure. Other plans were discussed rather than put into force.

After independent drugstore owners reorganized in 1898 under the name National Association of Retail Druggists, they soon gave priority to mitigating the aggressive price cutting. If the Association did not solve the problem permanently, it got results through a disciplined organization and persistence that was lacking in its ill-fated predecessor (the N.R.D.A. of 1883–1887).

Several different plans to curb price cutting were tried with more or less success, until finally the so-called "tripartite plan" resulted from an agreement among three parties, the National Association of Retail Druggists, the National Wholesale Druggist's Association and the Proprietary Association of America. This agreement intended to limit the distribution of many drug products to dealers who maintained established resale prices, but was nullified by legal counteraction by the United States Department of Justice.[17] The three associations were enjoined "from combining and conspiring to restrain trade, from fixing prices by agreement and blacklisting retailers, and from continuing in force the direct contract-serial numbering plan as heretofore enforced."[18] Other decisions seemed to abolish every possibility even for the individual manufacturer to maintain resale prices for his products.

Inasmuch as legislation had enabled the price-cutters to defeat their adversaries, the National Association of Retail Druggists "promptly entered the legislative field."[19] Until 1930 there was not much success. Then, in the throes of the great depression, small business men became more unified in their desire for resale price maintenance. The first "fair trade" law was passed in California (1931), and 45 other states followed suit by 1949. These laws were fortified by the Miller-Tydings Federal Enabling Act (amendment of 1937 to the Sherman Antitrust Act) and validation by the U. S. Supreme Court.[20]

The "fair trade" acts legalized contracts requiring a retailer to sell at or above the resale price set by his supplier (in the case of a pharmacist, it was the drug manufacturer). Eventually a "non-signer clause" was added to require compliance of *all* distributors in an area where a pricing contract was effective, even though all had not signed the contract (1933 in California, later in other states). This non-signer clause sparked periodic controversy during the ensuing years. Especially with the disappearance of a "seller's market" following World War II the low-margin distributors ("supermarkets" and "discount houses") found fair-trade restrictions increasingly galling. After one supermarket operator named Schwegman obtained a decision by the U. S. Supreme Court (May 21, 1951) that a non-signer clause could not be enforced in interstate commerce, supporters of the fair-trade concept tried to repair the damage by securing passage of the McGuire Act (1952) in Congress.

Although fair-trade laws were enacted for distributive occupations in general, pharmacy has received much of the credit—not always complimentary[21]—for the passage of many such state laws, under the leadership of the National Association of Retail Druggists.

One of the more formidable antagonists to the concept of "fair trade" has been the Federal Trade Commission, whose Chairman in 1975 urged Congress to "repeal of the two Federal statutes underpinning" the system, and reaffirmed that the FTC "has long supported repeal of State laws permitting resale price maintenance." Chairman Engman contended that, from the historical evidence, "it would be difficult to argue that the anti-trust exemptions granted by the Miller-Tydings Act and the McGuire Act have had the intended effect of protecting either small retailers or consumers from predatory pricing." Even without repeal of the Federal enabling legislation, the fair-trade structure by the early 1970's had been weakened through fair-trade laws having been repealed or declared unconstitutional in 10 states, and through the clause blanketing "non-signers" into the fair-trade agreements of suppliers having been struck down by the courts in 17 states.[22]

Amid the general concern over inflationary prices in these years, and the costs of medical care in particular, public opinion and public bodies no longer reacted as they had 30 or 40 years earlier, in a deflationary period.

The "fair trade" concept now came under increasing attack by consumer groups. Relabeled by its opponents as "resale price fixing," the system's legal supports were undermined by growing acceptance in mid-century America of "discount merchandising" as a form of price-cutting. The culmination came in 1976 when Federal legislation took effect that made it illegal for manufacturers and distributors, such as pharmacists, to agree on minimum resale prices, even in states still having fair-trade laws. A long chapter had ended in the chronic effort to balance the pharmacists' interest in protecting the dignity and quality of his services from the effects of predatory price-cutting and the public's interest in lowering the cost of medicines.[23]

In a sense, fair trade has run counter to the American commitment to "free enterprise." Yet, it supported an equally traditional concern for the life-chance of small, independent entrepreneurs. This concern had gained legislative strength as mass purchasing, mass distribution and mass promotion became linked into an increasingly efficient, powerful and impersonal mechanism for fulfilling consumer needs.

### Independent Pharmacy versus the Chain

While such commercial trends seem to be remote from the professions, American pharmacy has been particularly vulnerable, being for decades only a part-time profession for a majority of its practitioners. In the *non*-professional segment of his income-producing activities, the average community pharmacist has a tradition of selling small inexpensive products, often not of the highest quality so as to be subject to "bargain" merchandising.

Even health products warranting a pharmacist's professional or technical service attracted price cutters. When all but a vestige of laboratory manipulations (about 4% of prescriptions in 1961, about 1% in 1973)[24] had been withdrawn from American pharmacies into the large manufacturing laboratories, it became more difficult, despite the responsibilities inherent in prescription practice, for pharmacists to keep drug products isolated from commercial thought and ambition (among less thoughtful practitioners and non-pharmacist owners of pharmacies).[25]

Like "pineboard drugstores" of the early part of the century, many early supermarkets used the technic of stocking a limited number of best-selling products for self-medication, operating at the lowest possible cost, and making extreme price-cutting their principle. Others have gone farther by seeking out pharmacists willing to sell their services under grossly commercialized conditions, where prescription service is exploited through flamboyant advertising. Such tactics became more widespread in the 1950's, bringing pressure especially on urban pharmacists who tried to maintain full professional services and the standards that have given pharmacy its standing as one of the health professions. Although threatening the

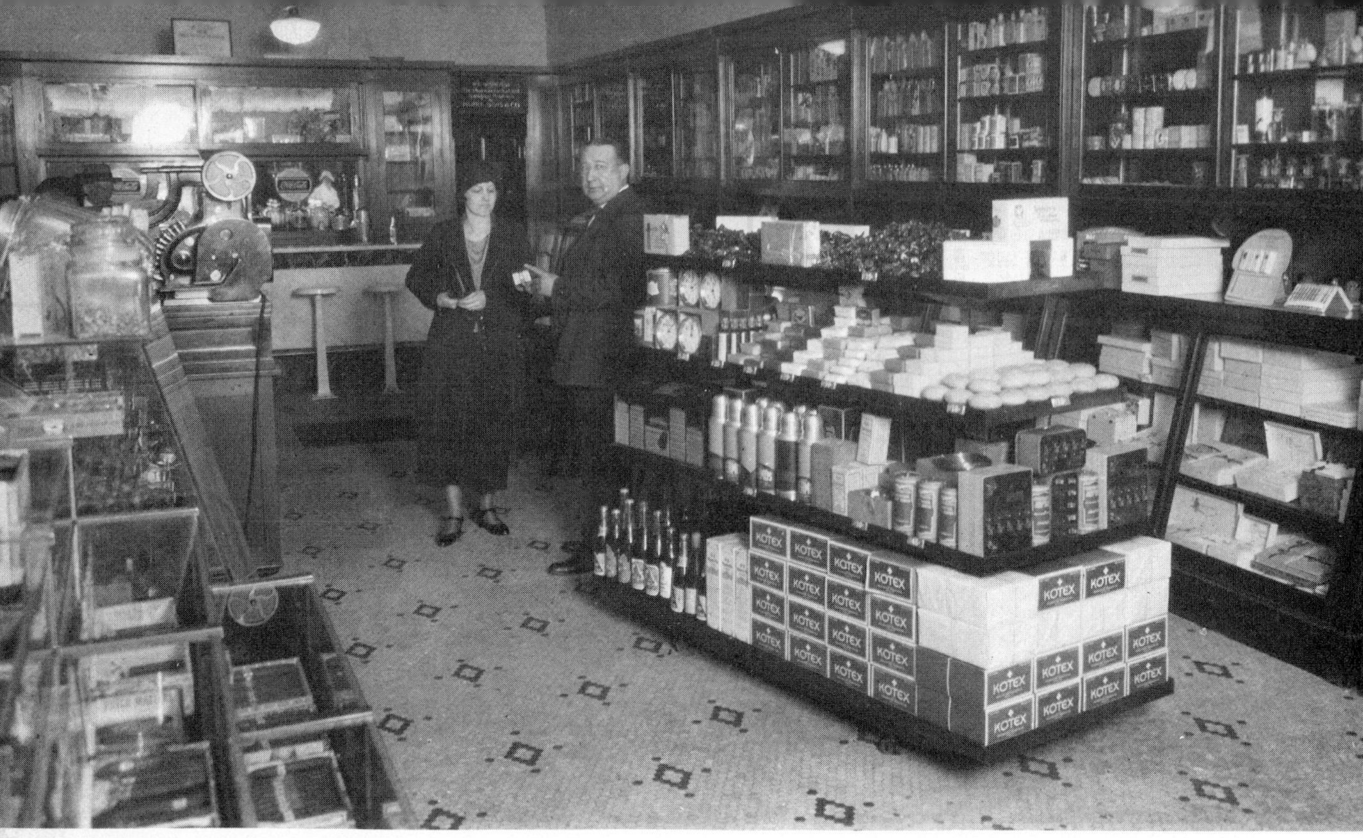


A scene typical of a neighborhood drugstore during the late 1920's in the United States. The front of the shop still had fixtures in fine, dark woods, although of simpler style than in the 19th century. A wide range of products was stocked, mostly in glass-fronted display cases, although limited "island" display had been common since at least the turn of the century. (From: *Drug Topics* Collection, AIHP)

economic base of professionally oriented establishments, the exigencies of economic life and public reaction were setting limits on the intrusion of "discount houses," and "supermarkets" by the 1960's.[26] Whereas the "supermarket" brought many kinds of small shops under one roof, the "chains" had emerged by linking together units of the same kind under many roofs but a single ownership. (This distinction has often been blurred in recent years, and large capital and high turnover are elements in common between the two types of enterprises, often giving them analogous characteristics.)

In large cities that developed in the late 19th century were pharmacists who owned two or even three drugstores in the community. However, they considered themselves to be "independent" pharmacists, like the owners of a single establishment. The suggestion that the term "chain stores" be used only for "four-store enterprises and sectional and national systems"[27] is arbitrary but to some extent makes the term more meaningful.

The first "chains" of drugstores were established in England and Scotland, where they were known as company-pharmacies, and developed to a remarkable degree by 1900.[28] Probably the American movement in its early growth was stimulated by the English example. The early development of chain drugstores in the United States is exemplified by firms such as Hegeman and Company of New York, Charles B. Jaynes of Boston, the Hall and Lyon Company of Providence, and Cora Dow of Cincinnati.

The rapid development of chain drugstores, however, arose just after the turn of the century with the bold empire-building by two men: Louis K. Liggett, who had initiated the founding of the United Drug Company (1907) and Charles R. Walgreen, who opened the first unit of the present chain in 1901.

By 1916 Liggett operated 45 drugstores, added to them the 107 drugstores of the Riker-Hegeman-Jaynes combination, and by 1930 the chain "touched its all-time peak of 672 stores." Grandiose plans of dominating community pharmacy in the Anglo-Saxon world ripened. "Combining with various large manufacturers to form Drug, Inc., the concern extended its operations to England, building up the drugstores of Boots, Ltd. there. At the height of the boom of the late 1920's 1000 drugstores in the two countries came under this single ownership. The Boots stores were disposed of in 1933, and Drug Inc. disbanded into several parts."[29]

The Chicago pharmacist Charles R. Walgreen, Sr., the other leader in the chain-store development, had acquired nine drug stores between 1901 and 1916. By 1922 the Walgreen establishments numbered 29; then multiplied 4-fold within 5 years; during the next 35 years multiplied 4-fold again (462 in 1961); and by 1973 totalled 580, besides 1800 franchised outlets.[30]

Drug-chain managers have always preferred urban districts and the best situated places within them (e.g., two-thirds of their units were in cities larger than 50,000 about 1947). Such drugstores have sales volume very different from that of their independent competitors, on the average. For example, while in 1935 "less than 4% of all independent drug stores did an annual business of over $50,000 . . . over 64% of chain stores did a business of over $50,000" per unit.[31]

During the next quarter century a dramatic increase in sales volume occurred, in both types of establishments, reflecting changes in the American economy and in the style of operating community pharmacies. Among independent drugstores (1960) an estimated 77 per cent, had an annual business of over $50,000, compared with about 96.6 per cent among chain stores. The result of the aggressive mass-merchandising that is characteristic of multiple-unit management comes into bold relief for this more recent period when considering drugstores with higher volume-levels. For example, three times as many chain stores took in over $125,000 annually as did independent stores (77.2% versus 26.5% of the total number operating in each category).

Although the sharp expansion in dollar volume obviously has not been restricted to multiple-unit operations, the average chain unit did have about twice as much volume as did its independent counterpart.[32] This has come about largely through the inexhaustible capacity of the chain drugstore for efficient purveyance of variety store merchandise. Often it makes pharmaceutical service so inconspicuous in "superdrugstores" that the term becomes incongruous and, to the public, even amusing.

"Sidelines" had been so much a part of the tradition of the average American pharmacy or drugstore since earliest times, such a widely varying supplement to the pharmacist's income, that it is hard to say when the tail began wagging the dog. Walgreen opened his first "gigantic store" in 1937 in Miami. A little more than a decade later when the firm opened a "superdrugstore" having almost 30,000 square feet, it already seemed part of a general American trend toward supermarket merchandising. Thus the 1940's appear to be the experimental period for using pharmacy and the pharmacist in exploiting the "superstore" concept. Other techniques of mass merchandisers, besides the one of scale and diversity, were introduced into such "drugstores" during the same period. Walgreen tested self-service in 1942–43, and opened a self-service unit in 1950 in Cincinnati. And declared already in 1962 that "Our drugstores are discount stores."[33]

Such enterprises, although in modern chrome-and-plastic dress, have a character strongly reminiscent of earlier profit formulas based on convenience, price, and volume: the vast Middle Eastern bazaars, which

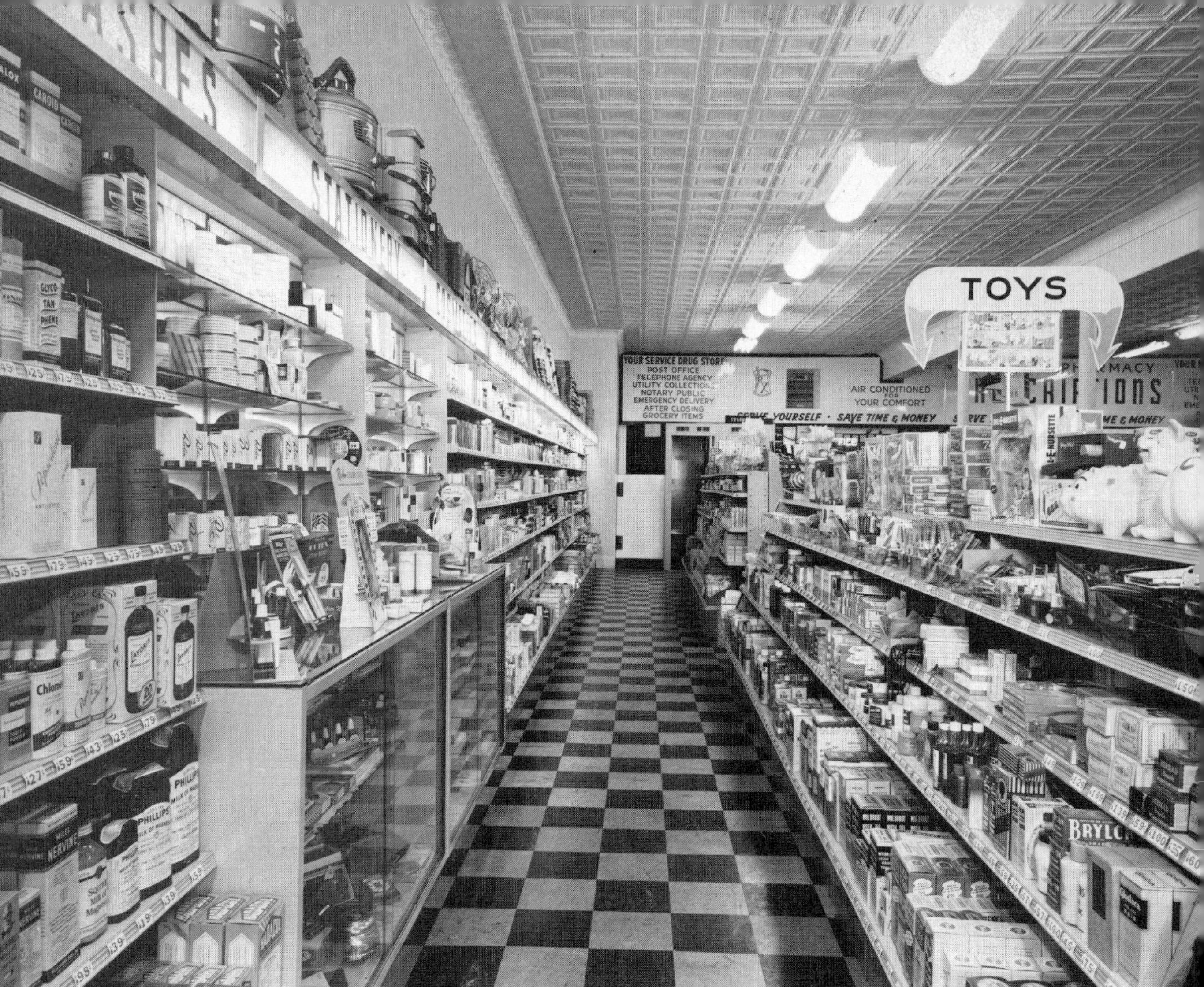

Diverging tendencies since the mid-20th century are illustrated by these photographs of two Ohio pharmacies in the 1950's. The establishment opposite reflects, through both the focus of professional effort and setting, a trend toward integrating pharmaceutical service with medical care. The one above reflects a simultaneous trend toward absorbing a pharmacist's practice into a supermarket or variety store, emphasizing the self-service concept.

often included small drug shops (prototype of the modern pharmacy); and in early America, the crossroads general store, which often included the only drug department within reach.

By 1973 about 22 per cent of American drugstores (pharmacies) were owned by 600 or more "chain" organizations and commanded about 41 per cent of the total dollar-volume of sales through American drugstores.

## The Cooperative in American Pharmacy

The "drug chain" exploited the advantages of scale in unifying as many units as possible under a single ownership, buying and adver-

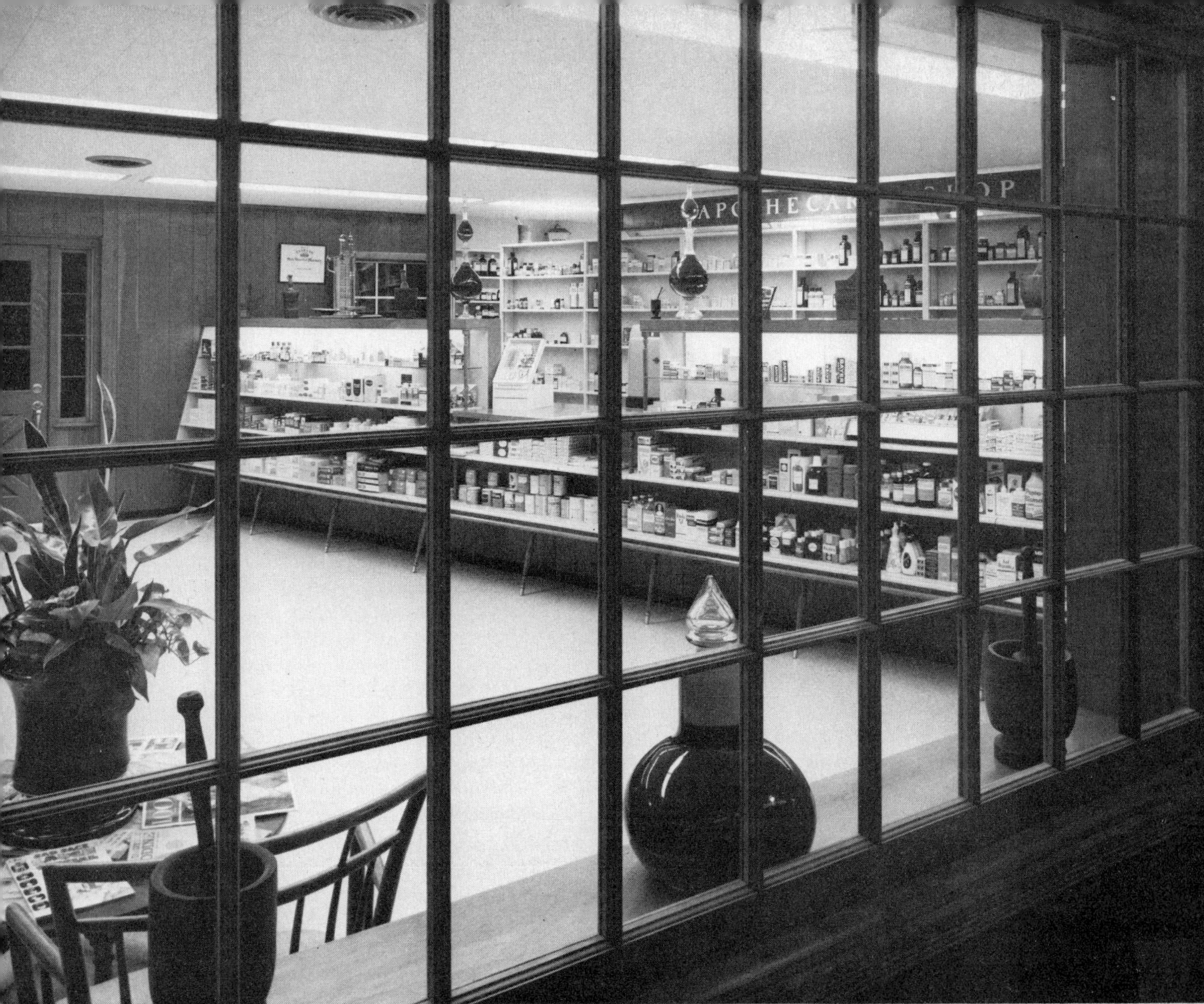

tising together and sharing common merchandising and management resources. This same prospect led the independent owners of pharmacies to turn to the cooperative movement as a means of defense against such powerful, often ruthless, competition. The pharmacist-sponsored "cooperative" and wholesaler-sponsored "voluntary" might almost fit a definition of multiple-unit organization, or "chain store," except for the varied arrangements of ownership.

Unlike the chain store—which has had a stable development in accord with a capitalist tendency toward agglomeration—the American cooperative movement had its ups and downs since the 19th century, in pharmacy as in other fields. The modern cooperative took its present mode in Britain and France as a form of mutual aid in economic enterprise during the early 19th century. It became a world-wide movement that took many forms; but as part of American pharmaceutical economics, the cooperative found its prototype in the old craftsmen's societies (combinations for the purchase of materials and for common marketing).

When Glenn Frank, President of the University of Wisconsin, addressed an audience of independent pharmacists of his state in 1930, he interpreted it as a time of

> the death struggles of an old individualism and the birth-throes of a new groupism throughout the economic life of America, a culmination that had its roots, of course, in earlier years. The symbol of the old America was the pioneer with his emphasis upon individualism. The symbol of the new America is the corporation with its insistence on group actions. . . . The America of tomorrow will act through highly organized groups. . . . That control can be either of two types. It can be a feudalized control or it can be a federated control.
>
> A feudalized control will mean an ever narrower control by the few . . . surrender to chain systems . . . [The alternative,] Federated control of group action means taking advantage of all the benefits of group organization without submitting to the tyrannies of a new feudalism.[34]

The audience was attentive, for the startling rhetoric spoke to a startling reality.

Beset by an oversupply of drugstores by most standards and apprehensive about "chains" as skilled price-cutters, independent pharmacists had first tried the simple defense of attempting to replace nationally promoted proprietaries with their own preparations or with products packaged under their own label by contracting with a drug manufacturer. The next step was cooperative manufacturing by groups of independent pharmacists, such as the Minnesota Pharmaceutical Manufacturing Company, the Empire State Drug Company at Buffalo and the Wisconsin Pharmacal Company. By 1896 "companies were formed in almost every section of the United States."[35] That year initiated the United States Pharmacal Company of Chicago as the first attempt to put cooperative drug manufacturing on a nationwide basis.

The next national undertaking, the United Drug Company of Boston, was not a defense measure of small pharmacies against aggressive "cutters" but rather cooperative manufacturing by community pharmacists, with that master organizer, Louis K. Liggett, as the initiator (1902) and general manager.[36] In 1933 United Drug was absorbed by Drug Incorporated, a Liggett vehicle for drug chains and proprietary manufacture, which thereafter produced the Rexall pharmaceuticals and toiletries for about 10,000 franchised Rexall drugstores. These have been independently owned drugstores, found "in every inhabited county of the nation," which "agree to purchase at least minimum amounts of Rexall products in exchange for discounts, local and national advertising advantages, and a distinctive window sign."[37]

After the dissolution of Drug Incorporated, a new Rexall Drug and Chemical Company also developed diversified operations of international scope, including the largest drugstore chain in the world (e.g., 553 units in 1947). Through a planned program the company then reduced the number of owned drugstores (e.g., 158 operating in 1961), and many that remained were expanded into self-service, large-volume supermarkets that include a pharmacy component. Pharmacy became only one part of the diversified retailing operations of the corporation; and these in turn were joined to diversified manufacturing operations. In a decade (1953–1962) Rexall Drug and Chemical had more than doubled both assets and earnings and increased the annual net sales from $189,244,000 to $280,850,000.[38]

Another nation-wide cooperative manufacturing corporation founded under the auspices of prominent price-cutting druggists was the American Druggists' Syndicate (established 1905).[39] In 1930, about 20,000 retail stores were purchasing from the syndicate, which had been taken over (1926) by the D. A. Schulte interests, operators of a large retail chain-store system."[40]

Thus a movement initiated to defend the independent small pharmacies to a large extent turned into a link between independent and chain drugstores, assisting also the chains by strengthening their manufacturing and buying power.

These cooperative manufacturing companies also did some cooperative buying. However, the mainstream of cooperative buying arose as a separate movement. It represented not so much a special means of defense against price-cutting as an attempt to economize by taking advantage of all the allowances, bonuses, etc., granted by manufacturers and wholesalers to big buyers. Members of the Independent Druggists' Alliance (founded 1930) were "alleged to reap all the administrative advantages and economies of chain store organization, but to retain independent financial status."[41] From the 1880's onward one "buying club" after another was founded. In 1905 it seemed to a pharmaceutical journalist that "The growth of this movement has been rapid, and its history is filled with fewer fruitless attempts and failures than that of co-operative manufacturing."[42] These were wholesale drug companies on a "coop" or "mutual" basis, often limiting the range of stock and brands that they distributed. Some grew to great size.[43]

The first attempt to put such a buying club on a national basis seems to have been the Associated Drug Companies of America (1906), which was superseded (1916) by the Federal Wholesale Druggist's Association (p. 324.[44] This national organization consisted of 20 local wholesale operations initially, under ownership of 12 per cent of the community pharmacies in the country; by 1930 FWDA had grown to 25 wholesale distributors, by 1973 to 50 (as well as branches and associate members in the manufacturing industry). The ownership of the stock of member firms originally was limited to licensed pharmacists; but after 1940 wholesale firms under other ownership were also eligible.[45] Another group of cooperative drug companies in 1929 organized a "chain system" under the name Mutual Drug Company. Pharmacists could become shareholders or profit by special discounts, according to the amount of their wholesale purchases. Remaining independent, they could gain certain chain-store advantages by joining the company and by identifying their establishments by the name "Ure Druggist, Inc."[46]

The wholesale "chain composed of former 'old line' jobbers" with which the Mutual Drug Company was competing was the combination brought into existence (1928) by McKesson and Robbins, Inc., which was founded (1833) as a small drug wholesaler. The new consolidation embraced 67 wholesale houses (1930). At this time, about 17,000 independent retail dealers had signed contracts to feature McKesson and Robbins products,[47] a system discontinued by McKesson in 1932. In 1949 each of the firm's 72 wholesale drug divisions represented a decentralized unit, operating under general policies formulated in New York, together claiming "more than 38,000 of the country's 49,400 independent drugstores are customers of McKesson Divisions." McKesson extended its wholesaling operations until sales totaled (1958) about $600 millions (almost a third in liquor), a 30-fold increase in less than four decades.[48]

Since the 1960's there has been a resurgence of cooperatives as an "affiliation movement," spurred by a trend toward decline of the independent drugstore in terms of numbers, volume, and profits. The newfound cooperation between N.A.R.D. and A.Ph.A. in "COPES" (p. 207) undoubtedly was fostered in part by this threat to the pharmacist's control of his own calling. The renewed initiative of old-line wholesale druggists thus to bolster the entrepreneurial pharmacist undoubtedly was fostered in part by the threat of large-scale purchasing power (whether superstore chains, government, or institutions), which tended to undermine their economic position as it did that of the independent pharmacies they serviced.

By 1972 more than 7000 single-unit pharmacies (about 14% of the U.S.A. total) were in the affiliated movement either as part of a pharmacist-sponsored "cooperative" (ca. 32% of the total movement) or as part of a wholesaler-sponsored "voluntary" (ca. 68%

of the whole). The journal *Chain Store Age* editorialized that the movement was "still in its infancy," partly because its members "realize as their predecessors never did, that affiliation is the only means of survival in an increasingly chain-oriented business."[49]

The typical "affiliated independent" of these years tended to be drawn into the struggle for larger volume and into merchandising strategies similar to those of chain stores in the effort to compete successfully with them. It was a commercialized milieu that seemed alien to the commitments and images held by younger pharmacists who considered themselves primarily "drug specialists" and "clinical pharmacists." If the rhetoric had sometimes outstripped the reality as American pharmacy continued to polarize, the interplay between pharmacy as an integral part of medical care and pharmacy as an integral part of a general or variety store was, on the other hand, a recurring theme in American history.

A historic question, still partly unresolved, perhaps implied an answer to the ambiguous position of the independent community pharmacist in the 20th century: Would the American pharmacist be given the right, as a social decision, to control ownership of his establishment, as had occurred in some other capitalist countries in their legal arrangements for medical care?

### The Question of Ownership

The need for capital and for financial skill under these conditions may override the importance of professional competence in the over-all operation, and hence often attract nonpharmacist ownership or control. In a field providing an important health service, this circumstance became a serious public question in some sections of the country earlier in the century. Several states (first New York and then Illinois, Michigan and Pennsylvania) attempted to prevent professional competition by nonprofessional persons, through legally restricting the ownership of pharmacies to registered pharmacists, following the continental European pattern. This was destroyed in 1928 when the United States Supreme Court declared the Pennsylvania law unconstitutional.[50]

Among the arguments presented in favor of pharmacist-ownership, J. H. Beal contrasted the psychological reality sharply with the legal fiction.[51] He emphasized that the professional manager is expected to obey the directions of the nonprofessional owner and therefore, for cogent personal reasons, may not meet the legal responsibility imposed upon him. For this reason legislation in Germany, for example, denied the right of pharmacists' widows and orphans, or of disabled proprietors to conduct their pharmacies personally or to exercise any influence on their management. Such pharmacies must be leased to registered pharmacists and must be conducted on their responsibility.

Despite constitutional handicaps to such restrictions in the United States, the issue remained alive, reinforced by some evidence that centering authority for the standards and the policies of pharmacy operation in the hands of pharmacists would be in the public interest.[52] However, the difficulties of doing so by state board regulation alone were exemplified as recently as 1962 by a court case in Minnesota.[53] Some organizations persisted in their interest, believing that modified legal precedent and philosophy made the old court decisions vulnerable.[54]

The issue has been somewhat confused by the fact that an increasing number of establishments legally defined and labeled as drugstores or pharmacies are misbranded, in that the main part of their operation has nothing to do with pharmacy. Such a circumstance led the Florida Supreme Court, for example, to strike down a statute in 1962 requiring that a "retail drug establishment" be supervised by a pharmacist, explaining, in part:

> It is only that part of the business of a retail drug establishment which deals with the preparation

and sale of controlled drugs which affects the public health, as the legislature intended to safeguard it in the pharmacy statute . . . . To require that [other parts of] such operations be supervised by a licensed pharmacist merely because done in a storeroom which also prepares and sells controlled drugs does discriminate against the owners and operators of such establishments without valid reason therefor and we cannot sustain the statute which requires it.[55]

To short-circuit such a line of reasoning and strengthen responsibility for pharmaceutical service by divorcing it from business enterprises of pharmacists, one statutory proposal (New Jersey, 1960) provided that "every registered pharmacy in this state shall be restricted to the sale of drugs, medicines, health aids and devices directly connected with health care as hereinafter defined."[56] Although the idea of thus devoting a pharmacy to activities related to the practice of pharmacy would have seemed an ordinary and traditional expression in various countries, within the American context it has seemed too radical to be adopted in any of the 50 states up to this time.

The degree to which pharmacy has been exploited commercially in the United States is perhaps unique historically, among highly civilized countries. This has practical consequences for both the pharmacist and the public, and can intrude even into these questions of legal control. For example, the Illinois Supreme Court looked back at the precedent-setting Liggett case and concluded that the chain "was conducting an ordinary business—namely, the operation of a drug store . . . ," while confirming, on a dental issue, that ". . . The law is well settled that the state may deny to corporations the right to practice professions and may insist upon the personal obligation of individual practitioners . . ."[57]

It was within this latter concept—to center responsibility upon the pharmacist for safe and effective control over drug use—that the North Dakota legislature required (1963) that at least a 51 per cent controlling ownership of pharmacies should be in the hands of qualified pharmacists. Acting on this mandate, the North Dakota Board of Pharmacy denied a permit to "Snyder's Drug Stores, Inc.," one enterprise of the Red Owl chain, which could not show that any North Dakota pharmacists were shareholders. Snyder contested the ruling on the ground that the state law was unconstitutional. When the case reached the North Dakota Supreme Court, it agreed that the state had violated the legal reasoning of the United States Supreme Court in the aforementioned case brought by Liggett's drug chain in 1928.

The Board of Pharmacy then obtained a hearing before the United States Supreme Court in 1973, arguing that its statute requiring majority ownership of a pharmacy by pharmacists was in the public interest, and was not a violation of the due-process clause of the Fourteenth Amendment of the Constitution. The A.Ph.A. and N.A.R.D. joined in filing a brief (*amicus curiae*) in support, a masterful 22-page sociolegal rationale for a law "to prevent the control of the profession of pharmacy by laymen and to assure professional guidance in the determination of pharmacy practices and policies." Before the highest court, organized pharmacy argued that, "When purely commercial interests wholly own or control pharmacies, the policies, practices and conduct of pharmacies have frequently been unduly influenced by commercial considerations. These abuses range from the creation of an unprofessional environment and adverse working conditions to serious infringements on the pharmacist's responsibility for the control and dispensing of drugs."[58]

It was a historic decision by the United States Supreme Court on December 5, 1973. It was a unanimous decision, that "The Liggett case, being a derelict in the stream of the law, is hereby overruled," agreeing in effect with arguments marshalled by counsel for the North Dakota Board of Pharmacy and by the supporting brief of the A.Ph.A. and N.A.R.D.[59]

The implications were far reaching; and the consequences could be assessed only through legislation and litigation of coming decades. Within 2 years about 15 states were considering the question of similar legislation on the ownership of pharmacies, and chain-store interests had given assurance of major opposition.[60]

The outcome desired by many pharmacists probably was voiced by one of the profession's thoughtful spokesmen, Donald E. Francke, when he said, "With the reversal of the Supreme Court's infamous Liggett decision, a dim light glows at the end of a long tunnel toward which community pharmacy may grope in an attempt to recapture a measure of its good name which has been effectively diminished by the blatantly arrogant merchandising practices of the chain drugstores—for the most part corporations owned by nonpharmacists."[61]

**Practitioners**

A correlate of the American reluctance to confine the economic control of pharmacies to pharmacists is the reluctance to limit the number of pharmacies or pharmacists by legal regulation. Even informal limitations (e.g., difficulties of obtaining education or license, capital or credit) have not curbed the number of establishments or practitioners as much as in most other countries.

Historical information on trends in personnel and facilities remain inadequate and may never be satisfactory because of the fragmentary, uncertain nature of statistics for periods prior to World War II. Still earlier, before the late 19th century, our view of the size and the distribution of the profession is fogged by the lack of a stable definition of what constituted a pharmacist or a pharmacy before the passage of modern pharmacy laws.

In terms of the pharmacy practitioner's establishment, one of the earliest quantitative reports is for Massachusetts, about 1850, when the number of drugstores in cities of 10,000 or more was 1 to 1,500 persons; in towns of about 6,000, the ratio was 1 to 2,000; and in "thickly settled districts," 1 to 3,000.

For the country as a whole in the half century before 1930, the available data suggest that there had been no dramatic change. The number of drugstores fluctutated narrowly at a ratio of about 1 drugstore to 1,850 to 2,250 persons.[62] In the years between 1930 and 1947, such factors as the great depression, increased educational standards and the impact of World War II combined to increase the ratio from, roughly, 1 drugstore to 2,000 to 1 drugstore to 3,000 persons. From 1948 (when more consistent statistics begin to be available) to 1960, the number of persons served by each pharmacy continued to increase, from an estimated 2,930 to 3,360. The long-range trend makes this number seem large, until it is compared with other countries—such as (in 1962) an estimated 5,000 persons per pharmacy in Italy, 3,000 in France, 6,300 in Germany and 13,000 in Holland.

During the quarter century after the late 1940's there was a slow trend toward proportionately more American pharmacists practicing for absentee owners, whether in chain units or institutional settings. The impact in terms of shortages of pharmaceutical service in community pharmacies has been partly cushioned by a 27 per cent increase in the number of active pharmacists between 1948 and 1974 (from roughly 94,800 to 119,500 nationally). Uneven distribution of graduates and uneven migration patterns have created periodic manpower problems regionally, especially in rural areas. The growing demand for prescription service—for example, a tripling of the number of prescription orders between 1940 and 1955 alone—produced no crisis in these decades, not only because of increasing personnel, but because a majority of prescription departments traditionally had not been operating at maximal capacity.[63]

The proportion of pharmacists in hospital

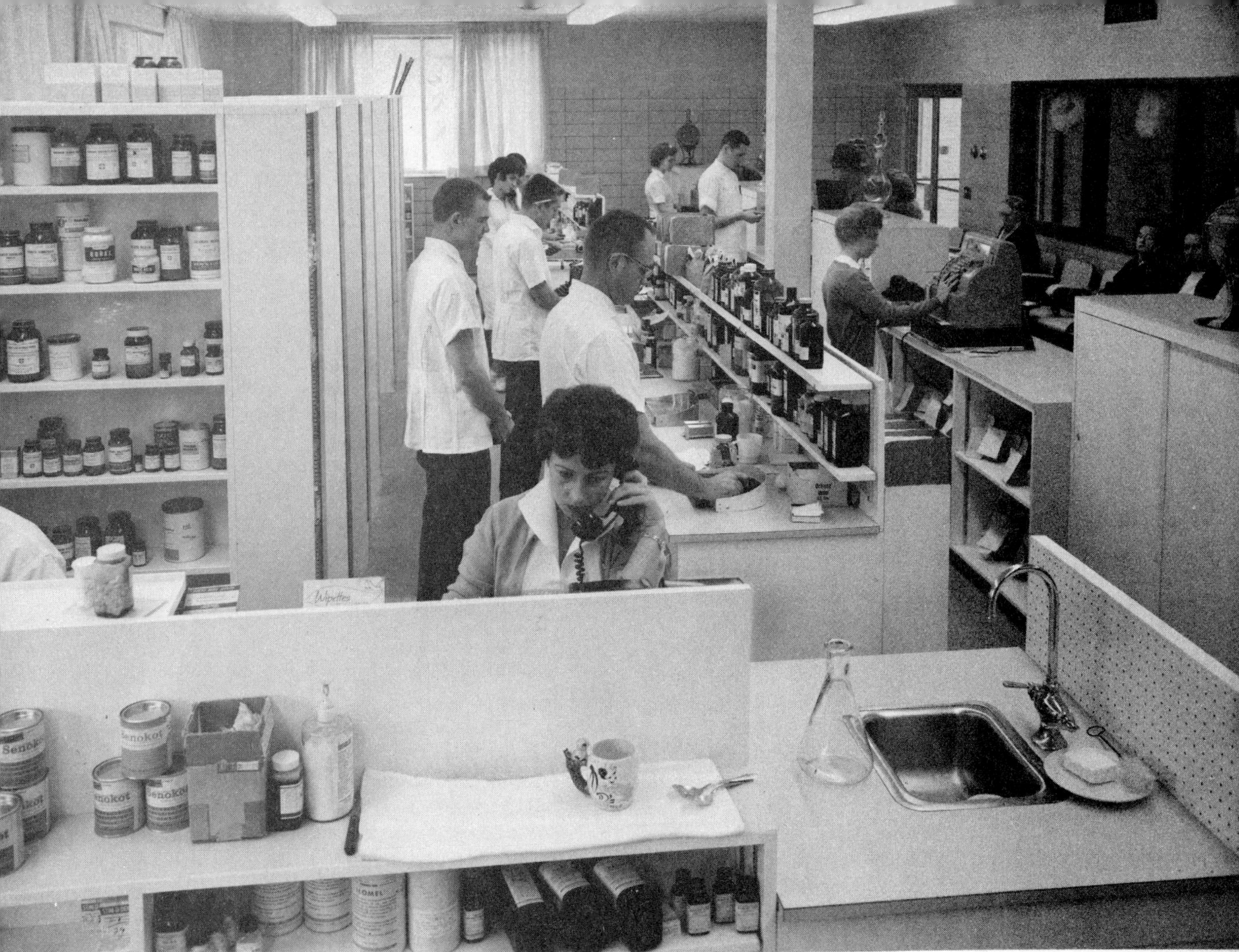


The impact of unionism was being felt in urbanized pharmacy during the 1960's—both through attempts to unionize employed pharmacists and through the operation of some pharmacies under the aegis of unions or under union agreements. This clinic pharmacy was dispensing about a thousand prescriptions a day to auto workers and other union members in 1961 at Toledo, Ohio. (From: *Drug Topics* Collection, American Institute of the History of Pharmacy, Madison)

practice appears to have stabilized at between 3 per cent and 4 per cent during the 1940's and 1950's, then surged upward to about 10 per cent by the end of the 1960's; and by 1974 totalled about 14 per cent of pharmacists in practice, if all types of hospitals, and nursing homes, are included. The proportion of the pharmacist-population reported employed by pharmaceutical manufacturers (in the home laboratories or in the field) appears to have remained within the range of 4½ per cent to 5 per cent between 1948 and 1974. While individual pharmacists have always found unusual uses for their special knowledge in government service, the number on duty outside of hospitals has been increasing, numbering in 1974 about 1.2 per cent of the pharmacists active.

A significant shift in the character or category of work-setting for many community pharmacists has been under way since the 1950's, and was quantified in the A.A.C.P.'s Pharmacy Manpower Information Project, which showed that in 1974 there were about 52,941 pharmacists practicing in single independent pharmacies, 29,860 in multiple-unit organizations (i.e., more than a single pharmacy under one ownership); and 4,267 in clinics and other outpatient medical buildings.[64]

In terms of professional personnel, the increased patronage per American pharmacy since World War II has fostered some decrease in community pharmacies operated by only a single pharmacist. From about 50 per cent of the total number, the one-pharmacist establishment dwindled to about 39 per cent by 1936, then apparently levelled off (e.g., about 41 per cent in 1969). The number of employed pharmacists (vs. pharmacist-owners) likewise has remained nearly constant, about 48 per cent or so of all active practitioners during the period 1948 to 1969.

The proportion of women as pharmacists had remained relatively constant at 5 to 6.5 per cent until the 1960's, during which the proportion of females in practice increased to about 9 per cent. The trend was to continue upward, since the percentage of female pharmacy students in American schools almost doubled during the 1960's (to 22%, although this still was less than half the proportion of female students in some European countries).[65]

In the early 1960's, Griffenhagen concluded that the United States had about 20 per cent of all pharmacists in the world (outside of Red China), serving less than 8 per cent of the world's population.[66] No country in the world except Japan has more pharmacists in relation to the population than does the United States.[67] The United States also has an unusually large number of pharmacies in relation to the number of people to be served, although there has been a tendency, since perhaps about 1900, toward a proportional decrease.

The number of American pharmacies has not needed to bear any quantitative relation to the demand for pharmaceutical services, as it has in some parts of the world by regulation. In the United States a pharmaceutical entrepreneur may simply continue adding income-generating sidelines (unrelated to pharmacy) to keep his pharmacy open and remunerative.

The pressures of competition upon the average American pharmacist, partly indicated in this chapter, more often than not prevented him from practicing pharmacy as a full-time occupation; and throughout history he has reached out for supplemental income—traditionally from necessity, in recent decades frequently just from custom.

## The Soda Fountain

Among side ventures unrelated to pharmacy it was the soda fountain that saved many drugstores from a more or less radical decline. It is a question of principle for American pharmacy, whether this rescue was to the advantage or disadvantage of the real task of the drugstore, its pharmaceutical services.

The development of the soda fountain as an integral and accepted part of the average American pharmacy seems to be unique in the world's pharmaceutical history. However, the manufacture of carbonated beverages as such was a European development, stemming from a fascination with the supposed medicinal value of natural mineral waters at spas. An English apothecary, Thomas Henry, is perhaps the earliest known producer of artificial mineral waters for public sale, albeit on a very small scale (sometime between 1767 and 1781). As early as the 1790's and through the 1820's, at least, "soda water" designated a particular type of carbonated water in which soda was a medicinal ingredient, one of a class of therapeutic artificial mineral waters. Deletion of soda water from the 1831 edition of the U. S. Pharmacopeia perhaps signaled a shift of attention from its status as a treatment to that of a treat.

A citrus-flavored carbonated beverage was

a European precursor of the fruit-flavored carbonated beverages of 19th-century America; but the ingenuity and the promotion that here popularized a wide variety of fizzy fruit drinks made them seem almost an American innovation. The U. S. Dispensatory gave recognition to such use in its first edition (1883), and a well-known drugstore (Smith and Hodgson in Philadelphia) was using fruit syrups by 1835.

While the famous chemist Benjamin Silliman of Yale University opened a "soda water concern" at New Haven in March, 1807, as did Joseph Hawkins at Philadelphia about the same time, the practical development and exploitation soon was taken up with particular effectiveness by pharmacists.[68] A former military pharmacist in the army of Napoleon, Elias Durand, operated in Philadelphia one of the first soda fountains in an American pharmacy (ca. 1825), and the apparatus he later used for bottling under pressure "was his own invention and superior to any used in France."[69]

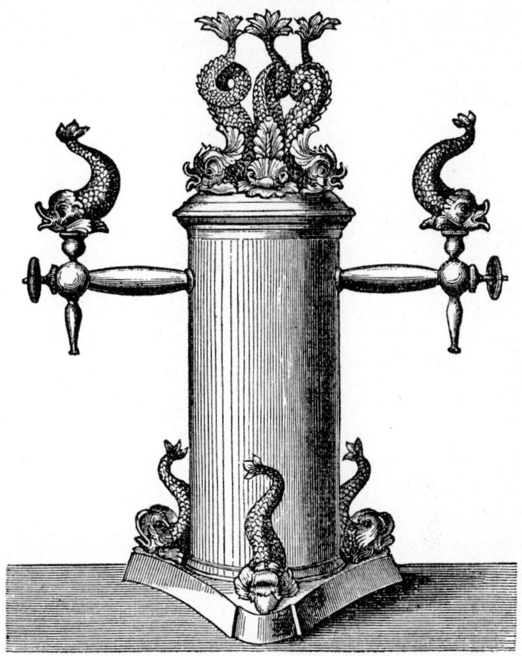

Nichols' Mineral Water Fountain typifies the simple counter device of the late 1850's which, by the end of the century, had developed into the elaborate soda fountain. The model shown has double draft tubes ornamented with dolphins disporting themselves. The top could be lifted off to repack in ice the block-tin coil of pipe inside the cylinder, for cooling the soda water. (From: Prices Current, for Druggists Only, T. Morris Perot & Co., Importers and Wholesale Dealers . . . Philadelphia, ca. 1858)

The dispensing of carbonated beverages by the glass from a small counter device soon became common in American drugstores, and more ornate fountains began to appear in the 1860's.

The soda fountain came into its own in the 1880's as a social institution, during the public's fight against the liquor business through the passing of local and state legislation banning saloons and liquor stores. When national prohibition under the Volstead Act became a fact (1919) the fountain business reached its climax.

"From 1919 to 1929 new installations went on to the tune of $19,500,000 a year." By 1929, of the 54,745 independent drugstores, 31,813 had fountains; of the 3,513 drug chain units, 3,031 had fountains.[70] In 1935 drugstores took in $121 millions from fountains, including meal service (6.8 per cent of the sales of meals for the U.S.A.), which had been introduced as a volume builder during the 1920's by Walgreen, and others.[71]

The soda fountain, often expanded into a second-class restaurant, became so important a feature of the average American drugstore that in the imagination of many people the concept of a drugstore included the fountain[72].

Within a quarter century the total soda fountain volume increased 5-fold in American drugstores (about $600 millions), despite a decline in both the number and the proportion of drugstores with fountains. This decline was due largely to shortages of fountain personnel and materials during World War II, when about one fountain in six closed.

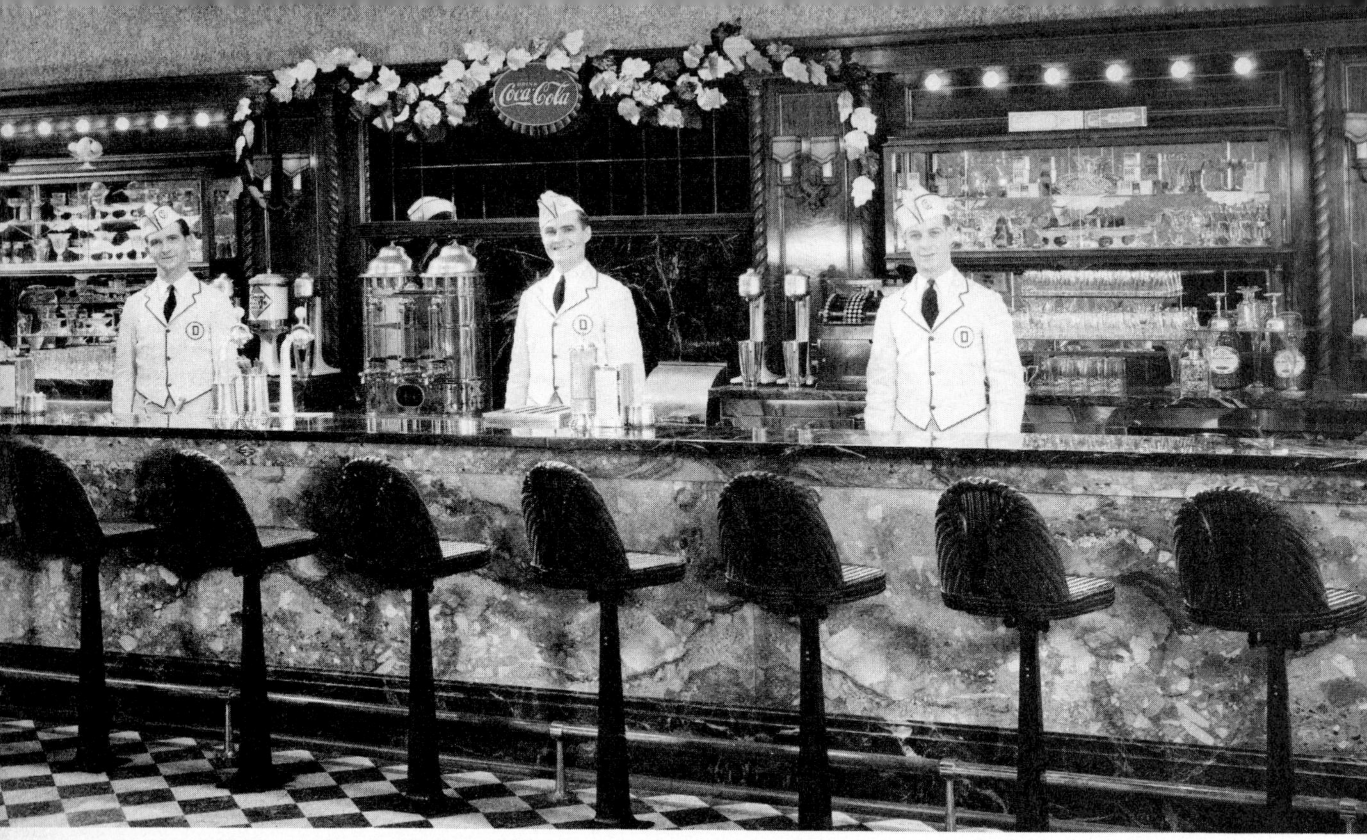


The soda fountain offered delights not available from the household "ice box" and served as a social meeting place for all ages. (From: *Drug Topics* Collection, AIHP)

Many pharmacy owners found meanwhile that the space could be used to better advantage. Estimates suggest that from about 1930 to 1960 the number of pharmacies with fountain and food service dropped from 58 per cent to about 46 per cent of the independent drugstores, and from 86 per cent to about 67 per cent of the drugstores in chains of more than three units. Thus a minority of American independent pharmacies any longer operated soda fountains by mid-century, and by the 1970's probably less than a third.[73]

### Growth and Character of Prescription Practice

Given the proper location, American pharmacists can earn a livelihood mainly from the profession for which they are educated. This has been evidenced, ever since the early 18th century by a small core of pharmacies devoted almost entirely to services related to pharmacy (sometimes miscalled "ethical pharmacies").[74] Some of the early Philadelphia pharmacies were well known for their exemplary professional standards as well as for their economic success (e.g., those of the Marshalls [1729–1825], of Durand [1825–1873], of Ellis and Morris, of Daniel B. Smith).[75] American practical pharmacy can be proud that many men who laid the foundation for American scientific and professional pharmacy, such as Procter, Parrish, Grahame and others, have been investigators and teachers while still operating as practicing pharmacists.

In New York the shop of John Milhau (1795–1874) was one of the best-known representatives of the older American pharmacies and of professional progress.[76] In

Boston the pharmacy of Theodore Metcalf (founded in 1837) became not only a well-known professional institution but also the rendezvous of eminent American people and European visitors.[77] The German influence on New York pharmacy, mentioned previously, found expression in a number of pharmacies (e.g., those of Alfred G. Dung, Adolph Heyl, and George A. Cassebeer) that commanded exceptional respect and clientele.[78]

But many pharmaceutical establishments that considered themselves professional between 1870 and 1920 were old-fashioned drugstores, not professional pharmacies. It was the type of old druggist of whom the chain store magnate, L. K. Liggett, ironically wrote that he sold all kinds of goods but "did not feature them," and displayed in his windows "festoons of dusty sponges, exhibits of cochineal bugs, rock sulphur and flyspecked cards announcing the 'Old Folks Supper' at the Methodist Church."[79]

While this somewhat fusty establishment can be disparaged from a later chrome-and-plastic vantage point, the fact remains that the late-19th-century pharmacy commanded considerable respect among the citizenry. The subsequent pharmaceutical literature is filled with apprehensions that new technologic and commercial currents would erode the professional foundations that a dedicated minority of earlier generations of pharmacists had helped to build.

Although having a professional function based on science, community pharmacies operated within the framework of business enterprise. As such they shared increasingly in the pressures felt by small specialty shops and family businesses during the present century. Under divergent influences, pharmacy tended to move off in all directions, becoming more varied than in other highly civilized countries.

On the one hand, some pharmacies have been incorporated into sprawling supermarkets, where prescriptions and other products related to health may require less than 5 per cent of the total floor area.[80] This infinitely variable mixture of pharmaceutical practice and variety-store merchandising has tended to cloud the "professional image" of pharmacy, especially when the entire establishment, and not just the pharmaceutical part, is labeled as a drugstore or pharmacy.

At the same time there has been a counter-trend toward more establishments that largely specialize in pharmaceutical services, including health-related supplies. In 1931 it was estimated that less than 1 per cent of all pharmacies (350 to 400) were "receiving 50 per cent or more of their total sales from their prescription departments."[81] Meanwhile, the number of professionally oriented American pharmacies has gradually increased, although there are differences of opinion about what constitutes a "professional pharmacy" and about what size and character of area will support one.

By 1935, about 3,200 pharmacies seemed to be primarily interested in prescription practice (but not necessarily 50% of volume), one analyst concluded.[82] Twelve years later a professional journal believed that about one pharmacy of every five could be called "professionally minded," with nearly 700 specialized to the extent of dispensing at least 75 prescriptions a day.[83] The number of pharmacies dispensing that many prescriptions increased sharply during the next 15 years if a 1962 estimate is comparable that places the figure at about 8,600 pharmacies (16% of the total). A further conclusion was that almost 25 per cent of American pharmacies derived at least half of their revenue from the prescription department,[84] in contrast with the 1931 estimate of only 1 per cent. However, another source contends that scarcely half as many pharmacies had such a large prescription practice.[85] Statistical disagreements have not been resolved, since sampling technics change from one investigator to another, and from one time to another, and sometimes have not been open

**EXPENDITURES FOR DRUGS AND DRUG SUNDRIES PER CAPITA, USA, 1929-1972***

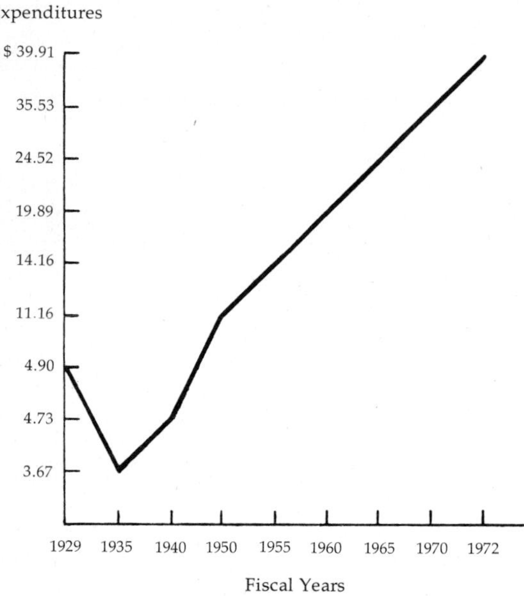


The per capita expenditure for all health services and supplies in 1935 totalled $22.65, in 1950 $81.86, in 1965 $204.61, and by 1972, $421.57. Of the aggregate personal health bill, nationally, by 1972 nearly two-thirds (estimated 64.4%) was being paid by third parties (government funds, private health-insurance funds, philanthropy, industry.) (Data from: B. S. Cooper et al.: National Health Expenditures, Calendar Years 1929-72. Research & Statistics Note No. 3-1974, Social Security Administration DHEW Publ. No. [SSA] 74-11701, Table 6).

*For selected calendar years, including research expenditures by manufacturers and including expenditures for eyeglasses and medical appliances. Figures are *not* calculated to a constant dollar.

to independent evaluation. However, there is agreement that the extent and the degree of professionalization has been growing in a widening sector.

Early in the 1960's the A.Ph.A. renewed its encouragement of this type of practice within a new framework of "patient-orientation." Many "oldtime druggists" also had been affectionately esteemed by the public for their patient-orientation (a term then unknown); but they usually lacked the work environment, the education, and the professional relationships and authority in medical care to move into the role of monitoring[86] and counseling patients' drug use as progressive elements in the role A.Ph.A. now envisioned. Pharmacist Eugene V. White of Berryville, Virginia, became one prototype for the practice of pharmacy in this mode. The compact professional-office type of installation that it required became routinely available (McKesson & Robbins), and well over 200 were in operation around the country by the early 1970's.[87]

Moreover, in recent decades an increasing amount of prescription service is provided in work settings other than the traditional corner pharmacy—clinics, "HMO" forms, and other group-practice environments for integrated medical care.

A more personalized pharmaceutical service in such settings remained a viable countertrend to making pharmacy just one aspect of a supermarket—partly because of a long-range trend toward increased usage of medications and other health supplies, and toward increased safeguards against their misuse.

The sharply increased demand for pharmaceutical services cannot be accounted for on the basis of population growth alone. More effective drugs, less dispensing by physicians and the tendency to prescribe individual drugs rather than compounds, probably all shared in increasing prescription totals.

The number of prescriptions dispensed in 1931 was estimated at "close to 165,000,000." Within 13 years the number had more than doubled (371 millions, representing a dollar volume of about $544 millions for 1948). After

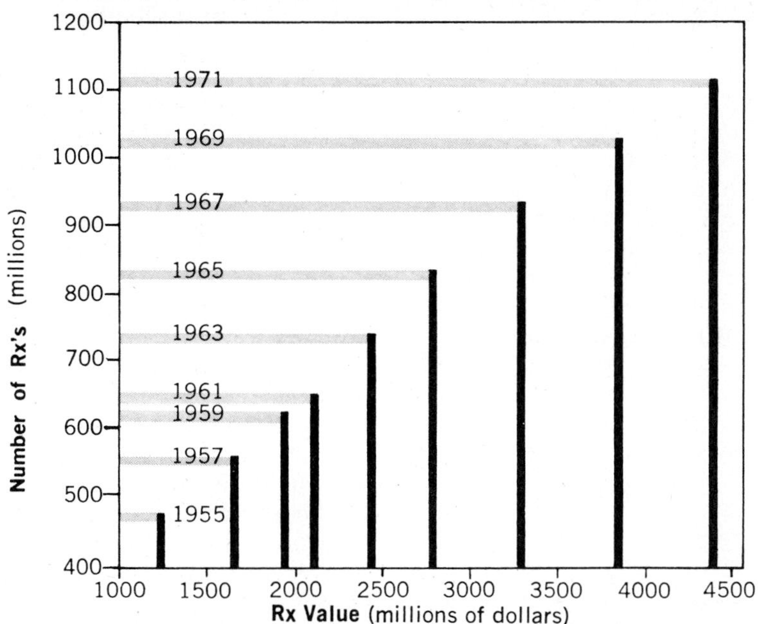


Prescription practice has increased during the past several decades for pharmacists in all types of work settings. The chart depicts this trend in terms of American community pharmacies 1955-1971. If pharmacy departments in supermarkets and discount stores were added to the 1971 figures, the total reportedly would be approximately 1,200 million. That is, while the U.S.A. population was growing by less than a fourth, the number of prescriptions dispensed almost tripled (in about 17 years). This can be attributed to therapeutically active substances being dispensed more often individually (rather than combined in a single prescription); to more effective medicaments becoming available, leading to their freer use and sometimes overuse; to a more affluent society in this period; growth of "third-party payment"; and other factors. If prescriptions dispensed in hospitals were added to the 1971 total, it would approximate 2 billion. National estimates of drug usage vary somewhat according to source. (From: Prescription Drug Industry Fact Book, p. 31, Washington: PMA, 1973)

a like period, the number of prescriptions had approximately doubled again and the dollar volume nearly quadrupled (729 millions, yielding a dollar volume of about $2,219 millions for 1960). These prescriptions, which were divided about evenly between new prescriptions and refilled prescriptions, represented on the average about 28 per cent of the drugstores' total dollar volume.[88]

The cost of pharmacists' services had not become a major issue in the American debate over medical economics in subsequent decades. Nor had the pharmacist's income been central to the escalation of the costs of medical care. Between 1967 and the end of 1971, for example, the government's Consumer Price Index rose 24 per cent for all types of items surveyed, while it rose only 1.7 per cent for prescription medications. Nonetheless, the pharmacist's services have been caught up in controversies surrounding "third-party payment" for health care in the United States since the early 1940's. The tradition of the patient's fee for services rendered by the health professions was breaking down, following a long-term international trend discussed previously (p. 129).

In the late 1950's pharmacists and consumer groups alike began to examine the implications of bringing prescription costs within the concept of health insurance or other third-party payment. The earliest American plan established solely to finance prepayment of drug charges, Campbell and Hammel concluded, arose in Windsor, Ontario in 1958, sponsored by area pharmacists as Prescription Services Incorporated. Within the United States itself, between 1964 and 1969 three different organizations developed to provide prepaid prescription programs and/or to assist other insurance companies in administering such programs: Paid Prescriptions, Prepaid Prescription Plans, and Pharmaceutical Card System Inc. By the late 1960's more than a third of Americans were covered for prescription expenditures as part of "major medical" insurance, but only 1 to 2 per cent held prescription insurance providing coverage on a "first-dollar basis." By 1974 some third party was paying at least part of the cost of one out of every four prescriptions dispensed in community pharmacies; and the upward trend was clear.

The decades-old debate, finally, seemed to have come to a decision: Americans would change their ways of paying for medical care, and many pharmacists felt pressures for new ways to cope with the rising volume of prescription service.[88a]

Not only had prescription practice grown, but its character changed profoundly since World War I, bringing far-reaching socioeconomic as well as professional consequences. Three prescription surveys at intervals of 20 and 15 years illustrate the transformation, if we pass by the question of comparability of exact figures to look instead at the general magnitude and character of the change. These surveys were made approximately in 1926 (sample of 17,577 prescriptions), 1946 (13,125) and 1961 (149,438).

Within these four decades "compounding" was swept away as a central function with which the profession was closely identified both by patients and by practicing pharmacists themselves. Disappearance of handmade multi-ingredient prescriptions was the combined effect of influences such as the full impact of the industrial revolution

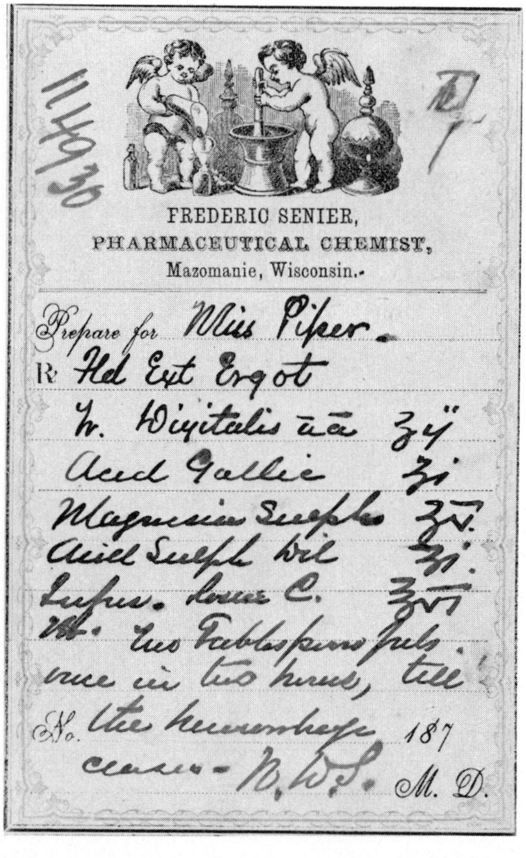

This prescription from the 1870's is typical of the compounding needed to dispense a majority of prescriptions received by practicing pharmacists until well into the present century.

applied to pharmacy, the discovery of medicinal substances individually effective as therapeutic specifics, and the mass promotion of trade-named prescription products.

Still in the late 1920's up to 80 per cent of prescriptions were not of sufficiently "simple nature" to make a "broad knowledge of compounding" unnecessary. This figure was corroborated by a government study that found 75 per cent of prescriptions requiring "the special skill and knowledge of a trained pharmacist to compound" (1930–1931). Within 20 years only a third as many (26%) required some combination or manipulation of ingredients. By 1962 only between 3 and 4 per cent of prescriptions required combining "two or more active medicaments"; and after 1973 this proportion dropped to a vestigial 1 per cent or less.[89]

As the compounding function moved from the prescription laboratory to the large-scale manufacturing laboratory, and expanding industrial research increased the number of drugs, an increasing number of different items was needed to dispense long runs of prescriptions. In the three illustrative surveys, the number of pharmaceutically different products or preparations drawn upon to prepare the prescriptions rose from 1,973 to 2,400, and then to 3,300. However, only 411 of the 3,300 appeared five times or more in each 10,000 prescriptions.

The massive shift away from a scientific or nonproprietary nomenclature toward the practice of prescribing by the trademarked proprietary name that each company creates for a drug occurred largely within the same time span (1920's to 1960). The analysis of prescriptions first showed 10 to 25 per cent prescribed by proprietary name, then 58 per cent, and finally about 88 per cent. As manufacturers continued their massive promotion of trade names for drugs in later years, physicians increasingly used trade names as a handy way of prescribing. Then, mounting social and professional criticism during the 1960's reversed the trend, and by 1973 the proportion of prescriptions ordered by trade-marked name had dropped back to about 89.5 per cent.[90]

Conversely, the proportion of prescriptions designating medicaments of the official drug compendia, as such, decreased. The U. S. Pharmacopeial drugs dropped from about 74 per cent, to 32 per cent, then to 12 per cent. National Formulary drugs specified in these prescriptions started at only about 7 per cent of the total, then dropped to 3 per cent, and finally to only 0.8 per cent.[91]

These and other changes since the 1920's were not peculiarly American. Yet, pharmacy changed more erratically and quickly here than it did in some older countries, as it was buffeted in the freer American economy without having fully developed moorings of professional maturity and traditions, or the same degree of government protection as part of a public health system. Not well organized, unclear about the broader socioeconomic forces changing pharmaceutical practice, and harassed by new forms of competition both within the licensed network of pharmacies and outside it, the average community pharmacist seemed less certain of his position and prospect—despite the upswing in demand for pharmaceutical services, which became obvious during the second half of the century.

## Dispensing Health Information

To reinterpret and bolster public understanding of pharmacists' professional function, cooperative projects were launched, such as National Pharmacy Week, an annual project (1924–1972) initiated by pharmacist Robert J. Ruth. This traditional observance established a pattern and a time for stressing the service rendered by professional pharmaceutical work to the American people,[92] although eventually it became obscured amid a welter of commercial "weeks" that crowd the American calendar.

The American Pharmaceutical Association tried to prevent commercial exploitation of National Pharmacy Week itself, but also shifted the emphasis from simply telling about the pharmacist's professional service to demonstrating the pharmacist's service. This objective was first made a reality (1947) by collaborating in the cancer-control program, under the leadership of Robert P. Fischelis, then the Association's Secretary.

Said the President of the United States, Harry S Truman,

> It is particularly gratifying to note that pharmacists are endeavoring to use their close contact with the community to help control major diseases through public education in cooperation with private and governmental health agencies.[93]

A precursor program was the A.Ph.A.'s collaboration begun 8 years before (1940) with the American Social Hygiene Association to help to motivate those with venereal diseases to undergo proper medical treatment.[94]

By 1948 the Association had adopted a long-range program of health education as official policy. Secretary Fischelis expressed the hope that

> in the planning of new pharmacies and in the renovation of existing establishments, a section will be set aside for permanent use in storing and distributing authoritative health information . . . available continuously for good health and civic programs in all pharmacies.

In extending this kind of effort from a special "week" to a periodic but year-round program, cancer control again was made the theme. Said an official of the U. S. Public Health Service, the collaborating agency,

> If pharmacists themselves are well informed, and if they use every opportunity to pass on their information to others, they have an extraordinary opportunity to make their establishments the health information centers of the entire community.[95]

This concept was valuable to pharmacists in creating good will, as well as in creating better health for the community. It attracted about 18,000 collaborating pharmacists, then faltered from insufficient funds, but remained alive as an objective through smaller-scale, sporadic projects.

The foundation for such service on a more systematic basis was developed by the American Pharmaceutical Association in 1963 through a grant from the U. S. Public Health Service "to evaluate the scope of the community pharmacy as a community health education center and formulate a procedure. . . ." Thus arose, beginning in 1964, the A.Ph.A.'s continuing project of having a unit for systematic dissemination of health information among subscribing pharmacies.[96]

The concept of making the pharmacist responsible for dispensing safe and effective health information, as well as safe and effective health products, began to move during the late 1960's from the status of an auxiliary service of the minority of practitioners to that of a core-function goal for the majority. The literature, the education, the aspirations of the American pharmacist were changing in the direction of something called "clinical pharmacy." It ranged from trying to minimize the misuse of prescription and non-prescription drugs across the counter of a village pharmacy to teamwork in teaching hospitals for designing drug regimens, monitoring drug actions, and mitigating drug interactions. The transition was slow, although the trend clearly led away from drug making (except as a specialty) and toward drug counseling and control based

→

The redoubtable Susan Hayhurst, pharmacist and physician (1820–1909), had charge of the pharmacy in the Woman's Hospital of Philadelphia for nearly three decades, and also conducted a community pharmacy on Locust Street. Although not the first woman graduate in pharmacy, she graduated as the only woman in a class of 152 at the Philadelphia College of Pharmacy and during her career encouraged young women in the profession. (From: Pharm. Era, p. 535, Nov. 19, 1903; *ibid.*, p. 432, Oct. 10, 1901) upon a new level and kind of expert information.[97] Often such innovations took root most readily in institutional settings of health care.

## INSTITUTIONAL PHARMACY

The pre-20th century hospital was all too often a stopover on the way to the burial grounds. It was so, not only for lack of aseptic and curative methods, but also for lack of an attitude making the hospital central for the medical care of its time. So while the hospital is medieval in origin, it came to America still largely as a charitable haven for passive recuperation or dying, especially for those who could not afford proper and costly attendance and medical care at home.

Early American hospitals thus could scarcely have offered either attractive scope or income to the most capable pharmacists for in-house careers. Much remains to be clarified historically about the place of pharmacy in such institutions. It would not be surprising to learn that pharmacy was fused with medicine, as it was in the public shops that we encountered previously on the streets of early American cities—in that hybrid tradition that had come to seem peculiarly British. Before the early 19th century at least, the scattering of hospital "apothecaries" in America as in England probably did "combine pharmaceutical with medical and nursing functions, such as caring for surgical instruments, administering medicines, visiting the sick; and, in the absence of the physician and surgeon, caring for emergencies."[98]

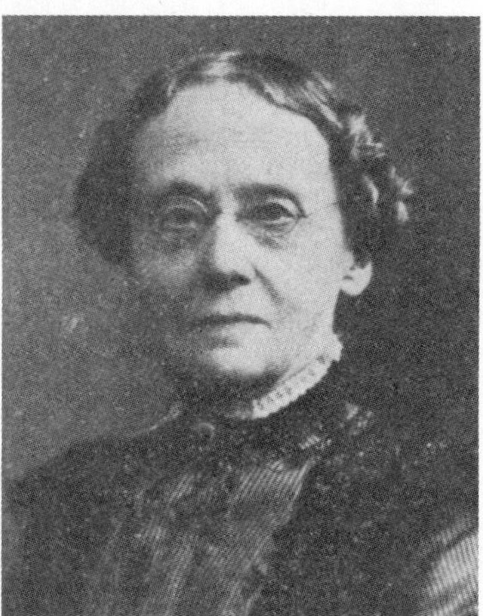

At the first American hospital, opened at Philadelphia in 1751, the attending physicians soon had an assortment of drugs sent over from London, as noted earlier. Having "opened an Apothecary's Shop in the Hospital, and it being found necessary, [they] appointed an Apothecary to attend and make up the Medicines daily, according to the Prescriptions. . . . " When the first apprentice was taken on at the Pennsylvania Hospital "to learn the art, trade and mystery of an apothecary," his indenture made clear that he was obligated not to fornicate, marry or gamble; but this was a standard for any indentured apprentice.[99]

At Old Blockley (which originated in an almshouse and later became part of Philadelphia General Hospital) the apothecary employed in-house, at least between 1788 and 1816, was expected to prepare medications prescribed by attending physicians, but also to "perform certain clinical work," such as "to cup and bleed in the medical ward."[100]

The second institution opened in America, the New-York Hospital, initially authorized an "apothecary," but apparently did not put one on duty until after 1790. His principal domain was an "apothecary's shop" 20 by 16½ feet in size; but he also had certain clinical duties, such as making rounds with the house surgeon, from which he had to "be prepared to report on the state of the patients to the visiting physicians and surgeons" (1804). Six years later this duty of the apothecary disappeared from the hospital's bylaws, becoming the duty of a physician. In 1811, when the hospital published its first formulary, the hospital's regulations set out a

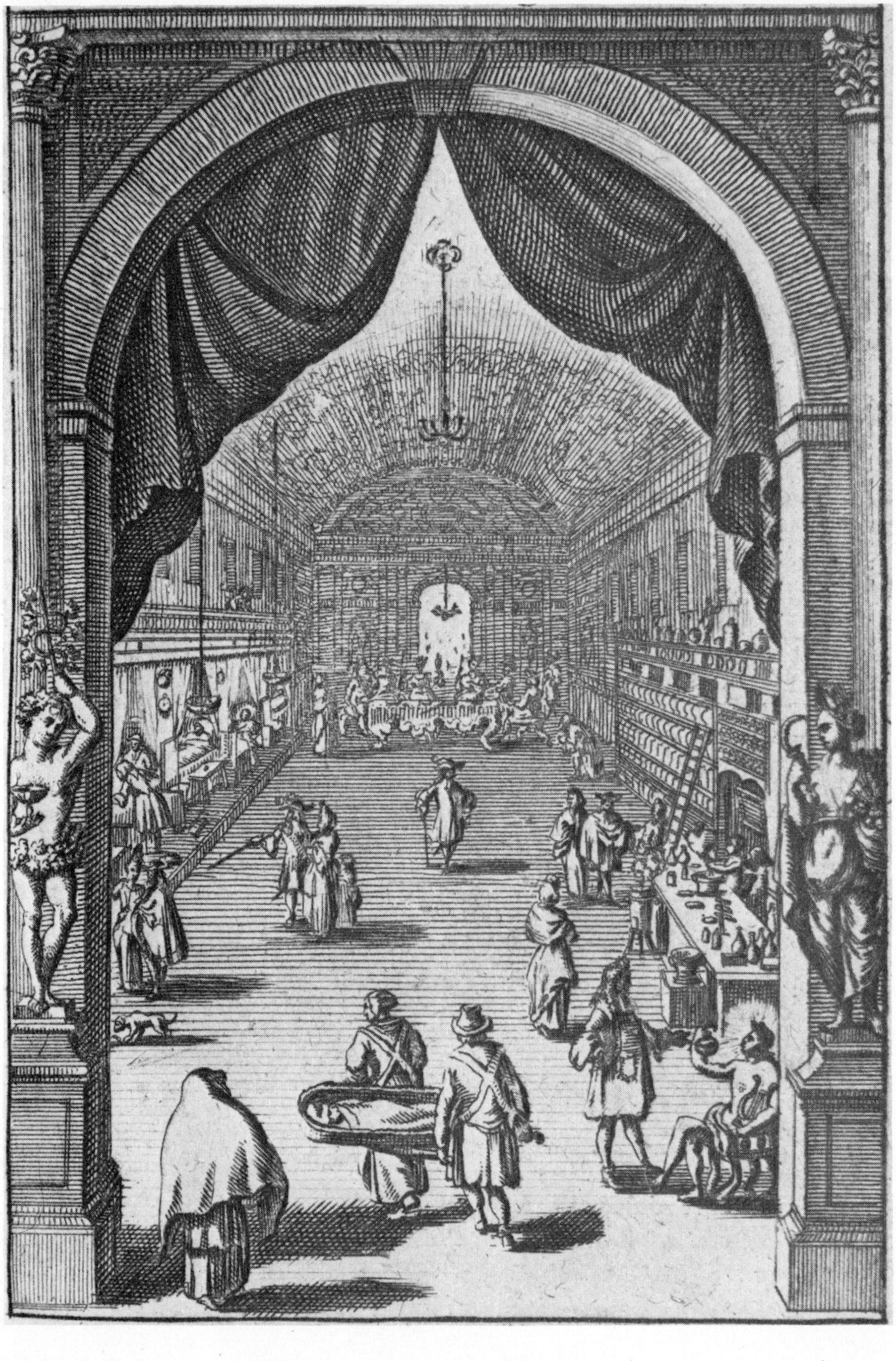

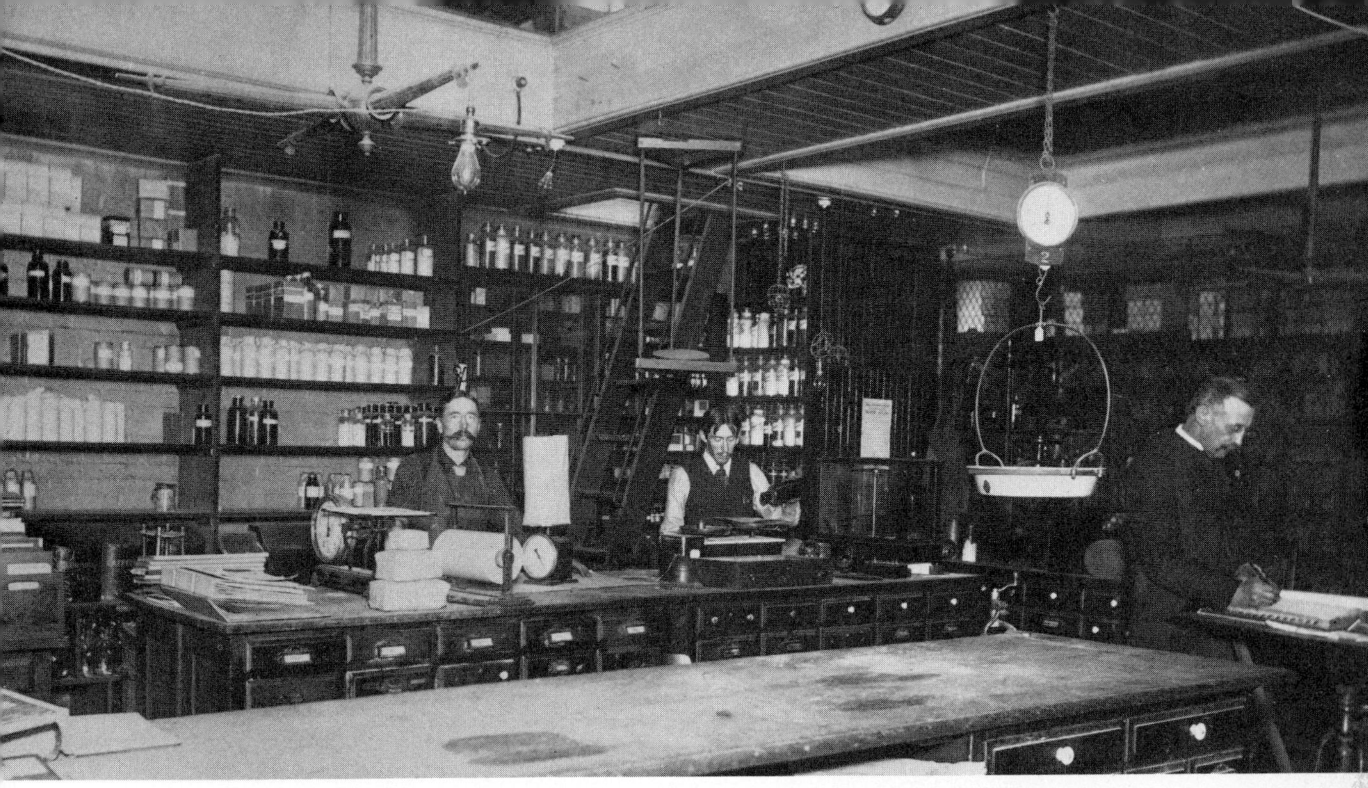

Part of the drug department of Bellevue Hospital, New York City, in the late 19th century, while Charles Rice served there as chemist. One of the most eminent American hospital pharmacists of the century, Rice headed three revisions of the U.S. Pharmacopeia, helped found the National Formulary, and influenced pharmacy by his writing and editing. (From: Pharmaceutical Library, University of Wisconsin, Madison)

rather clear picture of what was expected of such an apothecary, which said in part:

> The Apothecary shall compound and make up all medicines prescribed, agreeably to the formulae from time to time directed by the physicians and surgeons of the hospital. He shall deliver no medicines which are not ordered by the attending physicians or surgeons, and shall permit no medicines to be carried out of the house, except to out-door patients. He shall put up the medicines intended for each ward separately and shall annex to them labels, containing the names of the patients for whom they are respectively prescribed; and, when necessary, directions for taking them. And he shall send them to each ward by the orderly man, to be by him distributed to the patients.[101]

Whatever the qualifications of the pharmacists who staffed these early hospitals, few left a mark in history as did Charles Rice (1841–1901) of Bellevue Hospital in New York City and Martin I. Wilbert (1865–1916) of the German Hospital in Philadelphia; or, in her own way, Susan Hayhurst, Philadelphia graduate of 1883, who served the Women's Hospital as pharmacist for 33 years and was preceptor to many young women who otherwise found it hard to find places for training in pharmacy.[101a] Until after World War I, American hospital pharmacy appears to have remained a quiet tributary of the profession; and indeed many hospitals as then

←

The hospital setting nurtured professional development of pharmacy in Western Europe, as it had earlier in the Middle East, and would later under American conditions in the 20th century. In this idealized Dutch engraving of 1701, a pharmacy occupies most of the right wall. Beyond the work counter for compounding drugs stretch long rows of containers for bulk medicaments. Along the left wall are curtained cubicles for patients. (From: National Library of Medicine; frontispiece of N. Venette: Venus minsieke Gasthuis, Amsterdam, 1701) constituted got along without the pharmacist's services altogether.

During the early 20th century hospital pharmacy began to change, to come alive, partly because the hospital system changed. A new model had been set by hospitals following the prototype of the Johns Hopkins Hospital during the last quarter of the 19th century; the American Hospital Association began to make its influence felt after its founding in 1899. After the turn of the century the American Medical Association took up the cause of hospital reforms, and thrust beyond them to a new concept: that hospitals should be carefully organized for the best service of the patients, the training of personnel, and the progress of medicine.[102] The journal *Modern Hospital* became a vigorous exponent of the new American hospital—inspired by its social role, based on the cure and prevention of disease in every citizen, and supporting and being supported by burgeoning specialization. By the first World War, Lendefeld concludes, the foundation had been built and accepted, to be implemented in the postwar years.

The structure of this new hospital system—with its emphasis upon specialties, efficient management, and therapeutic effectiveness—created opportunities for hospital pharmacists of a different type as well as number. American pharmacy soon sensed the spirit of change. By the early 1920's hospital pharmacists became more visible in the journals of American pharmacy; pharmacist E. C. Austin of the Cincinnati General Hospital observed "that there has arisen a greater demand for hospital pharmacists" (1921) and good ones were scarce; the President of the A.Ph.A. spoke of "the exacting and responsible nature of their service, together with the fact that it is so largely along professional lines . . . ;" hospital pharmacists became active contributors to the A.Ph.A.'s Section on Practical Pharmacy and Dispensing, but it would be 1936 before a specific Subsection on Hospital Pharmacy organized. A number of state groups of hospital pharmacists also organized in the 1930's, for which the only precedent apparently was the Hospital Pharmacy Association of Southern California (f. 1925).

In 1932 Edward Spease, dean of pharmacy at Western Reserve University, foresaw a time "when hospitals will demand pharmacists trained in hospital pharmacy." Alex Berman has pointed out Spease's pioneer role in fostering special education and internships for institutional practice, and in working with M. T. MacEachern of the American College of Surgeons in developing minimum standards for hospital pharmacies accepted by the College in 1936, which met analogous response in the American Hospital Association.[103]

The American Society of Hospital Pharmacists emerged as an independent organization in 1942 (see p. 208)—then A.Ph.A.-affiliated but supplanting the Subsection—and signalled new stature and goals for this specialty. What could scarcely be foreseen was the transformation that would occur within a quarter century to bring the hospital pharmacist out of his basement "drug room" and into an unprecedented professional enthusiasm and stature in the history of American pharmacy. This trend gathered strength not only from farsighted leaders of the caliber of H. A. K. Whitney, Donald E. Francke, and others, but also from the expansion of facilities across the country made possible by the Hill-Burton Act, and the impact of voluntary and compulsory health insurance plans. Not the least factors in this trend were the environment and expectations to which many hospital pharmacists responded as the mainstream of medical care gradually shifted from private medical offices and pharmacy shops into structured, integrated, well organized work settings. These were not only hospitals, but clinics, group practices and extended-care facilities. Since the 1940's particularly it has offered American pharmacists an opportunity to return "to the basic purpose for the existence of pharmacy as their primary objective." Looking back from the early 1960's, the Audit of Pharmaceuticical Service in Hospitals expressed this purpose as essentially "to provide pharmaceutical services as an integral part of the total patient care concept in the interest, safety, and welfare of the public health . . . the only basis for the existence of pharmacy as a profession. It is because of this prime motivating force," the Audit suggested, "that we have realized tremendous progress in hospital pharmacy during the past two decades."[104]

Since 1957, the pharmacy has been included among the essential services of the hospital by the Joint Commission on Accreditation of Hospitals, and, indeed, has been described as "the most extensively used of the therapeutic facilities of the hospital."[105]

Moreover, the hospital pharmacist had moved by the 1960's into a position of considerable autonomy of professional planning and action, reflected in the respect accorded him by hospital administrators, which contrasts with his status before the 1930's.[106] The pharmacy had evolved from a storage room for medical materiel into, commonly, the focal point for all activities related to drugs, except their prescribing and administration to patients. By the 1970's even these latter two activities were becoming linked to pharmaceutical services, as "clinical pharmacists" trained to an advanced level moved out from the pharmacy itself onto the wards in close contact with other professional personnel and the patients themselves—especially in teaching hospitals where new role models and modified methods for medical care at large were being tested.

Although great progress had been made within a few decades in services, in physicial facilities and, not least, in *esprit de corps*, the Audit had shown concretely how wide the disparities, how great the range of pharmacy resources, even within hospitals of a given bed capacity.

In 1957 an estimated 5833 pharmacists were practicing in American hospitals (including 988 part-time). Of the hospitals having less than 100 beds only about 14 per cent had the services of a pharmacist, and during the ensuing years a trend developed for smaller institutions (nursing homes as well as hospitals) to have satellite pharmacies serviced either from a larger hospital or from a community pharmacy. A secondary role for the pharmacist as purchasing agent or as supervisor of central sterile supply in the hospital has made a full-time position for a pharmacist feasible in many small institutions.

About four hospital pharmacies in 10 of the early 1960's were still undertaking manufacturing or bulk compounding while it had disappeared completely from community pharmacies, and about the same proportion were preparing at least some of their sterile solutions for topical use.[107] This persistence of the traditional drug-making function has been related to institutional scale, a greater tendency in the institutional setting for physicians sometimes to utilize forms of medication not commercially available, and ths increasing availability of auxiliary personnel on pharmacy staffs in recent decades. The structure of institutional services since about midcentury has increasingly included pharmaceutical and therapeutic consulting services, which involves most hospital pharmacists, but to different degrees (mostly unquantified, although the trend seems clear). Such interactions with other health-care personnel often are much modified by the amount of printed information flowing from the pharmacy into nursing and clinic units as well as by the amount of "detailing" by manufacturers' representatives, which "has increased enormously during recent years as the percentage of the ethical drug market in hospitals has continued to rise . . . ," the Audit reported. By 1970 about four-tenths of all prescriptions dispensed in the United States were dispensed through hospital pharmacies, which numbered about one-tenth of all pharmacies.[108]

The dollar volume of hospital drug purchases from commercial laboratories had more than tripled between 1961 and 1973, but as a proportion of the total prescription-drug market in the United States, one study suggested, hospital usage remained during this period in the range of 22 to 25 per cent of the total.[109]

A balance wheel in the mechanism for pharmaceutical service in hospitals was the pervasive adoption of a formulary system, administered by a pharmacy and therapeutics committee. Several of the early pharmaceutical publications in America may properly be considered hospital formularies (see pp. 169 and 258); but only since the 1930's has the modern concept been widely applied. This hinged on a formal liaison between the hospital pharmacist and the medical staff. After the concept of a pharmacy committee (with a pharmacist as permanent secretary) became embedded in the Minimum Standard for Hospital Pharmacies of the American College of Surgeons (largely attributable to Edward Spease and Robert Porter of Cleveland), the systematic evaluation and selection of the medicinal agents and established policies of drug control and use within a particular hospital became more common. These policies were to be communicated and to become effective largely through the mechanism of a hospital formulary.

Substituting the group judgment of staff physicians and pharmacists, to some extent, for the free exercise of prescribing by the individual staff physician and for the free play of commercial selling techniques by drug manufacturers, the formulary system became periodically controversial both locally and nationally. A particular irritant to manufacturers during the 1950's and later was the concept by which a staff physician gave the hospital pharmacist "prior consent" to select the brand of a drug product to be dispensed, within the guidelines of the hospital's formulary. This culminated in a multi-society effort to ease the friction by generating "A Statement of Guiding Principles on the Operation of the Hospital Formulary System" (first version, 1960).[110]

Such activities perforce gave the most progressive hospital pharmacists a clinical orientation before clinical pharmacy emerged as a distinctive concept and program in academic pharmaceutical education. H. A. K. Whitney at the University of Michigan Hospital and Donald A. Clarke at the New York Hospital were on the cutting edge of this development, which was formalized after the late 1940's by the first graduate programs offering a Master's degree combined with a hospital residency.

The hospital as an interdisciplinary education center for the average student of pharmacy, however, did not become firmly linked to most schools until after the 1960's, with the help of federal funding of clinical faculties. From that base, institutional pharmacy moved off purposefully in a new direction.[111]

## WHOLESALE ESTABLISHMENTS

There is some doubt whether European professional pharmacies evolved from the early general store or from the pharmaceutical work done by monks in the monasteries. Probably both conjectures are true. However, there is no doubt that in continental Europe dispensing pharmacy existed before the specialized wholesale drug trade came into being. The North American continent offers the paradox that here the wholesale drug trade came first.

Like most paradoxes, this one surprises only when first presented. In Europe, with its comparatively early separation of medicine and pharmacy, the pharmacists from the 13th century on met the medicinal needs of the population. They were collectors of crude drugs and, on a small scale, manufacturers, buying limited amounts of imported drugs. It was not until the 17th century that the use of imported drugs had grown to a considerable extent, and not until the late

18th century that independent manufacturing on a large scale began to supersede the preparative work within the pharmacies. With this change, an organized wholesale trade in medicinals could establish itself.

This development could not take place in America. As noted previously, the medical and the medicinal needs of the populace in colonial times had to be met by the same persons. Although indigenous plants were collected and used, the official therapy of the colonies was that of Europe, more particularly that of England. This necessitated importation on a large scale. So a wholesale drug trade was organized at an early date, since most American medicopharmaceutical practitioners wanted to employ the same pharmaceutical products that the pharmacists in Europe at that time usually prepared themselves. Thus it came about that American professional pharmacy became the legitimate offspring of the wholesale business. The country doctors had to be supplied with necessary drugs by someone in a not-too-distant town. An opportunity thus arose for locally restricted wholesale trade in drugs usually in combination with retail trade.

This condition continued to a large extent until the Civil War. For example, it was not until 1868 that George A. Kelly of Pittsburgh disposed of his retail shops and devoted himself entirely to the wholesale business. Based on import, the American wholesale trade in drugs had its first centers in the great seaports in Philadelphia, New York, Boston, Baltimore and New Orleans. Later on the trade followed the inland waterways. Important establishments sprang up in cities farther south and west (such as Pittsburgh, Cleveland, Cincinnati, Detroit, St. Louis and Chicago and finally in California).

Some of the wholesale drug firms, founded between the end of the 18th century and the Civil War, survive today. The oldest was the Schieffelin Company in New York (founded 1794), which continued the wholesale part of its operation until 1963.[112] Henry H. Schieffelin, second in the long chain of members of the family heading the growing concern, was among the founders and early leaders of the College of Pharmacy of the City of New York.

As new territories were opened and rapidly settled, canals and railroads built, and the telegraph invented, the opportunities for wholesale trade seemed to be inexhaustible. However, this picture of progress had its reverse side. The period was over in which the retail or sub-wholesale druggist traveled once or twice a year to his wholesaler "in the East" to purchase a large stock. Now the broker entered the picture. A new kind of competition started. The Civil War interrupted the development, but only to give way to a new boom.

Tempted by short cuts to wealth, men rushed into business "imbued with the idea of 'getting there first.'"[113] Adulteration, short-weight and reprisals sometimes crept into business. In the wholesale drug field, destructive competition was the order of the day. Price, not quality, often governed. In 1876 representative wholesale druggists of the Middle West met in Cincinnati and founded the Western Wholesale Druggist's Association, which later became the present National Wholesale Druggists Association. The organization was created to "correct excessive and unmercantile competition" and remove "evils and customs that are against good policy and sound business principles."[114] Its members gained a key position in the drug trade, serving not only as a foremost supply agency for community pharmacy but as its advisor and promoter.

Between 1930 and 1958 the number of wholesaling drug merchants approximately doubled. By 1963 there were nearly 4000 (including both general-line and specialty-line houses). The total sales, about $2.8 billions in 1958, had nearly quadrupled in three decades, paralleling the growth in dollar volume noted in community pharmacies.[115]

The wholesaling margin has been kept relatively low—both in relation to earlier dec-

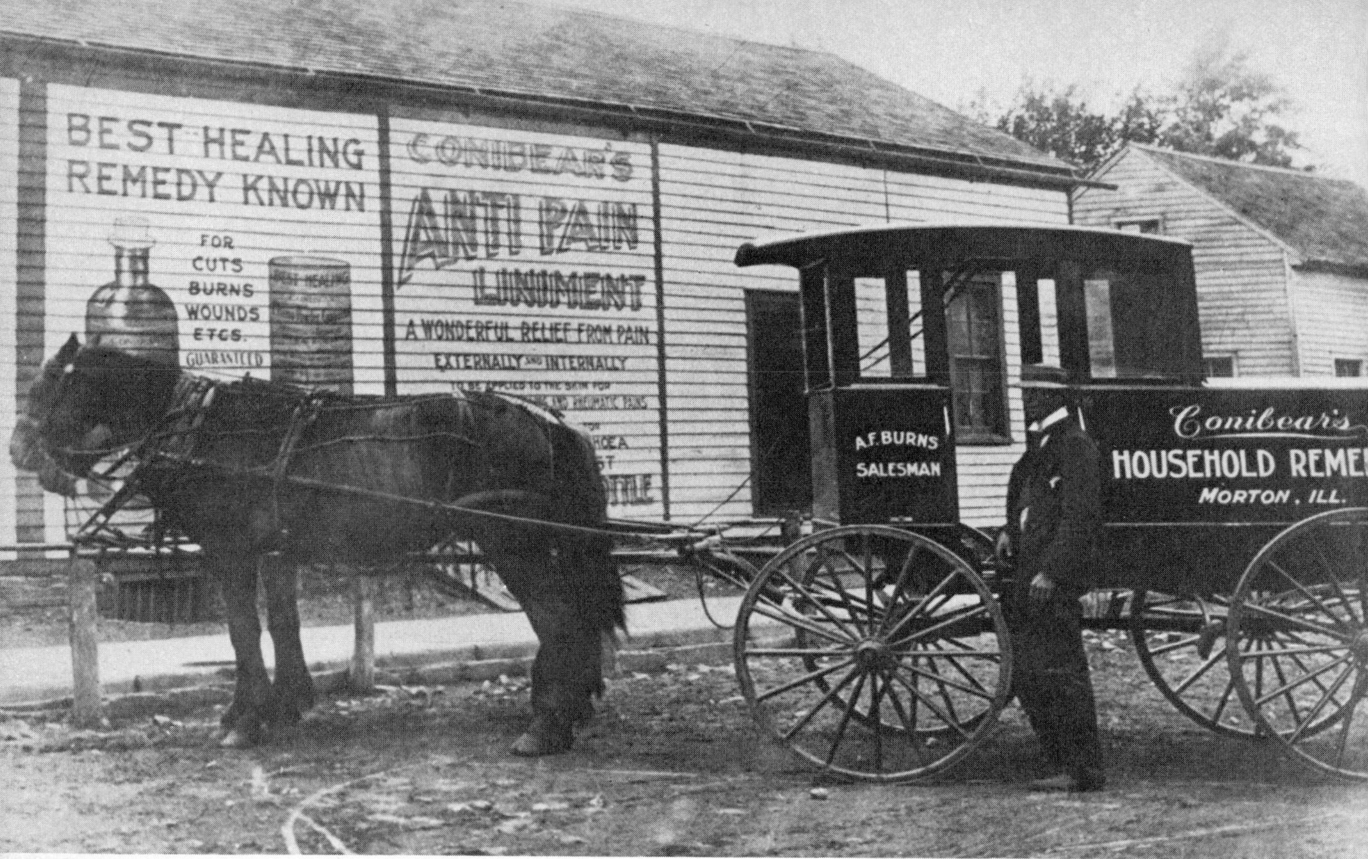


This old-fashioned delivery service contrasts with the illustration opposite. Probably photographed in the 1890's, the drummer's wagon was one of six that sold within a 30-mile radius about 275 products put up under the Conibear label. This regional enterprise grew out of the local Conibear Drugstore, and had its counterparts in other states. A majority of such regional distributors eventually disappeared rather than growing into a nationally known brand. (From: Edward Lewis, Jr., Canton, Ill.)

ades and to certain other fields of wholesaling—by various pressures. For example, wholesale houses that specialize in drugs and medical supplies (as contrasted with N.W.D.A.'s full-service wholesale druggists) developed as a distinct movement within the field, of which one evidence was the separate Pharmaceutical Wholesalers Association—which merged with the Federal Wholesale Druggists Association in 1974 under the title, International Pharmaceutical Distributors Association.[116]

Especially since World War II, more manufacturers had been establishing branch depots in major cities, not only to supply wholesalers but to increase direct selling to pharmacists (often offering price inducements). While some drug manufacturers were by-passing the wholesale druggist, others were reducing the discounts allowed to the wholesaler for his services. These shifts in marketing practices produced economic uncertainties and readjustments since the early 1960's in the drug distribution system. Had pharmaceutical products come to bear a disproportionate share of distribution costs in a commercialized system of pharmacy that embraced such a vast range of disparate types of products? Editor Wallace Werble, in 1961, expressed at least

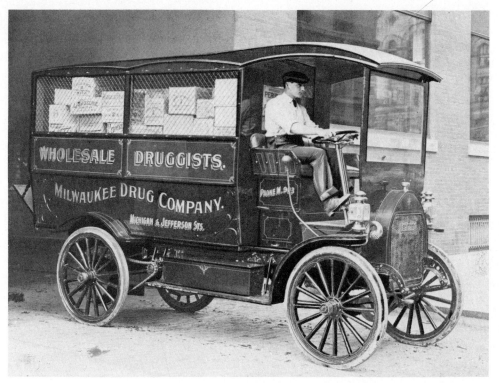


Ultra-modern service was represented by this delivery truck when it was put on the road (about 1912), reportedly the first used by a wholesale druggist in Milwaukee. The entire development of drug wholesaling has been based primarily on quick supply of health products in small quantities drawn from diverse, worldwide sources. (From: George A. Moule)

serious doubt that a marketing system in which life or death therapeutic agents are used to carry part of the costs of distributing other less vital products can survive in our present stage of economic and social development.[117]

However, whatever competitive experiments might be tried, there seemed to be little question that the system would continue to hold a place and function for the wholesale druggist. In 1880 proprietary drugs were on the market in 2,700 different items and sizes. A few years later, this amount had almost doubled, and thereafter increased enormously. "The industry assumed that it had reached an absolute limit in 1916 when the wholesaler was able to list some 38,000 different items and sizes," but by 1933 the total was 60,000. "This has meant that the retailer . . . has become increasingly dependent on the 'stockroom' facilities" of the wholesale druggist, offering immediate delivery in small quantity. Yet, the wholesale druggist has not been left complacent by the diversification, conglomerates, voluntaries, and mutuals that have scrambled established patterns and practices of pharmaceutical distributors during the late 20th century.

## MANUFACTURING PHARMACY

Changes since the mid-18th century have transformed the array of drugs available and the way of making them. This is rooted in fundamental changes undergone by the underlying sciences and technology, in some progress toward understanding the inner biological environment where drugs have their consequences, and in a transition from the handicraft of "little business" to a bureaucratized and mechanized "big business" dependent upon the interplay of large-scale production and large-scale promotion.

The modern manufacturing laboratory, with its big-business aura, had its beginnings to a large extent in that epitome of little business, the community pharmacy—in Europe and, later on to a lesser extent, in America. Two other types of small-scale preindustrial workshops had contributed knowledge of equipment and processes useful to pharmacy, but they were too preoccupied in other directions to constitute the main framework of a new form of drug manufacture. The alchemist's laboratory was oriented toward such "blue sky" ventures as astrological wizardry and the Elixir of Life. The mining-metallurgical laboratory had a contrasting orientation toward subterranean matters, with traditionally defined tasks. In the pharmacy, however, was the right combination of equipment, knowledge and experience that often provided a nucleus for industrialized production of drugs.

Already in the 17th century, and earlier, some individual substances used in medicine had been manufactured in Europe on a larger scale, but by neither intention nor potential were they to replace the compounding of drugs behind the pharmacist's prescription counter. In America before the 19th century, the majority of the drugs needed were imported from Europe, either intermediates or the finished drug products. Medicinal chemicals made in the American colonies before the Revolution are notable mainly as limited exceptions to customary imports. Glauber's Salt and Epsom Salt were being produced by selective evaporation (John Sears at Cape Cod) before the end of the 18th century, for example. Less a manufacturer but better known was the previously mentioned governor of the Connecticut colony (John Winthrop, Jr.), who made some medicinal chemicals in the mid-17th century, and ministered medically to the colonists. The Revolutionary War made it hard to import drugs, which stimulated home production on a small scale in a few of the better pharmacies.[118]

In 1778 Apothecary General Andrew Craigie initiated and later on managed "a general laboratory" in which medicines for the needs of the military hospitals and the fighting army were prepared. Only 3 years after the war (1786), the firm of Christopher, Jr., and Charles Marshall, wholesale and retail druggists in Philadelphia, "entered quite extensively into the business of making muriate of ammonia and Glauber's salt,"[119] being probably the first to produce pharmaceutical chemicals in this country on a large scale

The Marshalls were exceptional for the late 18th century. It was more particularly in the decades from about 1820 to 1840 that small beginnings of what would become large-scale drug manufacturing can be seen taking shape. A strategic combination of science, geography and economics made Philadelphia the focus for the new industry.

Transition of the famous Marshall pharmacy after 1825, under the management of Ellis and Morris, signalled the change. They

promptly expanded the laboratory, installing a boiler in the cellar and turning the second story into a drying room and storage warehouse. They equipped themselves with a jacketed copper pan, a filter press, and open furnaces and soon became makers of pharmaceuticals, specializing in solid extracts and a line of old English proprietary drugs. They improvised a series of oil barrels for coating 75 yards of cloth with adhesive plasters, a mechanism they later expanded to coat 2,000 yards in a single batch. In 1850 they moved into a real factory building, abandoning the retail business and introducing steam-driven stirring and grinding apparatus.[120]

The Philadelphia wholesale and retail druggist, Samuel P. Wetherill and Company announced in 1826, for example, that they were "now engaged in manufacturing on a large scale a variety of paints and drugs," among them "Tartaric Acid, Sup. Carb. of Soda, Rochelle Salt, Lunar Caustic, Red Precipitate, White Precipitate, Nitrate of Ammonia, Corrosive Sublimate, Blue Vitriol, Spirit of Hartshorn, Carbonate of Soda, Calomel, Sulphate of Quinine, Alcohol, Sulphuric Aether."[121]

In 1830 the Philadelphia wholesale and retail druggist John Elliott likewise offered "articles of his own manufacture," including some of the products mentioned above, and tartar emetic and Seidlitz salts.[122]

All these men were among the founders of the Philadelphia College of Pharmacy. John Farr, also a member of the College since its founding, established a manufacturing plant (1818). The firm of Farr and Kunzi commenced the manufacture of quinine (1822), only two years after its isolation from cinchona bark had been reported in France. After the druggists Thomas H. Powers and William Weightman became partners, the firm continued to gain in renown, and under the name Powers and Weightman (1847) it attained an international reputation for the manufacture of medicinal and other fine chemicals, at a time when American pharmaceutical industry in general was still in its infancy.[123]

Another early Philadelphia manufactory important to the development of pharmaceutical chemistry in this country was that of Rosengarten and Sons (f. 1822). The firm was the first to produce quinine sulfate in the United States. "They manufactured Morphine Salts in 1832, Piperine in 1833, Mercurials and Strychnine in 1834, Veratrine in 1835 and . . . Codeine, Bismuth and Silver Salts in 1836."[124]

The trend toward consolidation after 1900 brought about (1905) the amalgamation of Powers and Weightman with Rosengarten and Sons.[125] Then, Merck and Company of New York absorbed (1927) Powers-Weightman-Rosengarten Company.[126]

In 1841 another well-known Philadelphia pharmaceutical manufacturer, the Smith, Kline and French Company, got its start from a small pharmacy that had been founded by George K. Smith.[127]

Before the Civil War, Philadelphia thus was the most important center for manufacturing prescription products, but not the only one even then.

Some of the oldest manufacturing laboratories still producing are Caswell-Massey Co. Ltd. (beginning as a pharmacy) and Schieffelin & Co. of New York (beginning mainly as a wholesale house), the unusual Tilden Company (specializing in botanical drugs) and The Wm. S. Merrell Co. of Cincinnati (f. 1828). The latter firm, as well as the firm of H. M. Merrell and Company of Cincinnati (which later became Lloyd Brothers), worked successfully in the so-called eclectic field (see p. 175), using indigenous plants as the basis of manufacturing.[128] Tilden likewise grew to importance in eclectic medicine. The firm originated in the Shaker community at Lebanon, N.Y., organizing commercial production around 1847, when the Shaker religious community already had been marketing medicinal herbs for a quarter century.[129]

## Two Case Histories

Manufacturing pharmacy repeatedly has been stimulated by the medicinal needs of wartime, and it was largely in response to demands of the Civil War that the American industry took the decisive step into maturity. Two firms that will serve to illustrate the development were founded before the conflict, then proved their usefulness and improved their business during the war to such an extent that they became leaders in the field: Frederick Stearns and Company of Detroit (absorbed by Winthrop in 1944) and E. R.

Squibb & Sons of Brooklyn. The founders did more than create a prosperous business. By example and by incessantly emphasizing the ideal of purity, uniformity and reliability as the most important basis of manufacturing therapeutic products, they gave recognition to a pharmaceutical responsibility that goes beyond ordinary business. It was bold policy at a time when rugged individualism and unprincipled competition had reached virulent intensity in the business community.

The manner in which Stearns started his work was characteristic. His original "laboratory" was a 12 by 12-foot back room in his pharmacy in Detroit (f. 1855). Without capital he could not manufacture a stock of medicaments. Samples were, therefore, prepared, for him to show to druggists on trips through the state and, upon his return, the would-be manufacturer made the drugs for which he had orders.[130] It was the Civil War, in which Stearns acted as medical purveyor for the Michigan troops, that caused the small laboratory of his pharmacy to develop into a plant covering the entire floor space of a four-story building, equipped with steam power, milling machinery and extraction apparatus. Gradually the concern grew into an establishment known the world over. This success would have meant more to the owners of the firm than to pharmacy, had it not been the result of a new idea of general importance. This "new idea" (started in 1876 and fostered after 1879 by a house organ called the *New Idea*) was the creation of "popular non-secret family medicines" to counteract the branded nostrums—whose composition often remained secret from pharmacists and laymen alike, thus giving free reign to increasingly massive and dishonest promotional schemes.

> Disgusted with the rampant quackery of the time, Mr. Stearns resolved to offer a few simple preparations in popular-sized packages, bearing full directions for use and in addition a plain statement of the names and quantities of their ingredients. . . . Other druggists, lacking Mr. Stearns' manufacturing facilities, adopted the plan and had him manufacture and finish similar preparations for them, bearing their names. And from this beginning it spread over the country and within a few years had extended even to the Old World, so great was its popularity.[131]

The development of the Squibb firm differed from that of Stearns in much the same way as did the two men whose ideas were realized in the two manufacturing laboratories. Stearns was the practical druggist, not without scientific knowledge, but led primarily by his practical sense and by his desire to improve the practice of pharmacy. Squibb was an educated physician who had learned the practice of pharmacy through 5 years of apprenticeship before he took up the study of medicine.[132] He had a firm knowledge of pharmacy, but he was led primarily by his scientific interests and his desire to improve the practice of medicine. Stearns had created public formulas for medicaments, and placed them at the disposal of pharmacists for over-the-counter sale primarily. Squibb found new ways to prepare purer and more reliable products and placed this improved medicinal armament at the disposal of physicians for prescribing or dispensing.

In the naval service (1847 to 1857) Squibb had first been a surgeon and then (1852) assistant director of the pharmaceutical laboratory of the Navy. A year after his return to civilian life, Squibb was induced to establish (1858) a moderate-sized laboratory of his own by the Chief Medical Purveyor of the Army. However, it soon became evident that the medicinal needs of a peace-time Army of 25,000 men could not support even a laboratory of that size.

It was his medical friends who, recognizing the value to the medical profession of a drug manufacturer of his type, saved the young establishment from ruin in the first difficult years. When the laboratory building was entirely destroyed by fire (1858), these physicians furnished Squibb the capital necessary to rebuild.

Only 2 years later the Civil War broke out,

"The needs of the army became very large, and additional buildings were hired and equipped. . . . In 1862 another site was purchased and a large and commodious laboratory was erected." The description of what went on in this four-story building, with hand operations by upwards of 40 employees, survives from an inspection ordered by the Surgeon General of the Army, giving us one of the most concrete and vivid contemporary accounts of the pharmaceutical industry at that time.[133] A steam engine (25 h.p.) turned three mills for powdering the crude (basic) drugs, and probably it also powered grinding and sifting apparatus nearby. A steam-driven machine was utilized (not later than 1865) for triturating certain drugs. The traditional rows of copper kettles, percolators, and stills were there, to be gradually improved but not displaced.

Squibb's earliest and most valuable contributions to medicine were the new methods developed by him for the preparation of chemically pure ether and pure chloroform, products whose use almost completely rid anesthetization of the dangers which had been associated with it. One of Squibb's great services to pharmacy was his research on percolation, the results of which he published for the benefit of the profession at large.[134]

Frederick Stearns, as well as E. R. Squibb, actively supported the endeavor to elevate the general standard of American pharmacy. Stearns served the American Pharmaceutical Association as second vice-president and as president, Squibb as first vice-president then declined to be elected president, as he also declined the presidency of the American Medical Association.

## Revolution in Technology

The manufacturers of the late 19th century not only applied but helped to develop the machine technics that eventually removed from community pharmacies their age-old function of making drug products. American contributions to percolation (notably by E. R. Squibb, J. I Grahame and Wm. Procter, Jr., between 1845 and 1875) gave initial impetus to the development of processes of drug extraction that, although often adaptable to the prescription laboratory, were never considered very practicable by the majority of practitioners. The familiar hand plaster-iron gradually was laid aside after a Philadelphia pharmacist (Robert Shoemaker, 1838) "successfully developed a process for making plasters other than by hand and became a large manufacturer of this article.[135] Although sugar-coated pills, as well as gelatine capsules, were a French innovation of the 1830's, in America it was another Philadelphia pharmacist (William R. Warner, 1866) who became one of the first and certainly most successful of the large-scale manufacturers of sugar-coated pills.[136] Warner likewise introduced to American practice small pills ("parvules," 1879) that could be produced only on a large scale.

Compressed and coated tablets pushed the production of this form of medication still further beyond the range of the average prescription laboratory. The first compressed-tablet machine in America, a simple hand punch, was constructed by a Philadelphia druggist (Jacob Dunton, 1864; similar to an English invention by William Brockedon, 1843), although the first automatic power machines (single-punch and rotary) did not come into use until 1874–1875.[137] The biological products that came into use after the turn of the century, and the antibiotics from the 1940's onward, were still less suited to processing in a local pharmacy.

With each such innovation, the number of large-scale drug manufacturers grew. Although rather efficient apparatus for small-scale manufacture became available, few pharmacists outside hospitals could resist the blandishments and the economies proffered by mass-production laboratories. Indeed, a substantial proportion of practicing pharmacists were not well prepared by education for a modern manufacturing role until

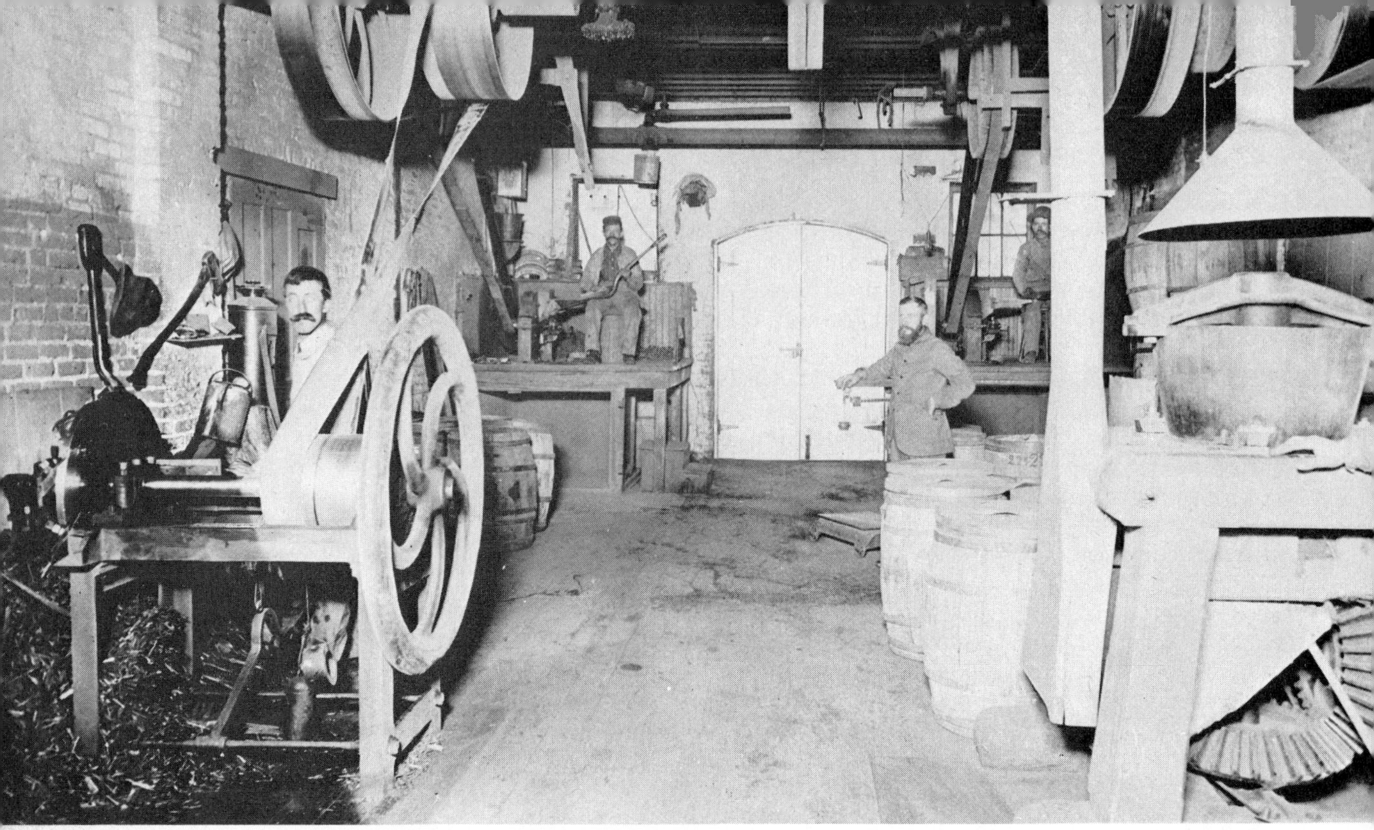

It seemed an exciting technologic advance when both the man-powered contusion mortar of centuries-old tradition and the horse-powered drug mill were outmoded after the mid-19th century, as steam engines were linked to high-speed grinding machines for medicinal barks, roots, and other parts of plants then still utilized. Machines in the foreground reduced woods *(left)* and barks *(right)* to a size small enough to feed through the drug grinders in the background (capable of 3000 rpm). (From: Pharmaceutical Library, University of Wisconsin)

after local production had become scarcely feasible economically. Moreover, successive changes in food and drug regulation during the present century made it increasingly difficult for small-scale manufacturing laboratories to meet all legal and scientific requirements.[138]

### After the Civil War

After the Civil War the number of pharmaceutical manufacturing firms increased rapidly. For example, S. P. Duffield formed a partnership (1867) with H. C. Parke, which after 4 years became Parke, Davis and Company. The Detroit firm, like most of its predecessors and many of its successors, started with the production of only "a few chemicals" and "a line of fluid extracts."[139] But as early as 1902, Parke, Davis and Company established its own research institute, one of the earliest in the whole of American industry.

One after the other, pharmaceutical manufacturing plants arose from modest beginnings to large establishments (ca. 1860–1880), some of them of world-wide importance. Often they traveled the same course, from the preparation of galenicals (often starting with fluid extracts), to the preparation of a few chemicals, progressing through research to a systematic production of certain groups of chemicals, biologicals, and antibiotics.

For example, when A. P. Sharp, Louis Dohme and Charles E. Dohme, all graduates of the Maryland College of Pharmacy, organized the firm of Sharp and Dohme (1860) in Baltimore, "they first undertook the manufacture of galenical preparations and did not enter the field of chemical manufacturing until 1886, when they began the production of pure plant principles." In 1929 the company absorbed the H. K. Mulford Company, in Philadelphia, then one of the leading producers of biological products in this country.[140]

The small laboratory opened by the pharmacist and colonel of Civil War fame, Eli Lilly, in Indianapolis (1876) "with cash capital amounting to $700 and goods . . . amounting to $600," started with the production of "fluid extracts, elixirs, syrups, a few wines and then-new liquid pepsine preparations."[141] Not only was the founder an educated pharmacist, his only son and successor, Josiah K. Lilly, graduated from the Philadelphia College of Pharmacy. Eli Lilly and Company became one of the great drug manufacturing laboratories of the world, and the first in America to establish a branch house (Kansas City, Mo., 1882). "What is now known as the scientific division had its beginning in 1886."[142]

Most of the establishments mentioned, constituting important assets of American scientific and commercial life, were founded by pharmacists, although the small laboratory of a pharmacy was not always the nucleus of the later plant.

The establishments emerging after the Civil War first devoted themselves, as previously shown, to the manufacture of galenicals. In their further development until 1917 they concentrated on medicinal plant research and, finally, on the production of biological products. The systematic synthesis and production of organic chemicals, particularly chemotherapeutic agents, came later. The reason was that in the second half of the 19th century, or at least after Kolbe's synthesis of salicylic acid (1874) and Knorr's preparation of antipyrin (1883) the field of pharmaceutical chemistry was dominated by the Germans. Synthetic organic chemistry began to change a large sector of drug manufacture and, ultimately, drug therapy. Exploiting these scientific and commercial weapons shrewdly, Germany kept much of the world, including America, heavily reliant upon her intermediate and finished medicinal chemicals. It required the exigencies of World War I to stimulate national pharmaceutical independence.

So far as there was American production of pharmaceutical chemicals before World War I, it was chiefly based on German research and conducted by people of German origin or at least German scientific education. The firm of Rosengarten and Sons, for example, was founded by German-Swiss people and based essentially on German and partly on French discoveries. It held its own through a whole century, finally amalgamating with Merck and Company.

The Mallinckrodt Chemical Works of St. Louis, one of the few important American firms which specialized from the beginning in the manufacture of "pure chemicals for use in medicine, photography, and the arts," was founded by three brothers of German descent (1867). Two of them had just returned from a four years' residence in Germany where they completed their chemical education.[143]

Some large German firms had their own factories in the United States long before America entered World War I. For example, the American firm of Merck and Company had been started as a branch of the old German mother concern (1891). Likewise, at the end of the 19th century the German essential-oil house of Fritzsche Brothers established laboratories in New Jersey. After separation from the mother concern, its own scientific research developed the American firm into one of the leading establishments of its kind in the world.

## After World War I

Until World War I most products of the German pharmacochemical industry were not manufactured in the United States, but only sold here under protection by American patents. The entrance of America into war against Germany led to legislation to seize these patents and to make them available to American industry.[144]

What these spoils of war meant to American pharmaceutical industry, economically as well as in the quality of the chemicals manufactured here, is exemplified by this comment in Abbott Laboratories catalog of 1925:

> For many years The Abbott Laboratories have manufactured fine medicinal chemicals; but this part of our business received a tremendous impetus during the World War, when we were asked by our Government to undertake the task of producing some of the synthetics formerly procurable only in Germany. The difficulties of making organic medicinals in America have been and still are very great but we are proud of the fact that in spite of the technical complexity of the problems to be dealt with, and in the face of destructive competition from sources intent on breaking the American chemical industry, we have gone steadily forward.

In the list following these remarks, several medicinal compounds of German invention are mentioned as first made in America by Abbott Laboratories (f. 1891, by a Chicago physician), such as chlorazene, dichloramine-T, arsphenamine, neoarsphenamine and sulpharsphenamine.

For a still more obvious example of the influence of the two World Wars (and of postwar politics!) on the American pharmaceutical manufacturing industry, consider the case history of Sterling Drug Incorporated.[145] This steadily and rapidly growing concern, amalgamating into its organization one firm after the other, got its start as a partnership organized in Sistersville, W.Va., for the purpose of manufacturing an analgesic called "Neuralgine" (1900). The founders were a pharmacist, W. E. Weiss, and a friend of his, A. H. Diebold, of Canton, Ohio. The concern grew by adopting advertising as "a guiding principle," and by "product diversification" through purchase of other existing firms, and in 1917 changed its corporate name to Sterling Products, Incorporated. There was progress, but it was slow. The great chance for the firm came after World War I, when the Alien Property Custodian offered for sale the stock of the Bayer Company, Inc., of New York, "created by the German Bayer Company to manufacture and sell Aspirin, physicians' drugs and dyestuffs."

More than a hundred American firms participated in the bidding at the public auction in 1918. Sterling topped all of them by a final bid of $5,310,000. The Aspirin business was continued under the Bayer cross trademark, while the Winthrop Chemical Company, Inc., was organized as a new subsidiary to manufacture the physicians' drugs which had been acquired. The dye business "was sold outright to another company." Trademark difficulties were settled "through a series of contracts with Farbenfabriken vorm. Fried. Bayer & Company of Leverkusen, Germany, the former German owners of American Bayer, and its successor, I. G. Farben . . . " For a time Sterling became a part of Drug Incorporated but resumed its individual identity when (1933) this product of mass amalgamation was dissolved "and its constituents went their several ways." On this basis, expansion assumed a rapid pace. The sales by Sterling in 1918 were $3,801,902; in 1944 they reached $47,678,024, in 1957, $198,703,000 and in 1961, $229,199,000, $594,412,000 in 1970.

Early in 1941, "the company agreed to cancel all contracts made by it or any of its subsidiaries with I. G. Farben, and also to dissociate from its employment all persons who had any previous connection with Farben." After the canceling of all limiting contracts with the Germans (and of all German interests in any of the products of the company),

> Sterling became the strongest competitor of I. G. Farben in the pharmaceutical markets of Latin America . . . . Winthrop's scientists cracked closely guarded German research secrets. It took them only a single year to learn how to make Atabrine on a commercial scale from raw materials

available in the United States. . . . In 1942 the corporate name was changed to Sterling Drug Inc. and the corporate structure revamped through the absorption of 16 domestic subsidiaries into the parent organization . . . to assume more effective operation of an enterprise serving a multiplicity of professions, businesses, countries and peoples.

### Concentration of Industry

The modern trend toward mammoth organization in industry at large has led also to a still-growing pharmaceutical edifice. With the growth of recent decades has come considerable restructuring of the pharmaceutical industry: heavier financial investments in the industry, notably from new outside sources, including the general public; more involvement of "outsiders" in management of the industry, often through purchase or merger; an increased merger movement, especially vertically;[146] and a trend toward diversification (especially amalgamation with producers of home remedies) by some companies formerly specializing in producing prescription drugs. Although the prescription-drug industry has not had as much of the market concentrated in the top companies as do many other industries, the 20 largest companies increased their share of the drug market from 63 per cent to 72 per cent between 1947 and 1956, and through the late 1960's were supplying about three-fourths of the drugs (in dollar value) for newly written prescriptions.[147] However, no single manufacturer has captured as much as 10 per cent of the drug market. The number of manufacturing laboratories has remained rather stable through recent decades, about 1,100 in 1939, nearly 1,400 in 1954 and 1,130 in 1967 (counting each plant location as a separate unit).[148] Comparisons over time are hazardous, however; and the number of separate American *firms* producing prescription drugs since the 1960's would not be more than 600 to 700. Many of these are relatively small; but increasingly high regulatory standards for their scientific resources and competitive pressures make their survival complicated and amalgamations frequent.

Cooperative effort and advancement of standards in the pharmaceutical industry are fostered through the Pharmaceutical Manufacturers Association ("P.M.A."), whose 115 members collectively produce about 95 per cent of the prescription drugs dispensed in America and upwards of half of the total "free world" output. Of about 80 committees and subcommittees functioning in the P.M.A. more than half are involved in scientific matters to some degree.

The P.M.A. organization was formed (1958) from two predecessor organizations.[149] The American Drug Manufacturers Association (f. 1912) had attracted particularly the producers of "official and other non-secret preparations to be dispensed by pharmacists on prescription, or to be used in compounding prescriptions." Its member-firms in 1931 produced more than 80 per cent of all "druggists preparations."[150] In contrast, the manufacturers who stressed the rising class of ready-made, trade-named prescription products had belonged either to this association or a second one, the American Pharmaceutical Manufacturers' Association (f. 1908). The latter tended to attract also the physicians supply houses (making drugs packaged particularly for dispensing physicians). As conditions of drug manufacture and distribution changed over the years, the differences between the two associations became more ill defined, while the duplication of efforts became more obvious, leading to their amalgamation in 1958 after more than 4 decades of separate existence.

The manufacturers of so-called "patent medicines" (not patented medicines!) or self medications, i.e., "medicines . . . bearing coined names protected by trademarks and intended primarily for self-medication,"[151] are organized as the Proprietary Association of America (founded 1881). The secret composition of most of these medicines was unmasked after 1938 when a declaration of "the common or usual name of each active ingredient'' was required by the revamped Federal Food, Drug and Cosmetic Act.

## Production Volume

The value of the products prepared and sold annually by the pharmaceutical industry has been increasing steadily. Amounting to $51,000,000 in 1905, it multiplied more than 6-fold within a quarter century ($325,000,000 by 1929). Divided by classes of medication, the 1929 figures are $120,000,000 for ''druggists' preparations,'' $56,000,000 for ''ethical specialties'' and $149,000,000 for ''patent medicines'' and other proprietaries sold to the general public, while sales of cosmetics and toiletries amounted to $161,246,000.[152]

In 1958, prescription-product manufacturers alone were estimated to have a volume of $1.8 billion (at producer's selling prices). By 1962 the estimate had soared past the $2 billion mark,[153] and a decade later the dollar-volume had more than doubled. While these figures are not directly comparable with those cited for the earlier period, there has been clearly a rather phenomenal increase in the production of drug and cosmetic products.

Part of this increase is due to the expansion of the foreign market. Between the end of World War II and 1957, drug exports increased roughly 2½ times, far more than American exports in general. Between 1960 and 1972, prescription drugs sold abroad by American companies (including exports) quadrupled.[154] Most of the large drug manufacturing plants in the United States had established footholds, subsidiaries and branches not only in North and South America, Australia, Africa and the Near and the Far East, but in Europe as well. The United States, a country which had long imported scientific ideas as well as most of the drug products based on them, has become an exporter of both to about 60 countries, as well as a producer of prescription drugs in 60 countries through American firms.

## Importance of Industrial Research

Scientific research gradually became an integral part of pharmaceutical industry between the late 19th century and the years following World War I. After the first quarter of the present century, the fruits of such research decisively transformed drug therapy. The American pharmaco-industrial investment in this endeavor, about $50 million annually by 1951, increased 4-fold during the ensuing decade, and increased almost another 3-fold during the next decade ($677 millions by 1971, or 11.9% of sales). This upsurge of pharmaceutical research was led, during the early 1970's by about 6,000 scientists with master's or doctor's degrees, mostly employed in a few dozen top companies.

To support research adequately—a speculative and costly enterprise—has become increasingly difficult for smaller manufacturers. For example, in 1961, the twenty-five largest of the manufacturing laboratories reporting (annual sales of more than $30 million each) had about 85 per cent of all the research employees and about six of every seven of the scientific men employed.[155]

One indication of the yield from industrial research efforts of this magnitude comes from a study covering three decades. From 1940 to 1971 United States manufacturers originated at least 557 single-chemical entities that were sufficiently useful to be regularly available on prescription, totalling almost two-thirds of the new medicinal substances brought into drug therapy here.

Among the additional new medicinal substances introduced (whose originating country was reported), the research of Switzerland, Germany, the United Kingdom and France accounted for more than all other countries combined.[156] Between 1948 and 1961 the number of single medicinal chemicals introduced nationally into prescription practice each year normally ranged between 30 and 50. Since then it has dropped to the range of 10 to 25 substances annually—at least partly attributable to far more demanding government regulations about both experimental and routine use of new drugs. A more welcome by-product of these controls has been to stem the previous flood of duplicate products and multi-drug mixtures of dubious rationale.[157] Indeed, one analyst estimated that 89 per cent of the hundreds of drugs put into prescription use during the decade before 1962 were later withdrawn, sometimes for commercial reasons; while in the decade after 1962 only about 37 per cent of the new drugs marketed had been withdrawn.

Despite the vitality and progress of the prescription-drug industry, it has undergone a recurrent drumfire of criticism since the 1950's, from Congressional committees, consumer representatives, government agencies and (to some extent) from the profession of pharmacy itself—involving promotional practices, profit levels and judgments of cost-to-benefit ratios on drug matters that were at odds with the social expectations of industry's critics.[158] The industrial manager often seemed nonplussed by the mushrooming responsibilities ascribed to him after mid-century, which involved an unusual mixture of professional, scientific and social considerations. These were not easy to harmonize with his commitments to business values and with his role as strategist of a business enterprise.

As for proprietary medicines and their advertising, conditions improved considerably, largely because of the unremitting efforts of the A.M.A., A.Ph.A. and other agencies in combatting pseudoscientific pretenders in the health field and because of effects of the Wheeler-Lea Act. The remodeling of the Food, Drug and Cosmetic Act in 1938 and 1962, with rigid regulation of drugs, medical devices, cosmetics and food-stuffs, and of the introduction of new drugs into therapy (dependent on examination of the claims and test data by the Food and Drug Administration) have advanced standards of operation still further.

The pharmaceutical industry has given the dispensing pharmacist a more effective drug armamentarium. Conversely, it was community pharmacy that provided a nucleus for the development of industrial pharmaceutical manufacturing. And the profession of pharmacy has always given some of its best men to the industry of pharmacy.

During the 20th century, the cumulative changes underlying drug manufacture—in the sciences, the methods of manufacture, and in the array and deployment of drugs—had far-reaching consequences not only for the industrialist, but for his uneasy allies, the physician and pharmacist, and for the patient himself.[159] How such a complex industrial organism—uniquely blending sciences and technologies, professions and business, management and labor—can best serve its reason for existence, the public health, has remained enigmatic.

PART FOUR

# Discoveries and Other Contributions to Society by Pharmacists

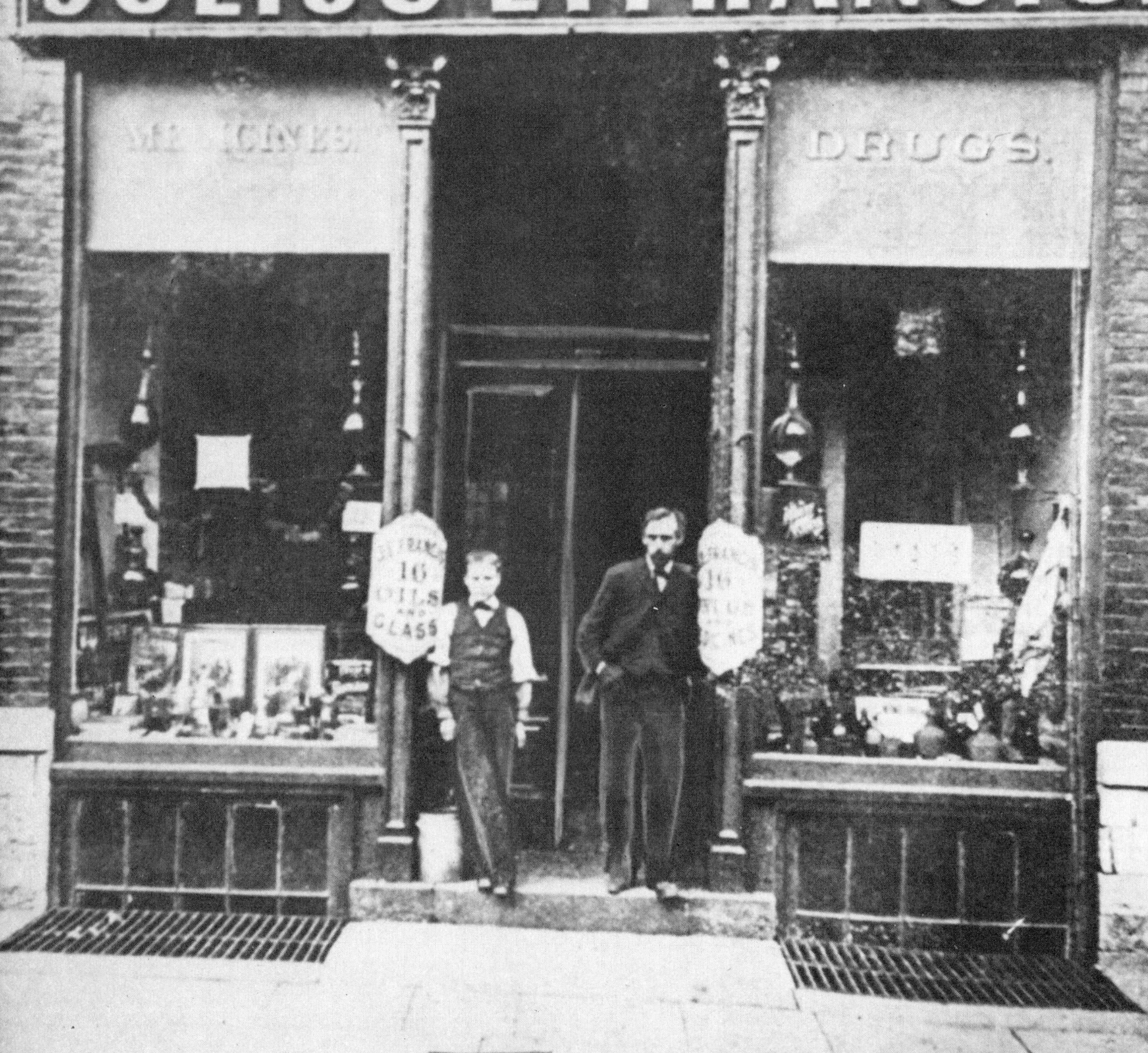
JULIUS E. FRANCIS.
DRUGS.
16
OILS
AND
GLASS
16

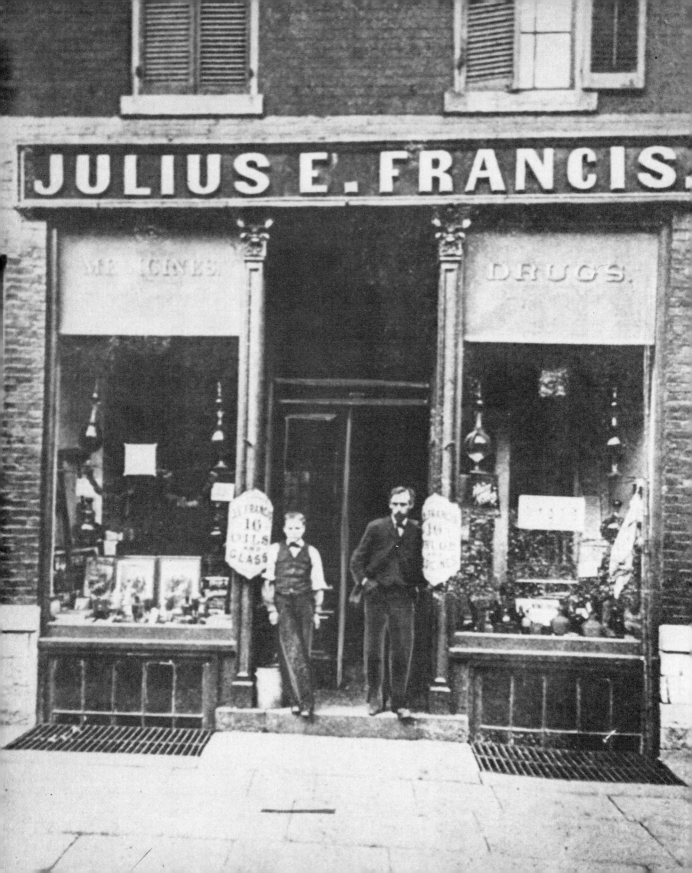

# 17

# The American Pharmacist in Public Service

## THE PHARMACIST IN CIVIC LIFE

### Philadelphians Set a Precedent

Pharmacists who founded the Philadelphia College of Pharmacy set an early example of social contributions from the profession. The first president of the college, Charles Marshall, was active in the Society of Friends, carried on various civic activities and is said to have been "one of the picturesque figures of the Revolution on the patriot side . . ." and "a deep student of Latin and Greek. The first vice-president, Peter Williamson, achieved the highest degree in American Masonry. The second president, William Lehman, was an active member of the Pennsylvania legislature and one of the leaders and benefactors of the Philadelphia Athenaeum.[1] The third president, Daniel B. Smith, "was elected a member of the Franklin Institute immediately after its organization in 1824 and was an incorporator of the Historical Society of Pennsylvania." He was elected a member of the American Philosophical Society (1829) and was also a member of the Academy of Natural Sciences. Furthermore, he was elected to the chairs of moral philosophy, English literature and chemistry at Haverford College (1834) and was made principal. He resigned to give increased attention to his pharmacy.[2] Henry Troth, whose energy did much to bring about the founding of the Philadelphia College of Pharmacy, is said to have been "one of the most progressive citizens of Philadelphia of his day . . . active in many philanthropic, business, and scientific organizations."[3] Later officers and teachers of the Philadelphia College of Pharmacy followed the example set by their early predecessors. The founding of the renowned Swarthmore College by the Society of Friends was largely due to the "personal exertions" of the pharmacist Edward Parrish, a professor at the Philadelphia College of Pharmacy (1864–1872). Parrish became the first president of Swarthmore College, and one of its buildings still carries the name "Parrish Hall."

To such men their profession of pharmacy must have seemed only a special aspect of their endeavor to render a particular service to society. This idea became more general as the professional status of pharmacy became more generally recognized. Thus American pharmacists participated to a remarkable extent in the development of American social life. People more and more took it for granted

←

Julius E. Francis (1822–1881), a pioneer in the movement to make Lincoln's birthday a national holiday, exemplifies the civic-minded role in which many community pharmacists have been cast. The photograph shows Francis *(right)* in the doorway of his small pharmacy typical of the late-19th century. Here in Buffalo, N. Y., the county historical society still preserves his Lincoln collection. (From: *Drug Topics* Collection, AIHP)

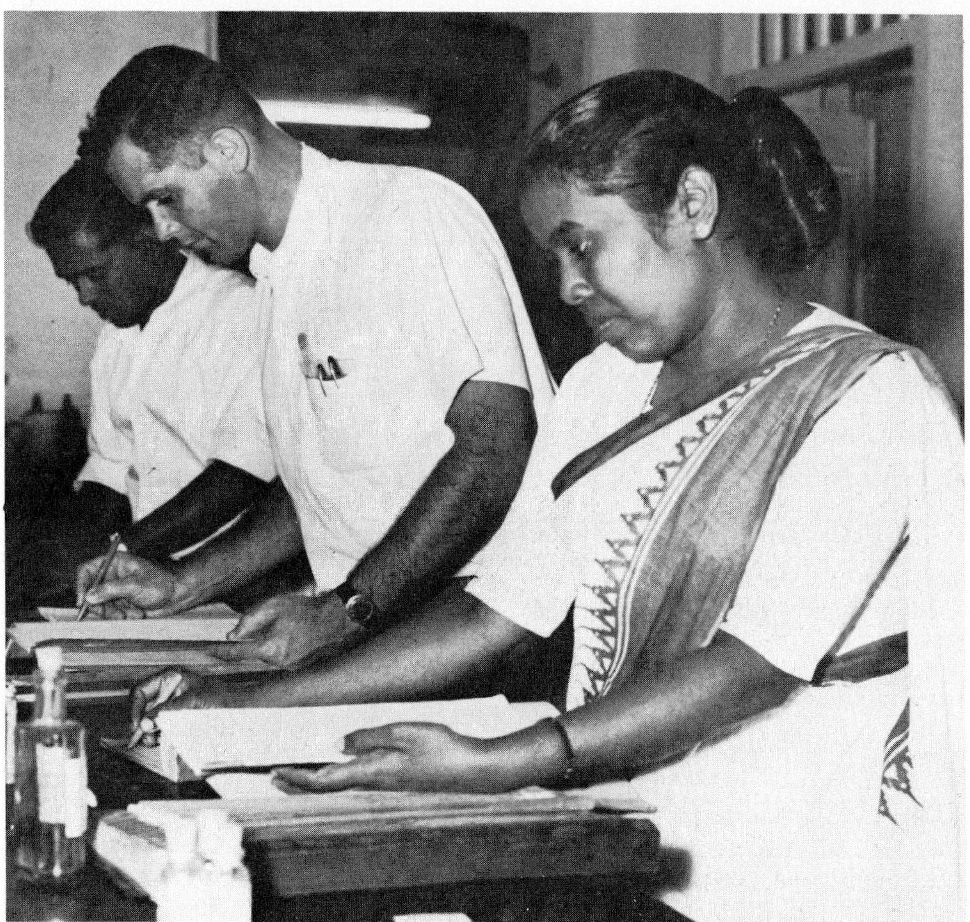

One of America's pharmacist-missionaries, Albert S. Bauman of Ohio *(center)*, brings the pharmacy's records up to date with the aid of two Indian associates at the day's end in Vellore. The work of such pharmacists epitomizes a humanitarianism traditionally associated with the health professions.

that the pharmacist was a well-educated man whose advice and assistance were at the disposal of his fellow citizens. Often he grew up with his business, in his home town. It was only natural that he enjoyed the confidence of his fellow citizens and sometimes became a guardian of the general cultural development in his place of residence.

In rural districts and smaller towns, the pharmacist has been now and again the mostly unpaid expert in questions requiring chemical and botanic knowledge. The method of the famous botanist G. H. E. Mühlenberg of asking "apothecaries . . . for the medicinal qualities and the trivial names of the officinal indigenous plants" he collected[4] has been followed in numerous noticed and unnoticed cases by other botanists as well as by laymen interested in botany, at least until pharmacists no longer needed to take such study seriously in their own education and work. Probably most sizable communities can recall examples of a pharmacist's contribution to social welfare growing out of his professional knowledge and ethical commitments—such as the work that earned pharmacist Abraham Fleisher of Wyncote, Pa., a Presidential Citation for Meritorious Service to the Handicapped (1962).[5]

### Humanitarian Endeavor

One of the least heralded of volunteer contributions has been humanitarian work by pharmacists, teamed with practitioners of the other health professions, in underdeveloped areas of the world. These representatives of the profession usually have served for little more than the satisfaction their work so richly yields. Often they leave secure positions at home to become part of a medical missionary team sponsored by one of the religious denominations. A secular counterpart, since the early 1960's, has been the scattering of pharmacists who have served in the Peace Corps. Among the first were the young pharmacists James McTigue in the Bolivian jungle, Daniel Goldsmith serving through the Bolivian Ministry of Health, Homer Butler in the Togolese hospitals and clinics on Africa's west coast, and Helene Johnson in Turkey for work in tuberculosis control.[6]

For various periods of duty, going back at least to 1910, American pharmacists have been working in field missions. Although at least some 30 individuals can be identified, their ministry to the poor and afflicted has been so unpublicized that we do not know how many more there have been. In addition to dispensing drugs, their work has included education, hospital management, drug manufacture and sanitation.

The selfless work of these missionary physicians, pharmacists and other health-care personnel has been reinforced in recent years by a voluntary agency called Medical Assistance Programs, Inc. (M.A.P.). Disaster aid is one of the more dramatic services provided by medical-care teams working under the sponsorship of 135 denominational and independent mission agencies in 82 countries (in 1972).

> When cholera struck unexpectedly in one African country, all available intravenous fluids were quickly exhausted. A missionary pharmacist cabled news of the disaster to MAP headquarters in Wheaton, Illinois, requesting 4,000 liters of IV fluids.
>
> MAP immediately telephoned the major manufacturers of these products and within 24 hours had a promise for gifts of 9,200 liters. The entire quantity, amounting to 17 tons, was airlifted to the epidemic area. . . . When the cyclone struck in East Pakistan (now Bangladesh) in November 1970 precipitating the worst natural disaster of modern times, an airlifted shipment from MAP brought the first medical supplies to arrive from the U. S.

These words are part of an appreciative account by pharmacist Donald Stilwell, who worked for MAP while on study-leave from his post as pharmacist (1958–1970) at the Ethiopian Mission Headquarters of the Sudan Interior Mission, in Addis Ababa.[7]

Still another variant of such humanitarian service is exemplified in the voyages of the S.S. Hope. Practicing pharmacists across the country contributed to this nonprofit (1960–1973) private venture, pharmaceutical manufacturers donated millions of dollars in drugs, and pharmacists, together with other health personnel, took tours of duty on the ship to bring services and models of medical care to developing nations in various parts of the world.[8]

## THE PHARMACIST IN PUBLIC SERVICE

Pharmacy as a profession is and has to be public service; therefore, each pharmacist honestly serving his profession is a public servant. In general, however, the label "public servant" is restricted to persons holding public office, either by appointment or by election.

In the offices open to all citizens of the United States, pharmacists have always served in city, state and federal administra-

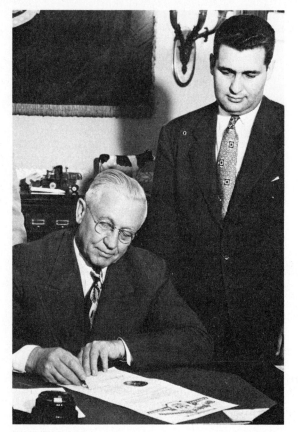

Pharmacist Oscar Rennebohm signs a document as governor of Wisconsin (1950). Looking on *(right)* is pharmacist William S. Apple, whose own work often has involved public-oriented service, since 1959 as Executive Director of the American Pharmaceutical Association. (From: Pharmaceutical Library, University of Wisconsin-Madison)

tions, and many have served in legislatures of their states and in the United States Congress. About 200 20th-century pharmacists have been identified by George Griffenhagen as having served in state legislatures, although the list is incomplete, as suggested by surveys in the 1960's indicating that an annual total of 47 to 57 pharmacist-legislators would be usual. There were also, in the late 1960's, "not less than 200 pharmacists who are serving or have recently served as mayors of their communities."[9]

For example, in 1927, Georgia had no less than nine pharmacists among its legislators, Idaho counted three senators and three representatives, and the Michigan legislature had two senators and nine representatives who had been pharmacists. In 25 states surveyed in 1945 not less than 51 pharmacists were serving in state legislatures. Furthermore, there were counted in the same states, without any pretense of completeness, nine mayors or city commissioners with pharmaceutical backgrounds, a state treasurer, and many members of public health committees. In 1955 a pharmacist was serving on the board of health in 23 states (including 16 states that made it mandatory). When further inquiry was made in 1961, incomplete data showed 25 pharmacists on state boards of health, 38 in state legislatures or cabinets, and 25 as mayor of their cities.[10]

Raleigh, North Carolina, offers an unusual example of the latter sphere of service, where pharmacists were mayors or other important municipal officials for more than two decades (excepting 2 or 3 years). "The people of Raleigh," wrote R. O. King, "recommend the 'pill rollers' to the world as honest, progressive, and efficient city officials."[11]

In Wisconsin, pharmacist Sarah Dean, formerly Assistant Administrator of the state's Division of Health Policy and Planning, attained cabinet level in 1975 as Secretary of the Department of Regulation and Licensing.

As early as 1860 a practicing pharmacist, John Gately Downey, was elected to the governorship of a state (California) by admiring fellow citizens, after his service as lieutenant governor. This pioneer and pharmacist had been the first person to establish a pharmacy in Los Angeles and "the first resident of Southern California to gain the highest position in the state. One of the lasting monuments commemorative of Downey's life is a town twelve miles southwest of Los Angeles that bears his name."[12] In more recent years the high office of governor has been occupied by men with pharmaceutical background in Arkansas, Arizona, Iowa, Maine and South

Carolina. While these men had left the profession before entering politics, a pharmacist of Wisconsin who became governor (1947–1951), Oscar Rennebohm, remained in the practice of his profession.

## In Washington

At the federal level, apparently only one pharmacist has achieved the rank of membership in the President's Cabinet, David Henshaw of Boston. As Secretary of the Navy he served less than a year (1843–44), because the Senate, out of deference to Daniel Webster and other Whigs, did not accept his appointment. However, he did serve long enough to prove his eminent qualifications, introduce a system of strict accountability for handling Navy funds and materials, and argue for the annexation of Texas. Henshaw had been an enterprising pharmacist, starting his own pharmacy at the age of 21. Within 13 years his clientele had grown to one of the largest in Boston pharmacy. In addition, he had become a banker, one of the directors of a railroad, and the founder and owner of a newspaper (*Boston Statesman*)![13]

At the rank of ambassador, Pharmacist Teodoro Moscoso of Puerto Rico (b. 1910) first served as United States representative to Venezuela, then was appointed by President Kennedy as U. S. Coordinator of the Alliance for Progress (1961), with the rank of Assistant Secretary of State. Moscoso served as the first president of the Colegio de Farmacéuticos de Puerto Rico while president of the Puerto Rican-American Drug Co. He gained prominence as the administrator (1942–1961) of the

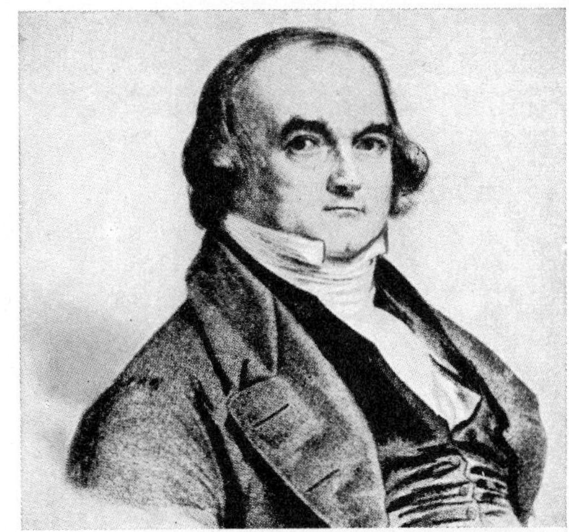

Druggist David Henshaw was appointed to the Cabinet of President Tyler, after giving up the world of drugs for the world of politics and entrepreneurist adventure. (J.A.Ph.A. *24*:858, 1935)

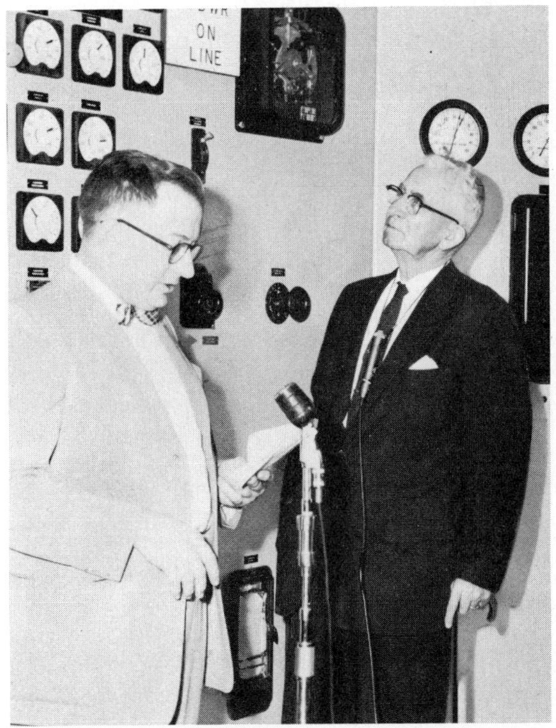


The pharmacist in civic life is exemplified by Congressman Carl T. Durham of North Carolina *(right)*, shown about to throw the switch starting the experimental boiling-water reactor at Argonne National Laboratory in 1957. Durham was serving as chairman of the Joint Committee on Atomic Energy. (Photo from Argonne National Laboratory)

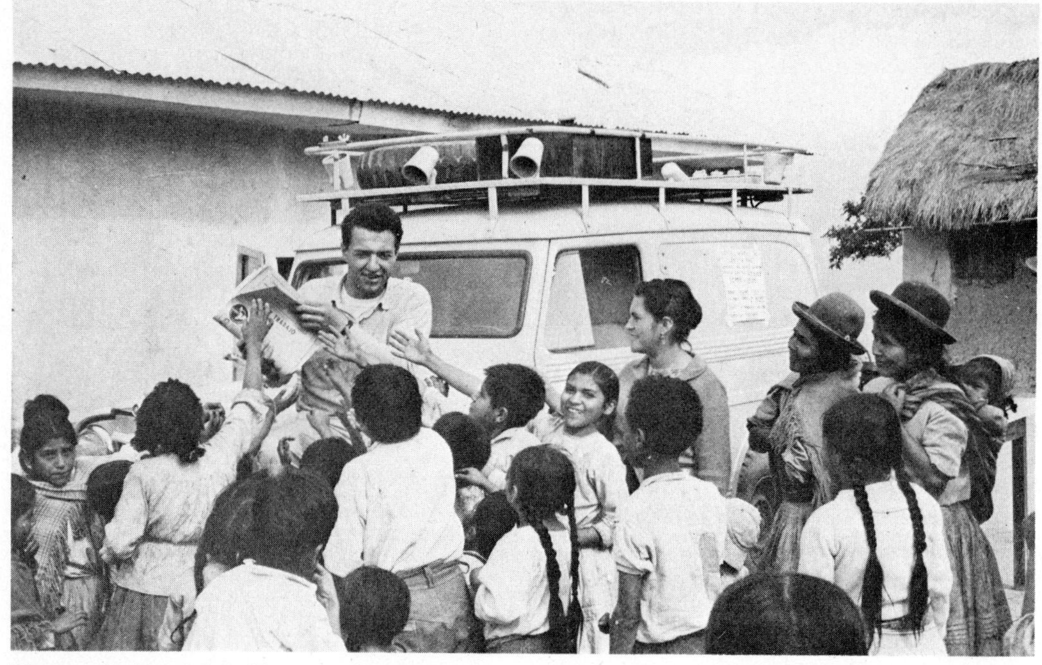

Pharmacist Daniel Goldsmith of Illinois, as a Peace Corps Volunteer (1963), exemplifies those in every generation of pharmacists who undertake humanitarian enterprises beyond routine practice. He is shown in the Bolivian back country distributing literature from his jeep, which is audio-visually equipped for health education purposes. (From: Foto Sacada, through American Institute of the History of Pharmacy, Madison)

highly successful "operation bootstrap" program for the economic development of Puerto Rico.

In Congress, pharmacists from time to time have taken their place alongside leading citizens from other walks of life in governing the country. Two examples are the representative and the senator who introduced the Durham-Humphrey amendments (1951) to the Federal Food, Drug and Cosmetic Act. Carl T. Durham had been a practicing pharmacist in North Carolina for 30 years before his election to Congress (1938), where he served with distinction for 22 years. He began his political career in 1922 as town councilman, and thereafter he held a continuous succession of public offices until he reached Washington. There he became noted particularly for his work as chairman of the Joint Committee on Atomic Energy of the United States Congress.

The second pharmacist, almost 20 years Durham's junior, has served in the United States Senate since 1948. Hubert H. Humphrey, the son of a pharmacist, practiced in the family pharmacy for 4 years before taking further studies to prepare for a career in public service and politics. His 3 years as mayor of Minneapolis served as a springboard to Washington, where he has been an energetic and articulate senator. He became majority leader of the Senate, in 1961, published two books on liberal goals and civil rights in the early 1960's and was Vice-President of the United States 1965–1969.

In the course of American history there have been at least 25 members of the United States Congress who came from the pharmaceutical field (up to 1965). Of these, nine had graduated in pharmacy, the earliest being Richard W. Guenther, a German immigrant (1866) who practiced pharmacy in Oshkosh, Wisconsin, was elected State Treasurer, then served three terms in Congress (1881–1889), and later was Consul General in Mexico.

While pharmacists thus have contributed their share to governance and leadership in America, the numbers turned up thus far do not suggest particular political awareness as compared with some other professions. This led the pharmacist W. Paul Briggs of Washington to observe (1962), "With the exception of a few far-sighted and dedicated men, pharmacy has suffered grievously from inattention to the science of government . . . . The future place of pharmacy will certainly be a reflection of its value and integrity as a profession, but its comparative status largely will be determined by its effectiveness on the political stage."[14]

## THE PHARMACIST IN THE ARMED FORCES

The election of pharmacists to political office suggests a public confidence in them, which doubtless is related to the part that pharmacy plays in the life and the minds of the people. But what of the role that pharmacy has been assigned in the armed forces of the United States? Here things have changed much since the Revolutionary War, to the detriment of pharmacy until comparatively recently.

In the Revolution the apothecary serving in the army of the patriots in his professional capacity held a rank equal to that of the surgeon, being a commissioned officer. This remained unchanged in the War of 1812:

> Economizing peacetime congressmen had not allowed the Army to utilize the experience which the medical [and pharmaceutical] officers had gained during the Revolutionary War. . . . It was not until 1813—when nine months of war had vastly aggravated the situation—that Congress took action. An act of March 3 provided that . . . a physician and surgeon general, as well as an apothecary general be appointed, with annual salaries of 2,500 and 1,800 dollars respectively. Dr. Francis LeBarron, a former Navy and Army surgeon was chosen for the position of apothecary general.[15]

More than a year later, a man whose former activities had been of a pharmaceutical nature was appointed assistant apothecary general of the United States Army. This man was James Cutbush.

> Concerning the "Apothecary General and his assistants" it was stated that they were "to receive and take charge of all hospital stores, medicines, surgical instruments and dressings, bought by the Commissary General of Purchases" and that they were to "account to the Supt. General of Military Supplies for all expenditures of the same." They were further directed "to compound and prepare all officinals and put up and issue medicines, etc., in chests or otherwise, conformably to requisitions."
>
> . . . The President directed in May, 1815 [after the war] that the apothecary general and two assistants be retained in the "Military Peace Establishment of the United States." The office of "Physician and Surgeon General," however, was abolished, and the Apothecary General became the ranking Officer of the Medical Department until 1818. In that year there was appointed the first officer to bear the present title of "Surgeon General."
>
> . . . In 1818, the office of the "commissary general of purchases" was abolished by the Army. Consequently, "that portion of his duties which pertained to the Medical Department" was transferred to the apothecary general and his assistants . . . . General Orders from the War Department, issued in September 1818, outline the new—and the old—duties at great length.
>
> In March, 1821, Congress had once more reduced "the military peace establishment of the United States." The budget did not allow for retention of the following grades, among others: assistant surgeons general, apothecary general, assistant apothecaries general. The holders of these offices were unceremoniously discharged.

In the period between 1821 and 1861 there was not much need for a regular pharmaceutical service in the insignificant army and navy of the United States. Moreover, pharmacists evinced little interest in this service. The existence of something like a pharmaceutical service in the armed forces of the United States was not commented on by representatives of organized American pharmacy before 1862 when the editor of the *American Journal of Pharmacy* commented:

> Occasionally, for many years, apothecaries have been employed on some of our naval vessels to facilitate the duties of the surgeons; but from the fact that no rank attaches to the position, we are told, it is but little sought after, as the "surgeon's mate" is socially ill situated on ship-board. We are not aware, that the apothecary has heretofore been employed in the medical department of the "regular" army of the United States. . . . To make this service more effective, it should be separated sufficiently from that of the surgeon to give a distinct standing and rank to the pharmaceutist, as in the French army, with clearly defined duties that his proper self-respect, and ambition to be eminent in his sphere, may have ample room for display. Unless such an arrangement can be made it is not probable that the better class of graduates in pharmacy would seek positions of this kind.[16]

A law of May 20, 1862, created a special group of pharmaceutical professionals in the military service, with the pay but not the rank of First Lieutenant, by adding "to the Medical Department of the Army, Medical Storekeepers, not exceeding six in number, who shall have the pay and emoluments of Military Storekeepers of the Quartermaster's Department, who shall be skilled Apothecaries or Druggists."

The duties of these men were "under the direction of the Surgeon General and Medical Purveyors, with the storing and safe keeping of medical and hospital supplies, and with the duties of receiving, issuing and accounting for the same according to regulations."[17]

This small group of pharmacists must be considered a civil rather than a military addition to the Army. It was in a similar civil rather than a military rôle that John M. Maisch served the United States during the Civil War by conducting the laboratory of the United States Army at Philadelphia after 2 years of collaboration with the drug manufacturer and former United States Navy Surgeon E. R. Squibb.

Insofar as pharmacists were engaged in their professional rôle within the regular military service of the Army and the Navy, they ranked as Hospital Stewards.[18]

With the close of the Civil War, serious attempts to better the position of the military pharmacists seem to have ended. In 1894, we find for the first time, among the committees of the American Pharmaceutical Association, a "Special Committee on the Status of Pharmacists in the Army and Navy of the United States." In the following year, this Committee reported a detailed survey concerning the regulation of the pharmaceutical service in the armies of all civilized countries, and two proposals for a legal change of the status of pharmacists serving in the United States Army and Navy.[19]

As early as 1898, the Committee could report a first success, and it may be assumed that the Spanish-American War provided the necessary favorable atmosphere. In the Navy the situation complained of during the Civil War still prevailed, and the naval apothecary had no legal status at all. Therefore, the endeavor of the Committee centered on this question. It succeeded, to the extent that the Hale Bill for the first time recognized pharmacists as representatives of a special profession with just claims to an appropriate designation, rank and pay. The bill established a Hospital Corps of the United States Navy consisting of "pharmacists, hospital stewards, hospital apprentices, and for this purpose the Secretary of the Navy is empowered to appoint twenty-five pharmacists with the rank, pay and privileges of warrant officers."[20] In 1902, the pharmaceutical "hospital stewards" too were granted the title of pharmacist.[21]

The year 1903 was noteworthy in the relations between organized pharmacy and the governmental agencies in which pharmacists should be working professionally, when the U. S. Navy and the Department of Agriculture both had official delegates at the meeting of the American Pharmaceutical Association. However, the United States Army declined to be represented, stating that "the position of pharmacist or apothecary does not exist in the Army," that "there are some graduates of pharmacy and many others competent to fill prescriptions . . . among our Sergeants . . . " and that "the Sergeant must be first a soldier, the dispensing of the 'ready-prepared tablets' or compounding of the 'simple medicines required' being only 'one of his secondary duties.' "[22]

No further progress was made until 1916, when two new grades, Master Hospital Sergeant and Hospital Sergeant, were created in the United States Army. In the Navy "the pay and allowances that are now or may hereafter be allowed a lieutenant in the United States Navy" were granted to the Chief Pharmacist on the active list.[23]

### After World War I

The experiences of World War I, in conjunction with the increasing educational attainment of pharmacists, began to take effect by 1922. There were at this time "about fifteen commissioned officers of the Medical Department [meaning the Medical Administrative Corps established in 1920] who are pharmacists, these being commissioned . . . in the grades of captain, first and second lieutenants" beside 69 pharmacists "already commissioned in the Medical Administrative Reserve." Two years later the number of pharmacists in the Reserve section of the medical service had increased to 89, and "twenty-five commissions have been granted with a rank above that of Captain in the Sanitary Corps."[24]

With a law that became effective in 1926 the requirements for pharmacists as applicants for professional public service became clearly defined, being "based upon the established principles of a profession or science and which requires professional, scientific, or technical training, equivalent to that represented by graduation from a college or university of recognized standing."

The difficulties that had to be overcome did not arise mainly from outside the profession. Once pharmaceutical education was on an equal footing with that of other professions, the pharmacist could expect a commensurate position in governmental service.

In 1936, a bill finally made graduation from a recognized 4-year school of pharmacy a prerequisite for appointment to the Medical Administrative Corps, appointees receiving the grade of second lieutenant. The number of these Regular Army pharmacist-officers, who had to pass an examination before appointment, was limited to 16. The development was epitomized in a report to the American Pharmaceutical Association:

> Ten years ago, pharmacy was still listed as a sub-profession. . . . To-day, pharmacy is recognized fully as a profession; pharmacists are classified in the professional as well as the subprofessional groups under the Civil Service. . . .[25]

This change was crowned by two acts of Congress creating a special Pharmacy Corps of the United States Army (act of July 12, 1943), and putting pharmacists in the United States Public Health Service on the same plan as other officers of the service (1944).

The Pharmacy Corps was created as a separate unit against the advice of the administration of the Army Medical Department, which contended that only by cooperation with the other medical auxiliary groups within one administrative unit could the greatest benefit accrue from the services of well-educated military pharmacists.

In pharmacy's view, however, this arrangement had restricted both the amount and the level of professional services in military pharmacy over the years. The concept of a separate and professionalized Pharmacy Corps therefore was pressed by organized pharmacy for at least nine years, through its Committee on the Status of Pharmacists in Government Service. Although U.S. Army resistance was overcome in Congress in 1943, the new Pharmacy Corps could not long survive the weight of military opposition. The role that commis-

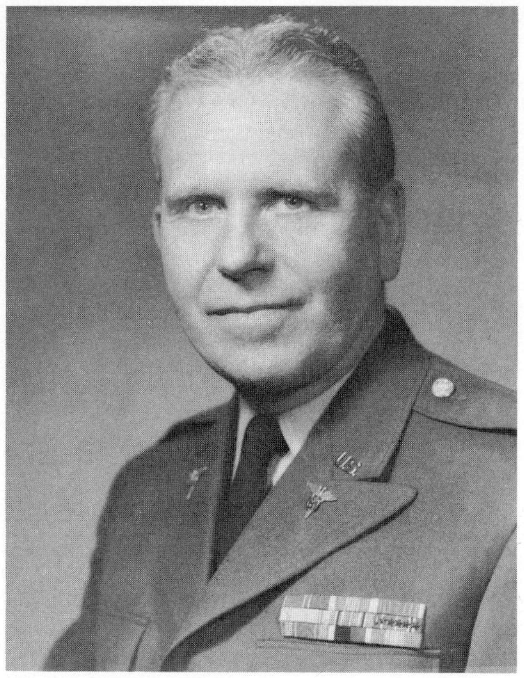

A former practicing pharmacist in Minnesota and Wisconsin, Bernard Aabel (1907–1968) is representative of those of his profession who have made distinguished contributions to governmental and military service. He headed a major departmental unit in the Army Surgeon General's Office; he served in the American Embassy at Helsinki (military attaché); he became Commander at the largest military medical installation during the Korean War. Later, Col. Aabel was responsible for procurement of Regular career officers for all six corps of the Army Medical Service Corps in 64 allied specialties. In 1962 he became Director of the Department of International Health of the American Medical Association. (Photograph from the U.S. Army)

sioned pharmacists could play survived, however, both in medical supply and in the coordination of medical auxiliary groups (because of the well-educated pharmacist's combination of a broad scientific knowledge and administrative skills). Therefore, after meeting some conditions set by organized pharmacy, opportunities for military pharmacists actually increased under a law (August 4, 1947) establishing a Medical Service Corps (of various health-related sciences, including pharmacy) in both the Army and the Navy, which at the same time abolished the long-contended Pharmacy Corps. With the upward stabilization of the pharmaceutical activities and rank in the United States Navy, the titles of "Pharmacists' Mate" as the designation of enlisted Hospital Corps personnel, and of "Pharmacist" as the designation of Warrant Officers were finally abandoned (neither title presupposing graduation in pharmacy).[26]

The highest rank to be achieved by a pharmacist in the Army is that of Colonel, in the Navy that of Captain. The Army Medical Service Corps had as its first Chief a pharmacist, Colonel Othmar F. Goriup. In the Navy at that time, Commander W. Paul Briggs was the highest ranking pharmaceutical officer, guiding the development of the pharmaceutical service of the U.S. Navy's Bureau of Medicine and Surgery.

In 1962 the Navy had 43 billets for pharmacy officers, the Army 93, the Air Force 252, although figures are not comparable because of variations in accounting for pharmacists serving in related capacities and for pharmacists with civilian status.

After another decade the U.S. Army had about 200 pharmacist-officers on duty. Most of them enter active service as first Lieutenant, after an initial orientation period in the Academy of Health Sciences at Fort Sam Houston. Pharmacy officers in recent years usually have been assigned as chief of Pharmacy Service at one of the Army hospitals (74 in 1974) or health clinics (13), or as a staff officer at one of the larger hospitals. Career officers (about 70 pharmacists, in the 1970's) pass through four stages of professional development in the Medical Service Corps, leading toward the rank of full Colonel. A pharmacy officer is encouraged to earn a master's degree; and a few are selected to earn, eventually, a doctorate. Still others undergo special training to develop their executive capacities, since mature officers ordinarily hold substantial supervisory or coordinating responsibilities within the Corps or elsewhere in the Medical Department.[27]

While technical pharmaceutical work has remained largely in the hands of noncommissioned and even non-pharmacist personnel, the armed forces have confirmed, on their own terms, the diverse positions in which selected commissioned pharmacists can serve to the advantage of military medical services.

### Veterans Administration

Although not a part of the armed forces of the United States, it is relevant to discuss the Veterans Administration here. Since World War II the "VA" developed into an important organization in which pharmaceutical activities play an essential part. Due to the initiative and the clear-mindedness of Commander W. Paul Briggs, Director of Pharmacy Service in the Veterans Administration through 1947, this service developed admirably within the veterans' hospitals. The increased utilization of pharmacists has been one example, rising from 450 to 615 Civil Service positions during the decade 1953–1962, in 168 V.A. hospitals. Inpatient or outpatient pharmaceutical facilities had been developed in every state, supplemented by contract-service from private "hometown" pharmacies. Despite periodic controversy over regulations governing the hometown service, millions of prescriptions have been thus dispensed to veterans with service-connected disabilities.

Organizationally, since 1946, pharmacy functions in the Veterans Administration "on a level with the other professional specialties." A Director of Pharmacy Service is responsible to the Chief of Professional Services; and an Assistant Director of Pharmacy Service has program responsibility, aided by pharmacy specialists in specific fields such as drug standards, personnel and operating procedures; while other pharmacists function as field supervisors of pharmacy operations.[28]

## PHARMACISTS IN THE PUBLIC HEALTH SERVICE

The United States Public Health Service originated in a law (July 16, 1798) creating the "Marine Hospital Service" for sick and disabled seamen. As additional duties fostering general public health were gradually imposed on this agency, its designation evolved into the "United States Public Health Service" (1912).

Beginning in 1897, graduation in pharmacy became a requirement for those appointed to pharmaceutical duties. When the U. S. Public Health Service was further authorized to commission pharmacists (1930), comparable to the commissioning of medical officers, it became a precedent that has since benefited pharmacists in other branches of government service.[29]

The duties and, still more, the performance of these men never have been limited to strictly pharmaceutical activities. They always have been both managerial and professional and have included quarantine procedure, supply and research. For example, one of the most remarkable pharmaceutical officers in the Public Health Service, Benjamin Holsendorf (d. 1944) devoted the greater part of his more than 40 years of service to a successful study of rodent control, which to this day affects the construction of ships and shore installations.[30]

> In 1944 the new Public Health Service Act lifted the promotion limitation and pharmacists can now be promoted to the director grade, which corresponds to an Army Colonel. . . . There was established in 1945 a Pharmacy Service with a Senior Pharmacist officer as its full-time chief. This pharmacy unit functions as part of the Hospital Division . . . which in turn is part of the

Bureau of Medical Services. . . . The Service Senior Regular Corps pharmacist officer has been assistant to the chief of the Bureau since early 1944 . . .[31]

The three pharmacists here quoted were among the most distinguished who have served the United States Public Health Service. Raymond D. Kinsey became (1949) the first pharmacist to receive the rank of Director (equivalent of Army colonel); and, subsequently, Thomas A. Foster and George F. Archambault both were likewise promoted to Director. Foster, originally a community pharmacist in Alabama, worked up through the ranks after 1933 to become Chief of Supply and Procurement for the entire service. On assignments with the Office of Defense Mobilization and in other government activities he rendered distinguished pharmaceutical service. Pharmaceutical progress in the Division of Hospitals was steady under the administration of George F. Archambault, pharmacist-lawyer from Massachusetts, who entered the Public Health Service (1947) to become Chief of the Pharmacy Branch and, from 1959 to 1967, to represent the Service in all pharmaceutical activities.[32]

By 1954 every pharmaceutical function in the Public Health Service was being "carried out by either a commissioned pharmacist or a Civil Service civilian pharmacist," in contrast to the history of more erratic utilization of pharmacists in the armed forces.

Pharmacists have been employed at U.S.P.H.S. posts in hospitals, clinics, quarantine and supply stations, Indian Affairs clinics, prisons, state health services and in the Washington office of the Surgeon General (e.g., 104 regular and 85 reserve officers in 1962). These duty-stations range from the most sophisticated research hospitals to rather primitive outposts. One pharmacist wrote of his experience that, "There is a unique challenge faced by the pharmacist . . . to cultivate the Navajo's change from traditional religious beliefs to the concept of health based on science. . . . "[33]

## INDIVIDUAL PHARMACISTS IN GOVERNMENTAL SERVICE

There always have been individual pharmacists in public service with authority and pay commensurate with the high standard of their special contributions—work not pharmacy as such but drawing on pharmaceutical knowledge and experience as well as other specialized training. Of the responsibilities assigned to such men, a few examples must suffice:

Lyman F. Kebler, who did particularly meritorious work while Chief of the U.S.D.A. Drug Division from 1907 to 1923 (forerunner of the Food and Drug Administration) was not only a pharmacist but a physician and chemist.

Frederick B. Power, head of the Phytochemical Laboratory of the United States Department of Agriculture (1916-1927), was a member of the National Research Council, and is apparently the only American pharmacist so far elected to the National Academy of Science.

Oswald Schreiner, the first pharmacy student to earn the Doctor of Philosophy on the basis of graduate work in a school of pharmacy of an American university (1902, Wisconsin), became Chief of the Soil Fertility Division of the U. S. Department of Agriculture.

Frederick W. Irish, a former community pharmacist (1921–1931), entered government service as a chemist, first for the Food and Drug Administration and then for the Federal Trade Commission. Then from 1951 to 1969 Mr. Irish was Chief of the Commission's Division of Scientific Opinions.

Henry L. Giordano left the practice of pharmacy for a career in government service devoted to the control of narcotics (1941–1969). Rising through the ranks, he became U.S. Commissioner of Narcotics in 1962, then Associate Director of the later Bureau of Narcotics and Dangerous Drugs in the Department of Justice.

Still other pharmacists have made notable contributions to the control of narcotics and addiction, such as Joseph M. Bransky, who served the Bureau of Narcotics for 43 years, both in this country and abroad. He was honored by the government of Japan for his aid in restoring order in the distribution of narcotics after World War II and in helping to organize the present Japanese Pharmaceutical Association. Mr. Bransky has been lauded for the "unique sense of personal dedication which he gave his public trust."

A quite different mission, designed to record rather than to carry out exploits of health-care professionals, occupies the Smithsonian Institution's Division of Medical Sciences. The succession of government pharmacists who have played a part in developing this aspect of our national museum depends upon their unique combination of personal qualities. Among the pharmacist-curators and historians there have been Charles Whitebread (1918–1948), George B. Griffenhagen (1952–1959), and Sami K. Hamarneh (1959–to date), and several others of shorter tenure.

Still another type of distinctive service by individual pharmacists is exemplified by Robert C. Gasen, a former community pharmacist from Illinois. The French government decorated him with the highest grade of the Order of Public Health, honoring the caliber of his medical supply work while attached to the Civilian Affairs Section of Allied Force Headquarters in Algiers during World War II. Mr. Gasen later served with the U. S. Foreign Economic Administration.[34]

M. Keith Weikel exemplifies the contribution to public life by exceptional pharmacists who specialize in social or economic aspects of health care. After experience in pharmaceutical education and industrial pharmacy, Dr. Weikel entered the Department of Health, Education and Welfare in Washington to become Director of the Division of Health Evaluation and then, in 1974, Commissioner of the Medical Services Administration. As "one of the government's leading authorities on third-party programs" for paying for medical care and on pharmaceutical

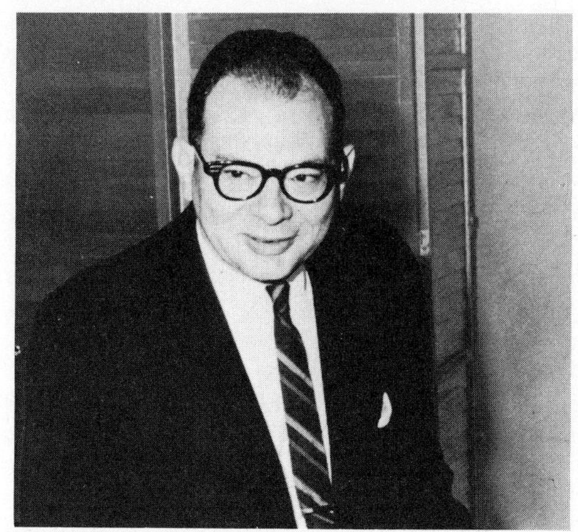

The former practicing pharmacist, Henry L. Giordano, as U.S. Commissioner of Narcotics in 1962, administrator of the entire national program of narcotics control.

costs under federally-funded programs, he has stood in an uncomfortable as well as prominent position between health-service providers and tax-paying consumers.[35]

## PHARMACEUTICAL EMERGENCY SERVICE

The rise of American pharmaceutical education produced a growing number of men offering the necessary scientific knowledge, as well as experience and administrative talents, needed in governmental agencies dealing with drugs and regulations concerning their production and distribution. These have included officials coming from pharmacy, such as Frank A. Delgado, who for a decade was chief of the Drug Section in the Bureau of Foreign and Domestic Commerce. During World War II he headed the Drugs and Fine Chemicals Unit, Chemicals and Drugs Branch, Office of Price Administration (1941–1943), subsequently serving as medical supply officer for the Office of Foreign Relief and Rehabilitation.

The war also brought others from pharmacy into government posts to help deal with special problems created in medical supply, a group perhaps most notably represented by Robert P. Fischelis as director of the Chemicals, Drugs and Health Supplies Division of the War Production Board, Office of Civilian Requirements (later Secretary of the American Pharmaceutical Association), and Fred J. Stock as chief of the Drugs and Cosmetics Branch of the Chemicals Bureau, of the War Production Board.

Besides the public service performed in the daily routine of a profession, or in fulfilling the obligations of a public office, there is a third service dictated by emergency, which requires an unqualified readiness to help. In great floods that this country has experienced now and again, American pharmacists have proved themselves equal to such tasks, as the tragic episodes of 1936 illustrated:

> Their selfless loyalty to the public trust will furnish a bright chapter in that grim tale of destruction and misery. . . . They worked by candle and lamplight in unheated stores with ice water slopping over their boot-tops. They braved treacherous currents in calling for and delivering prescriptions by boat. They saved biologicals, first aid supplies, flashlights, and foodstuffs. . . . They gave unstintingly of their professional knowledge, helping bacteriologists test water and food. . . . They manned relief centers. . . . They fought a successful battle for others against a rampant, hostile nature. . . . [36]

Another example would be the role of New Orleans pharmacists after a hurricane ripped through the city in 1965. A make-shift pharmacy was set up in the city hall by pharmacist William O'Brien and his associates, which was manned around the clock by 57 pharmacists during the emergency need for medical services and sanitation.[37]

This role of the pharmacist in combatting nature's disasters finds a logical extension in civil defense against the threat of man-made disasters. While every pharmacist has a potential role to play locally, selected pharmacists help to provide the leadership for preparedness within a larger framework, such as pharmacist Arnold H. Dodge, Chief of the U.S.P.H.S. Health Resources Branch in the Division of Health Mobilization (a field of work he entered in 1955). Of such responsibilities, the Surgeon General of the U. S. Public Health Service, Leroy E. Burney, has said:

> Because we recognize the planning abilities and diversified competencies of the pharmacist, we are presently placing heavy reliance on our headquarters pharmacists to develop plans and operational programs in the field of emergency medical supply, availability, stockpiling, distribution and utilization. However, it is only through disaster preparedness efforts of all pharmacists as members of the health profession team that we can hope to establish a firm basis for emergency medical care programs of the type anticipated under a post-nuclear attack situation.[38]

# 18

# Contributions by Pharmacists to Science and Industry

The profession of pharmacy has produced many scholarly representatives who applied to their calling the results of research in the sciences on which pharmacy rests. These representatives and their activities have been pointed out as part of pharmaceutical history in the countries concerned. Had they done nothing more, pharmacy would have led but a parasitic life. Fortunately for the calling, some of them made fundamental contributions to science. It is their story that is to be told here.

Writers on pharmaceutical history tend to claim as representatives of pharmacy anybody who spent even a brief period in this field. Thus Justus Liebig has been claimed for pharmacy, though he spent only 10 months as an apprentice in the pharmacy at Heppenheim. Thus Humphry Davy was "an apothecary's clerk at the beginning of his career,"[1] to be sure, spending 3 years as an apprentice to an apothecary-surgeon, John Borlase of Penzance.[2] The young man availed himself of the opportunity thus offered to conduct chemical experiments. No doubt he assisted in the preparation of remedies, but he can scarcely be regarded as having been a pharmacist. French writers on the history of pharmacy tend to claim famous men who taught at educational institutions of pharmacy,[3] but such men as Claude Louis Berthollet, Louis Pasteur[4] and Louis Jacques Thénard are not genuine representatives of pharmacy. Nor did the eminent Swedish chemist Joens Jacob Berzelius "first earn his living as apothecary."[5]

So many facets of science and technology have in fact been sustained by contributions coming from pharmacy that there is no need to claim or debate borderline instances.* The men and women to be mentioned here as pharmacists either practiced as such for a time or held a full legal qualification to practice pharmacy if and when they wished to do so. Hence we may speak of contributions coming from pharmacy, or contributions by pharmacists, even if in later life they devoted themselves to some specialized branch of scientific endeavor. Indeed, during the course of the 19th century, further specialization in education and effort became practically a prerequisite for memorable scientific achievement. The "pharmacist" thus often tends to become obscured in the modern context of science, even though the original profession of such creative men and women influenced, in widely divergent ways and degrees, their life choices and contributions.

## GENERAL CHEMISTRY

### Chemical Education

In modern times chemistry has been the science most closely related to pharmacy, so

*Discoverers mentioned in this chapter are not from pharmacy unless so identified.

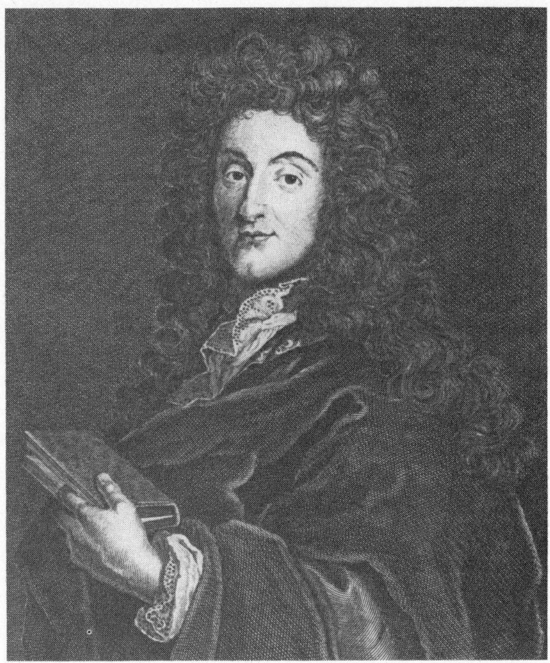

Pharmacist Nicolas Lémery of France (1645–1715), who later qualified also in medicine, was one of the founders of modern phytochemistry and one of the most-translated authors of his time. Lémery was elected to the French Academy of Sciences and other honors. (Engraving by N. Pitau; photograph from The Smithsonian Institution)

we should not be surprised to find that it is in this discipline that pharmacists have made their most significant contribution. Chemistry, of course, had always been associated with various practical arts. As Ferdinand Hoefer pointed out, the "first materials of chemistry . . . were to be met with in the shops of the smithy, the enameler, the painter in the botique of the pharmacopolist or druggist, as a matter of fact in the practice of all the useful arts, including the culinary art. In other words, science is born of the needs of life."[6] A wealth of chemical knowledge, processes and apparatus is to be found, for example, in metallurgical works such as the 16th-century *De Re Metallica* by George Agricola.

After the Paracelsians had succeeded in introducing many chemically prepared remedies into the European pharmacopeias of the 17th century (see Chapter 3), it became increasingly important for the pharmacist to become a skilled chemist. Pharmacy shops came to have chemical laboratories associated with them, containing equipment for distillation and for other procedures needed to produce the chemical remedies. Pharmacists were thus in a peculiarly appropriate position to contribute to chemical education and research. It must be remembered that chemistry itself was not yet a profession at this time.

At a time when there were no chemical laboratories in the universities, many aspiring young chemical researchers received laboratory training as apprentices in a pharmacy, such as the famous 19th-century chemists Justus von Liebig and Jean Baptiste Dumas.

A significant number of European pharmacists began to offer more formal instruction in chemistry through lectures and practical demonstrations in the laboratories of their pharmacies. Even when pharmacists, during the course of the 18th and 19th centuries, came to be appointed as professors of chemistry in the universities, they often continued to give their instruction (especially laboratory demonstration) in their pharmacies. Among the more noted of these chemistry teachers we may mention the Parisian pharmacist François Guillaume Rouelle (1703–1770), whose pupils included the great French chemist Antoine Lavoisier and the German pharmacist Carl Gottfried Hagen of Königsberg.

Pharmacists also wrote many of the first textbooks of chemistry. Two of the most popular of the early chemical textbooks were the *Traité de Chymie* of Nicaise LeFebvre, Court Apothecary of King Louis XIV of France and later of King Charles II of England, first published in 1660, and the *Cours de Chymie* of the French pharmacist Nicolas Lémery, first published in 1675. Lémery's book went through 20 French editions, and was translated into English, German, Dutch, Spanish and Italian. Through his *Cours de Chymie*, Lémery taught chemistry to untold numbers of students of the subject.

Pharmacists were also involved in the founding of many chemical journals, a fact reflected in the titles of some of these periodicals, such as the *Journal de Pharmacie et de Chimie* (founded in 1809 as the *Bulletin de Pharmacie*) and the *Annalen für Chemie and Pharmacie* (founded in 1832 as the *Annalen der Pharmacie*). These pharmaceutical and chemical journals, which began to make their appearance towards the end of the 18th century, helped to disseminate new knowledge in these disciplines.[7]

## Chemical Research

The contributions of pharmacists to chemistry involved not only the dissemination of established chemical knowledge through teaching and writing, but also the creation of new knowledge through research. Pharmacists possessed the knowledge and equipment that enabled them to engage in chemical investigations. Many of the famous chemists of the 17th, 18th and 19th centuries actually earned their living in the practice of pharmacy (e.g., Carl Scheele and Martin Klaproth).

Pharmacists made significant contributions to the emergence of chemistry as a modern science in the late 18th and early 19th centuries. One of the factors associated with the "chemical revolution" of this period was the development of the oxygen theory of combustion by the French chemist Antoine Lavoisier (1743–1794).

The phlogiston theory that had been suggested (by the German physician Johann Joachim Becher, 1635–1682, and elaborated by Georg Ernst Stahl, 1660–1734 was widely adopted to explain the phenomenon of combustion in the 18th century. According to this view, combustible substances must contain a material (called "phlogiston") which is transferred from the burning substance to the air during combustion. The German-Swedish pharmacist Carl Wilhelm Scheele believed that only a portion of the air was involved in accepting phlogiston; and he isolated that portion of air involved in combustion sometime prior to 1773 (probably in 1771 or 1772). Scheele called this substance, which we know to be oxygen, "fire-air."[8] Oxygen was discovered independently by the English clergyman Joseph Priestley in 1774. Priestly, like Scheele, interpreted his discovery in terms of the phlogiston theory, and so he called this substance "dephlogisticated air."

It was Lavoisier who recognized that combustion could be explained as the combination of a substance with oxygen, thus eliminating the need to postulate the existence of the elusive "pholgiston." He named the new gas "oxygine" ("acid former"). The isolation of oxygen by Priestley and by the pharmacist Scheele had played an important role in leading to the modern interpretation of combustion and respiration.

While the work of Lavoisier helped to give chemistry a new theoretical framework and a new nomenclature, there was still much to be done before chemistry gained the potential for today's science. One need was the development of improved analytical techniques. No single individual contributed more to this development than the German pharmacist Martin H. Klaproth (1743–1817). No less an authority than Berzelius, himself one of the greatest analysts, pronounced Klaproth "the greatest analytical chemist" of Europe. Unlike many of his contemporaries, Klaproth not only published his results but gave in detail the methods by which they were obtained, thus making his techniques available to others.

> Many manipulations which appear self-evident to the analytical chemist of today originated from Klaproth. He was the first to point out the necessity of drying at a definite temperature before weighing and to ignite precipitates until constant weight was obtained. He also took into account

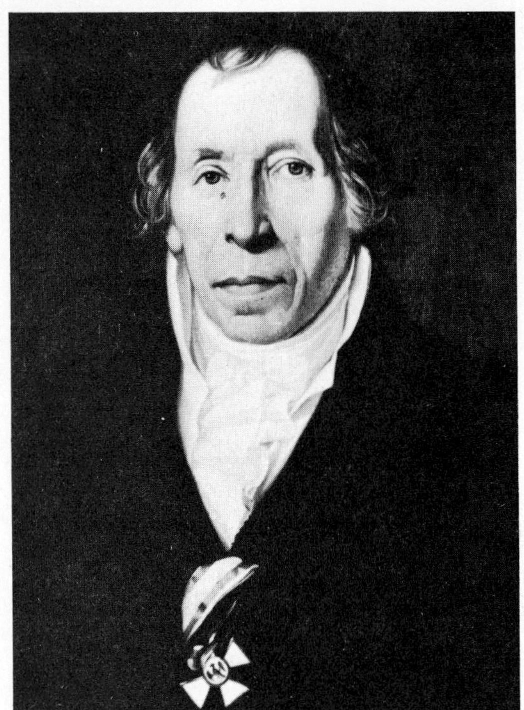

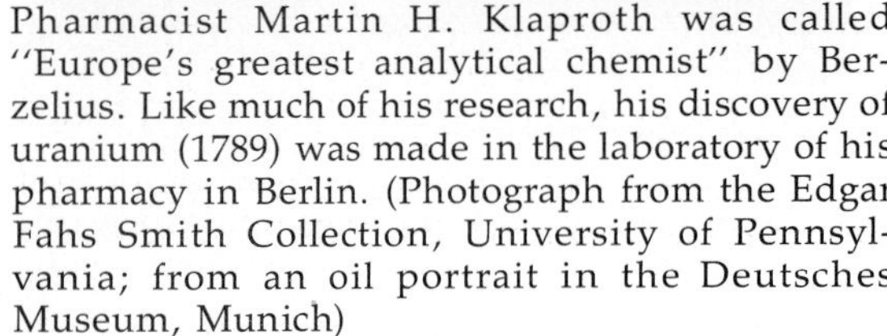

Pharmacist Martin H. Klaproth was called "Europe's greatest analytical chemist" by Berzelius. Like much of his research, his discovery of uranium (1789) was made in the laboratory of his pharmacy in Berlin. (Photograph from the Edgar Fahs Smith Collection, University of Pennsylvania; from an oil portrait in the Deutsches Museum, Munich)

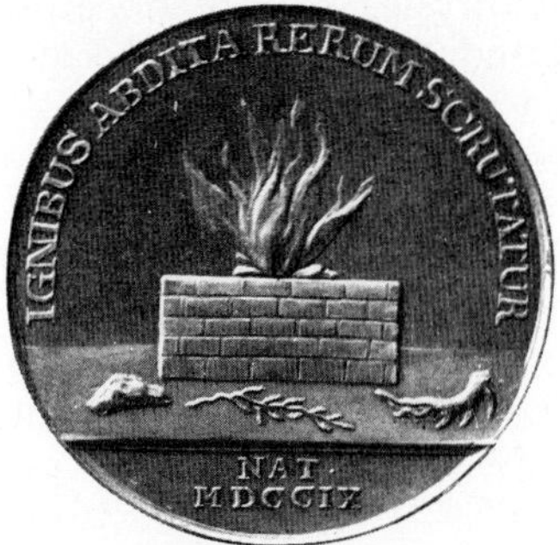


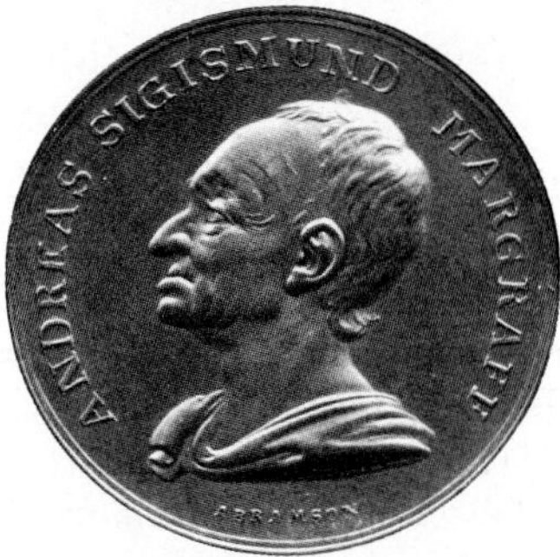


"Hidden things he searches out by fires," proclaims the Latin motto on a medal honoring a research pharmacist of the 18th century. Fire symbolizes the art of chemistry, since fire seemed indispensable in probing the secrets of the three natural kingdoms, which on the medal are represented before the chemist's hearth by a stone (mineral), a branch (vegetable) and an antler (animal). The obverse side shows a portrait of Pharmacist Andreas S. Marggraf, born the son of a pharmacist (1709), who discovered sugar in the sugar beet and advanced qualitative analysis.

the contaminations resulting from grinding hard minerals in iron mortars, prior to analysis. He realized the importance of analysing salts to determine the exact composition of precipitates, and he devised many efficient methods for preparing analytical reagents.[9]

Klaproth accomplished most of his remarkable experimental work in the laboratory of his pharmacy while busily engaged as a pharmaceutical practitioner. Not until he was 57 years old did he sell his pharmacy, to devote his entire time to research and teaching.[10]

The French pharmacist Louis N. Vauquelin (1763–1829) also played an important role in the reform of analytical chemistry. His laboratory became a practical school of chemistry, from which emerged a number of prominent chemists who followed in his footsteps. The famous Liebig, who is commonly credited with having established the first chemical laboratory at a university, worked for a time in the laboratory of Vauquelin.[11]

Another pharmacist who contributed significantly to the development of new techniques of analysis and isolation, as well as to other fields, was Andreas S. Marggraf (1709–1782).[12] A characteristic of Marggraf was that he never was content with having solved a specific problem; he tried in addition to find out all about it, regardless of its immediate practical value. He also avoided the fanciful generalizations so common during his time. He worked out an inexpensive method for the preparation of phosphorus and of phosphoric acid, thus providing the basis for important industries. He prepared and described phosphorus pentoxide and demonstrated that phosphorus is contained in urine as phosphates. When Marggraf first prepared potassium cyanide, he also showed its property of forming double salts with those of the heavy metals. He gave to chemistry the ferrocyanides and the ferricyanides as reagents for iron. His discovery of sugar in the sugar beet is one of those rare accomplishments that, influencing industry, have shaped the national economy. The use of ethyl alcohol as the solvent for extraction of the raw material paved the way for a new technic, as did his use of the microscope in the examination of the sugar crystals.

Marggraf had been thoroughly educated as a pharmacist and for several years assisted his father in the latter's pharmacy in Berlin. However, when 30 years of age, he became connected with the Royal Society of Berlin (known later as the Royal Prussian Academy of Science) and discontinued the practice of pharmacy.

The pharmacist Tobias Lowitz also contributed significantly to analytical chemistry, as well as to other areas of the subject.[13] Like Klaproth, he accomplished most of his results in a pharmacy, the laboratory of the Imperial Russian Court Pharmacy in St. Petersburg (now Leningrad). Here he served first as apprentice and then as assistant and, from 1776 until his death, as manager. This long experience was interrupted only by a 3-year absence, which he spent at the University of Göttingen in his native city.

Lowitz discovered mono- and trichloroacetic acids (1793). He first prepared absolute alcohol and pure ether (1796). He was the first to employ the seeding of solutions to induce the crystallization of the solutes. However, possibly his most important contribution to mankind was the discovery of the decolorizing and deodorizing property of charcoal (1785). Fully aware of the importance of this discovery, he made a thorough investigation of the subject. As early as 1794 he could report to the Russian navy that he was able to make impure water fit to drink. He introduced charcoal into the alcohol distilleries to remove fusel oil and developed other uses for this substance.

Although Lavoisier had offered a working definition of an element (as a substance which does not seem to be decomposed by any known chemical methods) and devised a table of elements, many of the elements were unknown at the beginning of the 19th century. Pharmacists played an important role in the discovery of many of the elements and of numerous important chemical compounds.

Pharmacists, for example, were responsible for the discovery of the four most important and most common members of the halogen family—chlorine, iodine, bromine and fluorine: the first by Scheele (1774), the second by Courtois (1811), the third by Balard (1826) and the fourth by Moissan (1886). All of these men came from the ranks of pharmacy. The discovery of this group of elements, individually important in themselves, brought about the overthrow of Lavoisier's oxygen theory of acids and thus gave rise to concepts that played so important a role in the development of the new chemistry: the actions of acids, bases and salts.

Elemental fluorine not only was discovered by the pharmacist Henri Moissan, but it was made known to the world before a pharmaceutical group, the *Société de pharmacie de Paris.*[14] Moissan was then professor at the École Supérieure de Pharmacie de Paris. He was awarded a Nobel Prize in 1906 for his research. It was also a pharmacist, A. S. Marggraf, who (1768) obtained hydrogen fluoride by distilling fluorspar with sulphuric acid. The resulting product attacked the glass retort he had used. Then, in checking Marggraf's results, Scheele made the same mistake. Johann Carl Friedrich Meyer, owner of a pharmacy in Stettin, in a detailed communication advised Scheele to use lead instead of glass. With this modification in the apparatus, the real nature of hydrogen fluoride could be revealed.

In like manner, the discovery of other halogen derivatives is attributed in no small part to pharmacists. Thus Antoine Balard (1802–1876), who had isolated bromine, also studied its compounds. The pharmacist George Simon Serullas studied derivatives of iodine as well as those of bromine. He prepared both iodoform (1822) and ethylbromide (1827).

If the discovery of iodoform is attributed to Serullas without question, that of chloroform has been claimed by three individuals: the American physician Guthrie, the German chemist Liebig and the French pharmacist Eugène Soubeiran (1797–1858). According to Max Speter, who made a thorough study of this question, it was the German pharmacist Friedrich Moldenhauer who first obtained (1830) a product which he, like Guthrie, regarded as a "chloric ether." Both Liebig and Soubeiran, however, pronounced the product obtained by them (1831) to be a new compound. The pharmacist Soubeiran correctly recognized it as a compound of carbon, hydrogen and chlorine, whereas Liebig overlooked its hydrogen content. The correct formula was assigned to it by J. B. A. Dumas, who replaced the designation "formyl chloride" with "chloroform."[15]

Research on halogens and their derivatives was not new to Dumas. While working in a Geneva pharmacy he was requested to look for iodine, which had been isolated by Courtois, in sponges. A local physician, Dr. Coindet, desired to use it as a specific against goiter. Dumas was successful; and he suggested that the iodine be used in the form of an alcoholic tincture or as potassium iodide (or combination of iodine and aqueous potassium iodide). With the publication of these results, Dumas made his first appearance in print.[16] Although Dumas left the profession he was always grateful to pharmacy. Wherever opportunity offered, whether as Senator of France or as Secretary of Agriculture, he promoted pharmacy.

As is well known, the metallic elements potassium and sodium, magnesium, calcium, strontium and barium were first isolated by Sir Humphry Davy, the father of electro-chemistry; however, the preparatory work leading toward their discovery had been done by German pharmacists. Thus derivatives of sodium and potassium, and magnesium, calcium and barium had been studied by Andreas S. Marggraf; those of barium by Carl W. Scheele; and, lastly, those of strontium by Martin H. Klaproth.

Klaproth has been acclaimed as one of the most gifted discoverers. He owed his discoveries, not to accident, but to his extraordinary skill in both qualitative and quantitative analysis, as has been previously noted. Although he did not isolate any of the elements enumerated above in a pure state (unlike Davy, he did not have the tools to effect their isolation), he has been credited with the discovery of uranium (1789), zirconium (1789) and cerium (1803). In addition, he has to his credit the verification of the elemental character of tellurium, strontium, titanium, chromium and yttrium.[17] However, it must be mentioned that cerium was discovered simultaneously and independently by Berzelius and Hisinger. Although Klaproth's announcement of the discovery of chromium was made several months later than that of Vauquelin (1797), the credit for its isolation nevetheless goes to pharmacy.

Elemental carbon, both as charcoal and as diamond, has been known since antiquity, although its elemental nature was not suspected at that time. However, the discovery of some of the most important properties of amorphous carbon was made by pharmacists. The German pharmacist Carl Gottfried Hagen[18] explained the adsorptive quality of powdered charcoal as a physical property (1793–1794). Whereas the German-Russian pharmacist Tobias Lowitz experimented exclusively with vegetable charcoal, the French pharmacist P. C Figuier published (1810) his results with animal charcoal, proving the latter to be superior to the vegetable variety in several instances. Lastly, the French pharmacist Tuéry demonstrated the antidotal properties of charcoal to the skeptical members of the French Academy of Medicine by swallowing a gram of strychnine after having previously taken 15 grams of charcoal.[19]

In 1844, the German pharmacist Heinrich Rose (1795–1854) announced the discovery of a new element which he named niobium. Some claim that it was but a rediscovery of columbium, which had been isolated from columbite by the English chemist Charles Hatchett. However, the prevailing opinion is that Hatchett did not discover niobium but tantalum, which is closely related to niobium and is commonly associated with it. (Columbium designates this element in the United States, whereas niobium, the name given to it by Rose, has been used in all other countries.)

The great Danish physicist Hans Christian Oersted (1777–1851), who paved the way for the isolation of metallic aluminum and established the laws of electromagnetism, worked as a youth in the pharmacy of his father and even managed, for a short time, a pharmacy in Copenhagen.

A number of European pharmacists also contributed to the formulation of certain theoretical concepts which were important in the development of chemistry as a modern science. In the early 18th century, for example, the French pharmacist Etiene-François Geoffroy presented his attempt to define the specific relationship existing between different substances. His chemical relationship table (published in 1718 in the *Mémoirs* of the Paris Academy of Science) represents an early attempt at a clarification of the principles of chemical affinity.[20]

Guillaume François Rouelle, also a French pharmacist, solved the problem of the nature of salts, a problem which had baffled the best chemical minds for centuries. In the period 1744–1754, he developed the modern definition of a salt as the product of the union of an acid with a base, and distinguished between neutral, acidic and basic salts.[21] Soon thereafter, Lavoisier, a student of Rouelle, defined an acid as the product of the union of a nonmetal with oxygen, and a base as that of the union of a metal with oxygen.

Just as the "*tables de rapports*" of the French pharmacist Geoffroy served as the starting point of numerous speculations, so the grouping of analogous elements as "triads" by Johann Wolfgang Döbereiner (1780–1849), a German pharmacist, was destined to become the forerunner of the periodic table of the elements.

But even before Döbereiner conceived his triads (1817, 1829; positing the atomic weight of the middle element as the arithmetic mean of the sum of atomic weights of the two extremes), another pharmacist had pronounced a mathematical rule. Joseph Louis Proust (1754–1826) pointed out, as a result of numerous investigations, that the elements combine with one another in definite proportions, which are constant. When the nonpharmacist John Dalton (1766–1844) demonstrated the law of simple, constant and multiple proportions, it was based partly on the experimental statements of Proust.

As this survey shows, there is scarcely a field of general chemistry without some important enrichment brought about by pharmacists. Thus it is only natural that they have also contributed to the development of chemical apparatus. The introduction of the microscope as a means of chemical research by the pharmacist Marggraf has already been mentioned. Less well known is the fact that is was the French pharmacist Nicolas LeFebvre who introduced the use of the thermometer into chemistry. The French pharmacist Antoine Baumé created with his hydrometers (or aerometers) (1768) the possibility of an easy and fairly exact determination of the density (specific gravity) of liquids, a method widely used up to the present. The German pharmacist Carl Friedrich Mohr (1806–1879) gave to volumetric analysis most of its auxiliary implements, among them the Mohr-pinchcock. The specific-gravity balance, likewise bearing his name, has been an important piece of laboratory apparatus. At the end of the 19th century the pharmacist Ernst Beckmann (1855–1923) presented chemistry with two different pieces of apparatus for the determination of boiling points and freezing points. Finally, the modern micromethods to a considerable extent owe their development and present status to pharmacists. The Austrian pharmacist Richard Wasicky (1884–1970), an honorary member of the American Pharmaceutical Association, constructed an apparatus for continuous extraction of microquantities of solids.[22] One of Wasicky's pupils, the Austrian pharmacist Ludwig Kofler (1891–1951), invented a melting-point apparatus for use on a microscope (in collaboration with Hilock, one of his students).[23] Finally, it was Wilhelm Carl Böttger (1871–1949), a man who started his career as a German pharmacist, to whom the world of chemistry is indebted for fundamental studies of potentiometric volumetric analysis and of the application of physicochemical laws to analytic problems.[24]

## PLANT CHEMISTRY

The vegetable kingdom, up to the 19th century, supplied more materia pharmaceutica than did the mineral and the animal kingdoms combined. The romance of these drugs held a particular charm, but later insight into their chemical constitution was even more intriguing.

The pharmacist Nicolas Lémery supposedly was the first to attempt to list separately from other drugs the vegetable substances whose chemical nature was supposedly known. However, this division in his *Cours de chimie* (1675) could name only a few individual chemicals: camphor, flowers of benzoes (benzoic acid) and sugar were almost the only ones. Even oil of turpentine (mostly pinene) could scarcely be regarded as an organic chemical.

The isolation of the constituents of plant drugs remained more of a goal than an attainment. In this endeavor pharmacists played an important and zealous role. The art of distillation of aromatic spirits and waters and, subsequently, of volatile oils was of importance in the practice of pharmacy, particularly during the phlogistic period of chemical history. Just as the distillation of aromatic waters (supposed to represent the quintessence of the plants) led to the isolation of volatile oils, so the storage and the observation of the volatile oils led to the isolation of the so-called camphors. Thus Caspar Neumann, administrator of the Prussian Court Pharmacy, in 1719 observed thyme camphor (thymol), and the pharmacist Johann Christian Wiegleb discovered mace camphor (myristic acid) in 1774.

Each observation constituted a notable contribution to the list of the few individual organic chemicals then known. The discovery of glycerin by Scheele, while making lead plaster, is a well-known instance. The French pharmacist Joseph Louis Proust isolated mannitol (1806), also leucin, gliadin and hordein.

Of far greater significance was the recognition of the acid character of the "flowers of benzoes," a name derived from production by the dry method of sublimation. It was in preparing the "flowers" by the wet method (extraction of gum benzoes with milk of lime, and precipitation of the acid from its calcium salt by means of hydrochloric acid) that Scheele recognized their acid character.

The application and the extension of this method led Scheele to the discovery of several new plant acids: tartaric acid (1769), citric acid (1784) and malic acid (1785). It also enabled him to demonstrate the wide distribution of oxalic acid in the vegetable kingdom. Scheele also obtained oxalic acid upon oxidation of sugar with nitric acid, an accomplishment of no mean significance later on, when the study of the structure of organic molecules by means of the "Abbau" method revealed many secrets of organic chemistry.[25]

A most important class of products (from the point of view of drug therapy as well as organic chemistry) were the alkaloids isolated from plant substances. The field of alkaloid chemistry was opened by the isolation of morphine from opium at the beginning of the 19th century. In 1805 and 1806 the German pharmacist Friedrich Wilhelm Sertürner published his first papers about his work on opium, leading to the discovery of what he then called the somniferous principle. Shortly before (1803) the French pharmacist Jean-François Derosne had reported on a crystalline precipitate—later considered to be a mixture of morphine and narcotine—isolated by him out of the same raw opium. Derosne stated that small amounts exerted the same physiologic effect as much greater quantities of the raw material, opium. It was likewise before the first publication by Sertürner that another Frenchman, the nonpharmacist Armand Seguin, reported finding (1804) "a very peculiar vegetable-animal material," but this report was not published until 1814. In contrast with Derosne and Seguin, Sertürner recognized immediately the alkaline character of the substance that he had found and the fundamental importance of this fact. However, his first statement received no attention. It was only after the appearance, in 1817, of a comprehensive publication (*Über das Morphium, eine neue salzfähige Grundlage . . .* in Gilbert's *Annalen der Physick*) that the real character of Sertürner's discovery and, hence, its full significance, was recognized. This paper included Sertürner's report that he had tested the pharmacological action of this drug in humans by using himself and three other young men as subjects. An accidental overdose led to symptoms of morphine poisoning in all four men, but fortunately they all survived the experiment.[26]

Here the salifyable property of this "plant base" was emphasized, and the organic analog to the inorganic base was supposed to have been found. It formed salts with organic acids (morphine acetate) as well as with inorganic acids (morphine hydrochloride). Thus organic systematics were supplied with a theory of acids, bases and salts, analogous to the inorganic classification. How this classification later gave way to the recognition of the alcohols as the true bases of organic chemistry is another story. It is sufficient here to point out that just as a technic had enabled Scheele to isolate a number of plant acids, so the new technic of Sertürner enabled others to isolate additional plant bases from crude drugs.

The very name alkaloid ("alkali-like" coined in 1818 by the German pharmacist K. F. W. Meissner) is suggestive of the rôle these substances played in organic theory and systematics. During the next 10 years no less than 10 alkaloids were isolated from vegetable drugs, most of them by pharmacists. To Joseph Pelletier and Joseph B. Caventou, two Parisian pharmacists, the world has been indebted for the discovery of strychnine (1818), brucine (1819), and, above all, quinine (1820). Cinchona bark had been brought from the Americas to Europe in the 17th century and was used to treat "intermittent fevers" and various other conditions. In the laboratory of their pharmacy, Pelletier and Caventou isolated the active constitutent quinine from the bark. Clinical tests by Paris physicians indicated that quinine sulfate was the most effective antimalarial agent.[27]

The history of alkaloids is a story by itself. Here only a few additional milestones may be mentioned. Pelletier and Dumas isolated narceine (1832) and thebaine (1833). The pharmacist F. F. Runge had isolated caffeine from the coffee bean (1821). A year later the same alkaloid was isolated independently by Pelletier, Caventou and Robiquet. The pharmacist Pierre Jean Robiquet had previously isolated narcotine (1817) and reported codeine (1832). The pharmacist Rudolph Brandes had isolated atropine in an impure state. Later, the pharmacist Philipp Lorenz Geiger, with the cooperation of the non-

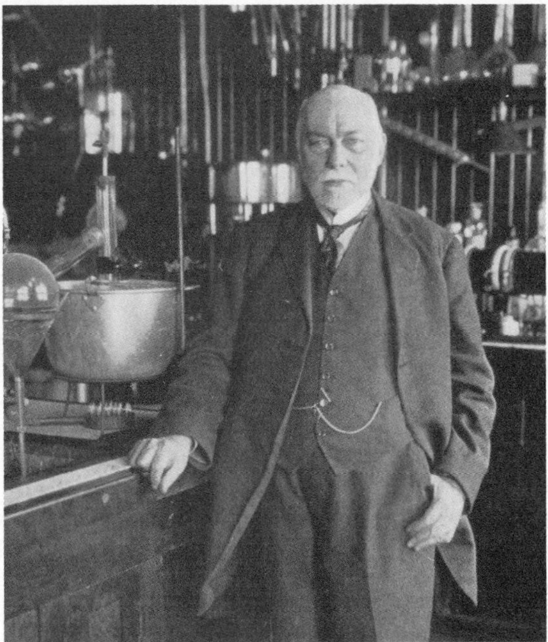

Frederick Belding Power, an American pharmacist who became a distinguished plant chemist, earned the Ebert Prize, the Flueckiger Medal, the Hanbury Medal and many other honors. (From the American Pharmaceutical Association)

pharmacist Hesse, obtained it in a pure state. They also isolated aconitine. Moreover, Geiger prepared pure coniine (1831), previously isolated by the nonpharmacist Carl Giesecke in an impure condition. The pharmacist Georg Franz Merck discovered papaverine; and the pharmacist F. Gaedcke isolated "small needle-shaped crystals" from "erythroxylon coca" (1855), a mixture of coca alkaloids, according to R. Zaunick. Finally the young pharmacist Albert Niemann, a student of the great chemist Wöhler, succeeded in isolating pure cocaine from coca leaves (1860). This promising young scientist died (not quite 27 years of age) only 1 year after receiving, on the basis of his work on cocaine, his degree of Doctor of Philosophy.[28]

The pharmacist E. Jahns synthesized arecoline (1890), an alkaloid which, with arecaidine and guvacine, he had isolated from the areca nut. These results he accomplished in the small laboratory of his pharmacy in Göttingen, the same pharmacy in which young Albert Niemann had served his apprenticeship. The German pharmacist Ernst A. Schmidt isolated scopolamine (1890). The German-American pharmacist, Ferdinand F. Mayer, may be credited with developing the so-called "Mayer's reagent for alkaloids" (mercuric potassium iodide test solution).[29]

Naturally, pharmacists have been interested in the study of glycosides as well as of alkaloids. The pharmacist Rudolph Brandes isolated delphinine (1817), the pharmacist Kahler discovered santonin (1830) and the pharmacist Sidney Smith isolated digoxin (1930). Possibly no drugs afforded greater difficulty in the unraveling of their constituents than digitalis and ergot. In the early study of both, pharmacists played a conspicuous part, although the decisive work in both cases was by a nonpharmacist, the great Swiss chemist, Arthur Stoll.

Important basic work in the study of essential oils was done by Sir William Tilden[30] (1842–1926), a pharmacist. He introduced nitrosyl chloride as a useful reagent for terpenes in the 1860's.

In the United States Frederick B. Power[31] (1853–1927) increased our knowledge of the volatile oils as well as other constituents of plants in a remarkable series of researches. Investigations begun in F. A. Flueckiger's Pharmaceutical Institute at the University of Strassburg, Power continued while at the Philadelphia College of Pharmacy and then at the University of Wisconsin. As Scientific Director of Fritzsche Brothers, in New Jersey, and later as Director of the Wellcome Research Laboratory in London, he and his colaborers published an epoch-making series of phytochemical papers. By no means least of these is his study of chaulmoogric and hydnocarpic acids, which not only contributed to the fight against leprosy, but made necessary a revised definition of the fatty acids. Upon Power's return to the United States, his phytochemical work was continued in the Bureau of Chemistry of the Department of Agriculture in Washington, and resulted in his election as a member of the National Academy of Science. At the University of Wisconsin his work on essential oils was continued by Edward Kremers (1865–1941), a disciple of Power as well as of Wallach.

It would scarcely be appropriate to refer above to Flueckiger without at least mentioning Daniel Hanbury of London (1825–1875), Alexander Tschirch of Bern (1856–1939) and Hermann Thoms of Berlin (1859–1931). All these men, who did meritorious work in examining and isolating the content of plants came from pharmacy. Flueckiger owned a pharmacy for some years, and Thoms managed one.

Last, it should be noted that the German-Russian pharmacist Johann Georg Dragendorff (1836–1898) contributed importantly to plant chemistry by developing a systematic process of plant analysis, based largely on solvent extraction procedures.

## PHYSIOLOGIC CHEMISTRY

Physiologic chemistry has been defined in a somewhat restricted sense as the application of chemistry to the study of the normal processes of the human body. In a broader sense, it covers the normal processes of all animal life, and the term may even be applied to the normal processes of plant life. Today its use has been largely replaced by biochemistry, which includes both.

Particularly in France, where clinical technology has been closely associated with pharmacy, many of the pharmacists who rise to the level of real scientific research have shown a bent toward the biologic aspects of chemistry. Such pharmacists in the early 19th century often studied medicine for advanced training. "This does not mean," Berman points out, "that these pharmacists practiced medicine, that they were clinicians, or that they had surrendered their identity as pharmacists, as the examples of Bouchardat, Méhu, Mialhe, Chatin, and Virey illustrate."[32]

Indeed, for some 23 years Apollinaire Bouchardat (1806–1886) had practiced hospital pharmacy while he conducted versatile investigations. His work in hygiene influenced the French etiologic approach to medicine. His research on diabetes provided the basis for what has been called "the most rational method of treatment up to his time."

In the opinion of the distinguished American biochemist, E. V. McCollum, the hospital pharmacist Camille Méhu (1835–1887) "made one of the most important discoveries in the entire history of protein investigations," notably that proteins precipitate from solution without changing their nature when saturated with ammonium sulfate.

Another French pharmacist, Louis Mialhe (1807–1886), isolated ptyalin and demonstrated the action of this enzyme on starch, among other contributions to physiologic chemistry. A contemporary who practiced hospital pharmacy in Paris for some 33 years, Gaspard A. Chatin (1813–1901) developed a micro-method for measuring iodine, on the basis of his studies of the iodine content of plants. He also advanced the view that a lack of iodine caused endemic goiter (1851–1852).

One of the most important products of animal metabolism, urea, was discovered in human urine (1773) by the French pharmacist Hilaire Marin Rouelle (brother of G. F. Rouelle, previously mentioned). At about the same time, Rouelle also discovered hippuric acid in the urine of cows and camels, but he believed it to be benzoic acid (an error later corrected by Liebig).[33] Another French pharmacist, Vauquelin, was one of the group of scientists who made a special study of urea, a substance which has played an important role, not only in physiologic chemistry, but also in the theory of vitalism.

H. M. Rouelle, furthermore, was the first to recognize the iron content of blood. The

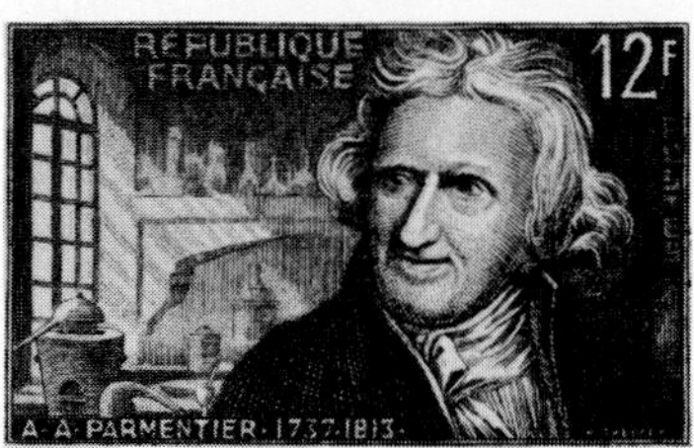


Commemorative postage stamps have been issued to help honor some of the pharmacists whose scientific contributions became significant. Pictured on this French issue is J. A. A. Parmentier, best remembered for his discoveries in the field of food chemistry.

pharmacist Antoine Baumé first pronounced milk an emulsion. Of the ten eminent early physiologic chemists who, according to Lieben, made important contributions to the study of milk, no less than six were pharmacists (Geoffroy, Baumé, Rouelle, Parmentier, Vauquelin and Scheele).[34] Among other observations, Vauquelin noticed that the addition of acid prevents fermentation.

The discovery of sugar in beets by the pharmacist A. S. Marggraf has already been mentioned. Proust isolated grape sugar from grape juice, and for a time was credited with discovering this substance. However, the pharmacist Tobias Lowitz had isolated it from honey 14 years earlier in pure crystalline form. Henri Braconnot, a pharmacist in Strassburg previous to his appointment as a professor at Nancy and director of the Botanical Garden, was the first to obtain grape sugar by treating sawdust with sulphuric acid, thus laying the foundation for an important chemical industry (1819). In addition, he discovered pectin and pectic acid (1824) and dextrin (1833). As early as 1820, he had obtained glycine, the first amino acid resulting from the hydrolysis of albumen with the aid of a mineral acid.[35]

The amino acid leucine had previously (1819) been discovered by the pharmacist Joseph L. Proust, whom Lieben regards as an "exact analyst" and as "one of the early albumen and nutrition investigators."[36] The first to characterize albumen was the English apothecary William Thomas Brande (1788–1866). The albumen reagent, an acetic acid solution of mercuric chloride in potassium iodide, was designed by the French pharmacist Charles Joseph Tanret (1847–1917), in the laboratory of his Troyes pharmacy.

It was pharmacist Scheele who first recognized the acid reaction of normal urine,[37] and it was his French colleague Proust who taught the prevention of the spontaneous fermentation of urine, which renders it alkaline and thus unfit for analytic tests by reagents. In the elaboration of the numerous reagents and methods employed in the analysis of urine, pharmacists or men trained in pharmacy have participated successfully. For example, the inventor of Fehling's solution (1850, used for the detection of inverted sugar in the blood as well as in urine), Hermann v. Fehling, practiced pharmacy for about 8 years before he gave up his profession to devote his life to scientific research.

## MEDICINAL CHEMISTRY AND PHARMACOLOGY

By the late 19th century, the various sciences had become highly specialized fields and advanced training (usually culminating in a doctoral degree) had become almost a prerequisite for performing significant scientific research. The practicing pharmacist who carried out research in the laboratory of his pharmacy gradually became a phenomenon of the past. Some pharmacists (or graduates of pharmacy schools), of course, elected to pursue graduate work in the sciences and to eventually enter a research career in the academic world or in government or in industrial research laboratories, thus continuing in a modified form the tradition of the pharmacist-scientist.

As pharmacy schools began to offer programs of graduate study, some pharmacists chose to undertake advanced work in the pharmaceutical sciences rather than in chemistry, botany or related fields. A report of the American Association of Colleges of Pharmacy indicated, for example, that there were 2,287 students (most of them probably graduates of pharmacy schools) enrolled in graduate programs in American schools of pharmacy in 1973. Most of these students were pursuing studies in the laboratory sciences, although a small number were studying in non-laboratory fields such as pharmacy administration.[38]

In this section, a few examples will be given of some significant contributions to the fields of pharmacology and medicinal chemistry by individuals who received their undergraduate training in pharmacy and then embarked upon careers in scientific research (research contributions directly in pharmacy itself, or pharmaceutics, will not be considered here, as the main focus of this chapter is the contributions of pharmacists to other, related sciences).

One of the most successful workers in the field of chemotherapy (i.e., the direct attack on the morbific agents in the cells by chemical substances having specific effects), the French medicinal chemist Ernest F. A. Fourneau (1872–1949), came from the ranks of pharmacy. For quite a while he combined his research activities with his service in his pharmacy. The arsenic compound Stovarsol was a child of Fourneau's genius. He also bared the secret of the effective drug Germanin by duplicating it with a preparation called Fourneau 309. From the Fourneau laboratories at the Pasteur Institute, as the fruit of Fourneau's initiative and under his guidance, came the important discovery that the astonishing effect of the German drug Prontosil was due to the sulfonamide part of the complex molecule. Furthermore, from the same place and under the same circumstances there emanated the first group of chemicals to earn the title of antihistamine agents, some of them carrying Fourneau's name.[39]

Another example of a medicinal chemist who began his career as a pharmacist is Friedrich Stolz (1860–1936). In 1904, Stolz synthesized adrenaline, the first hormone to be chemically prepared. In that same year, he also synthesized noradrenaline and recognized that it was as active as adrenaline in raising blood pressure in animals. The contributions of another important medicinal chemist, Fritz Hofmann (like Stolz a German pharmacist), are discussed in the section on "Industry."

Experimental pharmacology began to emerge as a separate discipline in the 19th century, as an offshoot of physiology. At first it found its academic home in schools of medicine and, while this tradition has continued, the 20th century has seen the science of pharmacology established in schools of pharmacy as well.

One of the most eminent 20th century pharmacologists, Ku Kuei Chen (born 1898), received his early training in pharmacy. Born in Shanghai, China, he obtained his B.S. in pharmacy from the University of Wisconsin (1920), his Ph.D. in physiology and pharmacology from the same institution (1923) and the M.D. from the Johns Hopkins University School of Medicine (1927). He became Director of the Pharmacological Division of Eli Lilly and Company (1929), a position he held until his retirement in 1963 (although he remained active as Professor of Pharmacology at the Indiana University School of Medicine).

Chen's contributions to pharmacology are numerous, and include studies on cardioactive drugs, synthetic analgesics and drugs that lower the blood sugar. His name is probably most closely associated, however, with the introduction of ephedrine into modern medicine. While working in the pharmacological laboratory of Carl Schmidt at the Peking Union Medical College in China in 1923, Chen decided to investigate the effects of the herb Ma Huang, which had been used in traditional Chinese medicine for centuries.

The alkaloid ephedrine had already been

isolated from this plant by the Japanese scientist W. N. Nagai in 1887, but it had not aroused much interest at that time. It was only after Chen had reisolated it, and he and Schmidt had investigated its pharmacology in detail, that the similarity of its effects to those of adrenaline (epinephrine) was clearly recognized. Clinical studies soon established its therapeutic value in the treatment of asthma, hypotension and various other conditions.

Chen received the Remington Honor Medal in 1965 for his contributions to the pharmaceutical field. In his award address, he discussed how he came to study pharmacy:

> In China sick people were treated with preparations of her native herbs on an empirical basis. When I was graduated from a junior college in Peking in 1918, I made up my mind to analyze these interesting herbs reputed to have healing properties. My teachers in China advised me to matriculate at the University of Wisconsin and wrote letters of recommendation. When I arrived at Madison, the registrar of the University did not know where to put me, so referred me to Professor Edward Kremers, the tenth Remington medalist. Professor Kremers mapped out my program with great emphasis on chemistry, including his own course on phytochemistry . . .
>
> After I obtained my bachelor's degree in pharmacy, Professor Kremers assigned to me a research problem on the essential oil of Chinese cinnamon leaves and twigs which he imported from China through the courtesy of the American embassy at Peking . . . While Professor Kremers urged me to concentrate on scientific pharmacy, I figured that I should know something about the profession of pharmacy. I got myself a part-time job in a drugstore. For the first few weeks my preceptor asked me to work at the prescription counter. Being satisfied with my work, he let me wait at the soda fountain.[40]

Chen's interest in pharmacology, a subject not then offered in most pharmacy schools, led him to pursue further graduate work in the medical school. While he never practiced pharmacy, he exemplifies the contributions made to science by those who have received academic training in pharmacy.

A pharmacist who has made significant contributions to both pharmacology and pharmaceutical chemistry is John C. Krantz, Jr. (born 1899), the son of a prominent Baltimore pharmacist. He received his bachelor's degree in pharmacy and his Ph.D. in pharmaceutical chemistry from the University of Maryland. During the course of his career Krantz taught at the University of Maryland School of Pharmacy (and was also simultaneously consulting pharmacist at the Johns Hopkins Hospital), served as Director of Research for Sharp and Dohme and as Chief of the Bureau of Chemistry of the Maryland Department of Health, and eventually became Professor of Pharmacology in the University of Maryland School of Medicine. His major research interests have centered about carbohydrate metabolism, general anesthetics and the mechanism of action of vasodilating drugs. Krantz is also the author of widely used textbooks in pharmacology and pharmaceutical chemistry.

## INDUSTRY

Scientific research has supplied the basis of industry in general and of special industries in particular to such an extent that each attempt at recounting the work of scientists and its effect on the development of industry of necessity entails some repetition.

Thus several industries, among them the manufacture of explosives (nitroglycerin), owe their existence to the discovery of glycerin by Scheele, mentioned earlier. Another discovery of Scheele, that of chlorine, became a basis for the bleaching and laundry industry. The importance of Scheele's discovery of the fruit acids, especially citric acid, for the foodstuffs industries (especially the production of beverages) is obvious. The decolorizing and purifying power of charcoal, discovered by Lowitz, plays an important part in the production process of a number of industries.

A few words more may be devoted to the discovery of beet sugar by Marggraf, already mentioned, since the discovery has become part of world history. It was Napoleon, in the course of his attempt to bar England from trading with those parts of continental Europe then under French domination, who recognized the importance of Marggraf's discovery in liberating Europe from the English monopoly in cane sugar. Furthermore, Napoleon appreciated the possibility, inherent in this discovery, of making sugar a general foodstuff for all, instead of a luxury for the rich. A famous Napoleonic edict (January 15, 1812), the basis of further development of the beet sugar industry, provided for training 100 young people in the manufacture of sugar, apprentices "to be chosen among the students of pharmacy, of medicine and of chemistry."[41]

Discoveries of pharmacists not yet mentioned also may be considered as of worldwide importance. The discovery of catalysis by the pharmacist Johann W. Döbereiner and the finding and characterizing of aniline in coal tar by the pharmacist Friedlieb F. Runge were of vital significance.

The scientific and industrial values of both discoveries proved to be almost immeasurable. In 1816, Döbereiner already had found that alcohol could be changed to acetic acid through catalysis by platinum. He obtained aldehyde in the same way. His memorable pamphlet (titled *"Über Neu Entdeckte Höchst Merkwürdige Eigenschaften des Platins"*) was about recently discovered highly peculiar qualities of platinum. In the year of publication (1823), now fully aware of the technical as well as of the scientific bearing of his invention, he constructed his famous tinder box. This was based on the catalytic capacity of spongy platinum to bring the hydrogen generated in the box into chemical union with oxygen from the air, hence to ignition. Döbereiner explained in detail the principles of its function and its manufacture. The historian of chemistry, H. Kopp, has commented appreciatively about the scientific unselfishness of this pharmacist:

> With the employment of it [catalysis] for the construction of his so widely used tinder box, Döbereiner presented it to his contemporaries, while frequently the practical employment of scientific discoveries of much less importance has been used as a private speculation in order to gain riches.[42]

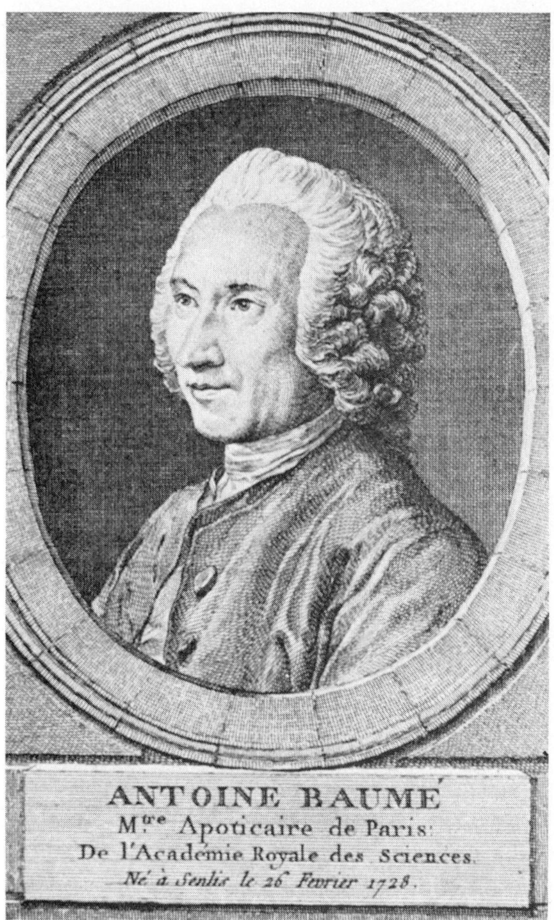
ANTOINE BAUMÉ
Mtre Apoticaire de Paris:
De l'Académie Royale des Sciences.
Né à Senlis le 26 Fevrier 1728.

Pharmacist Antoine Baumé of Paris, who established a pharmacy and laboratory that eventually marked him as one of the founders of modern pharmaceutical industry. His price list of 1775 reveals the range of this venture *(Prix courants des préparations de chymie et de pharmacie)*. The special hydrometer devised by Baumé still finds use in industry. Two of his influential works were textbooks on pharmacy and on experimental chemistry. (From: Illustrierter Apotheker-Kalender, Stuttgart, 1965)

The number of industries using, if not entirely dependent on, the process of catalysis is very large. A notable example is the "contact process" for the preparation of sulfuric acid. The entire industry of artificial fats, margarine, etc., is based on the coagulation of liquid oils to solid fats of the desired consistency by catalytic hydrogenation processes.

F. F. Runge published (in 1834) his classic essay *("Über Einige Merkwürdige Produkte der Steinkohlendestillation (Kyanol, Pyrrol, Leukol, Carbolsäure, Rosolsäure und Brunolsäure)")* concerning discoveries that included aniline (the "kyanol" of Runge) in coal tar. Thus the ground was laid for the entire industry of dyestuffs and synthetic organic remedies, using the aniline derived from coal tar as raw material. Runge's discovery of carbolic acid furnished the essential germicide for Lister's surgical antisepsis. Like Döbereiner, Runge was fully aware of the importance of his discoveries and took the first steps to prove them practically. He was the first to observe (1834) the blue color of aniline after the addition of chloride of lime and to find that by treating aniline with other oxidizing substances, dark green to black dyestuffs can be obtained. "He already had in his hands the emeraldin and the aniline black, so eminently important until to-day."[43] Furthermore, Runge gave the first impetus to the processing of cottonware with sulfonized oils, and was the first to produce the oxidation product of aniline on the textiles themselves. Because of this, some historians see in Runge the first to recognize and employ practically the principles of capillarity. The statement of Kränzlein that this pharmacist opened a new epoch with his discoveries is uncontested. "The world," says Kränzlein, "can consider Runge the first inventor of coal-tar dyestuffs without by this taking away anything of the immortal fame gained in the same field by A. W. Hoffmann and his pupils, and especially by W. H. Perkin."[44]

The genius of F. F. Runge was not exceeded, although perhaps almost paralleled, by another pharmacist, Adolf Frank (1834–1916), whose inventions establish him as the founder of several industries and who became, on the basis of his scientific findings, an industrialist himself. Frank invented (1882) the process of purifying water by filtration through infusorial silica (Berkefeld filter). Together with Caro, he discovered the possibility of binding free nitrogen to calcium carbide and thus laid the basis for the calcium cyanamide industry. The development of the calcium carbide and acetylene industry is to a large extent due to the technical inventions of this pharmacist, who likewise is considered to be one of the founders of the German potassium salts industry. Frank's studies on enamel and glasspastes laid the groundwork for the modern mosaic industry.[45]

A similar combination of scientific genius and commercial and administrative talent made the pharmacist Fritz Hofmann (1866–1956) one of the leading figures in modern chemical industry. His world fame derives from his successful work in the synthesis of caoutchouc (preceded by the manufacture of isoprene from turpentine by the English pharmacist William Tilden). This achievement was rewarded by a flood of honors—among them the Emil Fischer Medal, the highest proof of appreciation that organized German chemistry has to offer. In addition, Hofmann did much work in other fields of chemical research, including pharmaceutical chemistry. The following extract from a letter written by Hofmann conveys an idea of the man and his work. Having reported about his 6 years spent in practicing pharmacy and in pharmaceutical and post-graduate study and, finally, his appointment as a member of the staff of the Elberfelder Farbwerke (later the center of I. G. Farbenindustrie), Hofmann continued as follows:

> In Elberfeld I became director of the pharmaceutical scientific laboratory and vice-president of the concern. *My collaborators and I invented a long row of well-known synthetic remedies which belong until the present to the medicinal armamentarium.* Besides my activity in the pharmaceutical field the problems I worked on were those of the

> chemistry of perfumes, the chemistry of fermentation, that of light, and finally the search for chemical means against plant-diseases and vermin. . . . By 1909 I had succeeded in the synthesis of caoutchouc in the laboratory of the Elberfelder Farbenfabriken. . . . In Elberfeld I founded and conducted for six years the Institute for Chemotherapy which later under the leadership of Professor Hörlein reached the highest degree of perfection . . . and presented the world with Germanin, Plasmochin, etc.[46]

Hofmann remembered gratefully his work as a practicing pharmacist, to which he felt indebted for the general skill "which became so helpful to me in my later work."

"My collaborators and I invented a long row of well-known synthetic remedies." This statement by Hofmann is revealing. It reminds us why, in recent history, the invention of remedies usually has not been so closely connected with the name of single individuals as it was in earlier times. In this epoch of mass problems and mass production, even invention has become a matter of organization rather than of isolated genius. Yet, this organized research also requires men of ingenuity, talent and even genius, with ambition and vision as well as skill. In this army of relatively anonymous workers on the problems of joint research the contingent of people coming from pharmacy is still an important one. This has been proved now and again when, in cases like that of Hofmann, the impact of exceptional results has removed the obscurity that subordinates the individual research worker within the group of workers or within the complex of innovations from diverse laboratories on which a notable advance often depends.

Dulcine (phenetidine-urea), discovered by the pharmacist Hermann Thoms in the last decade of the 19th century, is 220 times as sweet as the sugar discovered in beets by Marggraf or that derived from sugar cane. This was a fact startling enough to end the anonymity of the inventor, although the discovery was made by Thoms while in the service of an industrial laboratory.[47]

Sometimes an individual pharmacist, besides making an important discovery outside of industry, has succeeded in utilizing it. E. Ritsert, a pharmacist who practiced in Frankfort-on-the-Main, found (1888) that the acetanilide then on the market was not chemically pure and invented a special process for manufacturing a pure product. In pursuing his private research, he prepared (1890) p-aminobenzoicacidethylester (benzocaine), which he called Anaesthesin because of its anesthetic effect. He made this product the basis of a factory of his own. Not only has benzocaine been used extensively the world over in external and internal therapy, but modern substitutes for cocaine, among them procaine, have been built on the basis of the invention by pharmacist Ritsert. Concluding a kind of autobiographic report, Ritsert wrote:

> I state with satisfaction that my observations . . . have laid the ground for an entire group of remedies of greatest importance. Even more satisfaction I take in the fact that, although being a pharmacist relying completely upon myself and without the means and the aid of big institutes or chemical plants, I was able to overcome all difficulties encountered and to carry the results of my work to victory.[48]

As indicated in preceding chapters, modern pharmaceutical industry has been derived to a substantial extent from community pharmacies. In Germany the laboratories of pharmacies developed in so many cases into industrial plants, which later on gained wide and sometimes international recognition, that it does not seem exaggerated to call German community pharmacy the nucleus or seedbed for the German pharmaceutical industry.[49] In other countries the situation has been similar, except that often instead of the laboratory of a pharmacy becoming a manufacturing plant, pharmacists have founded industries without using a pharmacy as a foundation.

As shown in the chapter on economics, however, there are in the United States several examples of pharmacies having served as nuclei for large present-day manufacturing

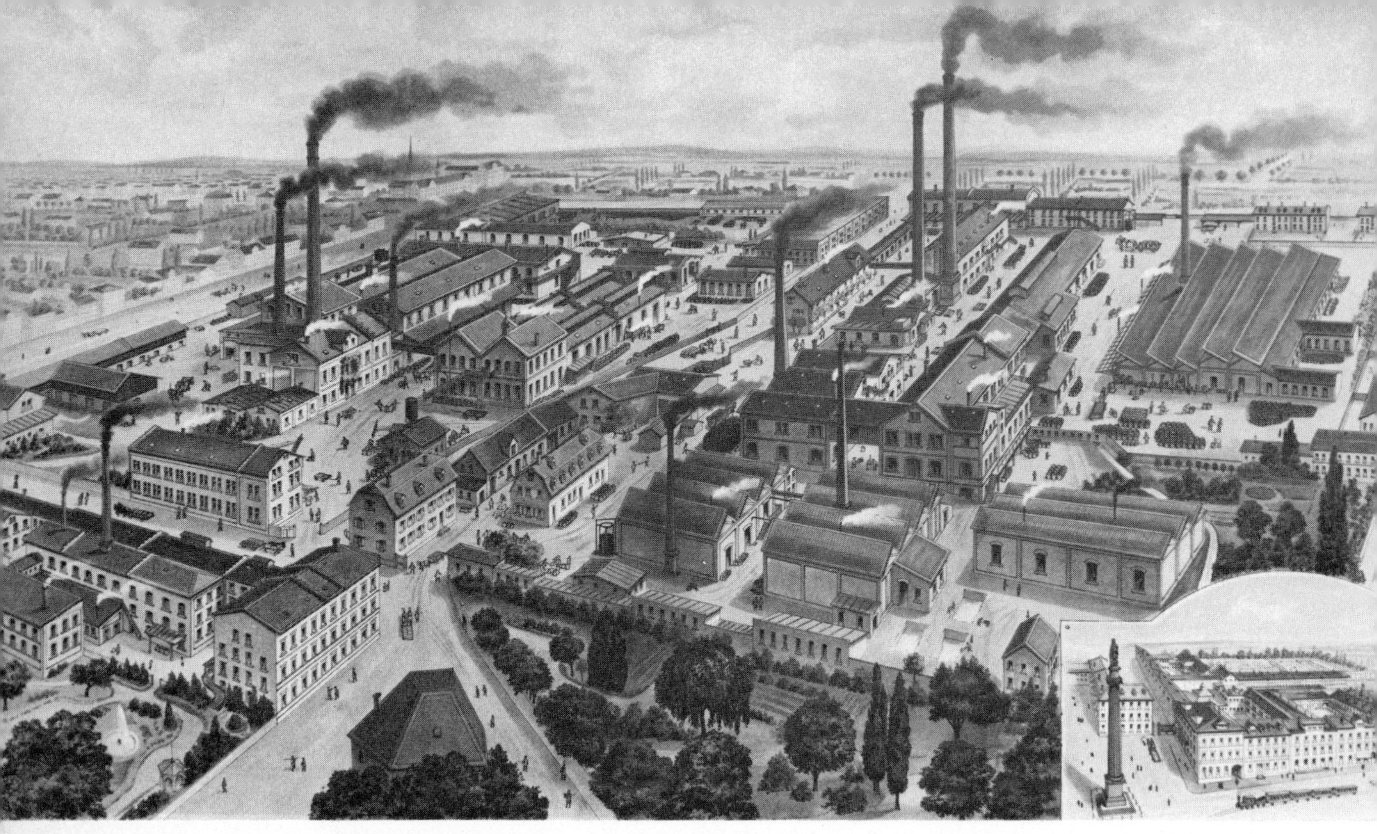

Large-scale production of drugs utilizing power-driven machinery often grew out of individual pharmacies that had utilized traditional techniques of hand-operated apparatus. This European (and later American) phenomenon is epitomized by this illustration: It shows the "laboratories and works" of E. Merck-Darmstadt in the late 19th century, which evolved from the Merck family's "Pharmacy at the Sign of the Angel," founded at Darmstadt in the 17th century. (From a company broadside, at The Smithsonian Institution)

laboratories. Furthermore, the success of some of the American pharmaceutical plants owned by pharmacists was sometimes to a significant extent due to the personal scientific research of their owners (e.g., Alfred Dohme of Sharp and Dohme, and Henry A. B. Dunning of Hynson, Westcott and Dunning).

## MISCELLANEOUS

Wherever we glance over the pages of the book of science, we meet the phenomenal figure of the pharmacist Carl Scheele. In describing researches concerning chemical effects due to the spectrum, the historian Friedrich Dannemann wrote:

> Already Scheele had proved that the parts of the spectrum show different chemical effects (1777). Knowing that silver chloride gets gradually blackened if exposed to light, he brought a piece of paper prepared with silver chloride into the spectrum and observed that it blackened much quicker under the influence of violet than by exposure to other colors. *This simple experiment may be considered the beginning of the spectral photography so highly developed in our days.*[50] [Italics added.]

The physicist who later (1801) proved the existence of chemically efficient rays beyond the violet, Johann W. Ritter, had worked in a pharmacy for 4 years before he devoted himself exclusively to science and became one of the best-known physicists of his time.[51] In the experiments by which he established with certainty the more powerful chemical effect of the rays—later to be called "ultraviolet" rays—he used Scheele's method of testing the differences in the rapidity of the destruction of silver nitrate.[52]

Early in the 18th century, Johann Friedrich

Böttger, who began as a pharmacist and who supposedly knew the alchemical mystery of the transmutation of base metals into gold, presented the precious invention of the manufacture of porcelain to the covetous King August II of Saxony, who kept him a prisoner. About this chemical invention Ferchl and Süssenguth wrote, "The greatest progress came to the European ceramic industry with the re-invention of the genuine Chinese porcelain, which we owe to the apothecary clerk Johann Friedrich Böttger."[53]

Of the many pharmacists who devoted themselves to botany, the "lovable science," we mention here as examples only six eminent men: the German Oskar Brefeld (1839–1925),[54] the Frenchmen A. L. A. Fée (1789–1874) and Emile Bourquelot (1851–1921), the Englishmen Edward Morell Holmes (1843–1930) and George Claridge Druce (1851–1932), and the German Ferdinand v. Müller (1825–1896).[55]

Of Brefeld's contribution to his special field of botany, J. R. Green wrote that "The work of Brefeld included a very careful study of the biology of many of the fungi and the nature of their dependence upon external conditions, together with the effect of the latter upon their pleomorphy and their reproductive processes."[56] It was Brefeld who introduced the method of cultivation into mycologic research. Likewise, it was in the field of mycology that E. Bourquelot contributed fundamental scientific and practical information. A. L. A. Fée was one of the foremost cryptogamists of his time, and also gained world-wide recognition by excellent historical research on antique materia medica and botany.[57]

The German Ferdinand v. Müller, educated as a pharmacist as well as in the science of botany, emigrated to Australia and became that continent's greatest botanist. His studies of the flora of Australia are recorded in 40 volumes. His advice was influential in the agricultural and horticultural development of his adopted country. One of Müller's services was his advice that the eucalyptus tree should be cultivated in the Mediterranean countries, South Africa and the United States, as a means of saving the soil from erosion. Thus he has been credited with preserving and even creating wide areas in which human and animal life may prosper.

While the French and German pharmacist-botanists mentioned above have devoted the greater part of their lives to academic research, after having completed their pharmaceutical education, their English colleagues E. M. Holmes and G. C. Druce for a considerable time combined the practice of pharmacy with their scientific pursuits. Holmes has been regarded as "probably the greatest expert on economic botany of his time,"[58] and Druce as "the greatest British field botanist of his day."[59]

The man whom Sigerist[60] has called the founder of the science of experimental hygiene, Max von Pettenkofer (1819–1901), was a pharmacist, although he also held a medical degree. Pettenkofer spent his life as pharmacist-in-ordinary to the King of Bavaria and director of the Royal Bavarian Court Pharmacy besides being professor of hygiene and director of the first Hygiene Institute at the University of Munich. He has stated his indebtedness to pharmacy for his acquiring accuracy in work and manual skill and for preventing scientific one-sidedness.

Pharmacists even may be mentioned among the pioneers of modern aeronautics. A French pharmacist, Pilâtre de Rozier, was the first human being who dared to make a balloon ascension (1783). Furthermore, he invented a new type of balloon, the so-called *rozière,* replacing the *montgolfière.* De Rozier was killed in a flight over the English channel.[61] Thus the first flyer as well as the first victim of aeronautics was a pharmacist. Moreover, a Dutch pharmacist and chemist, Johann P. Minkelers first replaced hot air or hydrogen in balloons with illuminating gas (1785) and pioneered in its manufacture.

One of the first scientists, if not the first who tried to examine experimentally the physical phenomena connected with aeronautics was likewise a pharmacist. Only one year after Pilâtre de Rozier's first flight, the young pharmacist M. H. Klaproth ventured a flight in a *montgolfière* balloon, armed with instruments for the determination of air pressure, etc. (1784). But the balloon was torn and rose only to a height of 10 meters, and thus the flight was without scientific results. More fortunate was the Brazilian pharmacist Paulo Seabra (born 1899), who did remarkable research on the biological and psychological effects of high-altitude flying. Moreover, one of the prerequisites to high-altitude flight itself was the invention of apparatus for oxygen inhalation by the French pharmacist Stanislas Limousin.[62]

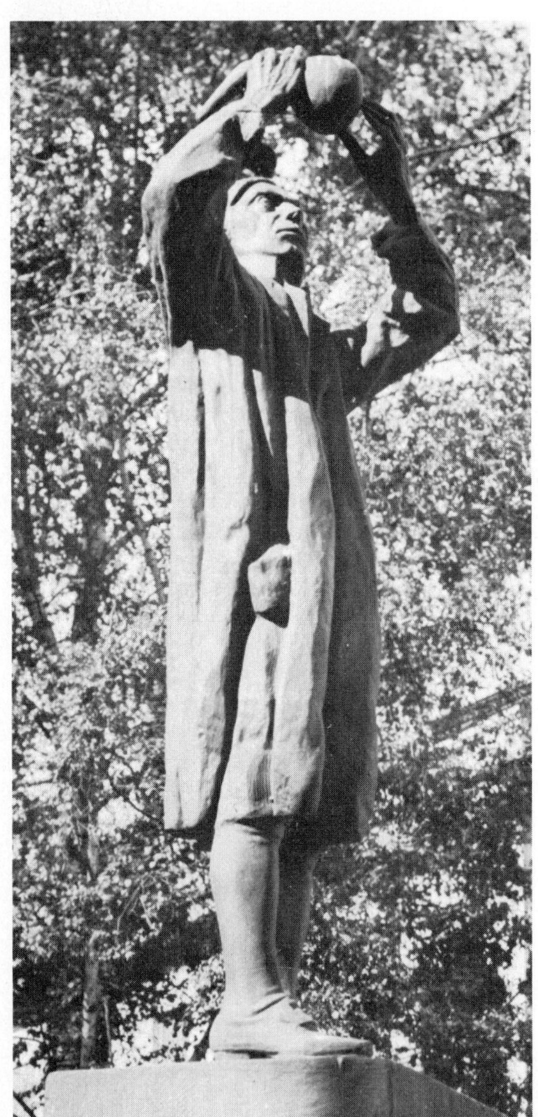

Carl W. Scheele of Sweden retains his place, after two centuries, as one of the great pharmacists of all time. This bronze statue by Milles at Köping (unveiled in 1912) shows the modest practitioner and experimenter in an attitude quite different from that of the glamorized monument at Stockholm. (Photograph from T. Lindham, Farmacevitiska Foreningen)

## CONCLUSION

Both contemporaries and posterity have shown their appreciation toward many of the men mentioned in this chapter. Monuments have been erected and medals have been coined in honor of many of the great pharmacists. In Stockholm and in the small town of Köping, statues commemorate the modest pharmacist Scheele, who passed his life in his profession while serving the world in his laboratory.

In Paris for more than 40 years, from 1900 until destroyed during World War II, one monument united in bronze the figures of Caventou and Pelletier, the two pharmacists whose joint work presented the world with so many important alkaloids, including quinine. Their undying renown is indicated by the fact that a second public monument to the same pharmacists has been erected on the same spot.

Sertürner is commemorated by tablets in Paderborn, Einbeck and Hameln, the places where this pharmacist practiced his profession, in Neuhaus where he was born and within the University of Münster. The bust of Klaproth adorns the peristyle of the University of Berlin, close to the busts of the brothers Alexander and Wilhelm v. Humboldt. The bust of another pharmacist, A. S. Marggraf, on the wall of the building in Berlin which once housed the laboratory of the Royal Prussian Academy of Science, bears witness to his work there for the benefit of humanity.

In Melbourne, Australia, the statue of the pharmacist-botanist F. v. Müller looks down rows of eucalyptus trees, *his* trees. In Canada, a monument in Quebec and a tablet in Annapolis Royal honor the memory of the pharmacist Louis Hébert (see p. 150).

All gratitude and honors naturally go to the individuals, rather than to the profession which these men practiced or in which they were trained. Yet every profession has some part in the bent of the efforts and the values of the work of its sons.

This survey of contributions by pharmacists to science and industry has necessarily been restricted to representative findings and experimental work of significance, and no person has been admitted on the basis of literary work alone. Even with this restriction, there is a need to select from among an abundance of individuals and scientific deeds. Such an abundance can scarcely be accidental. It must have some basis. Perhaps this basis can be found in the fact that hardly any other profession is committed like pharmacy to the study and the utilization of a number of sciences, and at the same time is closely connected with the desires and the needs of the daily life of society. From this arises an incentive to high attainment in the sciences and a dedication to work for the benefit of mankind.

The members of the profession derive pride from the deeds of their great colleagues. The younger generation may take these deeds and these men as models and as evidence of the opportunities open to everyone who attempts to honor his profession and himself in it. The world in general, and legislation and public opinion, should take cognizance of what pharmacy really means. Thus becomes clear a rational basis for public recognition and protection of pharmacy to help to assure the maintenance of professional vigor and creative spirit.[63]

# Appendices

# Appendix 1
# Representative Drugs of the American Indians

North American aborigenes had an extensive materia medica, varying somewhat from tribe to tribe. Here is a selective list of Indian drugs thought by Corlett to be "of special interest or of some distinctive value" because of official recognition once accorded in the white man's books of drug standards. For more comprehensive information, see especially V. Vogel: *American Indian Medicine*, Norman, Okla., ca. 1970, 583 pp. The list is abstracted from W. T. Corlett: *The Medicine-Man of the American Indian*, p. 318, New York, 1935.*

ANGELICA (*Angelica atropurpurea* L.)
ARBOR VITAE (*Tuja occidentalis* L.)
BALM OF GILEAD (*Populus candicans* Ait.)
BEARBERRY (*Arctostaphylos Uva-ursi* [L.] Spreng.)
BETH ROOT (*Trillium* species)
BLACKBERRY (*Rubus nigrobaccus* Bailey)
BLACK CHERRY (*Prunus serotina* Ehrh.)
BLACK COHOSH (*Cimicifuga racemosa* L.)
BLOODROOT (*Sanguinaria canadensis* L.)
BLUE COHOSH (*Caulophyllum thalictroides* [L.] Michaux.)
BLUE FLAG (*Iris versicolor* L.)
BLUE VERVAIN (*Verbena hastata* L.)
BONESET (*Eupatorium perfoliatum* L.)
BUTTERNUT (*Juglans cineria* L.)
CARDINAL FLOWER (*Lobelia cardinalis* L.)
CASCARA SAGRADA (*Rhamnus Purshiana* DC.)
CORN SMUT (*Ustilago maydis* Jul.)
CRANESBILL (*Geranium maculatum* L.)
CULVER'S ROOT (*Veronica virginica* L.)
DANDELION (*Taraxacum officinale* Weber)
DOGBANE (*Apocynum androsaemifolium* L.)
ELDERBERRY (*Sambucus canadensis* L.)
FLOWERING DOGWOOD (*Cornus florida* L.)
GINSENG (*Panax quinquefolium* L.)
GOLD THREAD (*Coptis trifolia* Salisb.)
GOLDEN RAGWORT (*Senecio aureus* L.)
GREEN HELLEBORE (*Veratrum viride* L.)
GUM PLANT (*Grindelia squarrosa* [Pursh] Dunal)
JACK-IN-THE-PULPIT (*Arisaema triphyllum* [L.] Schott)
JALAP (*Exogonium Jalapa* [Nutt. & Coxe] Baillon)
JIMSON WEED (*Datura meteloides* DC.)
JOINT FIR (*Ephedra antisyphilitica* C.A. Mey)
JUNIPER (*Juniperus communis* L.)
MANDRAKE (*Podophyllum peltatum* L.)
MULLEN (*Verbascum thapsus* L.)
NEW JERSEY TEA (*Ceanothus americanus* L.)
PARTRIDGE BERRY (*Mitchella repens* L.)
PASQUE FLOWER (*Pulsatilla paten* [L.] Mill.)
PEYOTE (*Lophophora Williamsii* [Lem.] Coult.)

*Among other lists, one holds particular interest because of the scientific methods of compilation and of testing the physiologic activity of some drugs thus identified: Train, Percy, *et al.*: Contributions Toward a Flora of Nevada; No. 45—Medicinal Uses of Plants by Indian Tribes of Nevada, rev. ed., with summary of pharmacologic research, by W. Andrew Archer. Herbarium, U. S. National Arboretum, Washington 25, D.C., 1957.

PLUERISY ROOT (*Asclepias tuberosa* L.)
POKE ROOT (*Phytolacca americana* L.)
PRICKLY ASH (*Zanthoxylum americanum* Mill.)
PRINCE'S PINE (*Chimaphila umbellata* [L.] Nutt.)
PUFFBALL (*Lycoperdon gemmatun* Batsch)
PUMPKIN (*Cucurbita Pepo* L.)
PURPLE CONE FLOWER (*Echinacea angustifolia* DC.)
RASPBERRY (*Rubus occidentalis* L. and R. *Strigosus* Michx.)
RED CEDAR (*Juniperus virginiana* L.)
RED ELDERBERRY (*Sambucus racemosa* L.)
SENECA SNAKEROOT (*Polygala Senega* L.)
SLIPPERY ELM (*Ulmus fulva* Michx.)
SMOOTH SUMAC (*Rhus glabra* L.)
SOLOMON'S SEAL (*Polygonatum biflorum* [Walt] Ell.)
SOUR DOCK (*Rumex crispus* L.)
STAGHORN SUMAC (*Rhus typina* L.)
SWEET FLAG (*Acorus Calamus* L.)
TOBACCO (*Nicotiana quadrivalvis* Pursh.)
VIBURNUM—MAPLE-LEAVED (*Viburnum Acerifolium* L.)
VIRGINIA SNAKEROOT (*Aristolochia Serpentaria* L.)
WAHOO (*Euonymus atropurpurea* Jacq.)
WHITE OAK (*Quercus alba* L.)
WHITE PINE (*Pinus Strobus* L.)
WILD LICORICE (*Glycyrrhiza Pepidota* Pursh.)
WILD BERGAMOT (*Monarda fistulosa* L.)
WILD CHERRY (*Prunus Virginiana* L.)
WILD INDIGO (*Baptisin leucantha* T. and G.)
WILD MINT (*Mentha arvensis* L.)
WINTERGREEN (*Gaultheria procumbens* L.)
WITCH HAZEL (*Hamamelis virginiana* L.)
YARROW (*Achillea millefolium* L.)
YELLOW DOCK (*Rumex crispus* L.)
YERBA SANTA (*Eriodictyon glutinosum* Benth.)

# Appendix 2
# Founding of State Pharmaceutical Associations, U. S. A.

1867 Maine
1869 California
1870 New Jersey
1870 West Virginia
1870 Vermont
1871 Mississippi
1873 Tennessee
1874 New Hampshire
1874 Michigan
1874 Rhode Island
1875 Georgia
1876 South Carolina*
1876 Connecticut
1877 Kentucky
1878 Pennsylvania
1879 Texas
1879 New York
1879 Ohio
1879 Missouri
1880 Iowa
1880 Kansas
1880 Wisconsin
1880 North Carolina
1880 Illinois
1881 West Virginia (reorganized)
1881 Alabama
1882 Virginia
1882 Louisiana
1882 Indiana
1882 Massachusetts
1882 Nebraska
1883 Maryland
1883 Mississippi (reorganized)
1883 Minnesota
1883 Michigan (reorganized)
1883 Arkansas
1885 North Dakota
1886 Tennessee (reorganized)
1886 South Dakota
1887 Delaware
1887 Florida
1887 Idaho
1890 Washington
1890 Oregon
1890 Maine (reorganized)
1890 Oklahoma Territory†
1890 Colorado
1891 Montana
1891 Mississippi (2nd reorganization)
1892 Utah
1893 New Mexico
1895 Indian Territory†
1902 Mississippi (3rd reorganization)
1904 Florida (reorganized)
1905 Idaho (reorganized)
1906 West Virginia (2nd reorganization)

---

*There is a notice in the Amer. J. Pharm. *44*:425, 1872, "That a pharmaceutical association in South Carolina is about being organized." However, there is no mention of the activity of such an association anywhere until March, 1876, the date of the incorporation.

†When, in 1907, the Territory of Oklahoma and the Indian Territory were formed into the State of Oklahoma, the respective pharmaceutical associations were merged into the Oklahoma Pharmaceutical Association.

1907 Oklahoma State†
1910 Arizona
1915 Wyoming
1932 Nevada
1945 Hawaii
1966 Alaska (reorganized)

# Appendix 3
# Passage of State and Territory Pharmacy Laws, U. S. A.

"Pharmacy Law" here refers to the statutory establishment of some qualifications for the practice of pharmacy and to the limiting of that practice to such qualified practitioners. *In many states legislation pertaining to poisons, abortifacients and adulteration preceded the statutes listed by many years.*

The list below is the Kremers and Urdang list (ed. 2, p. 276) with corrections and additions from subsequent research by David L. Cowen. Concerted study of this statutory history would likely reveal need for still further revision.

The date in square brackets is the year in which earlier legislation, still technically in effect, was superseded by a "modern" pharmacy law.

1808 Territory of Orleans (Louisiana)
1816 Louisiana, repealed 1852; new law, 1872
1817 South Carolina [1876]
1825 Georgia [1881]
1832 New York, for New York City; 1869 for State; 1871 for New York City; 1879 for Kings County; 1884 for Erie County; 1884 for all other counties; 1900 for State
1844 Mississippi, for Adams County; 1892 for State
1851 Kentucky, for Louisville; 1874 for State
1852 Alabama [1887]
1866 Pennsylvania, for Lycoming County; 1872 for Philadelphia; 1887 for State
1870 Maryland, for Baltimore; 1902 for State except Talbot County; 1906 for Talbot County; 1908 for State
1870 Rhode Island
1872 Florida
1872 California, for San Francisco; 1891 for State
1873 Ohio, for Cincinnati; 1884 for State
1873 Missouri, for St. Louis; 1881 for State
1875 New Hampshire
1876 Wisconsin, for Milwaukee; 1882 for State
1877 New Jersey
1877 Maine
1878 District of Columbia
1880 Iowa
1881 Connecticut
1881 Illinois
1881 North Carolina
1881 West Virginia
1883 Delaware
1885 Michigan
1885 Minnesota
1885 Massachusetts
1885 Kansas
1886 Virginia
1886 Wyoming*
1887 Idaho*
1887 Dakota Territory
1887 Nebraska
1887 Colorado

*An asterisk denotes passage of the original statute by the territorial government.

1889 New Mexico*
1889 Texas
1890 South Dakota
1891 North Dakota
1891 Arkansas
1891 Oregon
1891 Oklahoma Territory
1891 Washington
1892 Utah*
1893 Tennessee
1894 Vermont
1895 Montana
1899 Indiana
1901 Nevada
1902 Puerto Rico [1906]
1903 Arizona*
1903 Hawaii*
1904 Indian Territory
1909 Oklahoma
1913 Alaska*

# Appendix 4
# Schools of Pharmacy in the United States*

Including Some of the Better Known Extinct Schools and Arranged by Date of Organization

1821 Philadelphia College of Pharmacy and Science, Philadelphia, Pa. (called Philadelphia College of Pharmacy, 1822–1920.)

1829 Columbia University, New York, N.Y. (started as the College of Pharmacy of the City and County of New York, which became affiliated with Columbia University in 1904; discontinued in 1976.)†

1838 Tulane University of Louisiana, New Orleans, La.†

1840 University of Maryland, Baltimore, Md. (started as Maryland College of Pharmacy, which became a part of the state university in 1920.)

1859 University of Illinois, Chicago, Ill. (started as Chicago College of Pharmacy, which became affiliated with the University of Illinois in 1896.)

1865 St. Louis College of Pharmacy, St. Louis, Mo.

1865 Baldwin University, Berea, Ohio.†

1866 Medical College of the State of South Carolina. Charleston, S.C.‡ (a few occasional pharmacy graduates beginning 1867; separate pharmacy department 1882–84; reorganized as present School of Pharmacy 1894.)

1866 Medical College of Alabama, Birmingham, Ala.†

1867 Massachusetts College of Pharmacy (Between the founding of the College [association] in 1823 and the founding of the present school, short lecture courses were given occasionally.)

1868 University of Michigan, Ann Arbor, Mich.‡

1868 Howard University, Washington, D.C.

1870 University of Kentucky, Louisville, Ky. (started as Louisville College of Pharmacy, which became a part of the University of Kentucky in 1947.)

1871 University of Cincinnati, Cincinnati, Ohio (started as the Cincinnati College of Pharmacy in 1850, which sometimes organized instructional discussion groups; the College's regular school, f. 1871, affiliated with the University in 1945.)

1872 University of California, San Francisco, Calif. (started as California College of Pharmacy, which became affiliated

---

*Dates are intended to represent when organization was completed or instruction begun at the school in its *original* form (but consistent precision is difficult in a concise tabulation that involves so many mergers, suspensions and ambiguous records.)

†Discontinued school. A great many extinct schools are not listed.

‡College (or school) of pharmacy established as part of state institution (universities or colleges) before 1900.

with the University of California in 1872, and a part of the latter in 1934.)

1872 George Washington University, Washington, D.C. (started as National College of Pharmacy, which became affiliated with the George Washington University in 1906; discontinued in 1964.)†

1873 Tennessee College of Pharmacy, Nashville, Tenn.†

1878 University of Pittsburgh, Pittsburgh, Pa. (started as Pittsburgh College of Pharmacy, which became affiliated with the University of Pittsburgh in 1896, and a part of the latter in 1947.)

1879 Vanderbilt University, Nashville, Tenn.†

1881 Union University, Albany College of Pharmacy, Albany, N.Y.

1882 Western Reserve University, Cleveland, Ohio.† (started as Cleveland School of Pharmacy, which became affiliated with Western Reserve University in 1908 and a part of the latter in 1918; discontinued in 1949.)

1882 Iowa College of Pharmacy, Des Moines, Iowa (affiliated with Drake University in 1886.)†

1883 University of Wisconsin, Madison, Wis.‡

1884 Purdue University, Lafayette, Ind.‡

1884 Ohio Northern University, Ada, Ohio (formerly Ohio Normal University.)

1885 University of Iowa, Iowa City, Iowa.‡

1885 Ohio State University, Columbus, Ohio.‡

1885 University of Kansas, Lawrence, Kansas.‡

1885 University of Kansas City, Kansas City, Mo. (started as Kansas City College of Pharmacy.)

1886 Northwestern University, Chicago, Ill.† (The College of Pharmacy was merged with the University of Illinois College of Pharmacy in 1917.)

1886 State University of New York at Buffalo (formerly University of Buffalo), Buffalo, N.Y.

1886 Minnesota Institute of Pharmacy, Minneapolis, Minn.†

1887 Scio College, Scio, Ohio.† (amalgamated with Pittsburgh College of Pharmacy in 1908.)

1888 South Dakota State College, Brookings, S. Dak.‡

1889 Walden University (Meharry Pharmaceutical College), Nashville, Tenn.†

1890 Detroit Institute of Technology, Detroit, Mich. (started as a Department of the Detroit College of Medicine; independent 1905 to 1907; then part of the Detroit Institute of Technology.)†

1890 Highland Park College; from 1920 to 1927, Des Moines University, Des Moines, Iowa.† (See also Drake University, 1927.)

1891 Brooklyn College of Pharmacy, Brooklyn, N.Y. (since 1929 affiliated with Long Island University.)

1891 Ohio Medical University, Columbus, Ohio.†

1891 College of Physicians and Surgeons, Atlanta, Ga.†

1891 Shaw University, Leonard Schools of Medicine and Pharmacy, Raleigh, N.C.†

1892 Valparaiso University, Valparaiso, Ind.† (started as Northern Indiana School of Pharmacy, a Department of the Normal School and Business Institute of Valparaiso, which became Valparaiso University in 1906.)

1892 Rutgers, The State University of New Jersey. (College started as New Jersey College of Pharmacy, which became a part of Rutgers University in 1927.)

1892 University of Minnesota, Minneapolis, Minn.‡

1892 Louisville College of Pharmacy for Women, Louisville, Ky.†

1893 Ferris State College, Big Rapids, Mich. (formerly called Ferris Institute)

1893 State University of Oklahoma, Norman, Okla.‡

---

†Discontinued school.

‡College (or school) of pharmacy established as part of state institution (universities or colleges) before 1900.

1893 University College of Medicine, Richmond, Va. (absorbed 1913 by Med. Coll. Va.)
1893 University of Texas, Austin, Tex.‡
1894 University of Maine, Orono, Maine.†
1894 University of Washington, Seattle, Wash.‡
1895 Auburn University (formerly Alabama Polytechnic Institute), Auburn, Ala.‡
1896 Washington State University, Pullman, Wash.‡ (previously called State College of Washington, and, before 1905, The Agricultural College.)
1897 Medical College of Virginia, Richmond, Va. (From about 1876 on, medical students with certain pharmaceutical training were graduated in pharmacy. Absorbed in 1913 the pharmacy department of the University College of Medicine, q.v., 1893.)
1897 University of North Carolina, Chapel Hill, N.C.‡ (a pharmacy school existed from 1880 to 1886; revived in 1889, and again discontinued.)
1897 University of Notre Dame, Notre Dame, Ind.†
1898 Medico Chirurgical College of Philadelphia, Philadelphia, Pa.† (When, in 1916, the College and the University of Pennsylvania were consolidated, the department of pharmacy and chemistry of the College merged with the Philadelphia College of Pharmacy.)
1898 University of Tennessee, Memphis, Tenn.‡ (teaching started at Knoxville and came to Memphis in 1911.)
1898 College of Physicians and Surgeons, San Francisco, Calif.†
1898 Oregon State University [formerly College], Corvallis, Ore. (previously Oregon Agricultural College.)‡
1900 Marquette University, Milwaukee, Wis.† (founded as department of Wisconsin Medical College, with precursor in private tutorial school; affiliated with Marquette 1907.)
1900 Keokuk Medical College, Keokuk, Iowa.†
1900 Creighton University, Omaha, Nebr. (started as a Department in the Fremont Normal School, which became a part of Creighton University in 1905.)
1900 Loyola University, New Orleans, La. (started as the New Orleans College of Pharmacy, which became affiliated with Loyola University, in 1913, and became part of the latter in 1919.)†
1901 Baylor University, Dallas, Tex.† (originally part of the University of Dallas; taken over by Baylor University in 1905.)
1901 Temple University, Philadelphia, Pa.
1901 Illinois Medical College, Chicago, Ill.†
1902 North Dakota State University (formerly N.D. Agricultural College), Fargo, N.D. (organized as a Department of Chemistry and Pharmacy; a separate School of Pharmacy since 1919.)
1902 Tristate Normal School, Angola, Ind.†
1902 Rhode Island College of Pharmacy and Allied Sciences, Providence, R.I.;† see also 1957.
1903 Mercer University, Macon, Ga.†
1903 Southern College of Pharmacy, Atlanta, Ga.; merged in 1959 with Mercer University.
1903 University of Georgia, Athens, Ga.
1904 Butler University, Indianapolis, Ind. (started as Indianapolis College of Pharmacy, which became part of Butler University in 1946.)
1904 University of Toledo, Toledo, Ohio.
1905 University of Southern California, Los Angeles, Calif. (the College became an integral part of the University in 1922.)
1907 Montana State University, Missoula, Mont.
1908 University of Mississippi, University, Miss.
1908 University of Nebraska, Lincoln, Nebr.
1908 North Pacific College of Oregon, Portland, Oreg.†
1911 University of the Philippines, Manila, P.I. (the Philippines received their independence in 1945.)
1911 University of Colorado, Boulder, Colo.

1911 Fordham University, New York, N.Y.†
1913 University of Puerto Rico, Rio Piedras, P.R.
1914 West Virginia University, Morgantown, W.Va.
1918 The Idaho State College, Pocatello, Idaho (before 1947, University of Idaho, South Branch.)
1923 Wayne State University, Detroit, Mich. (until 1933 named College of the City of Detroit.)
1923 University of Florida, Gainesville, Fla.
1924 University of South Carolina, Columbia, S.C. (Earlier attempts at establishing pharmaceutical instruction were active from 1866 to 1877 and from 1884 to 1891.)
1925 Duquesne University, Pittsburgh, Pa.
1925 University of Connecticut, New Haven, Conn. (started as Connecticut College of Pharmacy, which became a part of the University of Connecticut in 1941.)
1927 Northeastern University (established as Meriano School of Pharmacy; incorporated 1940 as Boston School of Pharmacy; in 1949 re-named New England College of Pharmacy; in 1962 absorbed by the University.)
1927 Xavier University, New Orleans, La.
1927 Drake University, Des Moines, Iowa (started as Des Moines College of Pharmacy, 1927–1939; then became a part of Drake University; see also: 1882: Iowa College of Pharmacy and 1890: Highland Park College.)
1929 St. John's University, Brooklyn, N.Y.
1932 Samford University (until 1965 called Howard College), Birmingham, Ala.
1936 University of Grand Rapids, Grand Rapids, Mich.†
1939 Western Massachusetts School of Pharmacy, Willimansett, Mass. (not accredited)†
1941 Southwestern State College, Weatherford, Okla. (formerly Southwestern Institute of Technology.)
1945 University of New Mexico, Albuquerque, N. Mex.
1945 College of the Ozarks, Clarksville, Ark.†; discontinued 1951.
1946 University of Utah, Salt Lake City, Utah.
1946 University of Wyoming, Laramie, Wy.
1947 University of Arizona, Tucson, Ariz.
1947 University of Houston, Houston, Tex.
1949 Texas Southern University, Houston, Tex.
1951 University of Arkansas, Little Rock, Ark. (successor to College of Ozarks, f. 1945.)
1951 Florida A and M University, Tallahassee (called College until 1953.)
1955 University [formerly College] of the Pacific, Stockton, Calif.
1956 Northeast Louisiana State College, Monroe, La.
1957 University of Rhode Island, Kingston, R.I. (successor to Rhode Island College of Pharmacy, f. 1902.)

†Discontinued.

# Appendix 5
# Pharmacy's History—A Growing Awareness

Historical analysis becomes one tool to produce some semblance of order and logic out of kaleidoscopic events, and to make the pharmacist's place in society clearer to both the practitioner and his patients. In this enterprise the original authors of this volume, Edward Kremers and George Urdang (portraits, p. 388) became the most important pioneers in the Americas. Others played their part in developing a written history of pharmacy, in teaching the pharmacist's heritage as part of medical care as one learns to be a "pharmacist," in preserving and interpreting the working implements that previous generations of practitioners have left behind; and in organizing cooperative endeavor to do these things. The movement to make a serious effort to represent and understand pharmacy in this sense has come to some maturity just during the present century.

Men have always been curious about what's happened and their leaders in every generation (lacking clairvoyance) have paid their respects to the past as a source of gaining understanding and a sense of purpose in confronting the future. But until there is painstaking work and prolonged study and synthesis, the past remains a disassembled, and even disappearing, scatter of inert facts. The role of the historian therefore has been an ancient and demanding one. But until almost the present century, the role of the sciences and the professions based on science did not get much attention in historical accounts.

Pharmacy was no exception. This circumstance changed markedly in recent decades, with the growth of a specialized cadre of historians of the sciences (including many talented amateurs from these fields), new departments in universities, and specialized journals, museum collections and societies.

In terms of pharmacy, George Urdang expressed a two-fold purpose in 1941 upon founding the American Institute of the History of Pharmacy. One aim, he said, "is to equip the pharmacist for citizenship in the world of intellectual and moral responsibility by making him familiar with the non-technical aspects and humanistic ramifications of the profession." Another is "to do pharmacy's share in the cooperative endeavor for making the historical record of world civilization as complete as possible."

On this same ground, efforts have gone forward in other countries likewise; and the paragraphs below briefly characterize some of the previous work that helps make a volume such as this one possible.

### Written History

By the 18th century, pharmacy was sufficiently aware of itself, and sufficiently mature, to begin to capture what it had accomplished and experienced as a part of the recorded history of civilization. One early at-

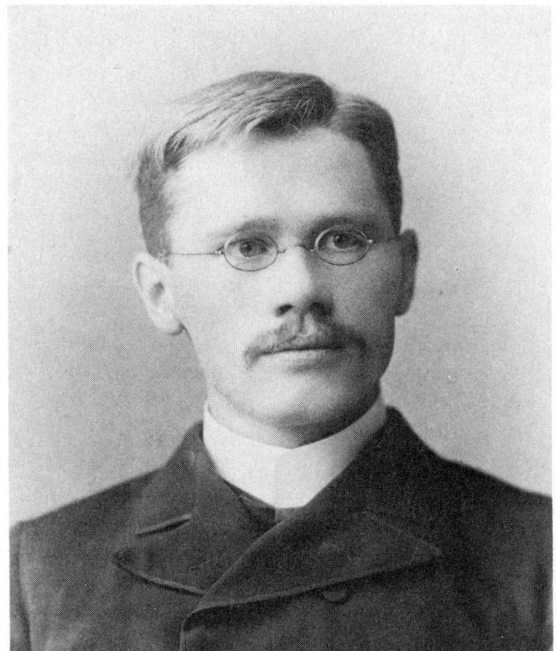

Edward Kremers as a young pharmacist about the time he embarked upon doctoral studies, leading to a career as educator, scientist and pioneer American historian of pharmacy (1865–1941). An idealist and reformer, Kremers became an influential mediator of change.

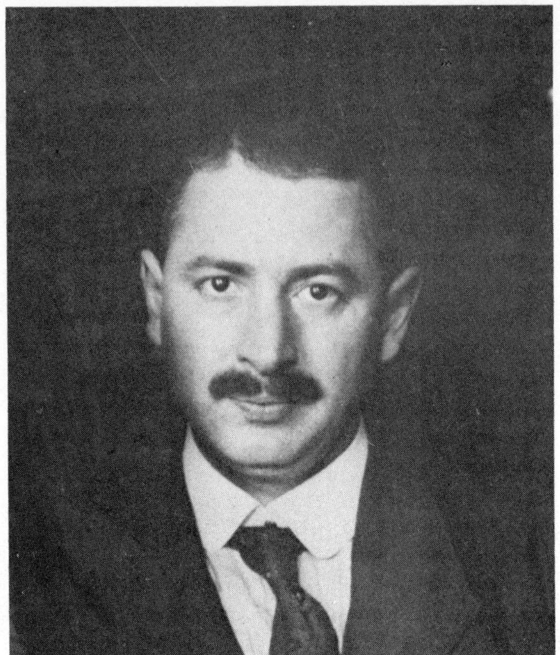

George Urdang as a young practicing pharmacist in Germany, about the time he became a pharmaceutical journalist, then historian of his profession (1882–1960). Arriving in Madison, Wisconsin, at the invitation of Edward Kremers in 1939, as a refugee from the Nazi regime, Urdang set about writing the first edition of this book on the basis of Kremers' historical collections and collaboration. (From: Kremers Reference Files, Pharmaceutical Library, University of Wisconsin-Madison)

tempt was a local history of pharmacy services for the imperial city of Nuremberg, although still earlier chronicles can be traced.[1] Shortly after 1800 essays on pharmacy's history appear as the introductory part of several German textbooks.[2]

The first comprehensive history of pharmacy was published by the Frenchman Adrian Philippe (1853; with a German version by J. F. H. Ludwig). However, the epoch of historical research and interest really began with the work of three great German pharmaceutical historians: Julius Berendes (1837–1914), Hermann Peters (1847–1920) and especially Hermann Schelenz (1848–1922), whose voluminous history of pharmacy (*Geschichte der Pharmazie,* 1904) presents such a treasury of information that the original edition was reprinted after more than a half century (1961). Since that time a flood of historical literature has appeared, including several national histories of the profession; biblio-

→

Several periodicals specializing in the humanistic side of pharmacy are published by organizations, the first founded by the French in 1913. This quarterly of the American Institute of the History of Pharmacy developed out of an earlier newsletter to members and has been in its present format since 1959.

# PHARMACY IN HISTORY

*Published by the*
*American Institute of the History of Pharmacy*

VOLUME 17 No. 1 1975 PAGES 1-40

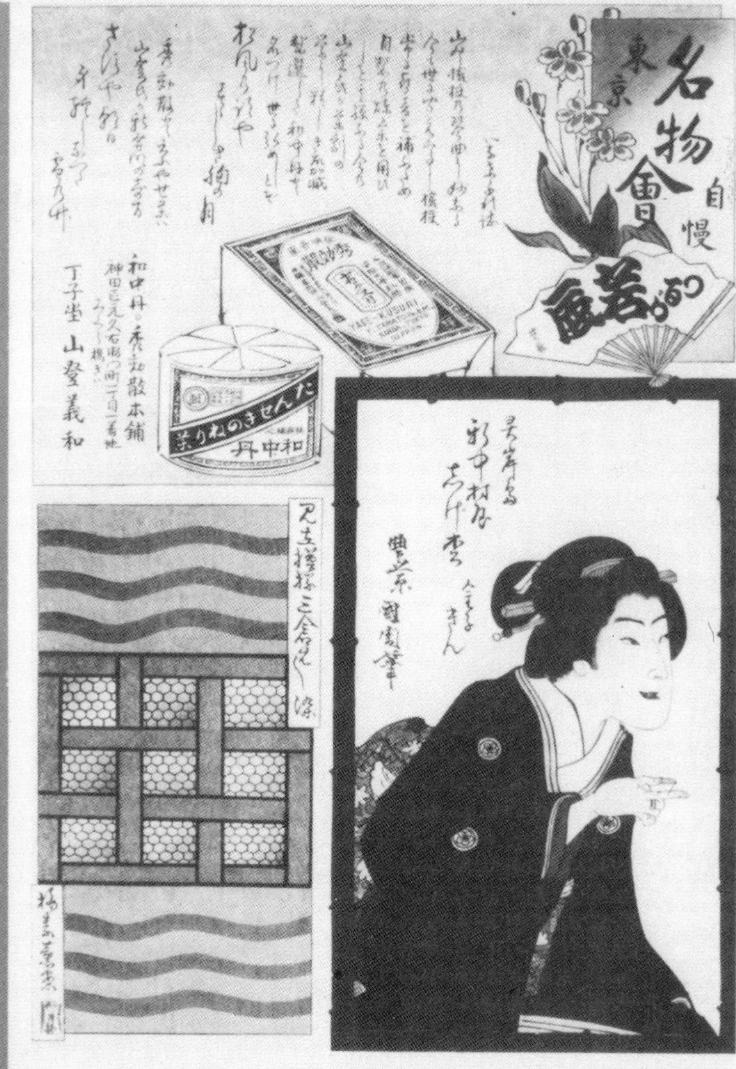


**See Inside Cover**

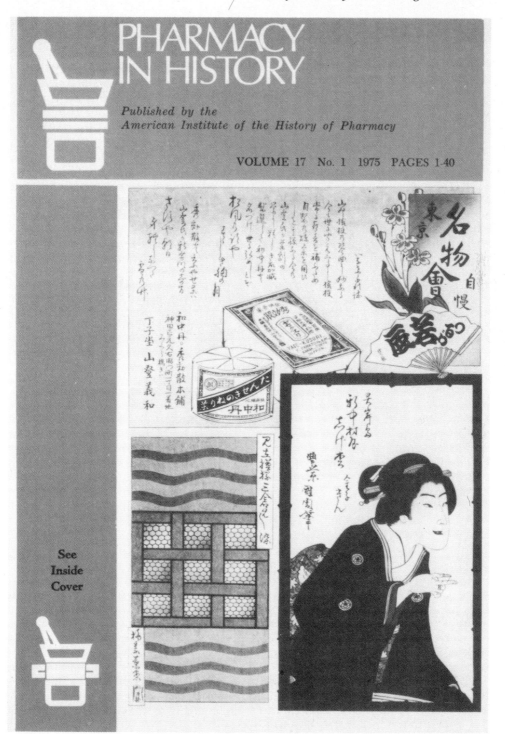

graphic guides are available to locate the historical accounts about the pharmaceutical profession, science and industry that are being built up.[3]

## Organized Endeavor

The first European society devoted especially to the history of pharmacy was founded in Paris in 1913 *(La Société d'histoire de la pharmacie)*. Since then it has published a remarkable *Bulletin*, which has appeared since 1930 under the title *Revue d'histoire de la pharmacie.*

Thirteen years later in 1926 an Austrian, three Germans and an American founded the Germanic *Gesellschaft für Geschichte der Pharmazie* (Society for the History of Pharmacy). This society took up the task of publishing books and pamphlets at a high standard. More or less dormant between 1939 and 1949, this society resumed with a meeting attended not only by Germans but also by French, English, Swiss, Dutch and Scandinavian pharmacists. This signalled an expanded international scope and recognition of its work and the unifying tendencies which it expresses and promotes. On this ground (1949) the *Gesellschaft* added the significant adjective "international" to its name *(Internationale Gesellschaft für Geschichte der Pharmazie)*. By the early 1970's this International Society consisted of nearly 1400 members from 30 countries (although only slowly outgrowing its Germanic flavor). Booklets are published annually on the history of pharmacy, including the proceedings of biennial congresses of historians and historically-minded pharmacists.

This kind of activity among individuals stimulated the founding of specialized national societies. As a founder of the original German society, which had evolved into international scope, George Urdang, at Madison, Wisconsin, envisioned a kind of world federation of such societies for "exchange of ideas, for publication and for world congresses every two or three years in one of the member countries, [and as] an incentive for the founding of historical associations in countries still without one. . . ."[4] Working with colleagues abroad—particularly two pharmacists and historians of Holland, P. H. Brans and D. A. Wittop-Koning—Urdang made this idea a reality in May 1952 with the founding of the World Union of Societies for Pharmaceutical History. Within four years the founding societies of France, Spain, the Benelux, and the United States of America had expanded into a "roof organization" linking pharmaco-historical societies of 12 countries. The World Union has been particularly useful in sponsoring historical programs associated with the biennial assemblies of the International Pharmaceutical Federation (q.v., p. 134), and in providing symbiotic contact among leaders of the societies devoted to the humanistic side of pharmacy in individual countries. That the productivity of the World Union has been less than its creators envisioned seems less attributable to a defective concept than to an underestimate of the strong international leadership growing out of the International Society of the History of Pharmacy (the old "Gesellschaft"). After all, in 1952, the "Gesellschaft" had barely revived and was perhaps thought of as too particularly Germanic (if not even Nazi-tainted) to provide the pharmaco-historical movement with a universally accepted framework.

The International Academy of the History of Pharmacy, likewise founded in 1952 (on the occasion of the 70th birthday of George Urdang, U.S.A.), has fulfilled a narrower, hence more manageable, function within the historical movement. The founding had been undertaken by Georg E. Dann, again with D. A. Wittop-Koning and P. H. Brans of the Netherlands as collaborators, mainly as an honorary body analogous to "academies" that serve many other areas of specialized intellectual endeavor. Full membership in the Academy always has been limited to not more than two historians of pharmacy in each country, besides selected associate

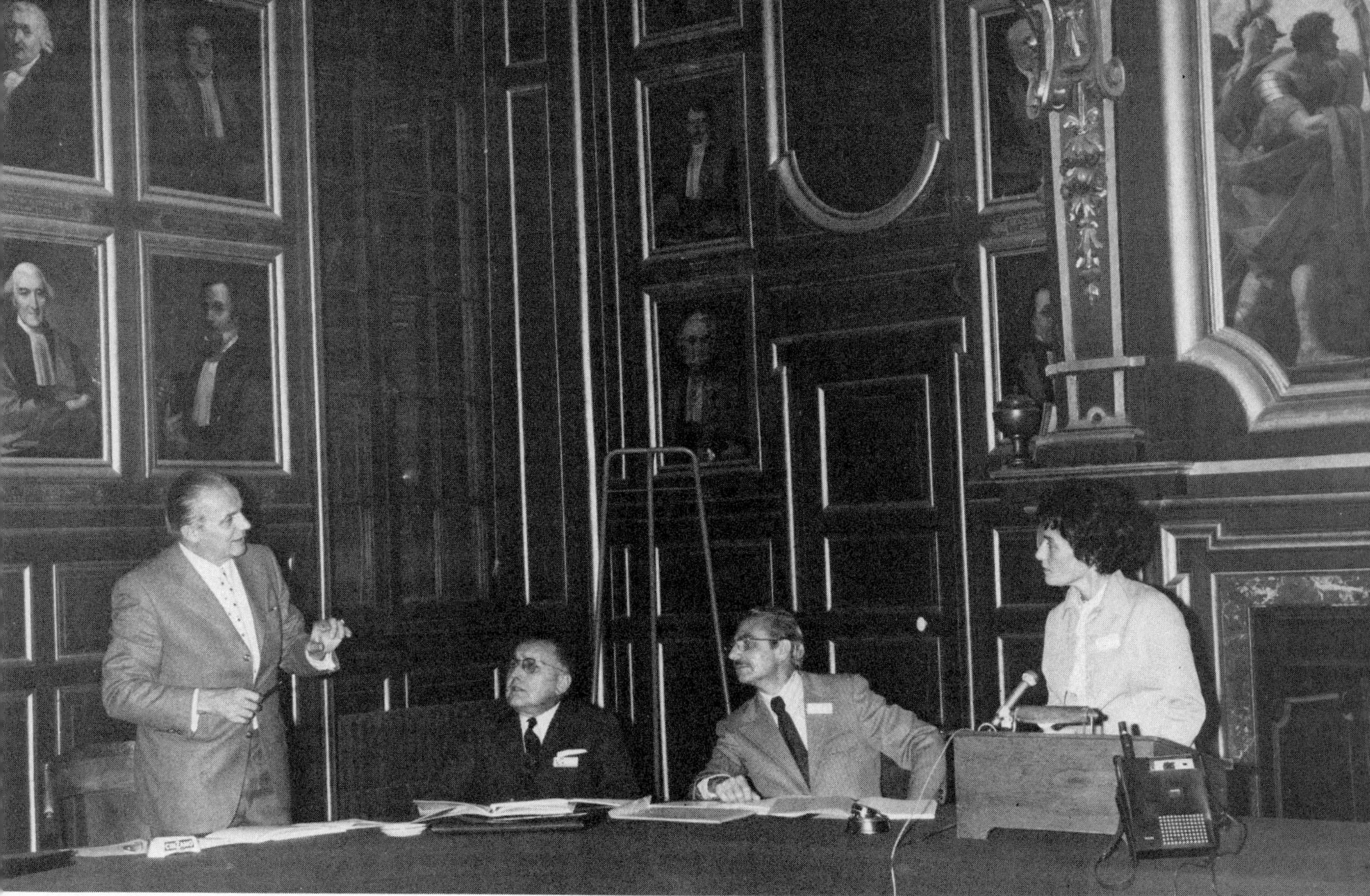

At a congress sponsored by the International Society for the History of Pharmacy, new findings are discussed at the speakers' table by historians of pharmacy from *(left to right)* West Germany, France, U.S.A., and Rumania. The setting is a room of the old Faculty of Pharmacy, University of Paris. (From: American Institute of the History of Pharmacy; photo by Actualités Mondial)

members. At international meetings in conjunction with other groups, the Academy honors distinguished achievements in work on pharmacy's history and sponsors invitational lectures and other special events, under the aegis of the Academy's members from 35 countries.[5]

How the international aspect of pharmaco-historical activities can best be served, organizationally, will be clarified and probably simplified by further experience in supranational collaboration.

Among national societies, the American Institute of the History of Pharmacy was particularly fortunate in having one of the great pharmacist-humanists as a founder and first Director (1941–1957). George Urdang had arrived at the University of Wisconsin in 1939 as a refugee from Germany, at the invitation of Edward Kremers. Even before there was a place for Urdang on the University faculty, the two pharmacist-historians were collaborating on the first edition of this book, which, as the only comprehensive survey of its kind in the English language, was to be both a textbook for students and a reference book serving the profession at large. They moved on to enthusiastic plans for other projects, but Kremers died in 1941, the same year that the American Institute of the History of Pharmacy came into being. Even before arriving on American shores, Urdang had in mind the establishment of such a society and work center, using as a model his

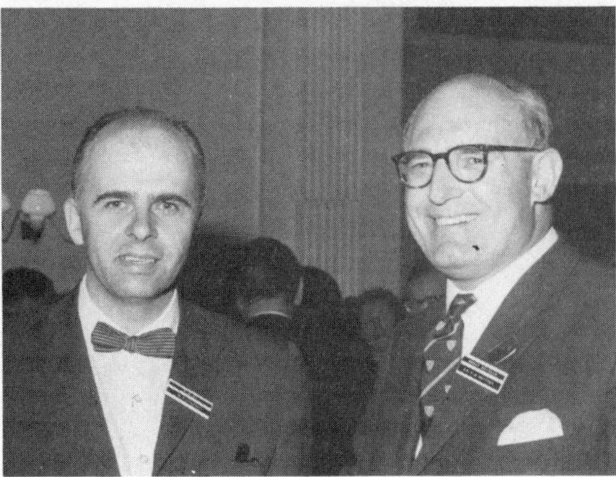

Two pharmacists who found unusual avocations in the history of pharmacy and made important contributions to it: William H. Helfand of New York *(left)*, Vice President of Merck Sharp & Dohme International (1974– ), America's leading iconographer and print collector on pharmaceutical subjects, and T. Douglas Whittet of London *(right)*, Chief Pharmacist in the Department of Health and Social Security (1967– ), who has written and lectured widely on his profession's history and encouraged humanistic activities in British pharmacy. (From: Pharmaceutical Library, University of Wisconsin-Madison; Fairlight Photographers Ltd.)

experience as one of the founders and leaders of the German society. Although the brillance of Urdang tended to identify the new American Institute with one man, after his death in 1960 the A.I.H.P. continued to grow in membership (about 1200 in the early 1970's) and diversify its activities. These include publishing the quarterly *Pharmacy in History* and other publications, setting historical markers, sponsoring awards, organizing programs and otherwise stimulating historical work, preserving the records of American pharmacy and providing a source of authoritative information.[6]

## Teaching History

On the ground that studying the profession's history invests pharmacy with broader meaning and sense of its professional place in society, instructional programs developed as specialized literature and historians became available to some schools.

The credit for having been the first country to make the history of pharmacy a part of the pharmaceutical curriculum (1852) goes to Spain. In 1923, the Austrian government made the history of pharmacy an obligatory part of the pharmaceutical curriculum. In Germany lectures on the history of pharmacy were delivered at the University of Berlin beginning in 1926. Meanwhile, significant programs in pharmaceutical history have developed in other German universities most notably at Braunschweig and Marburg, and in other countries, such as France, Holland, Yugoslavia, Czechoslovakia, England, Italy, Argentina, Brazil, Canada and the United States of America. At least half the American schools (including Puerto Rico) have offered some instruction in pharmaceutical history.[7]

The most substantial American efforts centered at the University of Wisconsin. As early as 1904 Edward Kremers instigated the establishment of a Section on Historical Pharmacy in the American Pharmaceutical Association, and in that forum propagandized for humanistic instruction in the curriculum of American schools. At Wisconsin he established (1907–08) both history of pharmacy and history of chemistry as officially recognized subjects of instruction.

The history of pharmacy has had an unbroken tradition at the University of Wisconsin ever since. In 1947, Urdang, whom Kremers had brought to Wisconsin earlier, was tendered the first full-time professorship in the subject on American soil and was authorized to train the first American pharmacists to the Doctor of Philosophy level as pharmaceutical historians.[8]

## History in Artifacts

The objects that pharmacists of other generations have left behind give a dimension to the history of pharmacy beyond what can be conveyed by the written word. Such artifacts are studied for what they tell about how the pharmacist worked, and about the historical stages of pharmaceutical technology and of drug therapy. This three-dimensional "lore of the apothecary" also has perennial public appeal. The early public museums of Europe often had at least a few pharmaceutical curiosities on display, such as unicorn horn and human mummy, two fabulous curatives of hoary repute. Besides individual remedies and objects from bygone times, "as early as the 17th century there was a restoration of a complete apothecary shop and laboratory in the Dresden Museum."[9]

Conversely, certain operating pharmacies of this time and onward functioned partially as a local museum, probably because of a pharmacist's lively interest in natural sciences as a source of medicinal substances, perhaps partly to attract and impress the townsfolk. An English traveller of the 17th century, for example, writes of what he saw in the collections of a pharmacist of Verona: "divers sorts of petrified shells, petrified cheese, cinnamon, spunge and mushrooms."[10]

Of more recent vintage, emerging in the 1880's, are the early museum collections of pharmaceutical antiquities that were brought together intentionally for study, as a way of supplementing our understanding of past civilization in general and pharmacy in particular. It was a time when general historical museums in Europe were growing vigorously, and this trend struck responsive chords in special fields such as pharmacy. In 1883 a move was launched by one of the pioneer pharmacist-historians, Hermann Peters, to set up a pharmacy museum within the German National Museum at Nürnberg. It is noteworthy that in this same year a curator of the Smithsonian Institution in the U.S.A. proposed to expand the materia medica collection to include also pharmaceutical and medical artifacts. Four years later Amsterdam and Copenhagen initiated collections of their own (1887).[11]

Other centers, such as Paris, London and Munich, were building collections by the early 20th century. This set up a chain reaction across national boundaries that yielded the remarkable array of pharmacy museums that Mr. Griffenhagen puts before us on the following pages. A majority of these collections are in Europe, but many may be seen in the United States (and elsewhere in the Americas).

The record of American pharmacy in three-dimensional objects mostly represents, of course, the 18th century and onward. It reflects the origins of the immigrants, for the fixtures and equipment of early American drugstores mostly were imported from England, France and the German states. As in Europe, some items of early equipment were preserved in general museums of Americana. The first instance of the preservation of an old drugstore as a museum unit probably is the one in the 17th-century Ward house in Salem, Massachusetts, although the Webb pharmacy there dates from the early 19th century.

As a colonial apothecary shop reconstructed in its community setting, the Williamsburg, Va., restoration (1760–1776) holds particular interest. Other examples of public restorations of pharmacies that have a setting or historical associations that add to their interest are the pharmacy attached to the Ephraim McDowell house at Danville, Ky., the Bringhurst shop exhibited at Mystic (Conn.) Seaport, and the historic apothecary shop of the physician and brigadier general of Revolutionary War fame, Hugh Mercer, at Fredericksburg, Va. The Mercer building is believed to be the oldest extant in the United States that was used as a pharmacy. A priceless reconstruction of a European pharmacy (Jo Mayer/Squibb collection) is on display at the Smithsonian Institution in Washington, together with a late-19th-century American pharmacy of exceptional quality. Yet, it is not in these restored pharmacies alone that the Smithsonian's Division of Medical Sciences finds its greatest import for pharmacy, but as the collector and protector of the only major general collection of pharmaceutical artifacts in the United States.[12]

Quite a number of American pharmacies from the second half of the 19th century have

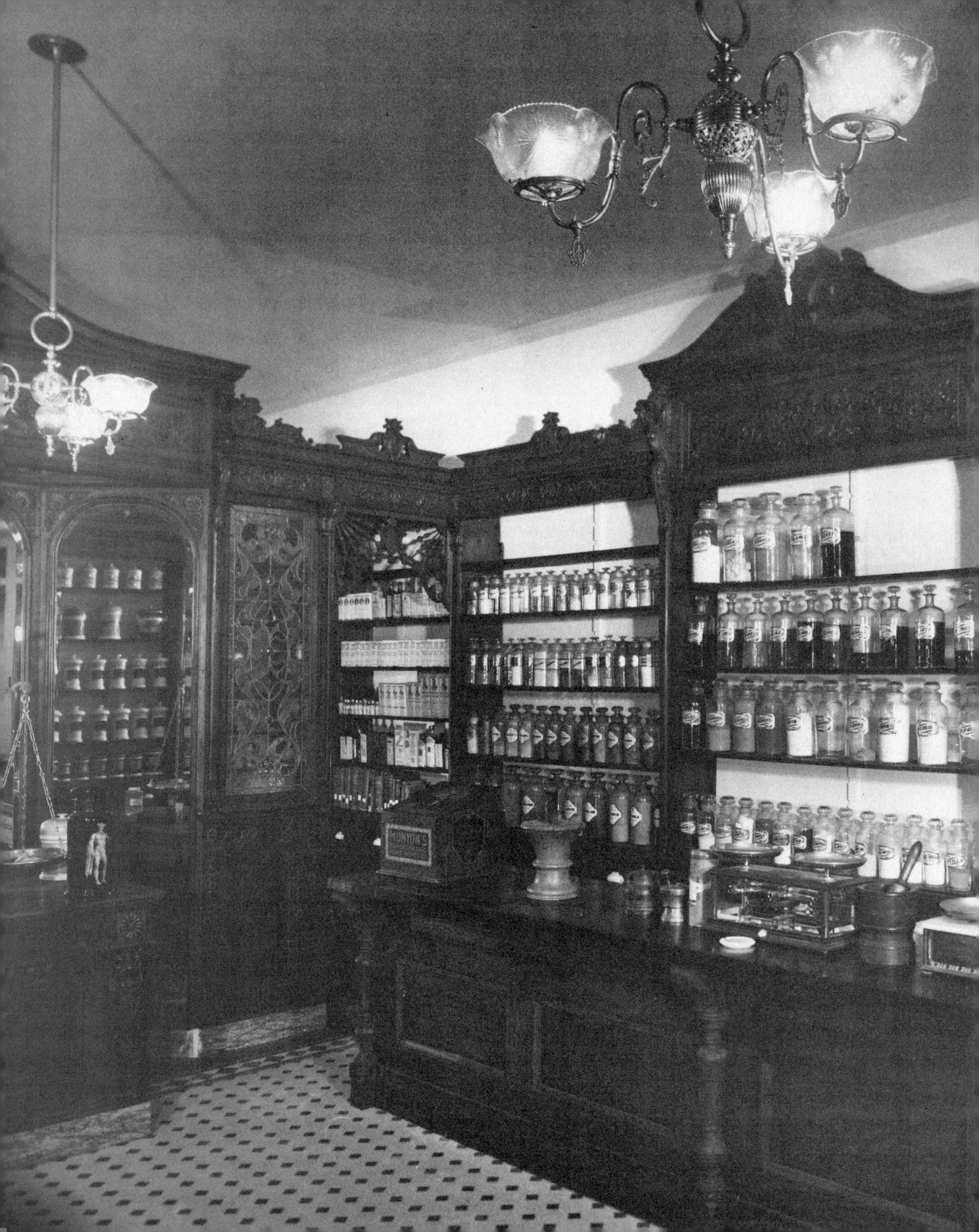
MUNYON'S

been restored (see "United States" in the guide to museum collections on following pages). One of the earliest period restorations of this type to be completed (1913) was brought together under the leadership of Edward Kremers and formerly exhibited at the State Historical Society of Wisconsin at Madison.

A restoration of this period holding still greater interest is "La Pharmacie Française" in the French Quarter of New Orleans, housed in an earlier building (1823) actually used for his pharmacy by Louis J. Dufilho, one of the first pharmacists to be licensed under a pharmacy law of this country.

Modern developments in American pharmacy brought forth as many types of fixtures and equipment as there are different types of drugstores or pharmacies: commercial or professional or mixed types, with or without soda fountains, with the prescription department as the center of the establishment, or in the rear, or not visible at all.

Varied as these drugstores and pharmacies have been, a great many throughout American history have used an old-fashioned Anglo-Saxon device to make obvious their character as pharmaceutical workshops, exhibiting "show globes" filled with colored liquids and illuminated after dark by lights placed behind them.[13]

While each generation has left behind some artifacts as characteristic tokens of its history, the broader significance of an epoch ending can be seen in new museum reconstructions of pharmacies from the late 19th and early 20th century. For in this period the community pharmacist was laying down his traditional tools for compounding drugs, which for centuries, though increasingly guided by science, had nevertheless served an art of the individual's own skilled hand. Then, primarily between the two world wars, these implements became little more than museum artifacts, except for a few still

←

Corner of a late-19th century American pharmacy reconstructed in the Smithsonian Institution, Washington. The Smithsonian's Division of Medical Sciences is unique in the United States for the broad range of its collections of artifacts concerning the evolution of medical care, in reference storage as well as on exhibit. At least one pharmacist usually has been on the Smithsonian staff during the present century—in the 1970's Sami K. Hamarneh as historian and Michael Harris as a museum specialist. (From: The Smithsonian Institution)

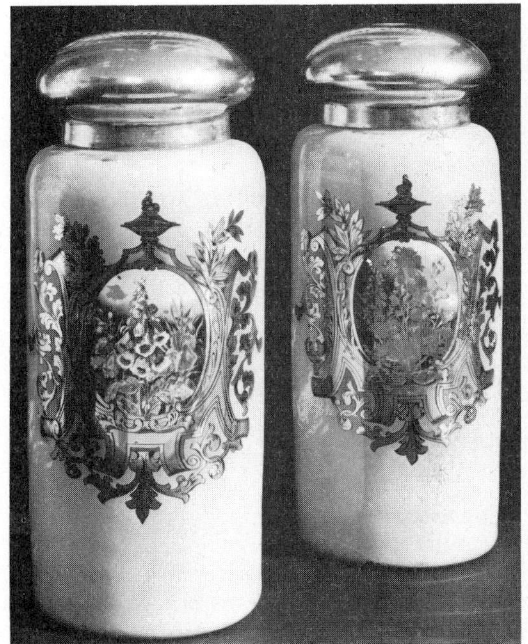

"Species" jars in matched sets held stock quantities of compound powders and (especially later on) comminuted botanical drugs and chemicals. As species jars became outmoded in use, individual specimens often were retained to ornament a pharmacy, both in the United States and abroad. These were glass jars, usually about 2 feet high, capped with a glass lid and richly ornamented with gold foil and colors. Because the 19th-century specimens shown lack drug names, they may have been made solely for ornament, although each cartouche does depict a medicinal plant. (From the Upjohn reconstruction formerly at Disneyland)

kept at hand to await the occasional prescription requiring their use.

The relics of few occupations co–mingle in such an appealing way the informative, the beautiful and the curious. This generates a perennial fascination among those laymen and health professionals in each generation who are susceptible to the allure, not only of historical collections, but of acquiring a personal collection as a pharmaceutical hobby. Publications readily available will help the interested reader get started, by providing information and particularly the bibliographic guidance needed to find other publications meeting specialized interests.[14] Perhaps the most pleasurable source of information will be visits to a few of the pharmaceutical collections on public exhibit; in the geographic guide on following pages, the annotations cite literature about collections that will open other doors to the world of pharmaceutical artifacts.

## INTERNATIONAL LIST OF PHARMACY MUSEUMS

**Compiled by George B. Griffenhagen**

The artifacts of pharmacy provide a kind of historical information not otherwise available. In design and ornamentation they often rise to a level that gives artistic expression to a segment of everyday life. This accounts for the rather remarkable number of pharmacy museums and collections that have been placed on public display, as here listed.

The public collections known to us around the world, and some outstanding private collections, are listed alphabetically by countries (and within the United States, alphabetically by states). References to published information are given wherever known, making it basically a bibliography of recorded historical pharmacy museums, as a guide for historians and students. However, some collections are no longer on public display (temporarily or permanently). Such instances known to us have been thus identified in individual entries, but the listings have been retained because such references may still help to locate either the artifacts once on display or information about them. It has not been practicable to list all collected pharmaco-historical artifacts, some of which may be found in a majority of historical museums, pharmacy schools, and in many pharmacies of the world.

One of the earliest worldwide listings of pharmacy museums was that published by Josef Anton Häfliger in *Pharmazeutische Altertumskunde* (Zürich, 1931). An annotated list of pharmacy museums worldwide was published by George Griffenhagen in *Pharmacy Museums* (Madison, Wisconsin, 1956). More recently Sami K. Hamarneh authored *Temples of the Muses and A History of Pharmacy Museums* (Tokyo, Japan, 1972); and various authors have published listings of pharmacy museums in specific countries. This "International List of Pharmacy Museums," originally appearing in the Third Edition of *Kremers and Urdang's History of Pharmacy*, has been updated as a supplement to the present volume, with the special assistance of Sami Hamarneh, Ernst W. Stieb and Glenn Sonnedecker.

### ARGENTINA

**Buenos Aires:** Museo de Historia de la Farmacia. "La Estrella" pharmacy restoration. Manual Farm. *10*:45, July, 1970.

### AUSTRALIA

**Melbourne:** University of Melbourne, Department of History. Pharmacy restoration, ca. 1915. Med. J. Aust. 2:540–542, 1971; Pharm. in Hist. *12*:20, 1970; Med. Hist. *15*:401, 1971; Hist. Med., Aust. & N.Z. Suppl. 3 (No. 4); 1972

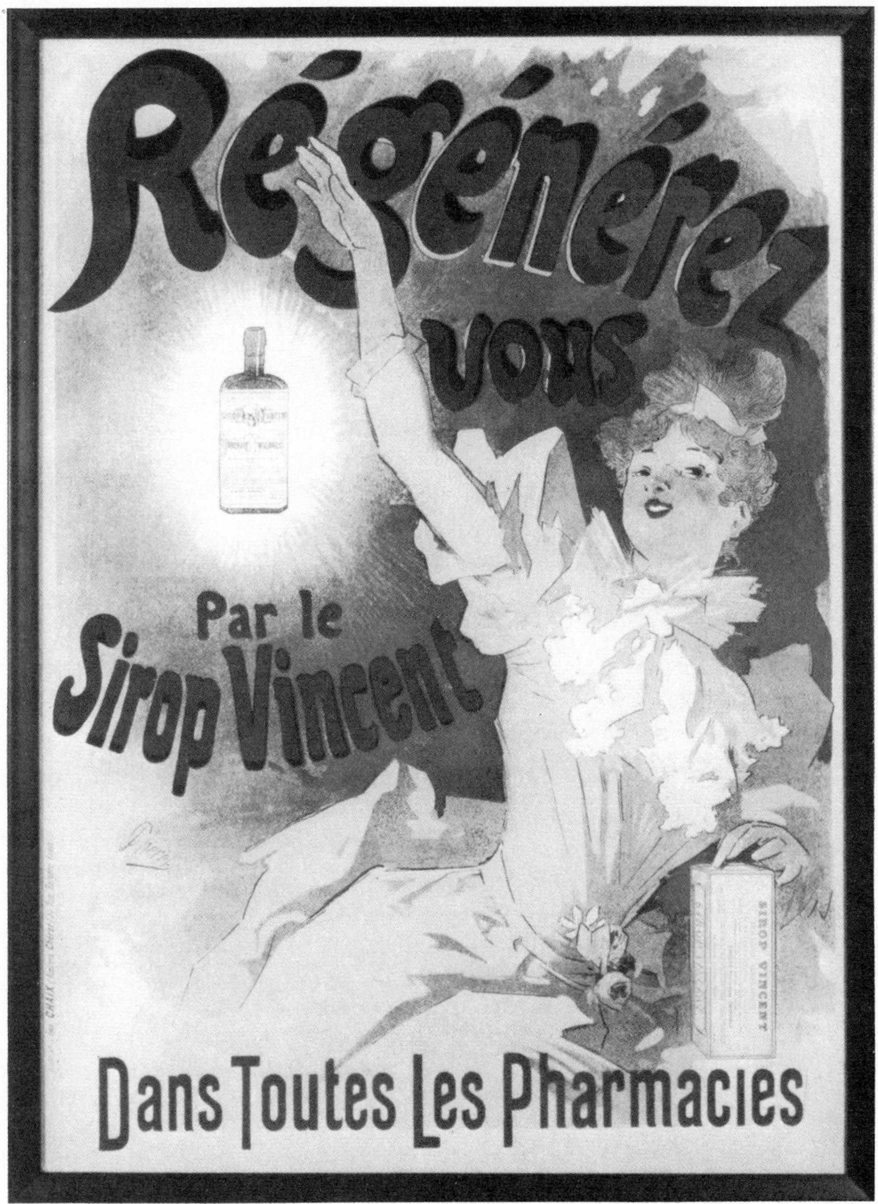


Not all "collectibles" in pharmacy are objects. Pharmaceutical posters and broadsides, for example, constitute a source for historians and a pleasure for collectors. The poster shown here is by Jules Cheret, who was important in raising posters to the level of an artform between 1880 and 1905. The young woman is inviting the viewer to be regenerated through use of Vincent's Syrup, a bottle of which glows with life-giving force! (From: W. Helfand, The pharmaceutical poster, Pharm. Hist. *15*:opposite 80, 1973)

## AUSTRIA

For general references to pharmacy museum collections in Austria, see Ganzinger, Kurt, Apotheken-Altertümer in Österreich, Internationale Gesellschaft für Geschichte der Pharmazie, 1951.

**Graz:** Landesmuseum. Pharmacy restoration. Ganzinger, l.c.*

**Innsbruck:** Winkler Stadtapotheke. Private collection. Winkler's Stadtapotheke zu Innsbruck, Gesellschaft für Geschichte der Pharmazie, 1928; Chemist and Druggist *102*:977, 1925; Apotheker-Kalender, 1935; Ganzinger, l.c.

**Linz:** Landesmuseum. Pharmacy restoration. Die Vorträge der Jubiläums Hauptversammlung in Salzburg, Internationale Gesellschaft für Geschichte der Pharmazie, 1951.

**Salzburg:** Hausapotheke des Benediktiner-Frauenstiftes Nonnberg. Österreichische Apotheker Zeitung *4*:458, 1950; *9*:759, 1955.

**Vienna:** Technisches Museum. Pharmacy restoration, alchemical laboratory. The Laboratory *21* (No. 1):2, 1951; Die Alte Apotheke, Paul Hartmann AG, Heidenheim/Brenz, 1954; Ganzinger, l.c.; Apotheker-Kalender 1956 (Sept. 1–10).

**Vienna:** Bildarchiv der Österreichischen National Bibliotek, Pharmacy manuscripts, illustrations, etc. Österreichische Apotheker Zeitung *9*:759, 1955.

**Vienna:** St. Elisabeth Hospital, 18th century pharmacy. Zeckert, Otto: Kunst in Medizin und Pharmazie (Vienna, 1955, pp. 55–56); FIP Program, 1962, p. 126.

**Vienna:** Barmherzigen Brüder Apotheke, Zeckert, Otto: Kunst in Medizin und Pharmazie (Vienna, 1955, pp. 40–43).

*To conserve space, only the last name of an author and "l.c." (*loco citato*) appears in this Appendix when a publication, once previously cited in full, is referred to subsequently in connection with another museum here listed.

**Vienna:** Institut fuer Geschichte der Medizin der Universität Wien. Hamarneh, l.c.

**Vienna:** Österreichischen Volkskundemuseums. The Austrian Folk Museum includes a restoration of an Ursuline cloister mid-18th century pharmacy. Zechert, Otto, Kunst in Medizin und Pharmazie, Vienna, 1962; Pharm. in Hist. *10*:111, 1968.

## BELGIUM

For general reference to pharmacy museum collections in Belgium, see Segers, E. G., and Wittop Koning, D. A.: Apothicaireries anciennes en Benelux, Deventer, Holland, 1958; and various numbers of the Bulletin du Cercle Benelux d'Histoire de la Pharmacie.

**Antwerp:** Musée du Folklore. Pharmacy and laboratory restoration. Catalogue du Musée de la Vieille Boucherie, No. 815–17; Segers and Wittop Koning, l.c.

**Assche:** Hôpital d'Assche. Ancient pharmacy. Wittop-Koning, Delftse Apothekerspotten, Deventer, 1954; Segers and Wittop-Koning, l.c.

**Bruges:** St. Jans Hospital. Ancient pharmacy. van Eyck, Jef: Wat wee og over den Apotheker, 1944; Bulletin du Cercle Benelux d'Histoire de la Pharmacie No. 8, 15 (April 1954); Segers and Wittop-Koning, l.c.; Prescriber (Sept., 1956).

**Brussels:** Musée de Cinquantenaire. Pharmacy restoration. Chompret, J.: Les Faiences Francaises Primitives, Paris, 1946; Wittop-Koning, D. A.: Delftse Apothekerspotten, Deventer, 1954; Bulletin du Cercle Benelux d'Histoire de la Pharmacie No. 3, 19 (Aug. 1952); Pro Medico *13*:17, 1936; Segers and Wittop-Koning, l.c.; Prescriber (Sept. 1956).

**Doornik (Tournai):** Musée de la Maison Tournaisienne. Pharmacy restoration. Segers and Wittop-Koning, l.c.

**Ghent:** Museum of Folklore. Pharmacy restoration. Pharmaceutisch Tijdschrift voor Belgie *28*:42, 1951; Vandewiele, L. J.: Inventaris der Apothekerspotten van het

Museum voor Folklore te Gent; Bulletin du Cercle Benelux d'Histoire de la Pharmacie No. 1, 6 (June 1951); Oostvlaamse Zanten, *49*:1951; Segers and Wittop-Koning, l.c.

**Louvain:** Pharmaceutical Institute. University of Louvain, Couvreur collection. Bulletin du Cercle Benelux d'Histoire de la Pharmacie No. 3, 19 (Aug. 1952); Segers and Wittop-Koning, l.c.

**Malines:** Musée Ville de Malines. Pharmacy restoration. Van Doorselaer: L'Ancienne Industrie de Cuivre a'Malines, 4 vols.; Catalogue de l'Exposition, Brussels, 1954; Segers and Wittop-Koning, l.c.*

**Orval:** Pharmacie de l'Abbaye l'Orval. Ancient pharmacy. Pro Medico *6*:88, 1929; annales Merck, 13 (1935); Segers and Wittop-Koning, l.c.

## BRAZIL

**Rio de Janeiro:** Antonio Lago Pharmacy Museum, Brazilian Pharmaceutical Assoc. Alfonzo, R. G., The Journal (Michigan) *39*:30 (May 1951); Raul Votta: Breve Historia da Farmacia no Brasil (Rio de Janeiro, 1965).

## CANADA

**Barkerville, British Columbia:** Gold Rush Pharmacy restoration. Canadian Pharm. J. *101* (No. 2): 70–72, Feb., 1968; Pharm. in Hist. *10*:89, 1968.

**Halifax, Nova Scotia.** Dalhousie University, College of Pharmacy. Museum. Can. Academy of the History of Pharmacy Newsletter, February 1974, 2–4.

**Niagara-on-the-Lake, Ontario:** Niagara Apothecary mid–19th century restoration. Bull. Ontario College Pharm. *17* (No. 2): 33–34, March, 1968; Pharm. in Hist. *10*:87–88, 1968; Ibid. *13*:149–150, 1971; Ibid. *14*:42, and 65–69, 1972; Bull. Ontario. College Pharm. *20*:33–51, 117, 1971.

**Port Royal, Granville Ferry, Nova Scotia.** Port Royal National Historic Park. Habitation, 1606 reconstruction includes quarters of Louis Hébert with drug chest and containers. Port Royal Habitation, Ottawa, 1970, 15 pp.

**Saskatoon, Saskatchewan.** Western Development Museum, Pioneer Village. Coad's Drug Store. Can. Pharm. J., *106*:22–24, 1973.

**Toronto, Ontario:** Academy of Medicine. Drake collection includes pill tiles, drug jars, mortars, coins and tokens, medicine chests, medicine spoons, pill boxes, prints, etc. Pharm in Hist. *12*:18–19, 1970; J. Hist. Med. *15*:31–44, 1960. Amer. J. of Diseases of Children, *39*:1–49–61, 1930; Canadian Med. Assoc. J., *25*:605–606. 1931; Ibid. *39*:585–588, 1938; Canadian Pharm. J., *72*:8, 10–11, 20, 1939; Bull. Hist. Med. *8*:128–132, 1942; Ibid. *12*:323–335, 1942; J. Hist. Med. and Allied Sciences, *1*:316–317, 1946; Ibid. *2*:48–50, 1947; Ibid. *3*:507–524, 1948; Ibid. *7*:68–78, 1952; Bull. Hist. Med. *29*:420–428, 1955; Chem. and Drugg. *165*:614–618, 1956.

**Winnipeg, Manitoba:** Museum of Man and Nature. Pharmacy restoration in Urban Gallery. Pharm. in Hist. *16*:79, 1974.

## CZECHOSLOVAKIA

For general references to Czechoslovakia pharmacy museums, see Hanzlicek, Z., Cs. Farm. *18*:212–217, 1969; Ibid. *21*:180–182, 1972; Duka, N., Farm. Obzor *40*:129–133, 1971.

**Bratislava:** Pharmacy museum. Zur Geschichte der Pharmazie 13, No. 2 (1962); Cs. Farm. (Slovak.) *21*:226–7, 1972.

**Brno:** Pharmacy collection, at Augustinian monastery (accessible basement storage).

**Kuks:** Merciful Brethren Hospital Pharmacy, founded 1743 and operated until the end of World War II. Restored 1956–64 to period of 1740's and now open to public. Hanzlicek, Z., Raltr, Z. and Rusek, V., Barokni Lekarna v Kuksu, Nakladatelstvi Kruh, 1971, 102 pp.

**Prague:** Technical museum. Alchemical

laboratory restoration. Sarton, George: A Guide to the History of Science, Waltham, Mass., 1952.

**Prague:** Pharmacy Museum. Rozpr. Naprodniho Techn. Muz. Rada Popul. Ved. No. *7*:150–153, 1963; Farm. Obzor. *33*:178–179, 1964.

## DENMARK

For general references to pharmacy museum collections in Denmark, see Andersen, Dannesboe, Gammelt Dansk Apotheksinventar, Copenhagen, 1944, with English supplement entitled Antique Furniture from Danish Prescription Pharmacies.

**Aarhus:** "Den gamle By." Pharmacy restoration. Andersen, l.c.; Købstadmuseet "Den Gamle By," Aarbog 16 (1942); *47* (1945); *31* (1949); Chem. & Drug. *167*:274 (1957).

**Copenhagen:** Medicinsk-Historiske Museum. Pharmacy restoration and collections. Københavns Universitets Medicinsk-Historiske Museum, Annual Reports, 1952–54; Medicine Illustrated *3*:134, 1949; München. med. Wchnschr. *81*:1436, 1934; Andersen, l.c.; Medicinsk Forum *3*:193, 1950; Archiv for Pharmaci og Chemi *102*:653, 1945; *103*:715, 1946; Chem. & Drug. *180*:666–667, 1963.

**Copenhagen:** Nationalmuseet. Majolica. Andersen, l.c.

## EGYPT

**Cairo:** Medico-Pharmaceutical Museum, Egyptian Ministry of Health. Opened in 1972.

## FINLAND

**Helsinki:** Pharmacy museum. Majolica and pharmacy material. Chem. & Drug. *102*:964, 1925; Zur Geschichte der Pharmazie *10* (No. 4), 1958; Farm. Obzor (Czech.) *33*:176–178, 1964.

**Helsinki:** Stads museum. Pharmacy restoration, period 1700. Karsten, Walter, Farmacins Historia Finland, Helsingfors, 1933.

## FRANCE

For general references to pharmacy museum collections in France, see Chem. & Drug. *72*:157, 1908; *102*:964, 1925; Bulletin de la Société d'Histoire de la Pharmacie, 1913–1929; Rev. Histoire Pharm. 1930–1955; Am. Drug. *67*:27, (Nov. 1919); Chompret, J.: Les Faiences Françaises Primitives, Paris, 1946 (includes a list of 79 hospital pharmacies possessing faience); Boussel, Patrice: Histoire Illustrée de la Pharmacie, Paris, 1949; "Apothicaireries de France," La Libre Pharmacie, Special No. (December 1961). See also Cotinat, Louis, Rev. Hist. Pharm. *21*:549–576, 1973, for a description of 28 museums of pharmaceutical interest in Paris and suburbs.

**Angers:** Hôtel-Dieu. Ancient pharmacy. Chem. & Drug. *102*:968, 1925; Chompret, l.c.; La Libre Pharmacie, l.c.

**Arles:** Hospital. Ancient pharmacy. Chompret, l.c.

**Avignon:** Augier Pharmacy. Pacific Drug Review *70*:16, Sept., 1958; El Farm. *34*:12, Nov., 1958; Drug Topics *101*:16, April 1, 1957; Modern Pharm. *38*:14, May, 1958; J.A.Ph.A. (Pract. Ed.) *20*:40, 1959.

**Bauge:** Hôtel-Dieu. 17th century pharmacy. Chompret, l.c.; La Libre Pharmacie, l.c.

**Bayeux:** Public museum. Faience. Chem. & Drug. *102*:968, 1925.

**Bazas:** Hôpital. Ancient pharmacy. Rev. Histoire Pharm. *41*:178, 1953.

**Besançon:** Hôpital St. Jaques. Louis XIV pharmacy. Chem. & Drug. *102*:968, 1925; Chompret, l.c.; Boussel, l.c.; La Libre Pharmacie, l.c.

**Carpentras:** Hôtel-Dieu. 18th century pharmacy, Chompret, l.c.

**Castres:** Musée Goya. Faience. Rev. Histoire Pharm. *43*:184, 1955.

**Chantilly:** Hôtel-Dieu. Ancient pharmacy. Guides touristiques, through Guitard, E. H., personal correspondence, Dec. 7, 1955.

**Dijon:** Hospital. Ancient pharmacy. Chem. & Drug. *102*:968, 1925; La Libre Pharmacie, l.c.

**Gayette:** Hospital. Ancient pharmacy. Chompret, l.c.

**Issoudun:** Hôtel-Dieu. 17th century pharmacy. La Presse Medicale *57*:32, 1949 (Jan. 5); Rev. Histoire Pharm. *38*:10, 1950; Robert, Louis: l'Ancienne Pharmacie de l'Hôpital d'Issoudun, 1950; Chompret, l.c.; La Libre Pharmacie, l.c.

**Limoges:** Musée de la porcelaine. Faience. Catalogues, through Guitard, E. H., personal correspondence, Dec. 7, 1955.

**Louhans:** Hôtel-Dieu. 17th century pharmacy. Chem. & Drug. *102*:968, 1925; Chompret, l.c.; La Libre Pharmacie, l.c.; Prescriber (Sept. 1956).

**Lyon:** Hôpital de la Charité. Ancient pharmacy. Chompret, l.c.; Bull. Soc. Histoire Pharm. No. 48, p. 129, 1925; La Libre Pharmacie, l.c.

**Lyon:** Bibliothéque et Musée d'Histoire de la Médecine, University of Lyon, Pharmacy material. Sarton, l.c.

**Mans:** Hôtel-Dieu. Ancient pharmacy. Bull. Soc. Histoire Pharm. No. 25, 159, 168, 1920.

**Marseille:** Hôpital de la Charité. Ancient pharmacy. Boussel, l.c.

**Montpellier:** Musée de la Société Archéologique. Faience. Chompret, l.c.

**Montpellier:** Museum of the History of Pharmacy. Rev. His. Pharm. *18*:515–518, 1967; Monspel. Hippocr. *11* (No. 39): 27–32, 1968; Rev. Hist. Pharm. *22*:91–92, 1974.

**Nancy:** Musée Historique Lorrain. 18th century pharmacy restoration, pharmacy material. Niklewski, Stefan: Biuletynu Farmaceutycznego *3*:118, 1948.

**Narbonne:** Hospital. 16th century pharmacy. Chem. & Drug. *102*:968, 1925; Chompret, l.c.

**Paris:** Musée d'Histoire de la Pharmacie, 4 Avenue de l'Observatoire. Henri Fialon faience collection and other pharmacy material. Bull. Soc. Histoire Pharm. No. 14, p. 240, 1916; No. 16, p. 279, 1917; No. 18, p. 313, 1917; No. 20, p. 369, 1918; Am. Drug. *67*:27, 1919 (Nov.); *69*:46, 1921 (April); *74*:12, 1926 (March); Chem. & Drug. *102*:964, 1925; Rev. Histoire Pharm. *36*:277, 1948; J. A. Pharm. A. (Pract.) *16*:600, 1955; Cotinat, l.c.

**Paris:** Musée de l'Assistance Publique et de la Pharmacie Centrale des Hôpitaux. Faience. Chem. & Drug. *72*:157, 1908; Am. Drug. *67*:27 1919 (Nov.); *102*:968, 1925; *74*:10, 1926 (March); La Presse Médicale *57*:19 (Jan. 5) 1949; Boussel, l.c.; Lothian, Agnes: "Pharmacy Jars," The Concise Encyclopedia of Antiques, Vol. II, Connoisseur, London, 1955; Cotinat, l.c.

**Paris:** Ordre National des Pharmaciens. Bouvet and Leclair collections. Rev. Hist. Pharm. *17*:61–71, 1964/65; Bull. Ordre Pharm. No. 118:349–351, Aug.–Sept., 1968; Ibid. No. 123:531–546, Aug.–Sept., 1969; Cotinat, l.c.

**Paris:** Musée du Louvré. Faience. Bulletin de la Société d'Histoire de la Pharmacie, No. 56, p. 453, 1927; Am. Drug. *67*:27, 1919 (Nov.); *72*:12, 1924 (Sept.); *74*:11, 1926 (March); Chem. & Drug. *102*:964, 1925; Chompret, l.c.

**Paris:** Musée de Sèvres. Faience. Bulletin de la Société d'Histoire de la Pharmacie, No. (1927); Chem. & Drug. *102*:964, 1925; Am. Drug. *75*:15 (Feb.) 1927; Chompret, l.c.; Boussel, l.c.; Rev. Histoire Pharm. *41*:147, 1953; Cotinat, l.c.

**Paris:** Musée de Cluny. Faience. Chem. & Drug. *72*:157, 1908; *102*:968, 1925; Am. Drug. *67*:27, 1919 (Nov.); *72*:13, 1924 (Sept.); Chompret, l.c.; Cotinat, l.c.

**Pont-Saint-Esprit:** Grand Hospital. Ancient pharmacy. Chompret, l.c.

**Rouen:** Musée de l'Hôtel-Dieu. Ancient pharmacy. Rev. Histoire Pharm. *38*:91, 1950; Boll. Soc. Ital. Farm. Osped. *18*:387–388, 1972.

**Rouen:** Musée céramique. Faience. Catalogues, through Guitard, E. H., personal correspondence, Dec. 7, 1955.

**Saint-Denis:** Hôtel-Dieu. Ancient pharmacy. Bull. Soc. Histoire Pharm. No. 35, p. 65, 1922; No. 43, p. 377, 1924; Am. Drug. *74*:10, March, 1926.

**Saint-Germain-en-Laye:** Hospital. Ancient pharmacy. Savare, Paule, l'Apothicairerie Royale de Saint-Germain-en-Laye, Paris, n.d.; Boussel, l.c.; Chem. & Drug. *102*:968, 1925; Am. Drug. *74*:12, March, 1926; Rev. Histoire Pharm. *34*:84, 1946; La Libre Pharmacie, l.c.

**Saint-Malo:** Hôtel-Dieu. Ancient pharmacy. Bull. Soc. Histoire Pharm. *97*:122 (No. 24) 1919; *97*:129 (No. 48) 1925; LeMarie, B., Contribution à l'Histoire de la Pharmacie dans la Bretagne Septentrionale, Rennes, 1946.

**Strasbourg:** Hirsch-Apotheke, West. Druggist *20*:220, 1898; Die Alte Apotheke, Paul Hartmann AG, Heidenheim/Brenz, Germany, 1954; J.A.Ph.A. (Pract. Ed.) *20*:40, 1959.

**Tarascon:** Hospital of St. Nicholas. Ancient pharmacy. Chem. & Drug. *102*:968, 1925.

**Toulouse:** Musée Paul-Dupuy. Bull. Soc. Histoire Pharm. No. 20, p. 392, 1918.

**Tournus:** Hôtel-Dieu. Ancient pharmacy. Chem. & Drug. *102*:968, 1925; Bull. Soc. Histoire Pharm. No. 40, p. 277, 1923; La Libre Pharmacie, l.c.

**Troyes:** Hôtel-Dieu. 18th century pharmacy. Chompret, l.c.; Bull. Soc. Histoire Pharm. No. 43, p. 377, 1924; Pinsolle, S., Contribution á l'Histoire de la Pharmacie en Champagne, La Garenne, 1937; La Libre Pharmacie, l.c.

**Versailles:** Hôtel-Dieu. Ancient pharmacy. Am. Drug. *74*:11, March, 1926; Rev. Histoire Pharm. *26*:436, 1938.

**Villefranche-sur-Saune:** 18th century pharmacy. La Libre Pharmacie, l.c.

**Yssingeaux:** Hospital. 16th century pharmacy. Chompret, l.c.

## GERMANY

For general references to pharmacy museum collections in Germany, see Apotheker-Kalender (July 1, 1932) and subsequent editions; the Apotheker-Zeitung *41*:1276, 1926; Pharm. Zeitung *81*:1287, 1936; Gesch. Deutschen Apotheke, No. 6/7 (April/May) 1937; Hein, Wolfgang-Hagen, Apotheken-Kostbarkeiten in Bayern, 1954; "Oeffentliche und private pharmaziegeschichtliche Sammlungen in Deutschland", a series commencing in Zur Geschichte der Pharmazie (Beilage to the Deutschen Apotheker Zeitung), hereafter cited as "Gesch. Pharm.," No. 3, p. 21 (1955); Gutmann, Siegfried, Alte Deutsche Apotheken, W. Spitzner Arzneimittelfabrik GMBH, 1972 (series of booklets describing "700 years of German pharmacy history with map locating over 500 old German pharmacies. Also see Conradi, Helmut Peter, Apothekengläser im Wandel der Zeit, Würzburg, Germany, 1973.

**Aachen:** Couven-Museum. Pharmacy museum. Felix Kuetgens, Das Couven-Museum in Aachen, Neuss, 1959; Gesch. Pharm. *15*:5, 1963.

**Braunschweig:** Vaterländisches Museum. Pharmacy restoration. Pharm. Zeitung *52*:151 (1907); Gesch. Deutschen Apotheke, No. 6/7 (April/May) 1937.

**Bremen:** Focke-Museum. Pharmacy restoration. Gesch. Pharmazie, No. 3, p. 21, 1955.

**Darmstadt:** Hessisches Landes-Museum. Pharmacy restoration. Apotheker-Kalender (1925); Gesch. Deutschen Apotheke, No. 6/7 (April/May) 1937; Gesh. Pharm. *22*:5, 1970.

**Eisenach:** Thüringer Museum. Pharmacy material. Apotheker-Kalender (Dec., 1933); Pharm. Zeitung *79*:1085, 1934; Fiek,

Wolfgang: Die pharmaziegeschichtliche Sammlung im Thüringer Museum zu Eisenach, Gesellsch. Gesch. Pharmazie, Mittenwald, n.d.

**Goslar:** Goslarer Museum. Pharmacy and laboratory restoration. Gesch. Pharmazie, No. 3, p. 21, 1955.

**Heidelberg:** Heinrici and Ferchl collections, among others. Gesch. Deutschen Apotheke No. 8, June, 1935; No. 9, July, 1935; No. 10, Aug., 1935; No. 11, Sept., 1935; No. 10/11, Aug./Sept., 1936; No. 2, Dec. 1937; No. 1/6, Jan./June, 1939; Deutsche Apotheker-Zeitung *91*:495, 1951; Neue Apotheken-Illustrierte No. 2, Feb., 1954; Die Alte Apotheke, Paul Hartmann AG, Heidenheim/Brenz, 1954; Am. J. Pharm. Ed. *14*:577, 1950; J.A.Ph.A (Pract. Ed.) *16*:600, 1955; Gesch. Pharm., vol. 9, No. 3, 1957; Deutsch. Apoth. Ztg. *95*:751, 1957; Schweiz. Apoth. Ztg. *95*:846, 1957; Führer durch das Deutsche Apothekenmuseum im Heidelberg (Frankfurt, 1959); Ibid., (ed. 2), (1962); Apotheker und Kunst, No. 7, p. 27, 1959; Pharm. Zeitung *105*:1421, 1960; Deutsch. Apoth. Ztg. *103*:1446–1447, 1963; Forsch. Prax. Fortbild. *17*:547–549, 1966; Gesch. Pharm. *28*:163–177, 1966; Guidebook to the German Pharmacy Museum in the Heidelberg Castle, 4pp., 1966; Pharm. in Hist. *10*:51–55, 1968; Orv. Hetil. (Hungarian) *112*:2293–2295, 1971; Poensgen, G. and Luckenbach, W., Das Deutsche Apotheken-Museum im Heidelberger Schloss, Springer-Verlag, Band 16, 1972.

**Heidelberg:** Kurpfälzisches Museum. Pharmacy material. Pharm. Zeitung *91*:647, 1955; Deutsche Apotheker Zeitung *95*:547, 592, 1955.

**Munich:** Deutsches Museum. Pharmacy and laboratory restoration. Bol. Assoc. Brasil Pharm. *11*:25, 1930; Am. Drug. *87*:44, Feb., 1933; Apotheker-Kalender (June 23-July 6, 1935); Gesch. Deutschen Apotheke, No. 6/7 (April/May) 1937; Hein, l.c.; Gesch. Pharm. vol. 9, No. 2, 1957.

**Nuremberg:** Germanisches Nationalmuseum. Pharmacy restoration. Peters, Hermann, Pharm. Zeitung *41*:183, 1896; *42*:765, 775, 783, 1897; Chem. & Drug. *112*:819, 1930; Apotheker-Kalender (1936); Deutsche Apotheken-Altertümer, Germanisches Nationalmuseum, Nurnberg, 1936; Veröff. Int. Ges. Gesch. Pharm. *22*:133–151, 1963.

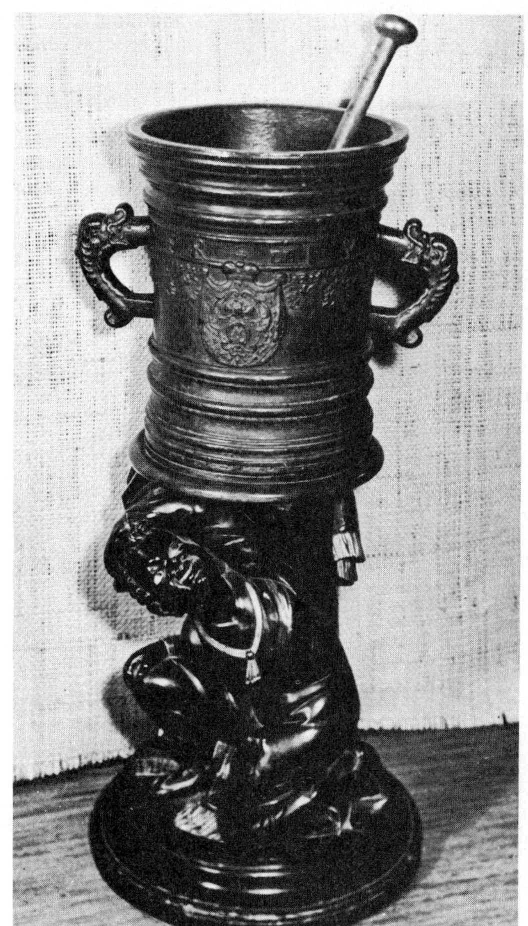

A crouching Moorish boy serves as a stand for this heavy bronze mortar with dolphin handles (made in 1704). On the front, the mortar bears the coat of arms of the prince-bishop at Mainz, in whose court pharmacy it stood. (Photograph from Verbandstoff-Fabriken Paul Hartmann AG, Heidenheim/Brenz)

**Ulm:** Gewerbemuseum. Pharmacy material. Apotheker-Kalender (1925); Gesch. Deutschen Apotheke, No. 6/7 (April/May) 1937.

**Waldenbuch:** Uhland-Apotheke, Schwäbisches Apothekenmuseum. Walter Dörr collection. Sammlung Walter Dörr, Stuttgart, 1933; Süddeutsche Apotheker Zeitung *89*:949, 1949; Apotheker-Kalender (June 1933); Dörr, Walter: Das Schwäbische Apotheken-Museum zu Waldenbuch, Stuttgart, 1933; Kostbarkeiten aus der Apotheke, Paul Hartmann AG, Heidenheim/Brenz, 1954; J.A.Ph.A. (Pract. Ed.) *16*:629, 1955.

**Wülfrath:** Niederbergischen Museum. Apothecary shop restoration. Gesch. Pharm. *24*:4, 1972.

## GREAT BRITAIN

For general reference to pharmacy museum collections in London, see Chem. & Drug. *159*:584, 1953 and Matthews, Leslie G., Antiques of the Pharmacy, London, 1971.

**Leeds:** Kirkstall Abbey House Museum. Taylor and Mason pharmacy. Chem. & Drug. *164*:189, 1955 and *165*:580, 1956; J.A.Ph.A. (Pract. Ed.) *16*:540, 1955.

**London:** Wellcome Historical Medical Museum, 183–193 Euston Road. Extensive pharmacy material: Henry S. Wellcome collection. Historical Exhibition of Rare and Curious Objects Relating to Medicine, Chemistry, Pharmacy and Allied Sciences, Wellcome, London, n.d.; J.A.Ph.A *16*:161, 1927; *20*:238, 1931; Am. Drug. *82*:30, Dec., 1930; Pharm. Zeitung *79*:214, 1934; Underwood, E. A.: Catalogue of an Exhibition Illustrating the History of Pharmacy (May 4-Sept. 28, 1951), London, 1951; Chem. & Drug. *159*:584, 1953; *164*:338, 373, 1955; J.A.Ph.A. (Pract. Ed.) *16*:662, 1955; *21*:86, 1960; Pharm. J. (4th ser.) *183*:129, 116, 1959; Chem. & Drug. *72*:27, 1959; Brit. Med. J. *2*:253, 1959; J.A.Ph.A. (Pract. Ed.) *21*:86, 1960. Med. Hist. *11*:215–227, 1967; Crellin, J. K., Medical Ceramics: A Catalogue of the English and Dutch Collections in the Museum of The Wellcome Institute of the History of Medicine, London, 1969; Trans. English Ceramic Circle *7*:191, 1970; Crellin, J. K. and Scott, J. R., Glass and British Pharmacy, London, 1972; Med. Hist. *17*:266–287, 1973.

**London:** Pharmaceutical Society of Great Britain Museum, 17 Bloomsbury Sq., Lambeth delft collection. Holmes, E. M., Catalogue of the Collections in the Museum of the Pharmaceutical Society of Great Britain (Materia Medica), London, 1878; Chem. & Drug. *159*:584, 1953; Pharm. J. 115, Jan. 31, 1970; Ibid. 205, Feb. 28, 1970; Ibid. 325, March 28, 1970; Ibid. 438–439, April 25, 1970; Ibid. 728–729, June 27, 1970; Pharm. in Hist. *12*:182, 1970.

**London:** Victoria and Albert Museum, South Kensington. Majolica. Rackham, Bernard: Catalogue of Italian Majolica, London, 1940; Chem. & Drug. *159*:584, 1953; J.A.Ph.A. (Pract. Ed.) *16*:540, 1955.

**London:** Society of Apothecaries, Black Friars Lane. Lambeth delft. Ann. Roy. Coll. Surgeons England *7*:497, 1950.

**London:** British Museum. Ancient pharmacy material. Chem. & Drug. *106*:797, 1927.

**London:** London Museum. Lambeth delft. Chem. & Drug. *128*:755, 1938.

**Oxford**: Museum of History of Science. Pharmacy material. Chem. & Drug. *126*:747, 1937; *161*:666, 1954.

**York:** Castle Museum. Pharmacy (chemist shop) restoration. Lewis, A. B.: The Parish of York Castle, A Description of the Museum 'Street,' York, 1949; J.A.Ph.A. (Pract. Ed.) *16*:540, 1955; Prescriber, Sept. 1956.

## HUNGARY

**Budapest:** National Technical Art Museum. Pharmacy restoration. Chem. & Drug. *112*:818, 1930; *102*:978, 1925; Apotheker-Kalender (Feb. 4–6, 1932); Bull. Soc. Histoire Pharm. *20*:136, 1932. Present status unknown.

**Budapest:** Iprarmuveszeti Muzeum.

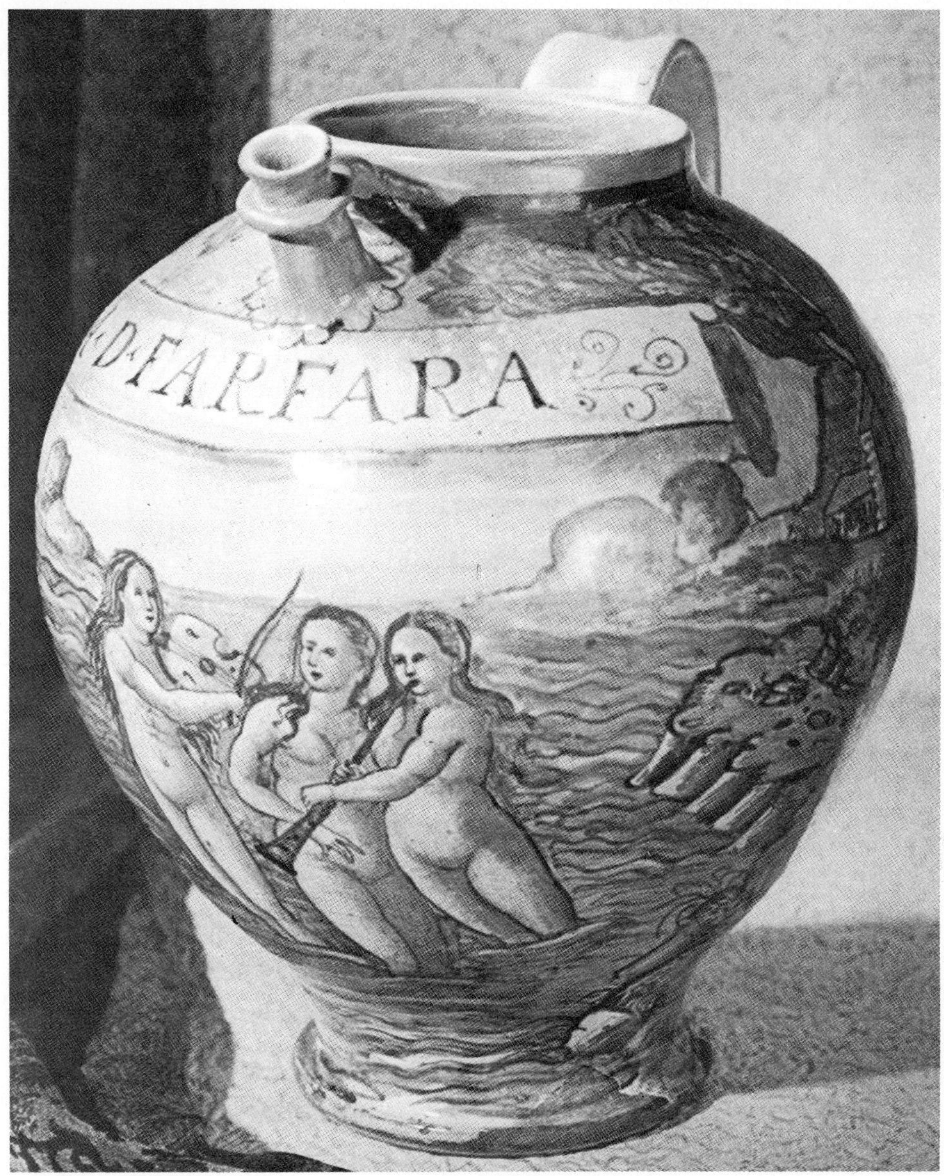


Potteries of Italy, especially between the 16th and 18th centuries, created many of Europe's most artistic drug jars for stock quantities on the pharmacists' shelves. The example shown is from Urbino, probably made in the late 16th century. (From: Medico-historical Collection of Hoffmann-La Roche & Co., Basel)

Majolica. Acta pharm. Hungarica, vol. 132, June, 1955.

**Budapest:** Arts and Crafts Museum. Köszeg Jesuit Monastery pharmacy restoration. Grünenthal Waage 7:95, 1968.

**Budapest:** Pharmaceutical Museum. Commum. Bibl. Hist. Med. Hung. No. 36:209–212, 1965; Gesch. Pharm. *38*:129–134, 1972.

**Debrecen:** Deri Museum. Hungarian apothecary shop restoration. Gesch. Pharm. *17*:10–12, 1965.

## INDIA

**New Delhi:** Institute of History of Medicine and Medical Research. Museum includes pharmacy artifacts of the Middle East with emphasis on the Eastern (Greco-Arabic) system of medicine, Pharm. in Hist. *12*:16, 1970.

## ITALY

**Faenza:** Musée Ceramique de Faience. Castiglioni, Arturo, La Farmacia Italiana del Quattrocento nella storia dell'arte ceramica, Faenza, 1922; Chompret, l.c. (much destroyed by war but collection being rebuilt).

**Florence:** Museo di Storia della Scienza. Pharmacy material. Catalogo Degli Strumenti del Museo di Storia della Scienza, Firenze, 1954; Pharm. in Hist. *9*:91–92, 1967.

**Florence:** Antica Farmacia del canto alle Rondini. Die Vorträge der Hauptversammlung der Gesellschaft für Geschichte der Pharmazie, Basel, May 17–20, 1934.

**Naples:** Museo Nazionale di Napoli. Ancient pharmacy material. Tergolina, Umberto, La Farmacia, Rome, 1939.

**Parma:** Museo Nazionale. Restoration of pharmacy of S. Giovanni Evangelista. La storica farmacia di S. Giovanni Evangelista, 1951; J. Hist. Med. & Allied Sciences *11*:227, 1956.

**Pavia:** Museo di Storia della Farmacia. La Chimica, No. 8, 1943; Scienza e Lavoro, No. 7, 1949; la Teriaca *10*:3, April, 1954.

**Rome:** Accademia di Storia dell'Arte Sanitaria. Pharmacy restoration. Apotheker-Kalender (Sept. 11–13, 1932); Il Farmacista *2*:347, 1948; Tergolina, l.c.

**Rome:** Instituto di Storia della Medicina dell'Universita di Roma. Pharmacy material, alchemical laboratory, Humana Studia, vol. 7, Series II, 1955; Rivista Ospedaliera, No. 9–10, 1955.

**Venice:** Pharmacie Santa Fosca (Farmacia Ponci 1730) Bull. Soc. Histoire Pharm., No. 40, p. 277, 1923.

**Venice:** Farmacia "Daniele Manin." Pharm. in Hist. *9*:104–105, 1967.

## JAPAN

**Tokyo:** The Naito Museum of Pharmaceutical Science and Industry. Finest museum of pharmacy related to the Orient. J. Jap. Hist. Pharm. *6* (No. 1): 10–11, 1971; Pharm. in Hist. *14*:43–44, 1972; Hamarneh, l.c.

## THE NETHERLANDS

For museum collections in The Netherlands, see various numbers of the Bulletin du Cercle Benelux d'Histoire de la Pharmacie; Wittop-Koning, D. A., Nederlandse Vijzels, Deventer, 1953; Wittop-Koning, D. A., Delft Drug-Jars, Deventer, 1956; Segers, E. G., and Wittop-Koning, D. A., De oude apotheek in de Benelux, Deventer, Holland, 1958 and Wittop-Koning, D. A., De Oude Apotheek, Van Dishoeck, Bussam, 1966.

**Amersfoort:** Museum Flehite, Pharmacy restoration. Wittop-Koning, D. A., Delft Drug-Jars, Deventer, 1956; Segers and Wittop-Koning, l.c.

**Amsterdam:** Medisch Pharmaceutisch Museum, Koestraat. Pharmacy and laboratory restoration; pharmacy material. Pharmaceutisch Weekblad *39*:764, 1902; Bull. Soc. Histoire Pharm. No. 30, p. 349, 1921; Apotheker-Kalender (1929); Pharmaceutisch Weekblad *88*:354, 710, 1953; The Laboratory *23*:56, Dec. 1953; Endeavor *13*:128, July, 1954; J.A.Ph.A. (Pract. Ed.) *16*:600, 1955; Bulletin du Cercle Benelux d'Histoire de la Pharmacie, No. 6, p. 14, Nov., 1953; Segers and Wittop-Koning, l.c.; Prescriber (Sept. 1956); Ned. Tijdschr. Geneesk., No. 13, 1955; Gesch. Pharm., vol. 9, No. 3, 1957.

**Gouda:** Museum Catherina Gasthuis. Pharmacy restoration. Wittop-Koning, D. A., Delft Drug-Jars, Deventer, 1956; Segers and Wittop-Koning, l.c.

**Haarlem:** Frans Hals Museum. Pharmacy restoration. Pharmaceutisch Weekblad *74*:775, 1937; Segers and Wittop-Koning, l.c.

**Leeuwarden:** Fries Museum. Pharmacy restoration. Pharmaceutisch Weekblad *75*:729, 1938; Segers and Wittop-Koning, l.c.

**Leiden:** Rijksmuseum voor de Geschiedenis der Natuurwetenschapen. Pharmacy material. Pharmaceutisch Weekblad *82*:185, 1947; J.A.Ph.A. (Pract. Ed.) *16*:600, 1955.

**Oldenzaal:** Musée d'Antiquités. Pharmacy restoration. Pharmaceutisch Weekblad *77*:273, 1940; Segers and Wittop-Koning, l.c.

**Rotterdam:** Museum Boymans. Majolica. Catalogus Oud-Aardewerk van 1250–1650 (1940).

## NORWAY

**Grimstad:** Grimstad Bymuseum og Ibsenhuset. Restoration of pharmacy where Henrik Ibsen worked. Grimstad Bys Historie, pp. 624–26, 1926; Prescriber (Sept. 1956).

**Oslo:** Universitetets farmasøytiske Institutts museum. Pharmacy material. Jermstad, A.: Personal correspondence, Dec. 14, 1955.

**Stavanger:** Stavanger Museum. Hygeia pharmacy restoration. Jermstad, A.: Personal correspondence, Dec. 14, 1955.

## PERU

**Lima:** Museo Maldonado de Farmacia, Laboratorios Maldonado, S.A. Angel Maldonado pharmacy collection. Museo Maldonado de Farmacia, Lima, 1951; Terreros, N.: personal correspondence, April 10, 1956.

## POLAND

**Crakow:** Muzeum Historycznym Aptekarstwa Polskiego. Pharmacy material. Farmacja Polska *8*:111, 193, 229, 263, 315, 1952; Rev. Hist. Pharm. *150*, 1958; J.A.Ph.A. ns *4*:392–393; Amer. J. Hosp. Pharm. *21*:268–273, 1964; Counterscope *2* (No. 26): 4–6, 1964; Pron, Stanislaw, Musaeum Poloniae Pharmaceuticum Seu Artis Pharmaceuticae Experimentalis Spectrum, Warsaw, 1967; Pharm. in Hist. *13*:46–47, 1971; Rev. Hist. Pharm. *21*:191–192, 1972; Roeske, W., La céramique de Pharmacie Polonaise dans la Musée de la Pharmacie dà Crocovie, 1973.

## PORTUGAL

**Lisbon:** National Library. Special exhibition of Portuguese faience and related pharmaceutical equipment, Sept. 4–9, 1972, during 24th General Assembly of FIP, assembled from various museums and private collections in Portugal. Exposicao de Faiancas Portuguesas de Farmacia, Lisbon, Portugal, 1972. See review in Pharm. in Hist. *15*:101, 1973.

## PUERTO RICO

**Rio Piedras:** Colegio de Farmacia, Universidad de Puerto Rico, Pharmacy Museum. Porcelain drug jars. Torres-Diaz, Luis. Breve Historia de la Farmacia en Puerto Rico, Amer. Inst. Hist. Pharm., Madison, Wisc., 1951; Pharm. in Hist. *11*:71–72, 1969; Hamarneh, Sami, Pharmacy Museums USA, AIHP, 1972.

## ROMANIA

**Bucharest:** National Institute of the History

of Medicine. Pharmacy material. Sigerist, H. E.: A History of Medicine, vol. I, Oxford Univ. Press, 1951.

**Cluj:** Institute of the History of Medicine and Pharmacy. Culture Cluj *1*: No. 3, 1924; Archeion *9*:517, 1928; Clujul Med. *11*:19–20, 1930; Gesch. Pharm. *9*: No. 4, 1957; Deutsch. Apoth. Ztg. No. 4, 29–31, 1957; Actas del XV Congreso Internacional del Historia de la Medicina, vol. 2, pp. 281–288, Madrid, 1958; Pharm. J. No. 4939, 477–479, 1958; Gesch. Pharm. *21*:1–3, 1969.

## SOUTH AFRICA

**Johannesburg:** Museum of the History of Medicine, University of Witwatersrand. Includes pharmacy artifacts. Pharm. in Hist. *11*:73, 1969; Hamarneh, l.c.

## SPAIN

For general reference to pharmacy museum collections in Spain, see Folch Jou, D. Guillermo: Historia de la Farmacia, Madrid, 1972.

**Barcelona:** Farmacia Museo del Pueblo Español. Bol. Soc. Esp. Hist. Farm. *20*:145–153, 1969; Gonzales, Ramon Jordi, Muy Ilustre Colegio Oficial de Farmaceuticos de la Provincia de Barcelona, 1972–73.

**Barcelona:** Museo de Arts de Cataluna. Pharmaceutical ceramics. Gonzales, Ramon Jordi, Muy Ilustre Colegio Oficial de Farmaceuticos de la Provincia de Barcelona, 1971–72.

**Madrid:** Museo de Historia de la Farmacia Hispana, Faculty of Pharmacy. Pharmacy restoration, majolica. Bol. Soc. Españ. Historia Farmacia *2*:171, 1951; Farmacia Nueva *16*:543, 1951; *17*:573, 1952; Rev. Farmaceut. Peruana *23*:14, Sept., 1954; Chem. & Drug. *175*:649, 1961; Folch Jou, G., Catalogo de los Botes de Farmacia, Madrid, 1966; Folch, La Colleccion do Morteros del Museo de la Farmacia Hispana, Madrid, 1966; Folch, Museo de la Farmacia Hispana, Madrid, 1972. Pharm. in Hist. *11*:77–78, 1969; Acofar No. 80, Dec., 1972.

**Madrid:** Antigua Farmacia de la Reina Madre. Farm. Neuva, 209, 1953.

**Madrid:** Museum of Military Pharmacy. Chem. & Drug. *175*:649, 1961.

**Masnou (Barcelona):** Museo Retrospectivo de Farmacia y Medicina, Laboratorios del Norte de España. Pharmacy restoration. Apotheker-Kalender (Aug. 1933); Museo Retrospectivo de Farmacia y Medicina, 1952; J.A.Ph.A. (Pract. Ed.) *16*:504, 1955; Prescriber (Sept. 1956).

**Santo Domingo de Silos:** Monastery pharmacy. Anal. Real Academia Farmacia *6*:40, 1940.

**San Juan Evangelista de Burgos:** Hospital. Ancient pharmacy. Jimeno y Jimeno, Pascual Domingo: La antigua y famosa botica del hospital de San Juan Evangelista de Burgos, Madrid, 1934.

**Toledo:** Tavera Hospital pharmacy. Chem. & Drug. *175*:649, 1961.

## SWEDEN

**Stockholm:** Farmacihistoriskt Museum. Svensk Farmaceutisk Tidskrift *57*:449. 465, 1953; Gesch. Pharm. vol. 9, No. 4, 1957.

**Stockholm:** Nordiska Museum (Skansen). Pharmacy restoration, where Carl Wilhelm Scheele carried on early research. Kockum, Arnold, Nordiska Museets Farmaceutiska Afdelingen, Stockholm, 1916; Apotheker-Kalender (1929); J.A.Ph.A. *19*:103, 1017, 1930; Urdang, George: Pictorial Life History of the Apothecary Chemist, Carl Wilhelm Scheele, Am. Inst. Hist. Pharm., Madison, Wisc., 1944; Modern Pharmacy *39*:16, May, 1954.

**Monsteras:** Pharmacy Museum. Svensk. Farm. T. *68*:723–726, 1964.

## SWITZERLAND

**Basel:** Schweizer Pharmazie-Historisches Museum, 3 Totengässlein. Outstanding collection, including two pharmacy restorations. Häfliger, Joseph Anton; Pharmazeutische Altertumskunde, Zurich, 1931; Schweiz. Apotheker Zeitung *65*:439,

1927; *66*:440, 1928; *657*:401, 1929; *68*:332, 1930; J.A.Ph.A. (Pract. Ed.) *16*:600, 1955; Prescriber (Sept., 1956); Schweiz. Kunstführer, 16 pp., June, 1968; Mez, Lydia, Die Sammlung, Basel, c. 1974, 119 pp.

**Basel:** Medizinhistorische Sammlung (Arturo Castiglioni collection), Roche; Antike Apotheken-Gefässe, Basel, n.d.; J.A.Ph.A. (Pract. Ed.) *16*:600, 1955.

**Lausanne:** University Museum. Burkhard Reber collection, formerly in Geneva. Deutsche Apotheker Zeitung *9*:289, 297, 305, 315, 325, 1894; Therapeutische Monatshefte *20*:419, 1906; Pharm. Rev. *25*:161, 1907; Reber, B.: Considérations sur ma Collection d'Antiquités, Geneva, 1909; Bull. Soc. Histoire Pharm., No. 2, p. 17, 1913.

**Zurich:** Landesmuseum. Pharmacy restoration. Häfliger, l.c.; J.A.Ph.A. (Pract. Ed.) *16*:600, 1955.

## TURKEY

**Istanbul:** Topkapi Seraglio Museum. Pharmacy material. Ünver, A. Süheyl: Kekimlik ve Eczcilik Tarihi Hakkinda, Istanbul, 1952.

**Istanbul:** Museum of the History of Pharmacy, University of Istanbul. Pharmacy artifacts largely from the Sultan's Palace. Rev. Hist. Pharm. *20*:314–316, 1971.

## U.S.S.R.

**Lvov:** Pharmaceutical Museum. Farm. Zh. (Ukrainina) *23*:91–96, 1968; Ibid. *24*:83–86, 1969; Ibid. *26*:88–93, 1971.

**Moscow:** Pharmaceutical Museum of the Central Pharmaceutical Scientific Research Institute J.A.Ph.A. *24*:429, 1935; Pharm. J. *80*:487, 1935; Farm. Obzor (Czech.) *33*:264–265, 1962; Farmatsiya *2*:51–54, 1971; Pharm. in Hist. *15*:90–93, 1973.

## UNITED STATES

For general references to pharmacy museum collections in the United States, please see: Winters, S. R., Drug Stores of Colonial America, Travel *92*:22–24, 32, Oct. 1948; Winters, S. R., N.A.R.D. Journal *75*:677–679, 700, May 4, 1953; Griffenhagen, G. B., Early American Pharmacies, Am. Pharm. Assoc., Washington, D.C., 1955; Griffenhagen, George, Pharmacy's Historical Collections, AIHP, 1957; Griffenhagen, George, and Sonnedecker, Cleo, Ibid. 2nd Edition, 1965; Stieb, Ernst, "The Past Recaptured," series in Pharmacy in History; Hamarneh, Sami, Pharmacy Museums USA, AIHP, Madison, Wisc., 1972. See also Zook, Nicholas, Museum Villages USA, Barre, Mass., 1971.

### ARIZONA

**Tucson:** Arizona Pharmacy Museum, College of Pharmacy, University of Arizona. 1875 "Botica" restoration and 1920 period room. Hamarneh, Pharmacy Museums USA, l.c.

### CALIFORNIA

**Anaheim:** Disneyland. Upjohn drugstore restoration, period 1900. J.A.Ph.A. (Pract. Ed.) *16*:276, 1955; Drug Topics *99*:52, Aug. 22, 1955; Louisiana Pharmacist *14*:6, Sept., 1955; Michigan Drug J. *43*:12, July, 1955.

**Bakersfield:** Kern County Pioneer Village, western-style drugstore restoration. J.A.Ph.A. (Pract. Ed.) *21*:489, 1960; A Journey Into the Past, Kern County Historical Society Official Museum Guidebook (1959); Harmarneh, Pharmacy Museums USA, l.c.

**Buena Park:** Knott's Berry Farm Ghost Town. 12 foot store front of 1890 desert mining town drugstore. J.A.Ph.A. (Pract. Ed.) *14*:454, 1953; Early American Pharmacies, l.c.; Hamarneh, Pharmacy Museums USA, l.c.

**Columbia:** State Historic Park. Mother Lode Pharmacy restoration. Calif. Pharm. Assoc. news release, Sept. 29, 1966; Hamarneh, Pharmacy Museums USA, l.c.

**San Fernando:** Southern California Pharmaceutical Association, 1066 N. Maclay

Ave., "Room of Memories," and early California drugstore restoration. Pacific Drug Rev. *63*:84, Sept., 1951; J.A.Ph.A. (Pract. Ed.) *15*:368, 1954; Early American Pharmacies, l.c.

**Stockton:** San Joaquin Pioneer Museum. E. S. Holden drugstore restoration, period 1900. J.A.Ph.A. (Pract. Ed.) *14*:454, 1953; Early American Pharmacies, l.c.; Hamarneh, Pharmacy Museums USA, l.c.

**Stockton:** University of the Pacific, School of Pharmacy. Lovotti majolica collection. Hamarneh, Pharmacy Museums USA, l.c.

## CONNECTICUT

**Mystic:** Mystic Seaport Marine Historical Association. Bringhurst pharmacy restoration from Wilmington, Del., and Karsh collection; founded 1793. Modern Pharmacy *31*:10, Sept., 1946; Northwestern Druggist *55*:34, July, 1947; J.A.M.A. *152*:36, 1953; J.A.Ph.A. (Pract. Ed.) *14*:732, 1953; Early American Pharmacies, l.c.; Apothecary Shop (Mystic brochure) n.d.; J.A.Ph.A. ns *4*:538, 1964; Hamarneh, Pharmacy Museums USA, l.c.

**New Canaan:** New Canaan Historical Society. Pharmacy restoration. New Canaan Hist. Soc. Annual 4 (No. 4): 37–53, Nov., 1966; Pharm. in Hist. *10*: No. 1, 45, 1968; Hamarneh, Pharmacy Museums USA, l.c.

**New Haven:** Yale Medical Historical Library, 333 Cedar Street. Edward Streeter collection and old apothecary shop. First Annual Report of the Historical Library, Yale Univ. School of Medicine, June 30, 1941; Ciba Symposia *6*:2083, 1945; J.A.Ph.A. (Pract. Ed.) *14*:732, 1953; Early American Pharmacies, l.c.; Hamarneh, Pharmacy Museums USA, l.c.

**Noroton (Darien):** Milestone Village Apothecary Shop, private collection of Lurelle Guild. Tile and Till *19*:102, 1933.

**Storrs:** University of Connecticut, School of Pharmacy. Edward Mogull Collection. Bridgeport Sunday Post, July 16, 1967, C3, 6.

**Waterbury:** The Mattauck Museum. Late 19th century apothecary shop restoration. Hamarneh, Pharmacy Museums USA, l.c.

## DELAWARE

**Dover:** Delaware State Museum, Pharmacy exhibit. Delaware State Museum News *3*:1, Oct., 1953.

## DISTRICT OF COLUMBIA

**Washington:** U.S. National Museum, Smithsonian Institution. Division of Medical Science. Pharmaceutical historical exhibits, national materia medica collection (commenced in 1881) and Old World Apothecary Shop. Pharm. Zeitung *75*:19, 219, 487 & 735, 1930; J.A.Ph.A. *28*:1055, 1939; *29*:36, 41, 1940; Urdang, George, and Nitardy, F. W.: The Squibb Ancient Pharmacy, New York, E. R. Squibb & Sons, 1940; J.A.Ph.A. (Pract. Ed.) *6*:184, 1945; *7*:157, 227, 1946; Drug Topics *90*:2, 97, July 8, 1946; Am. Druggist *115*:82, Feb., 1947; Squibb News *1*:14, May, 1950; Washington Star Pictorial Magazine, Feb. 14, 1954; for general review of pharmacy collections, see J.A.Ph.A. *19*:1125, 1930; Meyer Druggist *75*:8, June, 1955; Prescriptionist *2*:37, Aug., 1955; Gesch. Pharm., vol. 10, No. 4, 1958; Contributions from Museum of History and Technology, pp. 269–300, U.S. National Museum Bulletin 240, Smithsonian Institution, Washington, D.C., 1964; Amer. J. Hosp. Pharm. *23*:604, 1966; Pharm. in Hist. *9*:55–64, 70–71, 1967; Hamarneh, Pharmacy Museums USA, l.c.

## FLORIDA

**Pensacola:** Pensacola Historical Museum and Historical Preservation Society. Quina

Apothecary Shop restoration, period 1890–1920. Hamarneh, Pharmacy Museums USA, l.c.

GEORGIA

**Athens:** University of Georgia, School of Pharmacy. Historical pharmacy exhibits. Hamarneh, Pharmacy Museums USA, l.c.
**Columbus:** The Pemberton House Apothecary Shop. Pharm. in Hist. *16*:26, 1974.

ILLINOIS

**Chicago:** Chicago Historical Society, North Avenue at Clark Street. Early Chicago drugstore restoration, period 1850. J.A.Ph.A. (Pract. Ed.) *14*:388, 1953; Early American Pharmacies, l.c.
**Chicago:** Museum of Science and Industry, 5th Street and South Lake Shore Drive. Philo Carpenter drugstore restoration, period 1900. J.A.Ph.A. *22*:579, 593, 1933; J.A.Ph.A. (Pract. Ed.) *14*:388, 1953; Early American Pharmacies, l.c.; Hamarneh, Pharmacy Museums USA, l.c.
**Chicago:** Museum of the International College of Surgeons. Sackett and Taber 19th century pharmacy restoration. Pharm. in Hist. *9*:110–111, 1967; Hamarneh, Pharmacy Museums USA, l.c.
**Junction City:** McMaster Prescription Shop apothecary restoration. J.A.Ph.A. ns *1*:498, 1961; Hamarneh, Pharmacy Museums USA, l.c.

INDIANA

**Evansville:** Evansville Museum of Arts and Science. Medical Evansville in the Nineteenth Century, a physician's office with pharmacy artifacts. (Mead Johnson and Co., Evansville, n.d.); J.A.Ph.A. (Pract. Ed.) *21*:488, 1960; Hamarneh, Pharmacy Museums USA, l.c.
**Indianapolis:** Eli Lilly and Company, Restoration of Colonel Eli Lilly's first manufacturing laboratory founded 1876. Tile and Till *21*:52, 1935; J.A.Ph.A. (Pract. Ed.) *16*:402, 1955; Louisiana Pharmacist *14*:6, Oct., 1955; Hamarneh, Pharmacy Museums USA, l.c.
**Indianapolis:** Hooks Drugs, Historical Drug Store and Pharmacy Museum, Indiana State Fair Grounds. Late 19th century restoration. Indianapolis Star Magazine, 64–66, 68, Dec. 4, 1966; Pharm. in Hist. *9*:65, 1966; Tile & Till *53*:8–11, March, 1967; Pharm. in Hist. *12*:85, 1970; Hamarneh, Pharmacy Museums USA, l.c.
**Mitchell:** Spring Mill State Park. Spring Mill Village pharmacy restoration, period 1830–50. Saturday Evening Post, June 12, 1943; J.A.Ph.A. (Pract. Ed.) *15*:172, 1954; Early American Pharmacies, l.c.; Hamarneh, Pharmacy Museums USA, l.c.

IOWA

**Algona:** Druggists Mutual Insurance Company Museum. Pharmacy restoration, ca. 1909. Pharm. in Hist. *14*:77, 1972.

KANSAS

**Lawrence:** University of Kansas, School of Pharmacy. Restoration of B. W. Woodward drugstore, period 1870. Tile and Till *27*:128, 1941.

KENTUCKY

**Danville:** McDowell Apothecary Shop restoration. Courier-Journal Magazine, Sept. 13, 1959; J.A.Ph.A. (Pract. Ed.) *20*:603, 1959; Hamarneh, Pharmacy Museums USA, l.c.
**Richmond:** Eastern Kentucky State College, Jonathan Truman Dorris Museum. Collection of apothecary jars and pharmacy artifacts. Hamarneh, Pharmacy Museums USA, l.c.

## LOUISIANA

**New Orleans:** La Pharmacie Française, 514 Chartres St. Museum housed in original building erected by Dulfilho, 1823. Restoration of pharmacy, period 1880, on ground floor. Drug Topics, vol. 94, No. 24, 1950; Louisiana Phar. *9*:3, Oct. 1950; Am. J. Pharm. Ed. *15*:126, 1951; N.A.R.D. Journal *76*:36, April 5, 1954; J.A.Ph.A. (Pract. Ed.) *15*:245, 1954; Early American Pharmacies, l.c.; Pharm. in Hist. *8*:79–81, 1966; Hamarneh, Pharmacy Museums USA, l.c.

## MAINE

**Poland Springs:** Shaker Museum. Pharmacy artifacts. Hamarneh, Pharmacy Museums USA, l.c.

## MARYLAND

**Baltimore:** Maryland Pharmaceutical Association, B. Olive Cole Pharmacy Museum. Hamarneh, Pharmacy Museums USA, l.c.

## MASSACHUSETTS

**Abington:** Dyer Memorial Library. Exhibit of 19th century pharmacy artifacts. Patriot Ledger, Oct. 2 and 5, 1970; Pharm. in Hist. *13*:89, 1971; Hamarneh, Pharmacy Museums USA, l.c.

**Boston:** Massachusetts College of Pharmacy. Joseph S. Lindemann collection of Smith, Miller and Patch, Inc. Hamarneh, Pharmacy Museums USA, l.c.

**East Bridgewater:** The Standish Museums and Unitarian Church. Early 19th century apothecary shop restoration. Hamarneh, Pharmacy Museums USA, l.c.

**Salem:** Essex Institute: Restoration of an old New England pharmacy, period 1830–50. J.A.Ph.A. (Pract. Ed.) *14*:660, 1953; Early American Pharmacies, l.c.

## MICHIGAN

**Dearborn:** Henry Ford Museum and Greenfield Village. Restoration of Phoenixville, Conn., pharmacy, period 1850. 1890 drugstore period room restoration in Museum. Greenfield Village Guide Book, 1951; J.A.Ph.A. (Pract. Ed.) *2*:216, 1941; *15*:172, 1954; Early American Pharmacies, l.c.

**Detroit:** Historical Museum. Pharmacy restoration, ca. 1900. Pharm. in Hist. *12*:180–181, 1970; Hamarneh, Pharmacy Museums USA, l.c.

**Detroit:** Howard Mordue's "Apothecariana," Wayne State University. J.A.Ph.A. (Pract. Ed.) *21*:489, 1960.

**Grand Rapids:** Public Museum. Pharmacy restoration. Drug Topics *99*:34 Oct. 17, 1955; Pharm. in Hist. *15*:40–41, 1973.

**Manistee:** Manistee County Historical Society. Lyman-White pharmacy restoration. Hamarneh, Pharmacy Museums USA, l.c.

## MINNESOTA

**Minneapolis:** College of Pharmacy, University of Minnesota Museum. J.A.Ph.A. *21*:1162, 1932; Hobbies, vol. 59, Nov., 1954; Ivory Tower (U. Minnesota daily), April 1, 1957.; Hamarneh, Pharmacy Museums USA, l.c.

**South St. Paul:** Dakota County Historical Society Museum. Apothecary shop restoration. Hamarneh, Pharmacy Museums USA, l.c.

## MISSISSIPPI

**University:** University of Mississippi, School of Pharmacy. Collection of pharmacy artifacts. Pharm. in Hist. 135, 1973.

## MISSOURI

**Hannibal:** Grant's Drug Store restored in

building once occupied by Mark Twain. J.A.Ph.A. ns *1*:498, 1961; Hannibal, Mo., Chamber of Commerce (brochure), n.d.; Hamarneh, Pharmacy Museums USA, l.c.

**Point Lookout:** Ralph Foster Museums, School of the Ozarks. Pharmacy exhibit suggesting 1880 apothecary shop. Missouri Pharm. *28*:18, Sept., 1954; Springfield News and Leader, April 18, 1954; The Ozarks Mountaineer, 31, Sept., 1970; Pharm. in Hist. *13*:181, 1971.

**St. Louis:** St. Louis Wholesale Drug Co. Pharmacy restoration. Hamarneh, Pharmacy Museums USA, l.c.

**St. Louis:** St. Louis Medical Society Museum. Two pharmacy restorations. Hamarneh, Pharmacy Museums USA, l.c.

**St. Louis:** St. Louis College of Pharmacy. Early pharmacy exhibits. Hamarneh, Pharmacy Museums USA, l.c.

## MONTANA

**Stevensville:** St. Mary's Mission. Restoration of Rev. Anthony J. Ravalli's pharmacy, period 1845. J.A.Ph.A. (Pract. Ed.) *15*:678, 1954; Modern Pharmacy *11*:18, No. 4, 1955; Hamarneh, Pharmacy Museums USA, l.c.

## NEBRASKA

**Minden:** Harold Warp Pioneer Village Pharmacy restoration, period 1900. Antique Automobile *19*:43, Summer, 1955; J.A.Ph.A. (Pract. Ed.) *16*:662, 1955; Hamarneh, Pharmacy Museums USA, l.c.

## NEW JERSEY

**New Brunswick:** Kilmer Museum of Surgical Products, Johnson and Johnson, Inc. Johnson and Johnson Bull., vol. 12, Feb., May, Dec., 1953, and vol. 13, Oct., 1954.

**Princeton:** Historical Society of Princeton. William Bainbridge House with room used as clinic and apothecary restored. Hamarneh, Pharmacy Museums USA, l.c.

**Smithville:** Old Towne of Smithville. 1890 pharmacy restoration. Newark Evening News, Jan. 19, 1967; Pharm. in Hist. *13*:35, 1971; Hamarneh, Pharmacy Museums USA, l.c.

## NEW YORK

**Albany:** Albany College of Pharmacy. Restoration of Throop drugstore of Schoharie, N.Y., founded 1800. Tile and Till *24*:90, 1938; J.A.Ph.A. (Pract. Ed.) *15*:306, 1954; Early American Pharmacies, l.c.; Hamarneh, Pharmacy Museums USA, l.c.

**Brooklyn:** The Brooklyn Museum. Collection of pharmacy artifacts. Hamarneh, Pharmacy Museums USA, l.c.

**Brooklyn:** Long Island University, Brooklyn College of Pharmacy. Collection of pharmacy artifacts. Hamarneh, Pharmacy Museums USA, l.c.

**Buffalo:** Buffalo and Erie County Historical Society. Pharmacy restoration. J.A.Ph.A. (Pract. Ed.) *15*:505, 1954; Hamarneh, Pharmacy Museums USA, l.c.

**Clinton:** Park Row Pharmacy. Apothecary shop restoration, ca. late 19th century. Hamarneh, Pharmacy Museums USA, l.c.

**Cooperstown:** Farmer's Museum, New York State Historical Association. Restoration of New York druggist's shop, period 1820–40. N.Y. State Pharmacist *28*:34, July, 1953; American Cyanamid Monthly News Bulletin *18*:12, Dec., 1953; J.A.Ph.A. (Pract. Ed.) *15*:124, 1954; Early American Pharmacies, l.c.; Hamarneh, Pharmacy Museums USA, l.c.

**Monroe:** Old Museum Village of Smith's Clove. Restoration of the Vernon drugstore, founded in Florida, N.Y., 1886. New York Herald Tribune, June 26, 1950; J.A.Ph.A. (Pract. Ed.) *15*:306, 1954; Early American Pharmacies, l.c.; Hamarneh, Pharmacy Museums USA, l.c.

**New York City:** Columbia University College of Pharmacy. Restoration of an early New York drugstore. Merck Report *38*:100, July, 1929; Columbia Alumni News, *35*:5, April, 1944; Ballard, C. W.: A History of the College of Pharmacy, Columbia University, N.Y., 1954; J.A.Ph.A.(Pract. Ed.) *15*:438, 1954; Early American Pharmacies, l.c.; Hamarneh, Pharmacy Museums USA, l.c. Dismantled.

**New York City:** J. Leon Lascoff and Son, Inc. Apothecaries, Lexington Ave. and 82nd St. Private museum. Coronet, Sept., 1947; Pharmacy International, Dec., 1952; J.A.Ph.A. (Pract. Ed.) *15*:744, 1954.

**New York City:** Schering Apothecary Restoration. Freedomland, U.S.A., J.A.Ph.A. (Pract. Ed.) *21*:488, 1960.

**New York City:** Smith, Miller and Patch Apothecary, 902 Broadway. J.A.Ph.A. (Pract. Ed.) *21*:489, 1960.

**New York City:** Museum of the City of New York. Restoration of John Carle drugstore period 1852. J.A.Ph.A. (Pract. Ed.) *15*:505, 1954.

**New York City:** New York Historical Society. Restoration of New York drugstore, period 1850–1900. This Week, Sept. 3, 1939; J.A.Ph.A. (Pract. Ed.) *15*:505, 1954.

**New York City:** Metropolitan Museum of Art. Majolica. Am. Prof. Pharm. *13*:163, 1947; Hamarneh, Pharmacy Museums USA, l.c.

**New York City:** Mary Chess, Cosmetics, 601 Fifth Ave. 17th–century Florentine pharmacy fixtures. Drugg. Circ., vol. 29, June, 1935.

**New York City:** Hispanic Society of America Museum. Majolica. Frothingham. A. W.: Catalogue of Hispano–Moresque Pottery, New York, 1936; Notes Hispanic *1*:101, 1941; Hamarneh, Pharmacy Museums USA, l.c.

**Old Chatham:** Shaker Museum. Restoration of Shaker medicine manufacturing plant, period 1850–70, originally located at Mount Lebanon, N.Y., J.A.Ph.A. (Pract. Ed.) *16*:402, 1955; Hamarneh, Pharmacy Museums USA, l.c.

**Pearl River:** Lederle Laboratories. Restoration in main entrance lobby of early American pharmacy. J.A.Ph.A. (Pract. Ed.) *15*:438, 1954; Early American Pharmacies, l.c.; Louisiana Pharmacist *14*:6, Oct., 1955; Hobbies, vol. *59*, No. 8, Oct. 1954.

**Rochester:** Rochester Museum of Arts and Industries. Restoration of Benham Pharmacy, period 1865–75. J.A.Ph.A. (Pract. Ed.) *15*:124, 1954; Early American Pharmacies, l.c. Hamarneh, Pharmacy Museums USA, l.c.

**St. James, Long Island:** St. James General Store and Hartz Drug Museum. Collection of pharmacy artifacts. Hamarneh, Pharmacy Museums USA, l.c.

## NORTH CAROLINA

**Bailey:** The Country Doctor Museum. Apothecary shop restoration. Hamarneh, Pharmacy Museums USA, l.c.

**Chapel Hill:** University of North Carolina School of Pharmacy Library and Museum. Pharmacy material. Carolina J. Pharmacy *36*:35, Jan. 1955; vol. 37, cover, Feb., 1956; Hamarneh, Pharmacy Museums USA, l.c.

**Greensboro:** Greensboro Historical Museum. Restoration of Porter drugstore, in which William Sydney Porter (O. Henry) was apprenticed, 1876–81. Drug Topics *91* (No. 21):72, 1947; Rexall Ad-Vantages, vol. 34, 1948; J.A.Ph.A. (Pract. Ed.) *14*:752, 1953; Early American Pharmacies, l.c.; Hamarneh, Pharmacy Museums USA, l.c.

## OHIO

**Cincinnati:** University of Cincinnati College of Medicine. Partial restoration of 15th century Italian pharmacy. Drug Topics *97*:28, Feb. 9, 1953; Hamarneh, Pharmacy Museums USA, l.c.

**Cleveland:** Howard Dittrick Museum of Historical Medicine. Wall case and equipment from Smithknight drugstore, founded 1857, Bull. Hist. Med. *8*:1214, 1940; Northern Ohio Druggist *19*:14, Jan., 1941; Bull. Cleveland Med. Library *6*:15, 1959; Ibid. *11*:51, 1964; Hamarneh, Pharmacy Museums USA, l.c.

**Cleveland:** The Western Reserve Historical Society. 19th century pharmacy restoration. Hamarneh, Pharmacy Museums USA, l.c.

**Columbus:** Columbus Center of Science and Industry, Durell Street of Yesteryear. Apothecary shop restoration, ca. 1865. Hamarneh, Pharmacy Museums USA, l.c.

OKLAHOMA

**Norman:** University of Oklahoma, College of Pharmacy. Prescription desk, period 1885–90, and equipment. Drug Topics *98*:40, June 14, 1954; Hamarneh, Pharmacy Museums USA, l.c.

PENNSYLVANIA

**Bethlehem:** The Apothecary (formerly Simon Rau) 420 South Main St. Partial restoration of Apotheke, founded 1743. Drugg. Circ. *71*:1093, 1927; Am. J. Pharm. *111*:234, 1939; Merck's Report *41*:22, Jan. 1932; Tile and Till *25*:67, 1939; Dow Diamond *12*:6, Oct. 1949; Travel *91*:22, Oct. 1948; J.A.Ph.A. (Pract. Ed.) *14*:468, 1953; Drug Topics *99*:64, Feb. 21, 1955; Early American Pharmacies, l.c.; Moravian Historical Tours (brochure) Central Moravian Church, Bethlehem, n.d.; Hamarneh, Pharmacy Museums USA, l.c.

**Doylestown:** Bucks County Historical Society Mercer Museum. Collection of pharmacy artifacts. Hamarneh, Pharmacy Museums USA, l.c.

**Philadelphia:** Philadelphia College of Pharmacy and Science. Partial restoration of Glentworth pharmacy, founded 1812; and museum. Catalogue of the Historical Exhibition, Semi-Centennial Anniversary of the American Pharmaceutical Association, Philadelphia, Sept. 8–13, 1902; Am. J. Pharm. *98*:646, 1926; J.A.Ph.A. *25*:230, 1936; England, J. W.; The First Century of the Philadelphia College of Pharmacy, 1922; LaWall, C. H.; Four Thousand Years of Pharmacy, Garden City, 1927; Philadelphia Section of the Era Album, p. 100, 1908; J.A.Ph.A. (Pract. Ed.) *14*:468, 1953; Early American Pharmacies, l.c.; Hamarneh, Pharmacy Museums USA, l.c.

**Philadelphia:** Temple University, School of Pharmacy. Kendig Memorial Museum. Hamarneh, Pharmacy Museums USA, l.c.

**Philadelphia:** Franklin Institute. Pharmacy replica. The Museum News, Feb. 15, 1955.

RHODE ISLAND

**Newport:** Newport Historical Society. Original window from Charles Feke's pharmacy, founded 1796. The Rhode Islander, March 14, 1948; Modern Pharmacy *35*:19, Jan. 1950; Cosmopolitan, Nov. 1951; J.A.Ph.A. (Pract. Ed.) *14*:660, 1953.

SOUTH CAROLINA

**Charleston:** Charleston Museum. Restoration of Apothecaries' Hall, founded by Jacob De la Motta, 1820's. Bennett, John; Apothecaries' Hall, Charleston Museum, 1921; Merck's Report *40*:104, 1931; Ann. Med. His. *2*:259, 1940; Hoch, J. H.: The History of Pharmacy in South Carolina, Charleston, 1951; J.A.Ph.A. *12*:663, 1923 (Pract. Ed.); *14*:752, 1953; Early American Pharmacies, l.c.; Hamarneh, Pharmacy Museums USA, l.c.

SOUTH DAKOTA

**Brookings:** South Dakota State University Museum and Heritages Center. Pharmacy artifacts. Hamarneh, Pharmacy Museums USA, l.c.

## TENNESSEE

**Morristown:** Roberts and Turner Drug Co. Gay Nineties Museum and Drug Store. Hamarneh, Pharmacy Museums USA, l.c.

## TEXAS

**Jefferson:** Ye Olde Apothecary Shoppe, 312 East Broadway. J.A.Ph.A. ns *1*:499, 1961; Hamarneh, Pharmacy Museums USA, l.c.

**San Antonio:** The University of Texas Institute of Texas Cultures. Pharmacy artifacts. Hamarneh, Pharmacy Museums USA, l.c.

## UTAH

**Salt Lake City:** Pioneer Village Museum. Pharmacy restoration. 1860–80. J.A.Ph.A. (Pract. Ed.) *15*:505, 1954; U.Ph.A. Bulletin News *64*:4, Nov. 1955; *70*:2, May, 1961; J.A.Ph.A. ns *1*:499, 1961: Hamarneh, Pharmacy Museums USA, l.c.

## VERMONT

**Burlington:** Shelburne Museum, apothecary shop restoration. J.A.Ph.A. ns *1*:498, 1961; Hamarneh, Pharmacy Museums USA, l.c.

## VIRGINIA

**Alexandria:** Stabler-Leadbeater Apothecary Shop, 107 South Fairfax St. Restoration of original shop founded in 1792 and operated by same family for 141 years. Washington Herald, July 20, 1933; J.A.Ph.A. *22*:705, 1933; *23*:1137, 1934; J.A.Ph.A. (Pract. Ed.) *3*:216, 1942; *14*:322, 1953; Am. Drug. *117* (No. 5):75, 1948; Travel *91*:22, Oct. 1948; Early American Pharmacies, l.c.; Today's Health *39*:52, Feb. 1961; Hamarneh, Pharmacy Museums USA, l.c.

**Fredericksburg:** Hugh Mercer Apothecary Shop, 1020 Caroline St. Restoration of original building operated as a pharmacy by General Hugh Mercer, 1761–77. Trenton Sunday Times-Advertiser, March 20, 1932; Tile and Till *18*:31, 1932; J.A.Ph.A. (Pract. Ed.) *2*:61, 173, 1941; *3*:216, 1942; The Commonwealth *8*:15, April 1941; Waterman, J. M.: With Sword and Lancet, Richmond, Va., Garrett and Massie, 1941; Travel *91*:22, 1948; Hygeia *26*:478, 1948; J.A.Ph.A. (Pract. Ed.) *14*:221, 1953; Builders *61*:7, Oct. 16, 1954; Early American Pharmacies l.c.; J.A.Ph.A. (Pract. Ed.) *20*:649, 1959; Drug Topics, March 13, 1972; Hamarneh, Pharmacy Museums USA, l.c.

**Richmond:** Roy Apothecary Shop, Medical College of Virginia. Pharmacy restoration. Tile and Till *26*:52, May, 1940; The Virginia Pharmacist, Convention Number, May 5–12, 1940; The Commonwealth, vol. 7, April 1940. Disposition unknown.

**Williamsburg:** Colonial Williamsburg. Restoration of the Pasteur-Galt pharmacy, period 1760–76. Official Guide Book of Colonial Williamsburg, 1951; J.A.Ph.A. (Pract. Ed.) *11*:680, 1950; Midwestern Druggist *26*:22, Feb. 1950; Northwestern Druggist *59*:35, 1951; Am. Drug. *128*:18, July 20, 1953; Quarterly of Phi Beta Pi, vol. 50, Jan. 1954; Early American Pharmacies, l.c. National Geographic, *106*:439, 1954; Clark, Herbert, The Apothecary of 18th Century Williamsburg, Virginia, 1966; Pharm. in Hist. *13*:36–37, 1971; Hamarneh, Pharmacy Museums USA, l.c. (A second reconstruction, the McKenzie Apothecary Shop opened in 1968, has been withdrawn from exhibition.)

## WASHINGTON

**Olympia:** Washington State Board of Pharmacy and Washington State Pharmaceutical Association. The Heussy Pharmacy restoration. Hamarneh, Pharmacy Museums USA, l.c.

## WEST VIRGINIA

**Morgantown:** West Virginia University, School of Pharmacy. Cook-Hayman Pharmacy Museum includes apothecary shop restoration, ca. 1863. Hamarneh, Pharmacy Museums USA, l.c.

**Harpers Ferry:** Harpers Ferry National Park. Apothecary re-creation, ca. 1850–1870. Pharm. in Hist. *16*:107, 1974.

### WISCONSIN

**Cassville:** Nelson Dewey State Park, Stonefield Village. Apothecary shop restoration. Hamarneh, Pharmacy Museums USA, l.c. Also a drug manufactory.

**Madison:** Wisconsin State Historical Society. Restoration of a pioneer Wisconsin drugstore, period 1848–98. The Pioneer Drug Store, Wisconsin State Historical Society, 1930; Pharm. Era *50*:45, 1917; Merck's Report *40*:14, Jan. 1931; Badger Pharmacist, special reprint, April, 1930; Tile and Till *19*:86, 1933; Northwestern Druggist *55*:28, 1947; Drug Topics *98*:24, Aug. 9, 1954; J.A.Ph.A. (Pract. Ed.) *15*:12, 1954; Early American Pharmacies, l.c. Now dismantled.

**Milwaukee:** Milwaukee Public Museum. Restoration of a Milwaukee drugstore, period 1900. Am. Drug. *113*:84, April 1946; J.A.Ph.A. (Pract. Ed.) *15*:12, 1954; Early American Pharmacies, l.c.; Tile and Till *41*:94, 1955; Hamarneh, Pharmacy Museums USA, l.c.

**Milwaukee:** County Historical Society. Pharmacy restoration, ca. 1880. Pharm. in Hist. *15*:66, 1973.

### YUGOSLAVIA

**Dubrovnik (Ragusa):** Franciscan Monastery Pharmacy. Chem. & Drug. *124*:784, 1936; Pharm. Zeitung *87*:634, 1951; Pharm. J. *113*:339, 1951; Die Pharm. Industrie *15*:233, 1953; Tartalja, H., Veteris Ragusae Medicina et Pharmacia, Zagreb, 1970.

**Sarajevo:** Municipal Museum. "Old Jewish Pharmacy," Museum *8*:79, 1955.

**Split:** Archeological Museum. Ancient pharmacy material. Farmaceutiski Glasnik *11*:359, 1955.

**Zagreb:** Pharmacy Institute Museum. Pharmacy material. Farmaceutiski Glasnik *11*:102, 269, 1955.

# Appendix 6
# Pharmaceutical Literature . . . Some Bibliographic Historical Notes

The written word has been called the memory of mankind. In this sense contemporary firsthand accounts of events significant to pharmacy can recapture the structure and feel of history as it was happening. This section offers one guide to finding such "primary" sources. It does not provide guidance to "secondary" writings (nor constitute a history of pharmaceutical literature); but a number of accounts by historians have been cited in the Notes and References to individual chapters of this book, and still others can be located through guides mentioned in a note on bibliography included in Appendix 7 (p. 445).

The bibliographic essay that follows does supplement what little has been said in the main text about the printed literature contemporary to pharmacy as it was discussed for these several countries: Italy, Germany, France, Great Britain and the United States. Since only fragmentary information is given on publications of each country,* a selection of more general bibliographic lists and commentaries is first noted. These can serve to open up an additional range of primary publications related to pharmacy and drug therapy within the cultural areas represented by this book.

The *Index-Catalogue of the Surgeon-General's Library*, Washington, D.C., 4 series, 1880–1943, remains unexcelled in America (internationally?) as a massive, accurate, widely available catalog. (The series, each A–Z, overlap in chronologic scope.) Besides journal articles, the Index-Catalogue cites about 397,650 books of all periods and countries that are related to health science, including pharmacy—with entries listed by author, title, and subject. More recent printed catalogs, general or special, of other Anglo-American medical libraries known for their historical depth can be bibliographic aids to readers and writers of pharmacy's history—such as catalogs of the Wellcome Institute of the History of Medicine (London), Francis A. Countway Library of Medicine (Boston), New York Academy of Medicine Library (New York), U. S. National Library of Medicine (Washington, D.C.; formerly called Surgeon-General's Library), Bibliotheca Osleriana of McGill University (Montreal), and the Harvey Cushing Collection of Yale Medical Library (New Haven). Noteworthy in pharmacy among specialized printed catalogs is J. Neu: *Chemical, Medical and Pharmaceutical Books Printed Before 1800; In the Collections of the University of Wisconsin Libraries*, Madison, 1965 (extensive additions have been made to the collection since these

*For the present purpose, this leaves out of account much of the ancient and medieval literature on pharmacy and drug therapy, whether in manuscript or later printed form. These literatures can be pursued through specialized bibliographies available; and some of the works cited in Part I and in the Glossary of this book have bibliographies that offer an entering wedge.

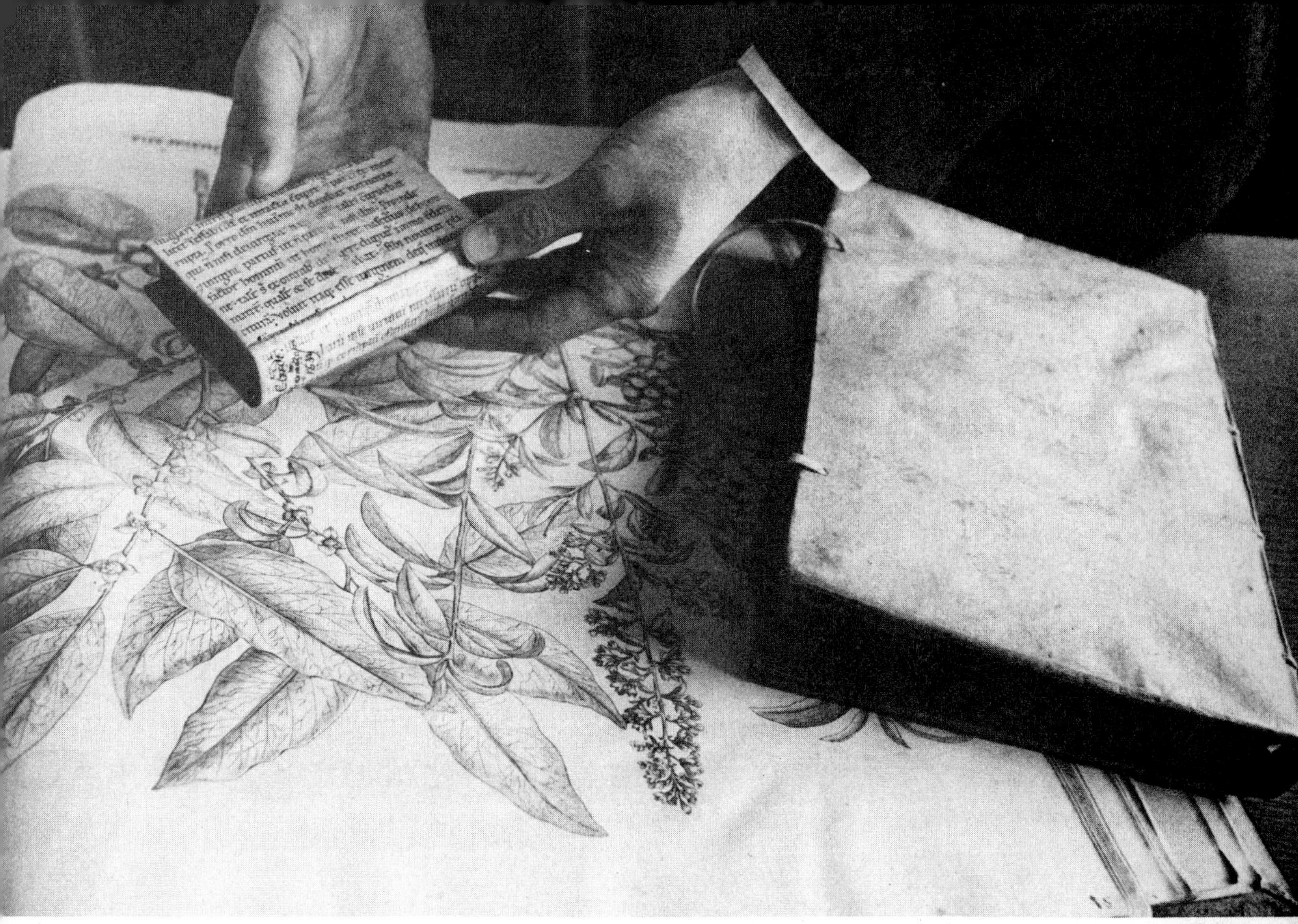

Rare books preserve firsthand testimony of the history of pharmacy. Among vellum-bound volumes in the University of Wisconsin's collection, one of the early legalized pharmacopeias (1559) is dwarfed when held against a magnificent herbal (1613) prepared by pharmacist Basil Besler, representing the botanical garden of his prince-bishop.

4,442 works were tabulated). See also J. U. Lloyd, (et al.): Catalogue of the pharmacopoeias, dispensatories, formularies and allied publications (1493–1957) in the Lloyd Library [Cincinnati], *Lloydia, 20*:1–42, 1957 (also available as a separate).

Among bibliographies, particularly useful in pharmacy is E.-H. Guitard: *Manuel d'histoire de la littérature pharmaceutique . . .et Biobibliographie pharmaceutique,* Paris, 1942, 138 pp., which is international before A.D. 1600, then French to 1860. (The same may be consulted, lacking minor additions and changes, in Revue d'Histoire de la Pharmacie, serially 1935–40.) A handy chronologic bibliography (with inaccuracies) is in the back of J. Volckringer: *Evolution et unification des formulaires et des pharmacopeés,* Paris, 1953. For a country-arranged list of mid-20th century pharmacopeias, see I. M. Strieby, and M. C. Spencer: national and international pharmacopoeias, a checklist, *Bull. Med. Library Assoc. 45*:410–20, 1957.

Pharmacy-related books of Europe of the 18th and early 19th centuries are especially accessible, bibliographically, because of five German works within this scope: D. A. N. A. Scherer: Literatura pharmacopoearum collecta, in *Codex medicamentarius Europaeus,* Section VII, Leipzig, 1822 (232 pp. covering

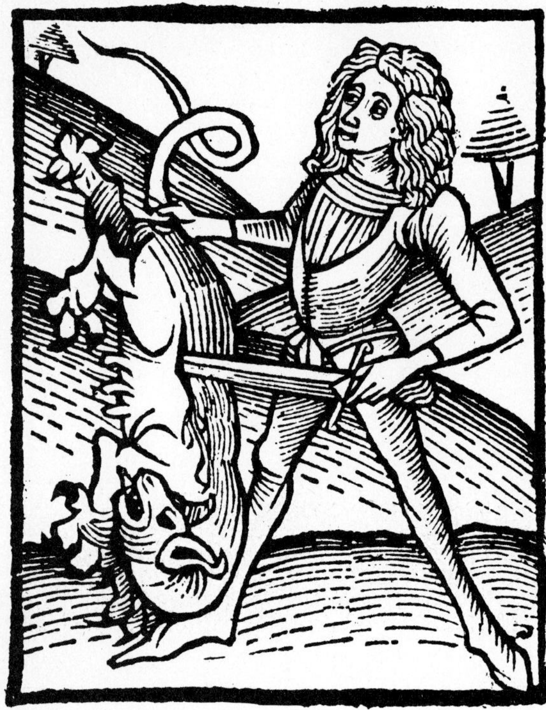

Early printed herbals were embellished with woodcuts showing the sources of drugs, animal as well as vegetable. Reflecting late medieval folklore, a dragon, "greatest of all serpents and beasts," is shown impaled on the sword of its conqueror. "If a dragon's tongue can be obtained, make a decoction of it in wine to anoint the body against various ills." (*Hortus sanitatis,* Strasbourg, about 1507, Chap. 48; from the University of Wisconsin Library)

15th to 19th centuries); E. G. Baldinger: *Litteratura universa materiae medicae, alimentairiae, toxicologiae, pharmaciae, et therapiae generalis, medicae atque chirurgicae, potissimum academica,* Marburg, 1793; W. Engelmann: *Bibliotheca medico-chirurgica et pharmaceutico-chemica, oder Verzeichniss . . . Bücher, welcher vom Jahre 1750 bis zur Mitte des Jahres 1837 in Deutschland erschienen sind,* 5th ed., Leipzig, 1838 (pp. 495–541 is an especially detailed A–Z listing of German pharmaco-chemical publications); a topical list of 8,243 publications between 1750 and ca. 1827 includes several pharmacy-related sections as published by K. Sprengel: *Literatura medica externa. . .,* Leipzig, 1829; an early chronologic list of pharmacy books still interesting is J. F. Gmelin: *Einleitung in die Pharmacie,* pp. 10–29, Nürnberg, 1781.

Two works comprehensively citing books and articles by European pharmacists from about 1780 to 1850 (although not limited to pharmacy or to Europe) are A. C. P. Callisen: *Medicinisches Schriftsteller-Lexicon der jetzt lebenden Aertzte, Wundärzte, Geburtshelfer, Apotheker, und Naturforscher aller gebildeten Völker,* 33 vols., Copenhagen-Altona, 1830–1845 (readily available in large American libraries since the reprinting of 1962–65), which includes literature contributed by pharmacists between 1750 and about 1830; and F. Ferchl: *Chemisch-pharmazeutisches Bio- und Bibliographikon,* Mittenwald, 1937, which cites literature (at the end of each biographical sketch, A–Z) published in the period between about 1500 and the mid-19th century. Of more selective pharmaceutical scope is J. C. Poggendorff: *Biographische literarisches Handwörterbuch zur Geschichte der exacten Wissenschaften,* Berlin, 1955 et seq. Among highly specialized bibliographies, it may be of special pharmaceutical interest to call attention to L. Winkelblech and E. Kremers: Book literature on new remedies, *J.A.Ph.A. 18*:354–356, 1929, which covers the period 1821 to 1922, as well as E. J. Waring: *Bibliotheca Therapeutica, or Bibliography of Therapeutics, chiefly in reference to Articles of the Materia Medica. . .,* 2 vols., London, 1878 and 1879 (3 indexes: diseases, authors, subjects), lists about 10,000 books and monographs of the 18th and 19th centuries, arranged chronologically within topical sections.

Of particular American interest and reliable guidance is R. B. Austin: *Early American Medical Imprints; A Guide to Works Printed in the United States 1668–1820,* Washington, D.C., 1961 (2106 items, A–Z by authors, including pharmacy and materia medica, with locations in 35 USA libraries; for addendum see *J. Hist. Med.* *20*:59 f., 1965). This annotated list is supplemented by the narrative essay by D. L. Cowen: *America's Prepharmacopoeial Literature* (i.e., pre-1820), Madison, 1961 and Francisco Guerra: *American Medical Bibliography 1639–1783 . . .*, New York, 1962.

It may be useful also to mention a little known bibliographic essay among highly specialized guides to primary literature by M. Randall, and E. B. Watson: *Finding List for United States Patent, Design, Trade-Mark, Reissue, Label, Print, and Plant Patent Numbers*, Berkeley, Calif., 1938, 31 pp., which is organized according to 3 main historical phases of the subject: 1790–1835, 1836–1871 and 1872–1938.

A general guide and useful finding-aid (in the absence of a pharmaceutical counterpart) is edited by J. B. Blake and C. Roos: *Medical Reference Works 1679–1966; a Selected Bibliography*, Chicago, 1967. This annotated list cites 2700 titles, a good many within the scope of our present interest, although the historical sections are necessarily highly selective and refer to secondary as well as primary sources. Finally, opening up a range of mid-20th century literature is a paperback compiled by the U. S. National Library of Medicine: *Drug Literature; a Factual Survey on the Nature and Magnitude of Drug Literature*, (Committee print of the Subcommittee on Reorganization and International Organizations of the Senate Committee on Government Operations, 88th Cong., 1st Sess.), Washington, D.C. 1963, 171 pp.

*Periodicals*. A journal literature of the professions and sciences developed from the 17th century onward, much later than some of the book literature abovementioned. Since this periodical literature represents the dynamic side of pharmacy's literature—finding later summation and synthesis in the books of its time the serious historical reader or writer also needs finding-aids to journal reportage in his subject field. For locating volumes of a specific title, it is understood that the *Union List of Serials in Libraries of the United States and Canada* remains the indispensable locator; but what about broader access to the old journals to which pharmacists contributed and from which some part of their lifework still draws?

The most useful historical list of American pharmaceutical journals, from the beginning (1825) until 1932 is M. Meyer and E. Kremers: The pharmaceutical journals of the United States, *J.A.Ph.A.* *22*:424–429, 1933 (classified by state in which published). Often overlooked is the availability (on microfilm from the F. B. Power Pharmaceutical Library, University of Wisconsin-Madison) of M. M. Meyer: *The Pharmaceutical Journals of the United States of America* (unpublished M.Sc. thesis, U. Wis.), Madison, 1934, 418 pp., mainly a single annotated, historical bibliography, A–Z by titles, which for some purposes is not as useful as the author's: *A History of Pharmaceutical Journals in the United States* (unpublished B.Sc. thesis, Pharmacy, U. Wis.), Madison, 1932, 177 pp., a chronological and geographical tabulation, etc. (but not actually a history). Also useful is the printed catalog of a single important collection such as, D. Nemec: *Periodicals and Serial Publications in Pharmacy and Related Subjects at the University of Wisconsin* (mimeographed), rev. ed., Madison, 1974, ca. 150 pp., which shows holdings A–Z by titles (comprehensive, although not entirely complete for early defunct serials held). Of historical writings, the best and most systematic work still is, E.-H. Guitard: *Deux siècles de presse au service de la pharmacie et cinquante ans de l'Union pharmaceutique'. Histoire et bibliographie des periodiques intèressant les sciences, la mèdecine et spècialement la pharmacie en France et à l'ètranger (1665–1860)*, 2nd ed., Paris, 1913, 315 pp. (emphasizes the French press).

For guides partly pharmaceutical or related, see the subsections on "Periodicals" and "Histories" of periodicals in, J. B. Blake and C. Roos: *Medical Reference Works 1679–*

*1966; A Selected Bibliography*, pp. 38–41, Chicago, 1967. For the modern period, use will be found for T. Andrews and J. Oslet: *World list of pharmacy periodicals*—revised and enlarged edition, 1975, *Am. J. Hosp. Pharm. 32*:85–122, 1975 (also available as an ASHP reprint-booklet). Still noteworthy are the cleverly designed chronological tables, which include pharmacy among the 8,603 titles in the back of H. C. Bolton: *A Catalogue of Scientific and Technical Periodicals 1665–1895 . . .*, 2nd ed., Washington, D.C. 1897. It should be kept in mind that the *Index-Catalogue of the Surgeon-General's Library*, Washington, D.C., (see above) constitutes almost a veritable universal index to the medical periodical literature encompassed (in addition to the books listed therein); see C. F. Mayer, The Index-Catalogue as a tool of research in medicine and history, in: *Science, Medicine, and History* (E. A. Underwood, ed.), V. II, pp. 482–493, Cambridge, 1953.

It may now be useful to turn from such bibliographic guides to mention some highlights of the pharmaceutical literature that evolved in countries represented by this book.

## ITALY

Of greatest influence on the practice of pharmacy among early Italian works was the *Ccmpendium aromatariorum* by the physician Saladin de Asculo,[1] written in the middle of the 15th century for the information of pharmacists. This book has been called "the first real treatise on pharmacy in a modern sense . . . which became the model for all later textbooks of pharmacy and for centuries was the indispensable vade mecum [reference book] of the apothecary."[2]

Mention should be made, among early similar books, of the *Lumen apothecariorum* (The Light of the Pharmacists), by the physician Quiricus de Augustus de Dertona;[3] the *Luminare majus* (The Greater Luminary), written toward the end of the 15th century by the pharmacist Joannes J. Manlius de Bosco,[4] and the *Thesaurus aromatariorum* (The Treasure Chest of the Pharmacists), written by Paulus Suardus in the first decade of the 16th century. Whether or not the treatise by the Spanish pharmacist, Petro Benedicto Mateo was written before that of J. Manlius de Bosco is an open question.

Among Italian books of the next 150 years the most notable was the *Nuovo et universale theatro farmaceutico* (1662), written by pharmacist Antonio de Sgobbis da Montagnana.[5] (Frontispiece reproduced p. 65)

After the close of the 17th century, scientific pharmaceutical treatises by Italian pharmacists and physicians seldom acquired renown beyond the borders of Italy.

### Journals

The earliest journals in Italy having relationship to pharmacy and publishing some pharmaceutical material were the *Biblioteca fisica d'Europa* (f. 1788) and the *Annali di Chimica* (f. 1790). The first Italian journal to give pharmacy its primary attention, however, appears to be the *Giornale di farmacia, chimica e scienze affini* (f. 1824). Two journals founded near mid-century became well known in the scientific world, *Il giornale di farmacia e di chimica* (f. 1852) and the *Bolletino chimico-farmaceutico* (f. 1861). Many other pharmaceutical journals have appeared meanwhile, including some specifically in the field of pharmaceutical manufacturing.

Among 20th-century periodicals directed more particularly toward the practicing pharmacist, the following are representative: The *Corriere dei farmacisti* (f. 1906; the official organ from 1945 of the "Ordini dei farmacisti e delle associazioni sindacali di categoria"), *Il Farmacista* (f. 1947), the official organ of the present Italian Pharmacists' Association ("Federazione degli Ordini dei Farmacisti Italiani") and *Farmacia* (f. 1950), the official organ of the largest Italian association of pharmacy owners. *La Farmacia Nuova* (f. 1945) is noteworthy here as the repository of articles published on the history of pharmacy from time to time.

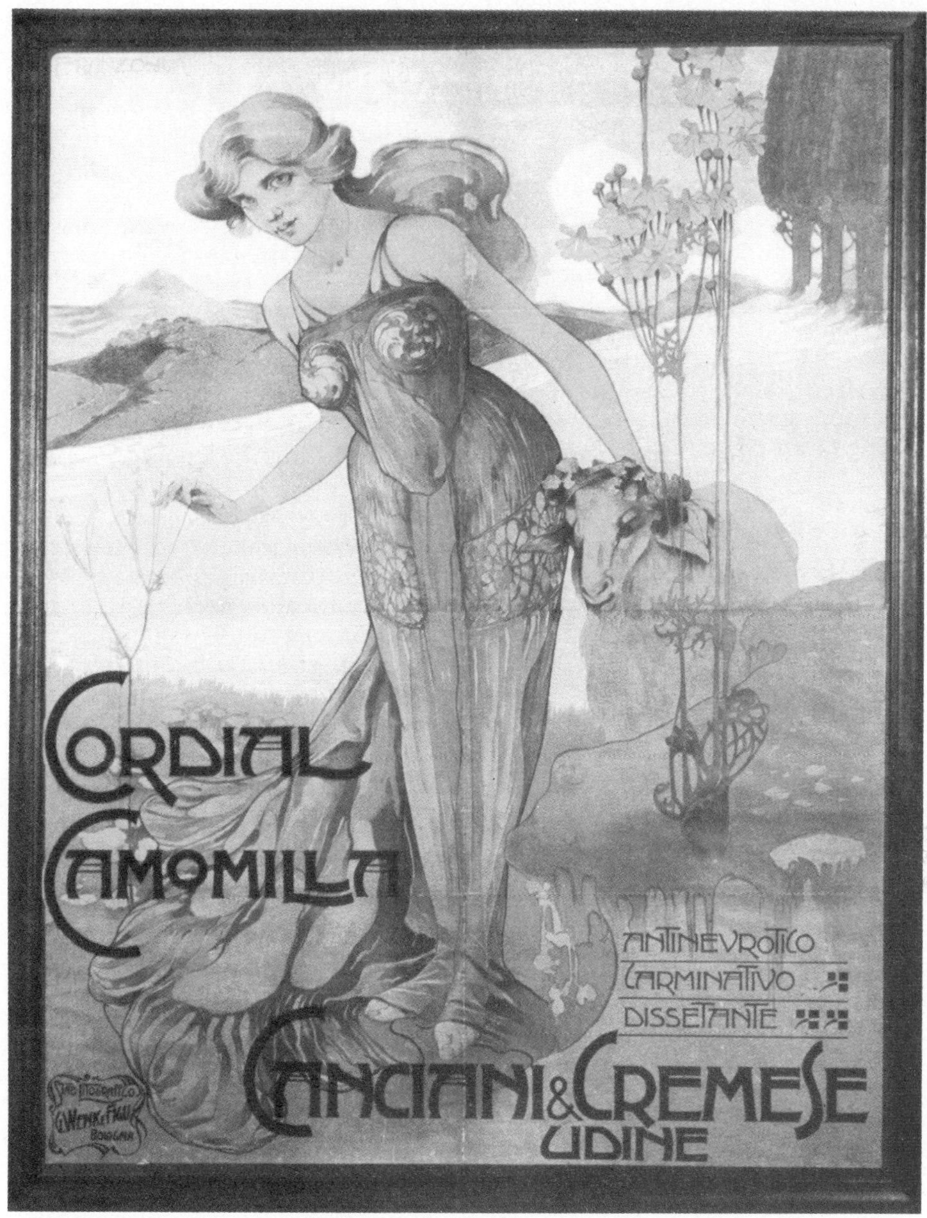


Posters promoting self-medications constitute an unusual form of literature, which collectors prize. In the example shown, an Italian poster by Franzoni (ca. 1900) invites a trial of a medicinal cordial containing extract of chamomile flowers. This plant (Anthemis nobilis L.) has been valued as a stomachic and tonic in the folk medicine of various countries since at least the late Middle Ages. (From W. Helfand: The pharmaceutical poster, Pharm. Hist. *15*: opposite 81, 1973)

### Pharmacopeias

In 1499 the medical members of the Florentine guild of physicians and pharmacists (*L'arte dei medici e speziali*) issued a pharmaceutical formulary entitled *Nuovo receptario*. Since this book was made obligatory for pharmacists by their guild, it sometimes has been considered the first European pharmacopeia. Lack of precise agreement on what constitutes a "Pharmacopeia" makes it a moot point. Recent research suggests that the Florentine book (88 leaves), like that of Barcelona 12 years later, could be characterized as containing the drug standards authorized by the guild. (The later Nuremberg dispensatory of 1546 received government sanction and support, which places its pharmacopeial status beyond question.)[6]

The *Nuovo receptario* followed the spirit of Arabic drug therapy, as we should expect. More than a half century passed before Mantua (1559) and, later, other Italian city-states[7] followed Florence's lead in issuing their own drug standards. Across Europe, the sequence and the circumstances of the founding of these early local pharmacopeias tend to reflect the standard of pharmacy and the nationalistic tendencies in the various political units.

The title "*Pharmacopoea*" was not used as such in Italy until 1580, at Bergamo, following an example set by the French physician Jacques du Bois (Sylvius) in 1548. However, Sylvius' *Pharmacopoeae libri tres* was a private book and not "official."

Not until 1892 did the government of the new kingdom of Italy (established 1870) issue the first official pharmaceutical standard for the entire country, the *Farmacopoea ufficiale del regno d'Italia*.

## FRANCE

### Treatises

Until the end of the 16th century, the works of Arabian authors and their European followers naturally dominated the libraries of the French pharmacists. To these treatises were added occasionally such books as the *Grand herbier*, a very free translation of the *Circa instans*. In the 16th century, books of French origin increased—at first written mainly by physicians.[8] In 1561 the first book in French written by a pharmacist on the art of pharmacy appeared. It was a manual of technic for pharmacy students (*L'Enchirid ou manipul des miropoles*) by Michel Dusseau of Paris.[9] During the following century the profession continued to generate its own literature.[10] Of particular influence on the practice of French pharmacy were the writings of Jean de Renou (1608), providing a formulary, a textbook and a guide to the preservation of drugs, the use of pharmaceutical equipment and to the rules of professional ethics. A similarity to instructions given by the Italian Saladino d'Ascoli in the 15th century can be discerned frequently.

After the middle of the 17th century the number of books by French pharmacists increased markedly, including among the authors such famous names as Moise Charas, Nicaise Lefebvre, Nicolas Lémery, Antoine Baumé and E. F. Geoffroy.[11] The chemical side of the literature began to be transformed after the late 18th century when Lavoisier—no pharmacist himself, but a pupil of the pharmacist Guillaume François Rouelle—published his famous experiments concerning the role played by oxygen in combustion. He thereby established the basis of the "new chemistry," the chemistry of our own time—and hence of scientific pharmacy.

### Pharmacopeias

The first local pharmacopeia or formulary of France appeared early in the 17th century (Lyons, 1628) and was followed by others.[12] The local approach to unifying drug standards was not superseded entirely until the first edition of the *Codex medicamentarius seu pharmacopoeia Gallica* became obligatory for the whole of France in 1818.

### Journals

The excellent men who formed the *Société libre des pharmaciens de Paris* created only a year later (1797) the first French pharmaceutical journal, the *Journal de la société des pharmaciens de Paris*. Two years later it was consolidated with the *Annales de chimie* (founded 1789), which had had several famous French pharmacists on its editorial staff. This initiated a rich journal literature that branched out diversely in the 19th century, reflecting the professional and scientific vigor of French pharmacy.[13]

Representative of the present century are the *Annales pharmaceutiques françaises,* its distinguished scientific antecedents dating from 1809 (and serving the Académie de Pharmacie since its founding in 1946), the *Bulletin de l'Ordre des Pharmaciens* (since 1947) as a professional journal, and *Le Moniteur des pharmacies et des laboratoires* (since 1947). An early and remarkable cultural offshoot of French pharmacy—the first journal of its kind—is the *Revue d'histoire de la pharmacie* (beginning in 1913 as the *Bulletin*).

## GERMANY

### Treatises

As in all European countries, the first scientific pharmaceutical knowledge came from Arabian sources via Italy. German original literature dealing with subjects of pharmaceutical interest, and influencing pharmacy, began with general books on natural history that included pharmacy. The earliest in German was the *Buch der Natur* by Conrad of Megenberg in the 14th century. From the 15th century on we find specialized books dealing with remedies and their uses (the *Arzneibücher*), with botanical drugs (the *Kräuterbücher*, or herbals), and with the complex art of distillation (the *Destillierbücher*), a process being utilized by the time of the Renaissance to prepare a host of medicinal products.[14]

The distillation books and the herbals often contained more than their names implied. For example, the herbals not only describe herbs but also animals and gems, with their assumed medicinal effects.

These books, written mostly by physicians, were intended to serve the colleagues of the authors as well as the pharmacists and, last but not least, laymen. H. Brünschwig wrote a renowned formulary on inexpensive medications for the poor (*Thesaurus pauperum*), to which there were many successors. Otto Brunfels wrote one of the most used herbals, as well as a book on the equipping and the managing of pharmacies (*Die Reformation der Apotheken,* 1536), similar to the book of the Frenchman Renou, which in turn was based on Saladin de Asculo. The famous commentary on Dioscorides by Mattioli was published in German as the *Neu deutsch Kreuterbuch,* 1563.[15]

Still in the 16th century, there appeared encyclopedic books that covered the entire scope of pharmacy, the ambitious counterparts of which still appear on pharmacists' shelves today. In 1561 the physician J. J. Wecker of Basel issued his *Antidotarium Generale,* which contains a comprehensive formulary, instructions on the art of filling prescriptions, directions for preparing galenics and for preparing the chemicals of that time.[16]

However, the universal textbook of German pharmacists for at least a century was another book, *Pharmacopoea medicophysica*, by the physician Joh. Christian Schroeder (1600–1664).[17] An important book in botany also appeared in the 17th century written by a pharmacist, Basilius Besler of Nuremberg, describing and cataloging the botanic garden in Eichstaett (*Hortus Eystettensis,* 1613).

Among the most important pharmacochemical books of the 17th century were three by German physicians: the *Basilica chymica* of Oswald Croll (1560–1609), an ar-

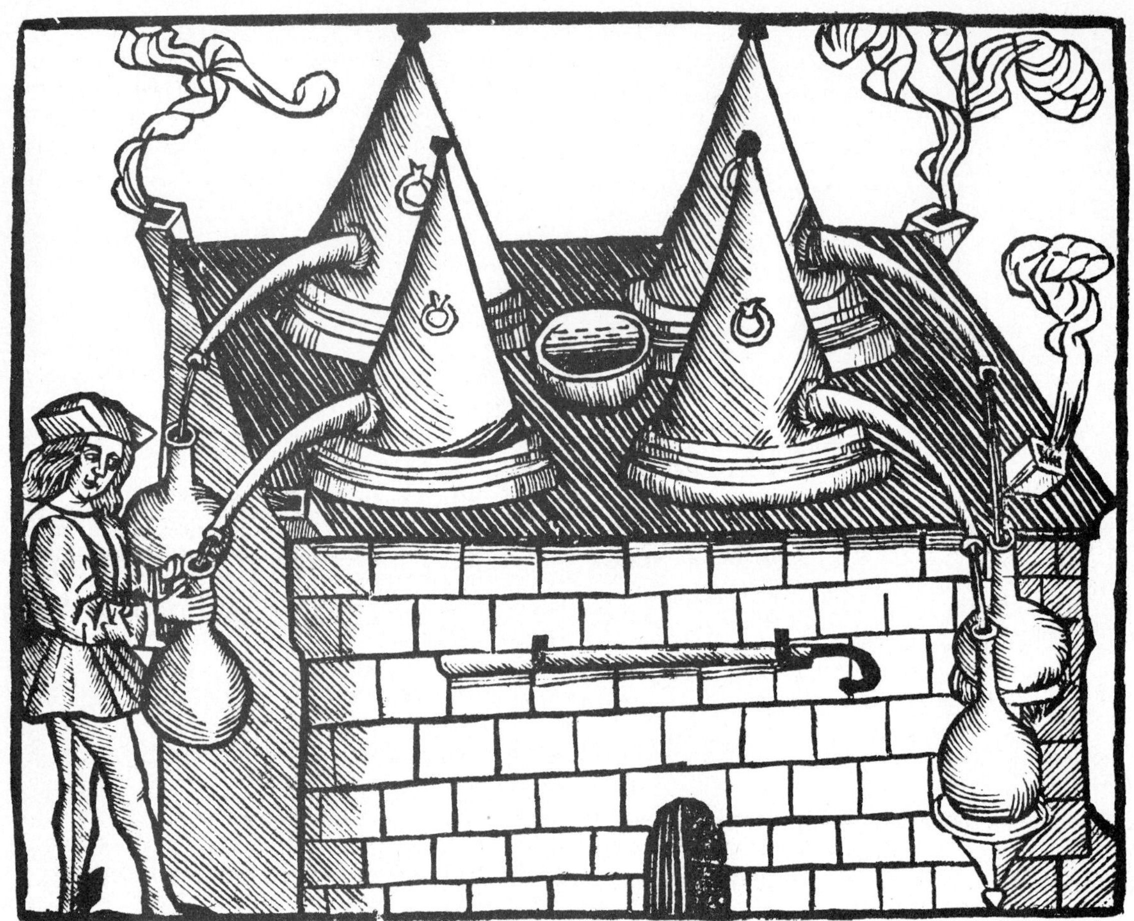

Medicinal distillates gained wide popularity after the early 16th century when this woodcut was published. Distillate is being collected from four cucurbits, each with a conical air-cooled alembic. An inner rim collected and guided the distillate to the delivery tube. At the corners of the furnace are four small chimneys, and in the center is a funnel for filling the water bath. This illustration comes from a book by H. Braunschweig, a Strassburg surgeon, whose works were enormously influential in making distillation technic an important part of the work of the pharmacist. (Photograph, University of Wisconsin, from 1517 edition; see also Forbes, Art of Distillation)

dent Paracelsist; the *Pharmacia moderno saeculo applicanda* (Pharmacy Applied to Modern Times) of D. Ludovici (1625–1680); the *Pharmacopoea spagyrica* of Joh. Rudolf Glauber (1604–1670), one of the first German chemists whose work helped to lay the foundations for German chemical industry.[18]

J. C. Sommerhof is credited with the first book on pharmaceutical subjects by a German pharmacist, his excellent *Lexicon pharmaceutico-chymicum* (1701). From the mid-18th century on, the number of such books by pharmacists increased extraordinarily. Almost without exception they set a high standard.[19] German scientific pharmacy had come of age.

The laboratories of German pharmacies were to a remarkable extent the precursors not only of the later university chemical laboratories but also of the large-scale pharmaceutical industry.[20]

## Pharmacopeias

The first official pharmacopeia in Germany was the *Dispensatorium* of Valerius Cordus, issued in 1546 and made official for the imperial city of Nuremberg.[21] Many consider it to be the first true "pharmacopeia" anywhere in the world, since it was enacted specifically as legally binding on all practitioners in the Nuremberg area, whereas the famous earlier book in Florence (1499) was made an authoritative standard only by the considerable power of the Florentine guild of physicians and pharmacists (rather than by documented enactment by civil authorities).

The Nuremberg book was followed within 20 years by pharmacopeias for Augsburg (compiled by Adolf Occo in 1564) and for Cologne (1565).[22] These three earliest German pharmacopeias represent three types of official books that recur later elsewhere. A good and concise compilation of old formulas, in a critical and progressive spirit but without elaboration, is the approach of Cordus. A more comprehensive approach was taken by Occo, with the interesting feature of a legal regulation that required pharmacists to keep in stock all drugs marked with an asterisk in the pharmacopeia. Most comprehensive of the three is the *Dispensarium Coloniense,* providing not only an official formulary but also a textbook type of information about the drugs. This latter concept became predominant among European pharmacopeias up to the end of the 18th century.

At the end of the 17th century, the *Dispensatorium Brandenburgicum* (1698), the first official pharmacopeia for a larger German political unit, appeared.[23]

In Austria, one of the most important parts of the German Empire until 1806, a peculiar situation arose when the medical faculty of the University of Vienna compiled a *Dispensatorium pro pharmacopoeis Viennensibus* (1570), but the sovereign did not give the necessary permission for publication! Eventually (1618), it was the *Pharmacopoeia Augustana* that became the official standard not only for Vienna but also for the Austrian provinces. From 1729 on, various pharmacopeias appeared in Austria, culminating with the first edition (1812) of the present *Pharmacopoea Austriaca.*[24]

Besides the Prussian-Brandenburgian dispensatory, the *Pharmacopoea Wirtembergica* was the official book of its time most esteemed and used, even beyond the German frontiers, representing the combined textbook and formulary style, the prototype of which was the *Dispensatorium Coloniense* of 1565. A special section gave good descriptions of the simple drugs. It was one of the most comprehensive pharmacopeias, supplying information about all drugs, new and old.

Both of these official books (Prussian-Brandenburgian and Würtembergian pharmacopeias) reflect the victory of the chemical or Paracelsian school of thought. The names of Arabian physicians, of Pseudo-Mesuë, and those of their European followers (e.g., Nicolaus, Fernel and Occo) have been dropped from the titles of the compound formulas of which they were the real or supposed authors. Instead, the Brandenburgian-Prussian pharmacopeia (1698) cites, in addition to the name of Paracelsus himself, the names of various paracelsists (Becher, Craanen, Croll, Ludovici, Mynsicht, Quercetanus, Rolfink, Sylvius, Wirtz and Zwelffer). In the *Pharmacopoea Wirtembergica* of 1771 this list of names is augmented by those of other chemically minded men (Camerarius, Dippel, Minderer, Schroeder, Stahl, Wedel and others).[25]

In consequense of the new theory of Lavoisier concerning the role of oxygen in

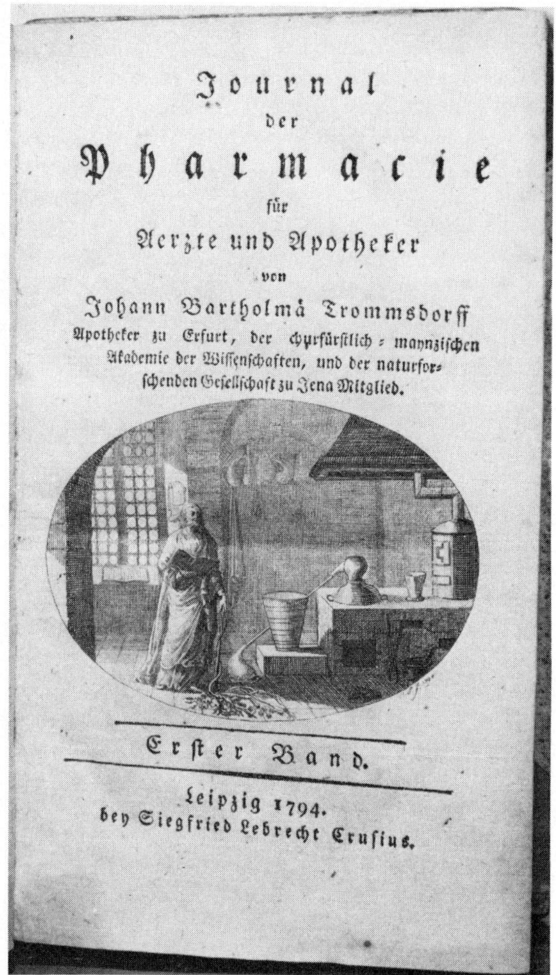

Journal
der
Pharmacie
für
Aerzte und Apotheker
von
Johann Bartholmä Trommsdorff
Apotheker zu Erfurt, der churfürstlich = maynzischen
Akademie der Wissenschaften, und der naturfor=
schenden Gesellschaft zu Jena Mitglied.

Erster Band.

Leipzig 1794.
bey Siegfried Lebrecht Crusius.

The earliest regular journal of pharmacy having a scientific character was issued between 1793 and 1834. Its pharmacist-editor, J. B. Trommsdorff, had a teaching laboratory for practical chemistry associated with his pharmacy, which may not have been unlike the pharmaceutical laboratory shown above on the title page of Volume 1. (From the University of Wisconsin)

combustion, the authorship of the German pharmacopeias underwent a decided change. The first *Pharmacopoea Borussica* represents an important milestone in the history of German pharmacopeias (1799). This book was one of the first official pharmaceutical formularies based on the new chemical theories, and was the first one in Germany prepared primarily and influenced decisively by pharmacists and not by physicians.[26] This was because the German development of chemistry, and more particularly of pharmaceutical chemistry, had been fostered by pharmacists since the middle of the 18th century. Their opportunity had come and it had found them ready. It was the triumvirate, M. H. Klaproth, S. F. Hermbstaedt and Valentin Rose, Jr., who elaborated the pharmacopeia, with the assistance of other pharmacists and the collaboration of physicians.[27]

The preparedness of German pharmacists proved to be of consequence in the next decisive stage in the history of German pharmacopeias. During the middle sixties of the 19th century, the general as well as the pharmaceutical situation in Germany demanded some kind of unification. Even before the German political unification became a reality in 1871 (not including Austria), the German pharmacists anticipated it by presenting to the German professional world a *Pharmacopoea Germaniae* (1865). The book had been elaborated exclusively by pharmacists under the sponsorship of their association.[28] It became official only for Saxony, but it paved the way for a pharmaceutical standard obligatory throughout the reunited Germany and showed how necessary such a standard was.

One of the first governmental acts of the new German Empire was to create such a standard. Only one year after the establishment of the new Empire, the first *Pharmacopoea Germanica* appeared (1872).[29] This book, as well as all later editions (published since 1890 in German instead of Latin), was elaborated by representatives of all interested professions and groups, but the decisive influence of the pharmacist has prevailed.

### Periodicals

The first periodical devoted primarily to pharmacy was German born: the *Almanach oder Taschenbuch für Scheidekünstler und*

*Apotheker,* an annual founded in 1780 by Johann Goettling.[30] It was followed by the first pharmaceutical publication appearing at more frequent intervals, hence having more the character of a journal, *Trommsdorff's Journal der Pharmacie* (1793). Since then a large number of scientific pharmaceutical journals have made their appearance.[31] Among independent journals (not affiliated with or supported by an association), the *Pharmaceutische Zentralhalle* (1859–1969) was best known. A new journal on drug research appeared in 1950 *(Arzneimittelforschung)*.[32]

Of the independent journals devoted to professional pharmacy as a whole—practical and socioeconomic aspects as well as scientific—mention should be made of the *Pharmazeutische Zeitung* (founded in 1856 by Hermann Mueller) and the *Süddeutsche Apotheker-Zeitung* (founded in 1861 as *Pharmaceutisches Wochenblatt).*[33] The *Pharmazeutische Zeitung,* a victim of the Nazi regime toward the close of 1937, was revived in 1947 (uniting in 1953 with the *Apotheker-Zeitung*). The *Süddeutsche Apotheker-Zeitung* (revived 1946) merged into the *Deutsche Apotheker-Zeitung* (1950). A counterpart journal of general circulation in East Germany, *Die Pharmazie,* has appeared since 1946.

Besides the independent journals others have appeared as the official publications of pharmaceutical associations.

Both the Deutscher Apothekerverein (professional) and the Pharmazeutische Gesellschaft (scientific) have issued their own publications. In addition to the *Archiv der Pharmacie,* the Apothekerverein since 1886 had published the *Apotheker-Zeitung.*[34] Its successor, the *Deutsche Apotheker-Zeitung,* is an independent weekly that covers the same subjects. The Pharmazeutische Gesellschaft, since its founding (1890), published the *Berichte der Deutschen Pharmazeutischen Gesellschaft,* which consolidated with the *Archiv der Pharmazie* (1924). Since then it has borne the dual title, *Archiv der Pharmazie und Berichte der Deutschen Pharmazeutischen Gesellschaft.* (Discontinued at the downfall of the Nazi regime, the *Archiv* was revived in 1950).

The journal of the Arbeitsgemeinschaft Pharmazeutische Industrie is *Die Pharmazeutische Industrie* (first issued in 1934, suspended after the Nazi downfall, then revived in 1950). As a more popular type of journal, the Pharmazeutische Gesellschaft has issued since 1972 *Pharmazie in unserer Zeit* as a bi-monthly.

The union or alliance of German employee-pharmacists (Verband Deutscher Apotheker, f. 1904) from 1905 issued the *Zentralblatt für Pharmacie.* In 1934 this employees' association and its journal were absorbed by the new totalitarian pharmaceutical association.

The important weekly, *Pharmazeutische Zeitung* (Frankfurt), covers scientific as well as professional and economic affairs as the official organ of the broad roof-organization uniting German pharmacy (ABDA, "Arbeitsgemeinschaft der Berufsvertretungen Deutscher Apotheker").

## GREAT BRITAIN

### Treatises

In Britain until the 16th century, the same books of the Galenic-Arabic school that formed the professional library of pharmacists in all European countries were used, such as the *Antidotaria Nicolai,* the *Grabadin* of the pseudo Mesuë, the *Book of Symon Januensis,* and the others. Later on, the most important French and German pharmaceutical literature was introduced.

Among English books issued in the early 16th century were *The New Herbal* (1551) by William Turner, physician to the court of Edward VI and Robert Recorde's *The Urinal of Physick* (1548). The popular *Herball* (1597) of John Gerard, a barber-surgeon, was based on a Belgian herbal by Dodoens; it was revised and much improved by the scholarly apothecary Thomas Johnson.

In the 17th century an English translation of *The Charitable Physician* and *The Charitable*

*Apothecary* by the French physician Guibert was popular.[35] The voluminous herbal *Theatrum botanicum. . .* (1640) was written by John Parkinson of London, one of the last representatives of a herbalist tradition soon to be pushed aside by modern botanists. In 1688, the apothecary James Shipton published a collection of formulas which he said were prescribed by the physician George Bate, and which he therefore titled *Bate's Dispensatory*. The book (usually known as the *Pharmacopoeia Bateana)* lived to see several editions in Latin and in English and was used as a book of reference until the end of the 18th century.[36]

Quincy's *Pharmacopoeia officinalis & extemporanea: or, A Compleat English Dispensatory* (1718) was so popular that it was issued in ten editions by 1736.[37] There were a few other compilations from Continental works and some commentaries on the London and the Edinburgh pharmacopeias—among them Salmon's New London Dispensatory,[38] Lewis' *New Dispensatory,*[39] Duncan's *Edinburgh New Dispensatory* and Thomson's *London Dispensatory*—but little sign of the lively, fruitful and sometimes creative acitivity so characteristic of the Continental pharmacists, the French and the Germans especially. However, the pharmacopoeia-related works of the English physicians George Bate, John Quincy, William Lewis and others—as well as the official pharmacopeias of Britain—were widely published abroad.[40]

Nineteenth-century books by pharmacists included *Practical Pharmacy* by the German Carl F. Mohr and the Briton Theophilus Redwood, *Pharmacographia* by the Swiss F. A. Flückiger and the Briton Daniel Hanbury and *Microscopical Examination of Foods and Drugs* and *Introduction to the Study of Materia Medica* by H. G. Greenish. Meanwhile, various books written by men from the ranks of British pharmacy currently serve aspects of the art, the science and the industry.

**Pharmacopeias and Formularies**

There were three official pharmacopeias in the United Kingdom until 1864, published in London, Edinburgh and Dublin, respectively. The first edition of the *Pharmacopoeia Londinensis* had an unusual fate, two "first" editions: one issued May 7, 1618, and another December 7, the latter replacing the earlier edition and becoming the basis of the editions that followed.

An epilogue in the later book blames the printer for withdrawal of the first issue, for having "snatched away from our hands this little work not yet finished off . . . " Actually, differences among the members of the College of Physicians of London about the scope of this first English pharmacopeia were responsible for replacement of the earlier book by the later one. In both issues the Galenic-Arabic school, which still dominated drug therapy, offered the main basis; however, the second issue represented the victory of baroque abundance over renaissance simplicity.[41] The first issue listed 680 simple and 712 compounded drugs compared with 1,190 simple and 963 compounded drugs in the second. The number of animals used pharmaceutically rose in the second issue from 10 to 31, and the number of parts of animals (among them various excrements and urines) rose from 47 to 162.[42] However, there were some signs indicating the dawn of a new era. Chemical preparations (among them calomel and preparations of iron and antimony for internal use) and others regarded as chemical at this period had been included in both issues of the new pharmacopeia. The French immigrant Theodore de Mayerne (1573–1655) almost certainly was responsible for the introduction of calomel—and probably the other chemicals also.[43]

Eight subsequent editions preserve for us a pharmacopeial picture of the state of pharmaceutical, chemical and medical knowledge and thought of their time.[44]

The first *Edinburgh Pharmacopoeia* appeared in 1699—a distinguished book that lived to see twelve editions (the last published in 1841).[45] The *Dublin Pharmacopoeia,* first published in 1807, lived only until the third edition (1850) and was supplanted by a pharmacopeia for the whole of the British Isles. While the *Dublin Pharmacopoeia* did not gain much attention beyond Ireland, during the 18th century the *Edinburgh Pharmacopoeia* ranked high among the internationally acknowledged pharmaceutical standards. Moreover, both the Edinburgh and London pharmacopoeias had been republished in Western Europe in numerous editions, which David Cowen interprets not only as a normal cultural diffusion but as a high compliment to the quality of British work in this field.[46]

The first *British Pharmacopoeia,* issued in 1864, replaced the London, the Edinburgh and the Dublin standards, but it disappointed the mass of the medical and the pharmacetuical practitioners because in it many of the preparations that they were in the habit of dispensing were omitted or changed.[47] Consequently, it already was superseded by a second edition in 1867.

After World War II, a long-delayed seventh *British Pharmacopoeia* appeared (1948), and, since then, a new revision has appeared every 5 years (parallel with the American revision schedule), plus an interim addendum.[48]

Until the end of the 18th century, the preparation of the official pharmacopeias in England was exclusively the work of the medical profession. Harbingers of pharmaceutical collaboration appeared as early as 1732 in work on the Edinburgh Pharmacopoeia and 1785 in work on the London Pharmacopoeia.[49]

The impossibility of editing such a standard treatise exclusively from the medical point of view and knowledge had become evident, and the necessity of pharmaceutical cooperation had become apparent. Neither the old apothecaries nor their successors, the chemists and the druggists, unorganized as the latter were at that time, had as yet produced the experts needed. However, a learned pharmacist, Richard Phillips, had criticized the edition of 1809 and the corrected reprint of 1815 with the utmost acrimony. It was he who was commissioned to translate the *Pharmacopoeia* of 1824 from Latin and to prepare a commentary. "Subsequently he assumed a more responsible position with reference to the work as editor as well as translator and commentator, in which capacities his name is associated with the editions of 1836 and 1851."[50]

The *British Pharmacopoeia* was edited by the GeneralCouncil of Medical Education and Registration until the Medicines Act of 1968, which passed this responsibility to a Medicines Commission of the government's Ministry of Health.

The British Pharmacopoeia Commission appointed by the government had essentially the same composition, however, as the preceding Commission. A striking feature of the resultant 1973 edition was its proclamation that the standards in the new *European Pharmacopoeia* would take precedence over the *British Pharmacopoeia* in the event of differences in specifications for the same drug.[51] This appears to be a further example of increasing involvement by British pharmacy in developments of the European Economic Community. The shift of authority for the British Pharmacopoeia from the professions to the government appears to be a further example of changes in Britain that more and more reflect the Continent.

After the appearance of the first edition (1864), a representative pharmacist, Peter Squire, "brought out a book called *A Companion to the British Pharmacopoeia* which proved a useful guide to medical practitioners, and acquired a great circulation."[52] In 1952 this book was absorbed into the *Extra Pharmacopoeia,* a comprehensive ready-reference work for practitioners (first edition, 1883). British pharmacists refer to this work informally as "Martindale" (as Americans refer to "Remington"), in remembrance of the original author, William Martindale, who was once chief pharmacist at University College Hospital in London and later founder of wholesale and retail pharmacies.

The Pharmaceutical Society has published at irregular intervals since 1907 the *British Pharmaceutical Codex.* More comprehensive than the *Pharmacopoeia,* it has included monographs on drug actions and uses and legal standards for surgical dressings in Great Britain. The *Codex* has appeared every 5 years, with increasing authority (from 1963, simultaneously with new editions of the *Pharmacopoeia*), although provisions of the 1968 Medicines Act for publishing the British Pharmacopeia and related publications have raised a question about continuation of the *Codex*. A *British Veterinary Codex* also is published by the Pharmaceutical Society (first edition, 1953).

A *National Formulary* was first issued for use in the old National Health Insurance plan and has been continued under the title *British National Formulary*, to avoid confusion with the *National Formulary* of the United States. As used in the universal National Health Service (government-paid services), it has been made into a comprehensive guide to prescribing, compiled by a joint committee of the British Medical Association and the Pharmaceutical Society of Great Britain.

### Journals

Apparently the first English journal connected with pharmacy was *The Chemist*, which existed for only 13 months (1824 to 1825). Around the mid-19th century, a number of other journals (now supplanted) helped to convey pharmaceutical information to the rising new class of practitioners of pharmacy, the "chemists and druggists."[53]

The oldest and professionally most influential journal in continuous publication is the weekly *Pharmaceutical Journal*, the official organ of the Pharmaceutical Society of Great Britain since the beginning in 1841. (Although it was founded on the private initiative of Jacob Bell, he presented the copyright to the Society in 1859). Until 1895 it was called *The Pharmaceutical Journal and Transactions,* then simply, *The Pharmaceutical Journal.* Coincidental with an official attempt to popularize the designation "pharmacist," the title was changed to *The Pharmaceutical Journal and Pharmacist* (1909). The designation "pharmacist," not having been adopted by the majority of the English dispensing "chemists," was dropped, and the title again reads *The Pharmaceutical Journal.*

*The Chemist and Druggist,* another important English pharmaceutical journal founded in 1859, has never changed either its name or its objectives. The main idea was to produce for the average practitioner a general and practical journal, whose aim was to be "simply useful—a trade journal."[54]

For pharmacists practicing in hospitals and similar institutions, the Guild of Public Pharmacists has published the *Journal of Hospital Pharmacy* since 1932 (titled until 1963 *The Public Pharmacist).*

The present monthly *Journal of Pharmacy and Pharmacology* (which includes the *Transactions* of the British Pharmaceutical Conference as a supplement) traces its lineage back to the beginning of the Conference as a scientific body. At first the *Transactions* (or *Proceedings*) of the Conference appeared in the *Pharmaceutical Journal* (1864) and as a reprinted booklet, later (1870) as part of a *Year-Book of Pharmacy,* which (1928) was divided into a *Quarterly Journal of Pharmacy and Pharmacology.* Expanding its scope, this quarterly became the present monthly *Journal* in 1950.

The work of a Committee on the History of Pharmacy in the Pharmaceutical Society during the 1950's developed into the British Society for the History of Pharmacy (1967), which issues serial notes, *The Pharmaceutical Historian* (f. 1967), and *Transactions* (f. 1970).

## UNITED STATES OF AMERICA

NOTE: For the principal discussion of American pharmaceutical literature see Chapter 15: "The Establishment of a Literature." Detailed information on just two aspects of Chapter 15 is given below for its reference value, without encumbering the narrative text of that chapter.

**Publications of the American Pharmaceutical Association**

| Annual | Monthly | | Supplemental |
|---|---|---|---|
| 1852 Proceedings of the A.Ph.A. through 1911* | 1906 Bulletin of the A.Ph.A. through 1911 | | Occasional monographs (e.g., *Handbook of Non-Prescription Drugs,* 1st ed., 1967; *Pharmacy and the Poor, a Report . . .,* 1971; *Evaluations of Drug Interactions* 1st. ed., 1971) |
| 1912 Yearbook of the A.Ph.A. through 1934 | 1912 Journal of the A.Ph.A. (new vol. numbers) through 1939 | | |
| | 1935 through 1948 Pharmaceutical Abstracts (monthly in Scientific Edition, but often bound separately) | | |
| | Scientific Edition (continuing vol. numbers) 1940 through 1960 | Practical Pharmacy Edition (new vol. numbers) 1940 through 1960 | |
| | Journal of Pharmaceutical Sciences (continuing vol. numbers) *50*:1961 to date | P. P. edition dropped from Journal title (New Series vol. numbering) *1*:1961 to date | The A.Ph.A. Newsletter *1*:1962, to date; Academy/GP *1*:1966; The Academy Reporter *1*:1965; S.A.Ph.A. News *1*:1971 |

*Although titled "Proceedings," the 1911 volume already had the character of subsequent "Yearbooks" (A report of the proceedings of the Annual Meeting is incorporated into the *Bulletin,* 1911.)

### American Pharmaceutical Association Press

*Because of the key position that publications of the American Pharmaceutical Association hold in the history of American pharmacy, the above chart has been prepared with the cooperation of Professor George E. Osborne of the College of Pharmacy, University of Rhode Island.*

**The National Formulary.** Published approximately every 10 years from 1888 to 1940; every 5 years from 1940 to date; numbered by editions. "N.F. XIV" (1975) was the last edition to be published by the Association; transferred to the jurisdiction of the U. S. Pharmacopeial Convention.

**Bulletin of the National Formulary Committee.** (Vols. 1 to 19, 1930–1951). Circulation at first irregular and restricted to Committee; took journal format with Vol. 7, 1938; continued under title *Drug Standards* from No. 5-&-6, Vol. 19 (1951) through Vol. 28 (1960), then absorbed into *Journal of Pharmaceutical Sciences.* After 1974 the function was substantially being fulfilled by a new serial, *Pharmacopeial Forum*, published by the U. S. Pharmacopeial Convention.

**The Pharmaceutical Recipe Book.** 1926, 1938 and 1943; now out of print.

**Proceedings.** From 1852, when the American Pharmaceutical Association was established, a volume of *Proceedings* of the meetings was issued annually, except for 1861 when no meeting of the Association was held. A useful *General Index to Volumes One to Fifty of the Proceedings of the American Pharmaceutical Association, from 1852 to 1902 inclusive* appeared as a separate volume.

In 1912 the *Journal* and the *Year Book* took the place of the separate *Proceedings.* After each subsequent annual meeting the proceedings usually were printed in the following 3 issues of the Journal. The *Year Book* provided a place for Association data (such as the official roster, the constitution and bylaws, the treasurer's report, and a list of members, alphabetically and geographically), as well as the abstracting service called "The Report of the Progress of Pharmacy."

The *Year Book* was discontinued with Volume 23, covering the calendar year 1934. Beginning with 1935 the annual "Report" was revamped as monthly "Pharmaceutical Abstracts," appearing as part of the *Journal*, but separately paged and indexed.

The proceedings later were published in one number of the *Journal* each year (rather than in three); and this number also included the Association data and list of members (which had appeared in the *Year Book*). In 1940 when the *Journal* began to be published in two editions, no proceedings number appeared, being combined with the proceedings for 1941. The Proceedings Numbers, which continued in the *Scientific Edition*, contained an abstract of the minutes of the various subdivisions of the Association and of its related organizations, and included addresses and reports (corresponding in part to the discontinued *Year Book*). Papers presented in the Sections and the later Academies (and their sectional substructure) have appeared, to the extent published by the Association, in other issues of the *Journal's* two editions.†

The Proceedings Numbers were discontinued with the 1945 issue and have not been revived (except for an abortive attempt in 1950, a separate issue covering only the General Sessions and the House of Delegates). In the ensuing years the proceedings have been "published in narrative form" (as summaries and principal addresses) in the *Journal* (Practical Pharmacy Edition prior to 1961).

Unpublished proceedings material has been classified into the Archive of the American Pharmaceutical Association (2215 Constitution Ave., N.W., Washington 7, D.C.), although some 20th-century material remains in storage. For a detailed topical outline, see: "Structure of the Archive of the American Pharmaceutical Association," *Pharmacy in History 7*:35–42, 1962.

A roster of the officials and subdivisions of the Association continued to be published in the *Journal*, expanding into a "Directory" (Pract. Pharm. Ed. *5*:187–193, 1944) that included addresses of other American associations, publications, state boards, and schools of pharmacy, which (after a hiatus) appeared annually in amplified form (*Journal* ns *1*:19–38, 1961, et seq.), then as a separate *Pharmaceutical Directory*, annually.

## Some Privately Published Journals

The first strictly independent journal of national circulation was *The American Druggist's Circular and Chemical Gazette* (after 1906, *The Druggist's Circular)*, the first number appearing in January, 1857. This journal was followed by a considerable number of independent journals published in various parts of the United States, particularly in drug centers such as New York, Boston, Philadelphia, Baltimore, Detroit, Chicago and Cincinnati.[55] Some appealed to a national audience; others were only regional in

†Based in part on J.A.Ph.A. (Sci. Ed.) *32*:313, 1943.

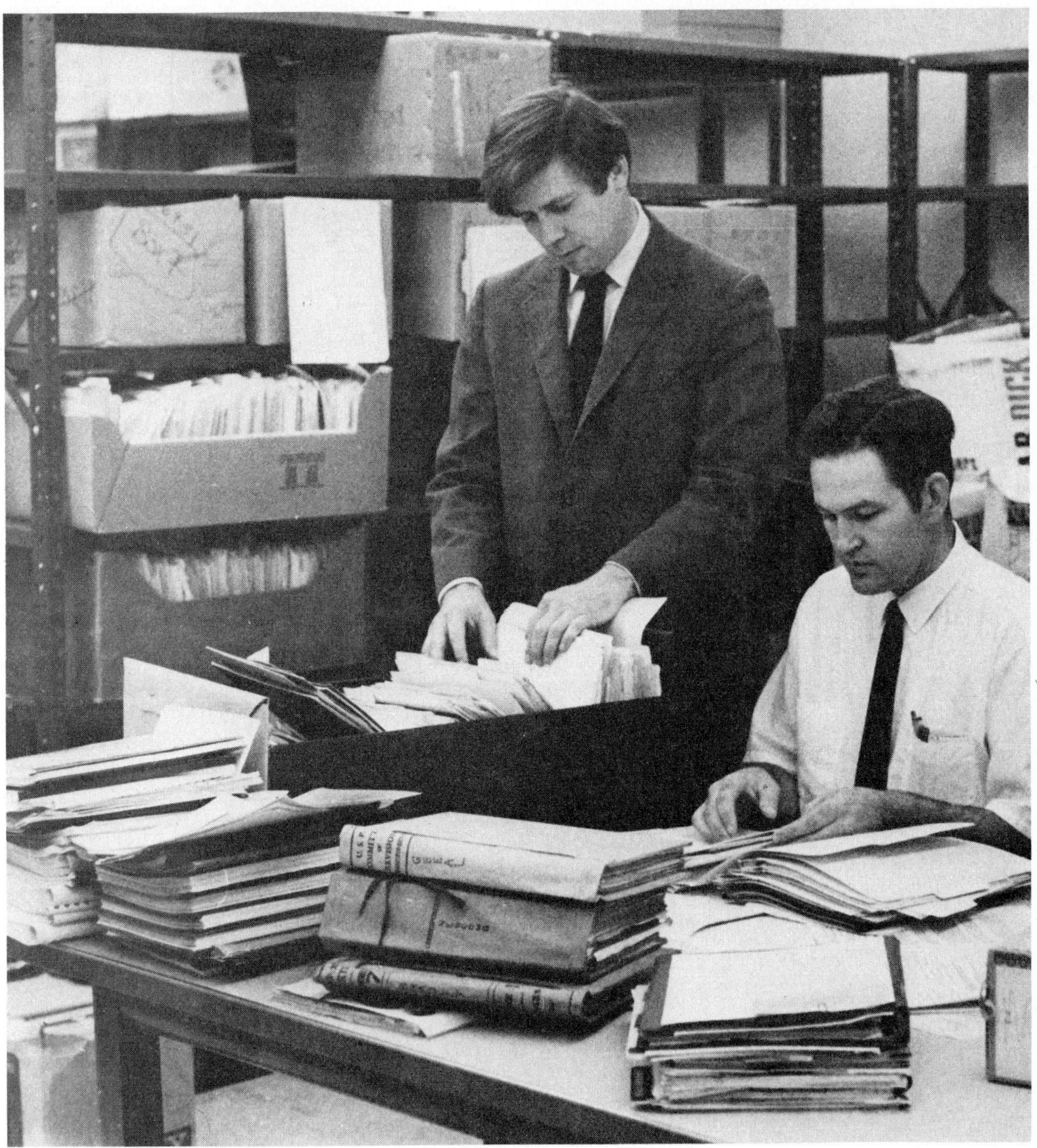

Supplementing printed publications are manuscript records of important persons and institutions that are preserved as sources for the history of pharmacy in depositories of various countries. Here, processing begins (1970) on the initial deposits of the American Institute of the History of Pharmacy Collection, as a cooperative project with the Division of Archives and Manuscripts of the State Historical Society of Wisconsin (F. Gerald Ham, chief archivist at left). (From: American Institute of the History of Pharmacy.)

scope[56] and came to be, as a class, relatively less prominent in pharmaceutical journalism of the late 20th century.

The position of *The Druggist's Circular* (1857–1940) in American pharmacy (at least until the death of its second owner and publisher, Vandeveer Newton, in 1880) cannot be indicated better than by the fact that Frederick Hoffmann rated it on the same level with the *American Journal of Pharmacy.* He stated that *The Druggist's Circular* differed from the *American Journal of Pharmacy*, but that among the earlier American pharmaceutical periodicals these two "will ever prominently stand forth as models of their kind at their time."[57] A journal of the same type and of like merits was the *Pharmaceutical Era* (1887–1933).

One of the most characteristic features of the American pharmaceutical press has been the incessant sequence of mergers and of changes in title, purpose and outer appearance. In the peculiar development of independent American pharmaceutical journalism, why was the dissemination of scientific-professional information left almost entirely to a few association journals and to one or two house organs published by pharmaceutical manufacturers? This cannot be explained entirely in terms of the general trend toward commercializing the entire field of human activity. More probably the journalistic stress on dollar appeal and entertainment value could be explained only by a more careful study of the tangled growth of independent journals and their influence. However, among influences at work can be inferred the effects of a further commercialization of thought and activities among the readers themselves; of more publishers competing to attract reader attention, and hence advertising dollars, by whatever means; and of editors who often were more at home dealing with the world of business than that of pharmacy.

A striking example of this development is *The American Druggist*. The first number of a publication then called *New Remedies, a Quarterly Retrospect of Therapeutics, Pharmacy and Allied Subjects* appeared (1871) under the editorship of the physician Horatio C. Wood, who was succeeded (1873) by another physician, Frederick A. Castle. The subtitle of *New Remedies* was changed (1876) to *A Monthly Trade Journal of Materia Medica, Pharmacy and Therapeutics,* and a pharmacist, Charles Rice became associate editor. The transformation from a predominantly medical journal to a pharmaceutical journal found expression (1884) in a further change of title. It now became the *American Druggist, an Illustrated Monthly Journal of Pharmacy, Chemistry, and Materia Medica* (the word "Trade" disappearing). Pharmacy now took the first place, with the intention of making the magazine representative of American pharmacy as a whole, including the allied sciences, and of putting it on a strictly professional footing.[58] After Rice died (1891) another pharmacist, Caswell A. Mayo, was made editor-in-chief. He changed the title to *American Druggist, a Journal of Practical Pharmacy,* thus expressing the intent to cultivate more the "practical" than the theoretical side of the calling. The *American Druggist* and the *Pharmaceutical Record* then consolidated (1893) under the title *American Druggist and Pharmaceutical Record,* the subtitle remaining unchanged. In 1923 the reference to the *Pharmaceutical Record* was dropped. Under a new proprietorship and editorship, the subtitle was changed (1927) to *The Pharmaceutical Business Paper* ("*Paper*" was replaced by "*Magazine,*" 1931, and 2 years later the subtitle disappeared entirely). By this time the paper had in fact become a typical magazine, a clever blend of features on business, professional and cultural aspects of pharmacy, besides some frankly for entertainment. This format of a popular magazine was carried through the 1940's under a succession of editors, mostly nonpharmacists. With Volume 125 (1952), *American Druggist* abandoned its staple, the popularized feature-length article, to become a pharmaceutical news magazine whose further commercialization was reflected in a change of title (1973) to *American Druggist Merchandising. American Druggist* had become directly competitive with the independent tabloid, *Drug Topics* (which began, 1884, as a house organ of McKesson & Robbins). The place accorded *Drug Topics* among independent pharmacists, which had been enhanced by its late chief editor, Robert L. Swain (1939–1960), attracted further competition with the founding (1961–1968) of another tabloid, *Drug News Weekly.*

Insofar as most such journals dealt with scientific progress in pharmacy and allied callings, an increased emphasis can be discerned toward mid-century on reporting scientific news, in contrast with evaluative, documented discussions of drugs and dosage forms. The case history of *American Druggist* (outlined above) illustrates this change, but it is even more striking in the history of the *American Professional Pharmacist.* Founded (1934) as an exponent of the movement of a segment of American pharmacies toward more strictly professional activity, this professional independent journal heavily stressed documented review articles on drugs and classes of drugs. Then, especially after a change of editors (1961), the *American Professional Pharmacist* turned sharply in the direction of capsule commentaries and semi-popularized digests and since 1969 has been titled *Pharmacy Times.*

This exemplified a seemingly anomalous circumstance of the 1960's: With an entire profession educated as specialists in the field of drugs, there was no longer a specialized journal, widely circulated among community pharmacists, that devoted itself mainly to professional and impartial discussion of drugs. However, *Drug Intelligence and Clinical Pharmacy* (founded 1967 by Donald E. Francke) appeared to have that potential, exemplifying as it did the American pharmacist's goal by the 1960's of a clinical orientation for the practice of pharmacy.

In the field of pharmaceutical research, an independent publisher launched (1959) the *Journal of Medicinal and Pharmaceutical Chemistry* (deleting "Pharmaceutical" from the title in 1963). Also, *Lloydia* (f. 1938) could justify a change of subtitle (1961) to "a quarterly journal of pharmacognosy and allied biological sciences."

Yet, perhaps no journal after mid-century was dealing with the application of science and technology at the community level of the health professions as well as did, in an earlier period, an American review journal called *Pharmazeutische Rundschau*, a journal that testified both to the level and the number of pharmacists who were from German immigrant families (founded by Frederick Hoffmann, 1882, in German until 1896, then in English as the *Pharmaceutical Review*).[59]

While the *Pharmazeutische Rundschau* was notable for its content, it was only one of various foreign-language journals published here,[60] one pharmaceutical reflection of the American "melting pot," especially before World War I.

The fact that many 19th-century practitioners provided both medical and pharmaceutical services created a market for journals covering both fields. Perhaps the earliest was the *American Lancet,* which began as the *Detroit Review of Medicine and Pharmacy* (1866–1876). As the health field in America matured and medicine and pharmacy more clearly separated, these journals also changed.[61]

An analogous change occurred in publications devoted to the wholesale trade in drugs, which sometimes were transformed into journals for practicing pharmacists, as a national network of pharmacies appeared and dispensing associated with wholesale houses disappeared. Consolidations also took place between journals of both types. The history of the *Oil, Paint and Drug Reporter,* once called by H. C. Kassner the "leading journal for manufacturers of drugs and pharmaceuticals and for wholesale distributors," is instructive in this respect. The paper (founded 1871) absorbed (1883) the *Oil, Paint & Drug Review* and (1885) the

*Weekly Drug News* (which in turn had consolidated [1883] with the *American Pharmacist* [f. 1882]). Since then it absorbed the journals *Drug, Paint and Oil Trade, New York Drug Bulletin, New York Druggist's Price Current, Soap Maker's Journal* and *International Petroleum Reporter.*[62] Since 1972 it has continued under the title *Chemical Marketing Reporter.*

In the field of pharmaceutical manufacturing, importance has been gained by *Drug and Cosmetic Industry*, started (1914) under the title *Weekly Drug Markets* (changed to *Drug and Chemicals Market* in 1916). After the journal was split into two separate periodicals (1926), *Chemical Markets* and *Drug Markets*, the latter was converted into the elegant and substantial *Drug and Cosmetic Industry* (1932). *Drug Trade News* (1925–1972), a trade newspaper, once held much the same position in the manufacturing field that its sister publication, *Drug Topics,* gained in the retail field.[63]

The general trend of independent pharmaceutical journalism in the United States has manifested itself in "trade" papers resembling magazines or newspapers, not only in their formats but also in their endeavor to devote themselves to the presumptive surface interests of their readers, stressing breadth of coverage rather than depth.

Striking features of American pharmaceutical journalism are the almost confusing abundance of the journals—of which only a few illustrative examples have been mentioned here—and the incessant changes they have undergone. A current list of national periodicals in, or directly related to, the pharmaceutical field is included annually in the *Pharmaceutical Directory* of the American Pharmaceutical Association (in 1975 numbering 45 titles, including 12 newsletters).

## Some 19th-Century Commentaries on Drugs

Books of similar character, but of less lasting influence than the dispensatories discussed in the main text are mentioned here for their reference interest. In their time they played a part in the evolving picture of American medical care. Failing to adjust to needs of new times, these publications have long since been discontinued.

One early volume of this kind was an American edition of Nicholas Culpeper's *Pharmacopoeia Londinensis or the London Dispensatory* (Boston, 1720).[64] It was well adapted to self-medication in a country where trained medical assistance was usually remote. More widely circulated and of greater professional influence were at least five different American versions of the *Edinburgh New Dispensatory* that appeared here between 1791 and 1818,[65] a work we noted had also formed the basis for Coxe's first *American Dispensatory* (1806). A more modest venture in the same direction was an American printing of Robert Graves' *Pocket Conspectus of the London and Edinburgh Pharmacopoeias* (Philadelphia, 1803). Another British book (Squire's *Companion to the British Pharmacopoeia*) quite possibly suggested a similar work to the Americans Oscar Oldberg and Otto Wall when the radically changed sixth revision of the U. S. *Pharmacopeia* appeared. The result was a *Companion to the United States Pharmacopoeia* (1884). Unlike its perennial British counterpart, this *Companion* went into only one more edition (1887).

These dispensatories and related commentaries all served the regular ranks of medicine and pharmacy. One of the more significant books that expressed the pharmaceutical views of a large clan of irregulars was the *American Dispensatory* (1852) edited by two physicians, John King and Robert S. Newton. They represented the "Eclectic" school of medical thought, a more modern and less dogmatic descendant of the American botanicomedical movement of the first half of the 19th century (see p. 174). King's *American Dispensatory* was, more precisely, a specialized formulary and commentary of eclectic drugs (not based on any pharmacopeia), but showed the character typical of the English and the American dispensatories. The book underwent four revisions, the rest of the 19 editions up to 1909 being mainly reprints. The demise of King's *American Dispensatory* reflected the decline of "eclecticism" as a self-conscious, separate segment of American medicine.[66]

Some 19th-century dispensatories were edited with the needs of physicians primarily in view. Illustrative of this class of dispensatories are a *Treatise on the Materia Medica* (1822; by Jacob Bigelow, author of the botanic part of the then new *U. S. Pharmacopeia*); *Dispensatory and Therapeutical Remembrancer* (1848, American version of the 2nd English edition, by John Mayne); *Dispensatory* (1848), American edition by R. Eglesfield Griffith of the English *Dispensatory* of Robert Christison, based on Duncan); and *The Dispensatory and Pharmacopoeia of North America and Great Britain* (1878; by John Buchanan and John F. Suggins).

# Appendix 7
# Glossary

**These pharmaco-historical notes are supplementary to topics of the text and not intended to be encyclopedic.**

**Aabel,** Bernard (1907–1968), American pharmacist who practiced in community pharmacies (1932–1941), then devoted his career to military and diplomatic posts. Col. Aabel rose to become Chief of the Army's Medical Service Corps (1955–1959), which included 64 allied medical and military specialties; then, after two years in the CIA, became Director of the A.M.A.'s International Health Department (1962–1968).

**Abbott,** Wallace Calvin (1857–1921), physician and founder of the Abbott Laboratories. See J.A.Ph.A. *10*:559, 1921.

**Abulcasis** or Abū al-Qāsim (ca. 936–ca. 1013), Arabic physician living in or near Cordova, Spain, whose 30-treatise encyclopedia (al-Tasrīf) conveyed much about Islamic pharmacy to Southern Europe. See S. K. Hamarneh and G. Sonnedecker: *A Pharmaceutical View of Abulcasis al-Zahrāwī in Moorish Spain* (Leiden, 1963).

**Alexander Trallianus** (525–605). The cognomen Trallianus refers to this Roman physician's native town of Tralles in Lydia. He wrote in Greek a *Materia medica* in 12 volumes.

**Allen,** William (1770–1843), English pharmacist, who became a well-known chemist. Allen was one of the leading English Quakers and a philanthropist of international importance. See E. C. Cripps: *Plough Court*, p. 25, London, 1927.

***Almanach oder Taschenbuch für Scheidekuenstler und Apotheker*** (1780–1829), one of the earliest serial publications directed particularly to pharmacists. Its title was changed in 1820 to *Trommsdorff's Almanach oder Taschenbuch für Chemiker und Apotheker,* and in 1822 to *Taschenbuch für Scheidekuenstler und Apotheker.* A French annual founded in the same year (1780) was the *Calendrier à l'usage du collège de pharmacie.*

**Anepu,** the apothecary of the Egyptian gods. He was considered the son of Isis and Osiris.

**Animal drugs.** Animal parts have always been used for medicinal purposes and folk medicine. Their bizarre use reached its climax in Joh. Jacob Wecker's *Antidotarium generale* (Basle, 1553) and in the *Neuvermehrte heylsame Dreckapotheke,* i.e., the newly augmented salutary dungpharmacy, by the German physician Franz Christian Paullini (1696 and reissued several times). See, e.g., L. Winkler: Animalia als Arzneimittel einst und jetzt. Innsbruck, 1908. 92 pp. and B. Hjalmar: Die Tierwelt in Heilkunde und Drogenkunde. . . . Berlin, 1925. 90 pp.

*Antidotarium.* See: **Pharmacopeia.**

**Apollo.** God of healing as well as of youth and beauty, of poetry and music, and of the wisdom of oracles. Gradually, he became identified with the sun god, Helios, and was considered the son of Zeus. Apollo was the first Greek deity to find a place in Roman religion, chiefly as a god of healing. See Ch. Kerényi: *Le médecin divin*, Basle, ca. 1948.

***Apotheca.*** Latinized form of *Apotheke, q.v.* During Roman antiquity it was commonly applied to the storage room for wine. Galen differentiated between his *apotheca* or storeroom and his *iatron, q.v.*, the room in which he saw his patients. The Roman *apotheca librorum* corresponds to our library or storage room for books. In the Middle Ages the term was more or less restricted to storerooms for spices and drugs, and thus the German *Apotheke, q.v.*, and the French *apothicairerie, q.v.*, came into general use. The French equivalent was replaced by *pharmacie, q.v.*, toward the close of the 18th century.

***Apothecarius,*** from Latin *apotheca, q.v.*, "storage room," and *-arius*, "pertaining to," literally the person in charge of a storage room. In terms of pharmacy, it came to refer to the person in charge of drugs and spices. See French *apothicaire*, English *apothecary*, and German *Apotheker* (spelled variously in different Germanic countries and at different times).

**Apothecary,** anglicized form of *apothecarius, q.v.* In England the designation became restricted to a combination medical-pharmaceutical practitioner after the middle of the 18th century.

**Apothecary shop,** outmoded English term for a pharmacy. See **Apotheca.**

***Apotheke,*** the Germanized form of the Latin *apotheca, q.v.* During the Middle Ages the name was applied to the German apothecary's establishment. French *apothicairerie, q.v.* and *boutique, q.v.*, Italian *botica, q.v.*, Spanish *botega*, English "apothecary shop," *q.v.*, and "pharmacy," *q.v.* The word also occurs in several forms of book titles and in various combinations, e.g. *Hausapotheke* ("medicine chest"), *Militarapotheke* ("regimental medicine chest"), and figuratively in *Seelenapotheke* ("medicine chest for the soul").

***Apotheker.*** German form of *apothecarius, q.v.* In Germany it is still the official designation of the pharmaceutical practitioner as opposed to the *Drogist, q.v.*

***Apothicaire.*** French form of *apothecarius, q.v.* At the close of the 18th century the word was replaced officially by *pharmacien, q.v.*

***Apothicairerie.*** Old French form for "pharmacy." See: ***Apotheca.***

***Apotteck.*** See: **Pharmacopeia.**

**Apple,** William S. (1918– ), executive director of the American Pharmaceutical Association since 1959 (Assistant Secretary, 1958); second American to hold Vice Presidency (1974– ) of International Pharmaceutical Federation; noted for advocacy of progressive professionalization of community pharmacy and pharmaceutical reforms. At the University of Wisconsin, Apple helped to develop the field of pharmacy administration (1952–58); and he himself earned the first Ph.D. awarded there in that specialty. *(Who's Who in America.)*

**Apprentice.** See: **Personnel.**

**Apuleius,** Lucius, or Pseudo–Apuleius, a late Roman medical author of uncertain identity (4th or 5th century A.D.), whose famous herbal introduced South-European medicinal plants to the English.

***Aquae aromaticae.*** In contrast to *aquae minerales* and other aqueous solutions (cf: **Spiritus aromatici**), the aromatic waters (aromatic spirits) were aqueous distillates of aromatic plants. Compare *Eaux des plantes odorantes* with *Eaux des plantes inodorantes* (in A. Baumé, *Elémens de pharmacie*). Rose water played an important role in Persian commerce as early as the 9th century, not only as a perfume but for the preparation of medicaments. Arnaldus de Villanova (died 1311) was important in introducing products of distillation into European therapy. Distillation and the products obtained thereby became so important that a new type of medicopharmaceutical treatise, the *Destillierbücher* ("books on distillation"), appeared. For

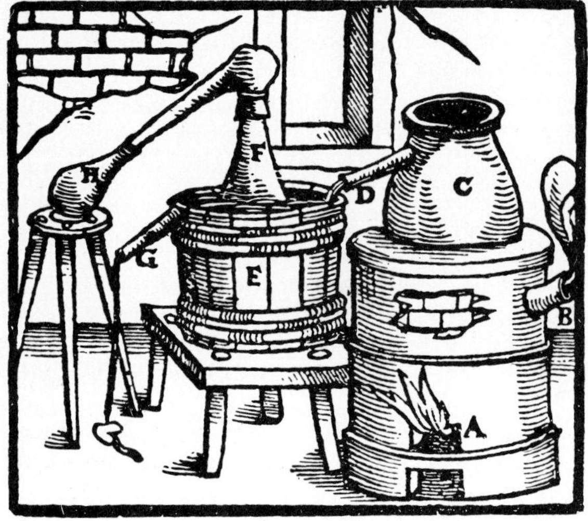


details see Gildemeister, Hoffman and Kremers: *The Volatile Oils, 1*:13, 1900. In modern pharmaceutical practice aromatic waters, for the most part, no longer are made by distillation, but by solution of volatile oils in water. For perfumery, however, such aromatic waters as rose water and orange flower water are still made by distillation.

**Archambault,** George F. (1909– ), distinguished hospital pharmacist, lawyer, teacher, editor, consultant. Commanding pharmacist, U.S. Public Health Service, 1947–1967); Editor, *Hospital Formulary Management,* 1967– . See *Who's Who in America.*

**Arny,** Henry V. (1868–1943), completed his scientific education in Germany; editor, author, professor and dean at the New York College of Pharmacy, 1911 to 1936. See *N.Y. State Pharm. 10*:9, 1936.

***Aromatarius,*** pl. ***-i,*** from Latin *aroma* ("spice"), and *-arius,* "pertaining to," i.e., dealer in spices.

**Aromatic waters.** See: ***Aquae aromaticae.***

***Asclepios,*** whose Egyptian antecedent was Imhotep, *q.v.* A culture hero considered to be a physician (Homer), he later became the Greek god of medicine and healing. The chief seat of his worship was Epidauros. His many sanctuaries not only were places of worship, but also centers of miracle-medicine. In Greek mythology Asclepios is the son of Apollo. The Romans also worshiped him, frequently with his daughter Hygieia as the god of health, calling him Aesculapius or Asklepias. See Edlestein, E. J., and L.: *Asculepius, A Collection and Interpretation of the Testimonies,* Baltimore, 1947.

**Assistant.** See: **Personnel.**

**Assistant pharmacist.** A subordinate class of practitioners common in late 19th-century America, which (because of lax practices) were being licensed by only a few states by the mid-20th century.

**Assyria.** During the era of its greatest expanse, ancient Assyria comprised the territory between the Euphrates and the mountain slopes east of the Tigris. At one time, during the reign of Ashurbanipal (668–626 B.C.), it extended to the Nile. Its history can be traced back to about 2300 B.C. Its civilization was borrowed almost wholly from Babylonia *(q.v.).*

**Atkins,** Henry (1558–1635), physician-in-ordinary to the English King James I. It was under the presidency of Atkins that the London College of Physicians issued the first *London Pharmacopoeia.* See *Dictionary of* (English) *National Biography, II*:220.

**Attfield,** John (1835–1911), English pharmacist, professor at the Pharmacy School of the Pharmaceutical Society of Great Britain and author of a textbook that was widely used in the United States as well as in England. See *Am. J. Pharm. 78*:102, 1906; Jos. P. Remington: *J.A.Ph.A. I*:490, 1912.

**Avenzoar,** or Abū Marwān Ibn Zuhr (1113–1162). A Spanish-Arabic medical author called by Sarton "the most famous physician of his time, not only among Muslims, but in Christendom." See George Sarton: *Introduction to the History of Science,* vol. 2, pp. 231–234, Baltimore, 1931.

**Avicenna,** or Abu 'Ali al Husain ibn 'Abdallah ibn Sina (980–1037), the most famous and the most influential Persian-Arabic physician of the classical period of Arabian (or Greco-Arabic) medicine. See W. E. Gohlman (ed. & trans.): *The Life of Ibn Sina,* Albany, N.Y., 1974; Soheil, M. A.: Avicenna, His Life and Work, London, 1957; and Wickens, G. M.: Avicenna: Scientist and Philosopher, London, 1952.

**Babylonia.** In the time of her highest glory (6th century B.C.), Babylonia extended from the Euphrates valley into Asia Minor and Egypt. It was a center of the world's commerce and of the arts and sciences. Its language can be traced back to about 3500 B.C. See L. Delaporte: *Mesopotamia, the Babylon and Assyrian Civilization,* London, 1925.

**Bache,** Franklin (1792–1864), physician; professor of chemistry at the Philadelphia College of Pharmacy and later at Jefferson Medical College; co-author of the *United States Dispensatory.* See J. W. England: *First Century of the Philadelphia College of Pharmacy,* p. 399, Philadelphia, 1922.

**Baitâr,** Ibn al (1197–1248), Spanish-Arabic medical author, physician-in-ordinary to the ruler of Egypt. See Tschirch: *Handbuch der Pharmakognosie,* vol. 1, Part 2, p. 600, Leipzig, 1910; George Sarton: *Introduction to the History of Science,* vol. 2, part 2, pp. 663–664, Baltimore, 1931.

**Balard,** Antoine Jérome (1802–1876), French pharmacist. He discovered bromine (from the Greek *bromos* = "stench") in the salt brine of the Mediterranean (1826). Of his further discoveries, that of amyl nitrite (1844) is noteworthy. See *Am. J. Pharm. 48*:287, 1876, and *Figures Pharmaceutiques Francaises,* pp. 89–94, Paris, 1953.

**Barton,** Benjamin Smith (1776–1815), American botanist and professor at the University of Pennsylvania. See *Bull. Lloyd Lib., 1,* 1900.

**Bartram,** John (1699–1777), American botanist. At Kingsessing he founded the first botanic garden in America. Linné termed him "the greatest natural botanist in the world." See *Am. J. Pharm. 80*:416, 1908; *Dictionary of American Biography, II,* p. 26.

**Bartram,** Moses (1732–1809), son of the famous botanist Bartram, *q.v.*, and pharmacist in Philadelphia. See Edward Kremers: "Two invoices of 1785," *J.A.Ph.A. 20*:691, 1931.

**Bastedo,** Walter A. (1874–1952), pharmacist, physician, professor of clinical medicine at Columbia University, president of the U.S. Pharmacopoeial Convention, 1930. See *J.A.Ph.A. 20*:199, 1931.

**Bastin,** Edson T. (1843–1897), started as a pharmacist in Chicago; became a teacher of botany and of materia medica, Northwestern College of Pharmacy and Philadelphia College of Pharmacy. See *Proc. A.Ph.A. 45*:32, 1897; England: *First Century of the Philadelphia College of Pharmacy,* p. 413, Philadelphia, 1922.

**Bate,** George (1608–1669), physician-in-ordinary to the English Kings Charles I and Charles II and to the Lord Protector Cromwell. His formulae were published by a London apothecary, J. Shipton, under the title: *Bate's Dispensatory,* or *Pharmacopoeia Bateana.* See *Dictionary* (English) *Natl. Biog., III, p.* 390.

**Bauhin,** Caspar, professor of anatomy and botany at the University of Basle, Switzerland (1560–1624), one of the most learned botanists of all time. His book, *Prodromus theatri botanici,* in which he describes about 6,000 plants arranged according to a kind of natural system, represents the best dictionary of botanic nomenclature of his period.

**Baumé,** Antoine (1728–1804). Baumé is among the important French pharmacist-chemists of the 18th century, who simultaneously enriched pharmacy and chemistry. He introduced the hydrometer (Baumé's degrees), improved the process of distillation and gave in his *Elémens de pharmacie théorique et pratique* a comprehensive description of pharmaceutical apparatus and manipulation, and manufactured many chemicals and galenics on a large scale.

**Bayen,** Pierre (1725–1798), French pharmacist. In 1774 Bayen published his observations on the "escape" of "*un fluide élastique*" (i.e., an air) when heating mercuric oxide. He is therefore supposed to have discovered oxygen before Scheele or Priestly, without, however, recognizing the importance of his discovery.

**Beach,** Wooster (1794–1868) founded the American "reformed school of medicine," which later on merged into the eclectic school. Beach's book, *The American Practice of Medicine*, was recognized all over the world as the standard work of the new movement. See A. Wilder: *History of Medicine,* p. 437, New Sharon, 1901; *Dictionary of American Biography, II* p. 85.

**Beal,** George D. (1887–1972), graduate in pharmacy and chemist, who made distinguished contributions in organized American pharmacy, especially through the American Pharmaceutical Association and U.S. Pharmacopeia. In the Mellon Institute for Industrial Research, Dr. Beal served as Assistant Director (1926–1951) and Director (1951–1958).

**Beal,** James Hartley (1861–1945), pharmacist, lawyer, educator and writer. The personality and the ideas of J. H. Beal were of great influence on the development of American pharmacy. See J. A. Koch, American contemporaries, *Industrial and Engineering Chemistry*, News Edition *13*:352, 1935.

**Becher,** Johann Joachim (1635–1682), chemist, polyhistorian, author and physician-in-ordinary to the elector of Bavaria. He was the first to determine the increase in weight after oxidation (calcination of lead). His mentioning of a principle of combustion inherent in all combustible substances laid the foundation of the phlogiston theory of Stahl, *q.v.*

**Beckmann,** Ernst Otto (1853–1923), pharmacist and professor of pharmaceutical chemistry at the University of Leipzig. His main work and merit lay in the field of physical chemistry. His apparatus for determination of the lowering of the freezing point and of the raising of the boiling point became indispensable tools in chemistry.

**Bedford,** Peter W. (1836–1892), New York pharmacist and (after 1873) professor at the New York College of Pharmacy; also editor of the *Pharm. Record.* See *Drug. Circ. 51*:82, 1907.

**Behring,** Emil von (1854–1917), German physician and academic teacher of hygiene in Marburg; inaugurator of serum therapy. See Sigerist: *The Great Doctors,* p. 372, New York, 1933.

**Bendiner,** Samuel J., Hungarian-born pharmacist in New York (1839–1897). See *Proc. A.Ph.A. 45*:33, 1897.

**Benger,** Frederick Baden (1840–1903), English pharmacist and manufacturer. See *Pharm. J. 70*:145, 179, 1903.

**Berendes,** Julius. German pharmacist and pharmaceutical historian (1836–1914). Berendes' most important books are *Das Apothekenwesen,* especially devoted to German pharmacy, and *Die Pharmacie bei den alten Kulturvölkern* (pharmacy during antiquity). He also translated the *Materia medica* of Dioscorides and the *Seven Books of Paulus Aegineta,* from Latin and Greek texts into German. See Häfliger: Biographicon in Tschirch's *Handbuch der Pharmakognosie,* Leipzig, 1932.

**Bernard,** Claude (1813–1878), French physiologist. Bernard began his scientific career as an apprentice to a pharmacist, and later studied medicine at Paris. His important physiological researches include the elucidation of the role of the pancreas in digestion, the discovery of the glycogenetic function of the liver, the recognition of the importance of the sympathetic nervous system in the regulation of metabolism, and the explanation of the mode of action of curare and carbon monoxide. See *Dictionary Scient. Biog.*; J. M. D. Olmsted: *Claude Bernard,*

*Physiologist,* New York, 1938; F. L. Holmes: *Claude Bernard and Animal Chemistry,* Cambridge, Mass., 1974.

**Berzelius,** Johann (Joens) Jacob (1779–1848), Swedish physician and one of the greatest chemists. He is the founder of the modern chemical nomenclature and was the first to observe and to describe isomorphism, polymorphism and allotrophy. An interesting controversy respecting nomenclature between Robert Hare of the University of Pennsylvania and Berzelius may be found in the *Am. J. Pharm. 9*:1, 1837. See Soederbaum: *Joens Jacob Berzelius* (biographical notes) English trans. by O. Larsell, Baltimore, 1934; George Urdang: Berzelius and pharmacy, *J.A.Ph.A. 37*:481–485, 1948.

**Besler,** Basilius, German pharmacist and botanist (1561–1629). His *Hortus Eystettensis* was one of the first botanic works to make use of copper etchings rather than woodcuts.

**Bevan,** Silvanus and Timothy, London wholesale druggist and apothecary. Silvanus Bevan (1691–1765) founded the establishment in 1715 and entered partnership with his brother Timothy between 1731–1736. This firm later became Allen and Howard; Allen, Hanburys and Barry; and, finally, Allen and Hanburys, Ltd., London. See E. C. Cripps, *Plough Court,* London, 1927; and D. Chapman-Huston and E. C. Cripps, *Through a City Archway,* London, 1954.

**Bibliography.** References have been given in the "Notes and References" to each chapter, of the text itself, and in Appendix 6. Unlike the latter, the following bibliographic note emphasizes keys to finding *secondary* sources related to pharmaceutical history (although not exclusively):

Glenn Sonnedecker, J. H. Hoch, and W. Schneider: *Some Pharmaco-Historical Guidelines to the Literature,* Madison, Wis., 1959 (also in *Am. J. Pharm. Ed. 23*:143–172, 1959); *Index-Catalogue of the Library of the Surgeon-General's Office, U. S. Army,* 1880–1936 four series; E.-H. Guitard, *Manuel d'Histoire de la Littérature pharmaceutique,* Paris, 1942 (see also *Revue d'Histoire de la Pharmacie* for this and other rich bibliographic material); *Current Work in the History of Medicine* (quarterly since 1954); *Bibliography of the History of Medicine* [and pharmacy] *of the United States and Canada, 1939–1960,* ed. G. Miller, Baltimore, ca. 1964 (cumulated from *Bull. Hist. Med.*); *Bibliography of the History of Medicine 1964–1969,* Bethesda, Maryland, ca. 1972, 1475 pp. (includes pharmacy; annual supplements of same title from National Library of Medicine); "Critical Bibliography" (including pharmacy) of *Isis* (99th in 1974; cumulative index in press); Glenn Sonnedecker and Alex Berman: *Some Bibliographic Aids for Historical Writers in Pharmacy,* Madison, Wis., 1958; David L. Cowen: *America's Pre-Pharmacopoeial Literature,* Madison, Wis., 1961; George Sarton: *Horus; A Guide to the History of Science,* Waltham, Mass., 1952; George Sarton: *Introduction to the History of Science,* Baltimore, 1927–1947; H. C. Bolton: *Chemical Bibliography,* Smithsonian Institution, Washington, D.C.; J. C. Poggendorff: *Biographischliterarisches Handwörterbuch zur Geschichte der exakten Wissenschaften,* Leipzig, 1863–; H. Schelenz: *Geschichte der Pharmazie,* Berlin, 1904; John Ferguson: *Bibliotheca chemica,* 1906; J. A. Häfliger: Biographikon, in Tschirch's *Handbuch der Pharmakognosie,* Leipzig, 1932; Adlung and Urdang; *Grundriss der Geschichte der deutschen Pharmazie,* Berlin, 1935; F. Ferchl: *Bio-und Bibliographikon,* Mittenwald, 1937; *Chemical, Medical and Pharmaceutical Books Printed Before 1800; In the Collections of the University of Wisconsin Libraries,* ed. John Neu, Madison, 1965, 280 pp. (a bibliography, dated but still useful); R. B. Austin, *Early American Medical Imprints; A Guide to Works Printed in the United States 1668–1820,* Washington, D.C., 1961, 240 pp. G. B. Griffenhagen and E. W. Stieb: *Tools of the Apothecary: A Selective Bibliography,* Madison, 1975; D. L. Cowen: *A Bibliography on the History of Colonial and Revolutionary Medicine and Pharmacy,* Madison, 1975; E.-H. Guitard: *Index des travaux d'histoire de la pharmacie de 1913 á 1963,* Paris, ca. 1968; G. B. Griffenhagen: *Bibliography of Papers Published by the American Pharmaceutical Association That Were Presented Before the Association's Section on Historical Pharmacy, 1904–1957,* Madison, 1958; *Pharmaziegeschichtliche Rundschau* (supplements to *Pharm. Ztg.;* compiled by G. Dann, 1954 to date); G. Mann, ed.: *Internationale Bibliographie zur Geschichte der Medizin 1871–1901,* Hildesheim–New York, 1970 (reprints 6 works in 1 vol.); W. Artelt, ed.: *Index zur Geschichte der Medizin, Naturwissenschaft und Technik,* Munich/Berlin, 1953; J. Steudel et al.: *Index zur Geschichte der Medizin und Biologie,* 1949–1952, Munich, 1966.

**Bigelow,** Jacob (1787–1879), physician in Boston, professor of materia medica at Harvard, a great educational reformer and one of America's most learned botanists. See Kelly and Burrage: *American Medical Biographies,* p. 100, New York, 1920.

**Biroth,** Henry (1857–1912), German-born Chicago pharmacist, one of the leading pharmacists and chemists of the Northwest in his time. Biroth wrote on pharmaceutical and general subjects. See *J.A.Ph.A. I*:776, 1912.

**Bliven,** Charles A. (1911– ), first full-time Executive Secretary of the American Association of Colleges of Pharmacy, 1961–1974. He had taught at the U. of Nebraska (1936–1938) and at George Washington U. (1940, and dean from 1947 to 1962) (Melvin R. Gibson in Am. J. Pharm. Edu. *23*:499–502, 1959).

**Bobst,** Elmer Holmes (1884– ), pharmaco-industrial tycoon who began as Pennsylvania pharmacist. In 1911 Bobst became a "detail man" with the American branch of Hoffmann-LaRoche and advanced rapidly to become General Manager. In 1945 he began a second career as President of William R. Warner Co., engineering a series of mergers that by 1970 made Warner-Lambert "the world's largest manufacturer of health products." Philanthropist, confidant of USA Presidents, art collector. See E. H. Bobst: *Bobst, The Autobiography of a Pharmaceutical Pioneer,* New York, 1973.

**Bock,** Hieronymus (1498–1554), German cleric, physician, and botanist. His *New Kreuterbuch* (1539) became well known, especially for its excellent illustrations.

**Boë,** François de le. See: **Sylvius.**

**Boerhaave,** Hermann (1668–1738). Dutch physician and academic teacher of medicine and of chemistry in Leyden. His medical writings were read all over the world, and his *Elementa chemiae* (Leyden, 1732) is considered the best book on the subject in the first half of the 18th century. F. Garrison: *History of Medicine,* p. 261, Philadelphia, 1929; Sigerist: *The Great Doctors,* p. 185, New York, 1933.

**Boettger,** Johann Friedrich (1682–1719), pharmacist's assistant and alchemist. Assisted by E. Tschirnhaus, he invented process of production of European porcelain.

**Bois,** Jacques du (Latinized as Silvius or Sylvius; 1492–1552), French physician and academic teacher at the University of Paris. In his *Pharmacopoeae, libri tres* (1548), he was the first to use the term "Pharmacopoe[i]a" as the title for a formulary.

**Bond,** Thomas (1712–1784), Philadelphia physician and one of the founders of the Pennsylvania Hospital. See *Dictionary of American Biography 2,* p. 433.

**Boogaerdt** (Bogart), Herman Meynders (or Myndertz) van den (1612–1648), Dutch-American surgeon. See John Shrady: *New York Med. Register 25*:231, 1887.

***Botica.*** Italian form of the Latin *apotheca, q.v.* See: ***Apotheke.***

***Bottega.*** Spanish form of the Latin *apotheca, q.v.* See: ***Apotheke.***

***Boutique.*** French form of the Latin *apotheca, q.v.* See: ***Apotheke*** and ***Apothicairerie.***

***Bowditch,*** Henry I. (1808–1892), physician,

author and one of the leading spirits of the antislavery movement before the Civil War. See *Dictionary of American Biography* 2:492, 1929.

**Boyle,** Robert (1627–1687), Irish-English aristocrat, one of the earliest eminent English chemists, a founder of the Royal Society of Great Britain and director of the East India Company. Boyle is one of the originators of analysis by precipitation. His general chemical knowledge was far ahead of his time. He formulated Boyle's Law and introduced the terms "analysis," "reaction" and "reagent" into chemical language. *Dictionary of Scien. Biog.*

**Boylston,** Zabdiel (1679–1766), American-born medical practitioner, taught by his father, who likewise practiced medicine. Without academic study or a medical degree, he achieved a high reputation in his profession. See *Dictionary of American Biography, 2,* p. 535.

**Braillier,** Pierre (sixteenth century), French pharmacist. See L. André-Pontier: *Histoire de la pharmacie,* p. 210, Paris, 1900.

**Brandes,** Rudolph (1795–1842), German pharmacist. He initiated the *Apothekerverein im Noerdlichen Teutschland,* discovered delphinine and hyoscyamine (both in 1819), and wrote many books and essays.

**Breasted,** James Henry (1865–1935), the first American to specialize in ancient history, especially Egyptian. He became an international authority. His importance for pharmacy was two-fold: First, he started his career as a pharmacist, graduating from the Chicago College of Pharmacy (1886); and, secondly, he translated, annotated and published the Edwin Smith Papyrus. See John A. Wilson: James H. Breasted, National Academy of Sciences of the United States of America, *Biograph. Mem. XVIII,* p. 95, 1938; *Alumni Rec.,* University of Illinois, 1921, p. 346.

**Bridges,** Robert (1806–1882), physician and professor at the Philadelphia College of Pharmacy (1842 to 1879). See J. W. England: *First Century of the Philadelphia College of Pharmacy,* p. 401, Philadelphia, 1922.

**Briggs,** W. Paul (1903–), Commander U.S. N.R., 1942–1945; chief, Pharmacy Section, Bureau of Medicine and Surgery, U.S.N., 1948–51; chief, Pharmacy Service, Veterans Administration, 1946–1947; teacher and writer; Executive Director, American Foundation for Pharmaceutical Education, 1951–1973. Before entering government service, Briggs had served on the pharmacy faculty of George Washington University, 1927–46. *Am. Men of Science.*

**Brockedon,** William (1787–1854), a principal inventor of compressed tablets. See L. F. Kebler: The tablet industry. *J.A.Ph.A.* 3:820, 1914, and description below.

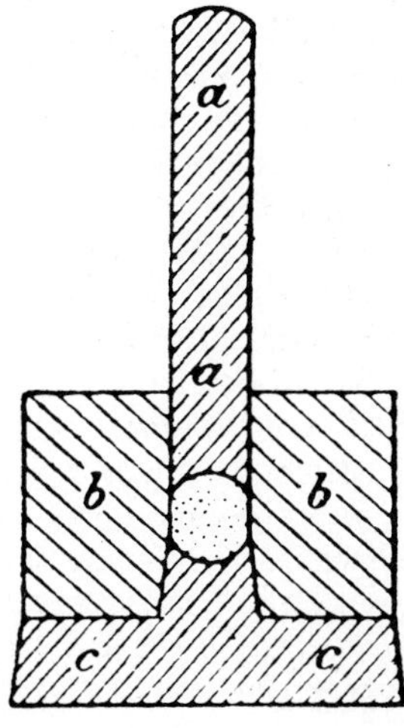


The compressed-tablet machine (1843) invented by an English watchmaker was hand operated and simple. First, the upper die *(a)* was removed and the lower die *(b, c)* was filled with powder by means of a patented measuring instrument. Then the upper die was reinserted and struck sharply with a mallet, thereby compressing the powder. The upper die was then removed to extract the tablet, and the process was repeated. A century after this invention, compressed tablets had become the most popular form of medication (about 1/3 of all American prescriptions). (See P. A. Foote: Tablets, Bull. Univ. Wis. No. 1566, Madison (1916?).)

**Brown,** John (1735–1788), Scottish physician. See F. Garrison: *History of Medicine,* p. 314, Philadelphia, 1929; Sigerist: *Man and Medicine,* p. 43, New York, 1932.

**Brown,** William (1752–1792), Scottish-born American physician, graduated at Edinburgh, of high professional and social standing. He wrote the so-called Lititz pharmacopoeia. See L. C. Duncan: *Medical Men in the American Revolution,* p. 240; Carlisle, 1931; John Kebler: *J.A.Ph.A. 16*:1090, 1927; *Badger Pharmac.* Nos. 22–25, 1938; *Dictionary of American Biography, III,* p. 157.

**Brown-Séquard,** Charles-Edouard (1817–1894). A native of Mauritius, he was chiefly associated with French medicine. He was professor of the Collège de France (1878) and in the Harvard and the Paris medical faculties. *Dictionary Scien. Biog.*

**Brunfels,** Otto (1500–1534), German cleric, physician and botanist. He not only wrote his famous botanic work, first in Latin as a *herbarium,* then in German as a *Kreuterbuch,* but also many other treatises. Among them was a dictionary of synonyms and his *Reformation de Apotecken,* published after his death in 1536. His *Reformation* presents an account of pharmaceutical duties and served as a guide to both pharmacist and government.

**Brunschwygk,** Hieronymus (also spelled Brunschwig, Brunschwyk, etc.; 1430–1512), German surgeon. His books on the art of distillation initiated a new period of pharmaceutical art. In addition, Brunschwygk wrote a *Thesaurus pauperum* (literally "treasury of the poor"), a popular medicine book designed for self-treatment.

**Buchner,** Johannes Andreas (1783–1852), German pharmacist and professor of pharmacy, first at the University of Landshut, later at Munich. He discovered salicine in willow bark, solanine in potato plant, berberine in Berberis, aesculin in ashtree bark, nicotine in tobacco, and also acrolein. Fron 1815 to 1852, Buchner edited the *Repertorium der Pharmacie.*

**Bulleyn** (also Bullein), William (d. 1576), English physician, botanist and rector of Blaxhall, Suffolk. See *Dictionary* (English) *National Biography, VII,* p. 244.

**Bullock,** Charles (1826–1900), Philadelphia pharmacist. See *Drug. Circ. 51*:82, 1907; *Proc. A.Ph.A. 48*:38, 1900.

**Burroughs,** Silas Maineville (1850–1895), American pharmacist and, together with Henry Wellcome, *q.v.,* founder of the English pharmaceutic firm of Burroughs, Wellcome and Company. See *Am. J. Pharm. 67*:433, 1895.

**Cadet de Gassicourt,** Charles Louis (1769–1821), French pharmacist. Of his books, *La chimie domestique* (8 volumes), *Pharmacie domestique* and his *Formulaire magistral et mémorial pharmaceutique* are noteworthy. See *Dictionary Scient. Biog.*

**Carney,** Charles T. (1832–1862), Boston pharmacist and teacher at the Massachusetts College of Pharmacy. See: *Drug. Circ. 51*:157, 1907.

**Carpenter,** Philo, Chicago's first pharmacist (about 1800–1850). See: Mrtek, M. B., et al., *Pharm. Hist. 12*:151–155, 1970; also, *Bull. Pharm. 16*:100, 1902.

**Caspari,** Charles J. (1850–1917), American pharmacist, professor at the Maryland College of Pharmacy and for 15 years general secretary of the American Pharmaceutical Association. See E. F. Kelly: *Am. J. Pharm. 89*:565, 1917.

**Cassebeer,** George A. (1817–1895), German-born and educated pharmacist of New York. See *Am. Drug. and Pharm. Rec. 27*:124, 1895.

**Caswell-Massey Co. Ltd.,** renowned pharmacy of New York City, has been referred to as "America's oldest pharmacy" because its pharmaceutical genealogy traces to an establishment founded in 1752 in Newport, Rhode Island. However, the pharmacy has had various locations and various owners. (Meras, P.: America's oldest apothecary shop, Providence (R.I.) Sunday Journal Magazine, n.d.; (ca. 1970), in Pharmaceutical Library, University of Wisconsin).

**Cataplasma,** Greek *kataplassein,* to spread over, hence a topical medication of gruel-like consistency.

**Catelan,** Laurent, pharmacist and lecturer at the University of Montpellier (16th and early 17th century). See J. A. Häfliger: *Das Apothekenwesen Basels,* p. 52, Mittenwald, 1938.

**Catesby,** Mark (1679–1749), English naturalist and artist, travelled 10 years in Southern North America and in the Bahama Islands, then wrote the books: *The Natural History of Carolina, Florida and the Bahama Islands,* and the *Hortus Britanniae Americanus.* See *Dictionary of American Biography, III,* p. 571.

**Caventou,** Joseph Bienaimé (1795–1877), French pharmacist and one of the earliest and most successful investigators of alkaloids. In collaboration with Pelletier, *q.v.,* he discovered strychnine (1818), brucine and, simultaneously with Meissner, veratrine (1819), quinine and, after Gomes, cinchonine (1820). Named chlorophyll (from Green *chloros* = light green and *phyllon* = leaf) for the green pigment of plants. Among his many publications was a textbook on pharmacy *(Traité élémentaire de pharmacie théorique). See Dictionary Scient. Biog.;* also *Am. J. Pharm. 49*:384, 1877.

**Chapman,** William Barker (1813–1874), Ph.G. and M.D., pharmacist in Cincinnati and professor of pharmacy in the Cincinnati College of Pharmacy. See G. Sonnedecker: *Am. J. Pharm. 126*:91–97, 1954; also *Am. J. Pharm. 46*:544, 1874; *Drug. Circ. 51*:82, 1907.

**Chaptal,** Jean Antoine Claude, Count of Chanteloup (1756–1832), French physician and chemist. His major field was chemical technology.

**Charas,** Moise, French pharmacist (1618–1698). His *Pharmacopée royale galenique et chymique* (1672) and other treatises (e.g., treacle and China bark) received much attention.

**Chiron.** A centaur (half man, half horse) in Greek mythology, who knew all mysteries, among them those of the art of healing, which he taught to Asclepios, *q.v.*

**Chemist.** Origin of the term, not undisputed, is assumed to be either the Arabic *Al-kimia* or the ancient name of the Egyptian country, *Kemi,* or the late Greek *chymeia.* "Chemist" as a designation for pharmaceutical practitioners is restricted primarily to the Anglo-Saxon world. Especially in the combination "chemist and druggist" (see: **Druggist**), it has become general since the early 19th century. After World War I, the chemists proper attempted to deprive pharmaceutical practitioners of the term "chemist" as their legal title, but attempts to introduce the designation "pharmacist" in Britain to replace "chemist" were not altogether successful. The designation "chemist's shop" for a pharmacy is common in England.

**Chemist and Druggist.** See: **Titles.**

**China.** On the early materia medica of the highly developed Chinese culture see especially the publications of Gottfried Schramm, e.g., in *Wissenschaft. Zeitschr. d. Karl-Marx Univ. Leipzig (Mathematisch-Naturwissensch. Reihe), 6*: Heft 5, pp. 481–503, and *Die Vorträge der Hauptversammlung der Internationalen Gesellschaft für Geschichte der Pharmazie,* Bd. 13, pp. 185–195, Eutin, 1958; A. Mosig and G. Schramm: *Der Arzneipflanzen und Drogenschatz Chinas and die Bedeutung des Pên-ts'ao kang-mu als Standardwerk der chinesischen Materia medica,* Berlin, 1955; also in H. Schelenz: *Geschichte der Pharmazie,* Berlin, 1904; I. Berendes: *Die Pharmazie bei den alten Kulturvölkern,* Halle, 1891; Tschirch: *Handbuch der Pharmakognosie,* Leipzig, 1910, *I,* Part 2.

On old Chinese medicine in general see Pierre Huard and Ming Wong: *La Médecine Chinoise au cours des Siècles,* Paris, 1959; a comparable book in English, but without illustrations is by Wang Yen Ming and Wu Lien Teh, *History of Chinese Medicine,* ed. 2, Shanghai, 1936; W. R. Morse, *Chinese Medicine,* New York, 1934; Wong Ch. and Wu, L.: *History of Chinese Medicine,* Chicago, 1936; K. L. Kaufman, a chronology of some events of pharmaceutical interest in ancient China and Japan, *J.A.Ph.A. 28*:544, 1939; I. Cameron and K. K. Chen, The old and the new pharmacy in China, *Pharm. J. 114*:633, 1925; H. E. Hume: *The Chinese Way in Medicine,* Baltimore, 1940.

**Christensen,** Bernard V. (1885–1956), American educator and pharmacognosist from 1927; dean of pharmacy at U. of Florida (1933–39) and Ohio State U. (1939–55). At Ohio State Christensen initiated the first required 5-year undergraduate curriculum in U.S.A. pharmacy. He served pharmacy nationally in many official positions. (E. P. Guth in *Am. J. Pharm. Ed. 20*:649–651, 1956; and *Amer. Men of Science,* ed. 8, p. 429.)

**Christensen,** H. C. (1865–1947), American pharmacist, in practice 1893–1911, who became influential in National Association of Boards of Pharmacy from the founding and served as Secretary 1914–1942. See P. H. Costello, Proc. N.A.B.P. 1954, pp. 81–90. also *J.A.Ph.A. 19*:315, 1930.

***Circumforaneus,*** pl. ***-i.*** See ***pharmacopolae circumforaneae.***

**Clyster** (also "ibis" or "enema"), term for a liquid injection into the lower intestine, from the Greek work *glyzein,* "wash off" or "out". According to Pliny, the ancient Egyptians learned the use of clysters from the bird called the "ibis," which was said to inject water into its bowel with its beak. Clysters or enemas—made from a variety of medicated formulas—had widespread use in antiquity and a continuous tradition into modern times. The clyster reached the height of therapeutic faddism about the 17th century in France and only in recent decades reached a low point in both professional and folk medicine. See Friedenwald and Morrison: *Bull, Hist. Med. 8*:68, 1940. For a sarcastic account of this chapter of French pharmaceutical history see Phillipe: *Histoire des apothicaires,* pp. 99 ff., 328, Paris, 1853; or Phillipe and Ludwig: *Geschichte der Apotheker,* pp. 119 ff., 923, Jena, 1855.

**Coblentz,** Virgil (1862–1932), American pharmacist, later professor at the New York College of Pharmacy. *J.A.Ph.A. 21*:425, 1932.

***Codex.*** See **Pharmacopeia.**

***Codigo.*** See **Pharmacopeia.**

**Coggeshall,** George D. (1809–1891), influential pharmacist in New York and one of the original members of the New York College of Pharmacy, as well as of the A.Ph.A. See J. W. England: *First Century of Philadelphia College of Pharmacy,* p. 127, Philadelphia, 1922; *Proc. A.Ph.A. 40*:18, 1892.

**Collyrium,** Greek *kollyrion,* poultice or eye salve, used as a designation for medicated applications for the eyes, now usually eyewashes.

***Compendium pharmaceuticum,*** by Coste. A formulary, compiled for the French forces in North America by Jean François Coste, chief physician of Rochambeau's French Expeditionary Forces in the American Revolution, printed in Newport in 1780. Republished in facsimile by John E. Lane in the *Bulletin of the Society of Medical History of Chicago 45*:214, 1930, and with a translation into English and annotations by Edward Kremers, in *Badger Pharmacist,* Madison, Wis., Nos. 27 to 30, 1940 (see also Kremers, E.: *American Pharmaceutical Documents, 1643 to 1780,* Madison, Wis., 1944). For an account of Coste's life see John E. Lane: *Americana 22*:51, 1928, reprinted in *Military Surgeon 63*:219.

***Composita,*** from the Latin *compositus* ("made up of parts") i.e., composite substance. In the system of humoral pathology, *q.v.,* in its Galenic form, *composita* were drugs with compound or composite effect, in contrast to *simplicia,* which exerted only the simple effects of warmth or cold, moisture or dryness. Pharmaceutically speaking, however, composita were preparations and simplicia, *q.v.,* was the generic term for simple drugs used unmixed or for making the composita. It became customary to divide pharmacopeias into two parts, the one giving directions for making the composita, the other giving a list of simplicia.

***Concordantia.*** See: **Pharmacopeia.**

***Concordia.*** See: **Pharmacopeia.**

***Confectio (nes).*** Lat. *conficio, -ere, feci, -fectum,* literally anything that is made. (Our word "factory," derived from *facio, facere, feci, factum,* implies a place where things are made.) In a more restricted sense, the term confectio designated certain preparations made by the pharmacist in his *officin* (from *opus,* "work," and *facere,* "to make"), particularly *confectiones* proper, *i.e.,* soft, semisolid or solid mixtures of powdered drugs with honey, syrup or sugared fruit juices. Modern English usage restricts the use of the word confection to candies and similar wares. See L. Winkler, *Dispensatorium des Valerius Cordus,* p. 13, Mittenwald, 1934. Compare ***Electuary.***

***Confectionarius,*** pl. ***-i,*** from *confectio,* "that which is prepared" (*con* and *facere,* "to make") and *-arius,* pertaining to a maker, in this case a maker of medicaments. The term appears in the **Law** of Frederick II of 1240, *q.v.* Cf. ***Pharmakopoeos*** and ***Medicamentarius.***

***Conservae.*** From Latin *con-servo, avi, atum.,* "to keep in existence, to preserve." One part of finely cut fresh flowers or herbs were mixed with two parts of sugar, the product representing sugary morsels or a sugary paste. Trommsdorff (See *"Konserven"* in his *Wörterbuch*) points out that they were subject to deterioration—the opposite of the property implied in the name! Hence, they were discontinued. Preparations resembling candied fruits (and prepared the same way) were likewise called *Conservae* or, by the more specific term, *Condita.*

**Constantinus Africanus** (1020–1087), the first to translate on a large scale Greco-Arabic works (particularly Arabic works) based on Galen or the Hippocratean Corpus, into Latin. He is said to have been a North African Christian monk before coming to Salerno. See *Dictionary of Scient. Biog.* L. Figuier: *Vies des savants illustres du moyen age,* p. 103, Paris, 1867; G. Sarton: *Introduction to the History of Science,* vol. 1, p. 769, Baltimore, 1927.

**Cook,** E. Fullerton (1879–1961) became chairman of the Committee of Revision of the U. S. Pharmacopeia in 1920 and served for three decades. He was the first U.S. chairman to take an active part (1937–1954) in international drug standardization problems and helped to prepare the first *Pharmacopoeia Internationalis.* He was professor at the Philadelphia College of Pharmacy (from 1903), with which he remained associated for a lifetime. Author, and coeditor of *Remington's Practice of Pharmacy.* (*Am. J. Pharm. Ed. 25*:478, 1961; and J. England: *First Century of the Philadelphia College of Pharmacy,* p. 421, Philadelphia, 1922.)

**Cook,** Roy Bird (1886–1961), American practicing pharmacist; Secretary of West Virginia Board of Pharmacy 29 years; prominent in organized pharmacy nationally; writer and exponent of state history.

**Cordus,** Valerius (1515–1544), German physician whose *Dispensatorium* made his name famous. It was compiled at the suggestion of the pharmacist Johannes Ralla, his uncle. In the laboratory of the pharmacy of Ralla, Cordus experimented with the distillation of ethereal oils, the results appearing in the writings which Conrad Gessner, *q.v.,* published after the death of the author. In *De artificiosis extractionibus* the first known formula for the preparation of ether has been given. See Winkler: *Dispensatorium des Valerius Cor-*

*dus,* Gesellschaft für Geschichte der Pharmazie, Mittenwald, 1934.

**Cosmas,** (d. a.d. 303), Arabic–Christian martyr, who, together with his twin brother Damian, is said to have given medical and medicinal help gratuitously to all who needed it. After their martyrdom both brothers became the favorite patron saints of medicine and of pharmacy in all Christian countries. See M.-L. David-Danel: *Iconographie des Saints médecins Come et Damien,* Lille, 1958 (bibliography pp. 235–244); also below under **Saints.**

**Coste,** Jean-François (1741–1819), chief physician of the French Expeditionary Army in the American Revolution; author of a brief formulary in Latin for the use of the hospitals under his charge, which was published under the title *Compendium pharmaceuticum,*" *q.v.*

**Costello,** Patrick H. (1897–1971), pharmacist and authority on pharmacy law administration. He was Secretary of the National Association of Boards of Pharmacy, 1942–62, and previously had been Secretary of the North Dakota Board of Pharmacy, 1927–1942. Costello acquired his first pharmacy in 1919, and in the ensuing years had held many professional and civic positions. See: *Who Was Who in America,* and *Proc. N.A.B.P. 1972,* p. xxiii.

**Courtois,** Bernard (1777–1838), French pharmacist, discovered (1811) iodine in the ashes of seaweeds. The name iodine (from the Greek iodes = "violet color," ion = "a violet") was given to the new element by Davy, because of its violet vapor.

**Coxe,** John Redman (1773–1864), American physician, professor at the University of Pennsylvania and author of the first dispensatory to be published in the United States. See. *Am. J. Pharm. 36*:275, 1864; J. W. England: *First Century of the Philadelphia College of Pharmacy,* pp. 44, 60, Philadelphia, 1922.

**Craigie,** Andrew (1754–1819). Served in the "Army of the Patriots," during the American Revolutionary War, with the title "apothecary general" (conferred January 1, 1777) and later as "apothecary" (October 6, 1780). After the war, he became a successful wholesale pharmacist. See L. F. Kebler: *J.A.Ph.A. 17*:63, 167, 1928; *Dictionary of American Biography, IV,* p. 497.

**Croll,** Oswald (1560–1609), German physician and one of the foremost followers of Paracelsus, *q.v.* His principal work, the *Basilica chymica,* contains numerous formulas for inorganic chemical remedies. See M. Klutz: *Die Rezepte in Oswald Crolls 'Basilica Chymica' (1609) und ihre Beziehungen zu Paracelsus,* Bd. 14, Veröff. Pharm. gesch. Seminar Techn. Univ. Braunschweig, Braunschweig, 1974.

**Culpeper,** Nicholas (1616–1654), an English medical practitioner, who had been apprenticed to an apothecary. He wrote an amazing number of books on herbs and on materia medica in the short time of his life. He brought himself into notoriety by publishing (1649) his unauthorized English translation of the London College of Physicians' *Pharmacopoeia.* His herbal was reissued in revised editions under his name until the late 19th century. Together with Culpeper's *The English Physician,* it was widely used for self-treatment, not only in England but also in the North American colonies.

**Curtman,** Charles O. (1829–1896), German-born American pharmacist and author; during the Civil War director of laboratories for manufacturing gunpowder and other products for the Confederate Army, professor of chemistry in the St. Louis College of Pharmacy. See *Am. J. Pharm. 68*:351, 1896.

**Cutbush,** Edward (1772–1843), physician, chief surgeon of the U. S. Navy, after 1829 professor of chemistry at Geneva College, Geneva, N.Y. See Kelly and Burrage: *American Medical Biographies,* p. 272, 1920.

**Cutbush,** James (1788–1823), Philadelphia pharmacist and chemist, first president of the Columbian Chemical Society, founded in 1811; and professor of chemistry in St.

John's College, Philadelphia, later at West Point. See *Dictionary of Am. Biog. V*, p. 10; H. G. Wolfe: *Am. J. Pharm. Ed. 12*:89–125, 1948.

**Cutler,** Manasseh (1742–1823), American clergyman and botanist. See *Lloyd Libr.*, Reprod. Ser. No. 4, 1903; *Dictionary of Am. Biog., V*, p. 12.

**Damian** (d. 303 A.D.), Arabic-Christian martyr and patron saint of medicine and particularly of pharmacy. See **Cosmas.**

**Dargavel,** John W. (1894–1961), Executive Secretary of the National Association of Retail Druggists, 1933–1961. He had been a practicing pharmacist in Minnesota from 1917–1933 and Secretary of the Minnesota State Board of Pharmacy, 1923–1934. As N.A.R.D. Secretary he gave pharmacy owners vigorous representation of their economic interests and worked relentlessly for Fair Trade Laws. (*Drug Topics 23*:2 and 16, Oct., 1961; *Who Was Who in America.*)

**Davis,** William (seventeenth century), apothecary in Boston. See *Bull. Mass. Coll. Pharm. III*:39, No. 4, 1914.

**Dealers in drugs, terms.** From antiquity to the European Middle Ages, the designations of dealers in drugs included:

In Greek literature: *migmatopoloi, myropoei, myrepsoi, pharmacopoeoi, pharmacolopoli* and *rhizotomoi.*

In Rome: *circumforaneae, pharmacopoei, pharmacotribae, pharmacotritae, pharmacopolea, pigmentarii, sellularii, seplasiarii* and *unguentarii.*

During the Middle Ages: *apothecarius, aromatarius, herbarius* and its modifications, *speciarius* and *stationarius.*

Most of the modern designations are derived from two Greek words, *pharmakon* or *apotheke.* From the former, the French *pharmacien,* the English *pharmacist* and *pharmaceutist,* and the German *Pharmaceut (Pharmazeut)* are derived; from the latter, the French *apothicaire,* the English *apothecary* and the German *Apotheker;* also the corresponding terms, with slightly modified spelling, in other Germanic languages. With the advent of the iatrochemical school, the terms *chemist* and later *pharmaceutical chemist* came into use. (Some terms used traditionally in Europe mostly for non-pharmacists were: *druggist, q.v.,* the French *droguiste,* and the German *Droguist* and *Drogist,* possibly the *Laboranten* and the *Olitätenhändler* or German peddlers of medicaments). For details look up each term; see also, Rudolf Schmitz: Über deutsche Apotheken des 13. Jahrhunderts; Ein Beitrag zur Etymologie des apoteca-apotecarius-Begriffs, Sudhoffs Archiv *45*:289–302, 1961, also Pharm. Ztg. *104*:871–872, 1959; M. Fialon: Histoire des mots "Pharmacien" et "Apothicaire," Bull. Soc. Hist. Pharm., Dec., 1920, No. 28, pp. 263–269; E.-H. Guitard: *ibid., 44*:383–384, 1956; T. D. Whittet: From apothecary to pharmacist: A study of changes of title, Chem. & Drugg., June 30, 1962, pp. 734–736; Oct. 6, 1962, pp. 385–386, et seq.; Wilkening: Zur Geschichte des Wortes "Pharmazie" und "Apotheker," Pharm. Ztg. *75*:225, 1930.

**Decoctio.** From Latin decoctus, "boiled down," an aqueous potion prepared by boiling vegetable drugs with water; one of the earliest modes of administration.

***Defectar.*** See: **Personnel**

***Defectarius.*** See: **Personnel.**

**Degrees in American pharmacy** for undergraduate or graduate studies, over the decades, have been: Bachelor of Pharmacy; Bachelor of Science (in Pharmacy); Doctor of Pharmacy; Doctor of Philosophy (with Pharmacy, Pharmacognosy, Pharmaceutical Chemistry, etc., as major); Graduate in Pharmacy; Master of Pharmacy; Master of Science (Pharmacy, etc.); Pharmaceutical Chemist.

**Deities** or deified persons to whom medicine, etc., is attributed.

1. Egyptian: Thoth, Osiris, Isis, Horus, Imhotep, Anepu (Anubis).

2. Greek: Apollo, Hephaistos, Herakles, Prometheus, Asklepios, Hygeia, Chiron.

As to replacement of these pagan deities, see **Saints, Christian, as Patrons of Pharmacy.**

**Demachy,** Jean François (1728–1803), French pharmacist. Besides his *Manuel de pharmacien,* he wrote several books about industrial pharmaceutical and chemical technic, among them one concerning the preparation of liquors.

**Derosne,** Jean-François (1773/4–1855), French pharmacist. As early as 1803 *(Annales de chimie 45*:257–285, 1803), he prepared opium alkaloids, without, however, isolating the individual ones and recognizing their alkaline nature. See *Dictionary Scient. Biog.* IV, 41 f.

**Dia-preparations.** Preparations designated by putting the word *dia* before the main constituent of the compounded medicine or *confectio, q.v.* Thus one knew that the most important constituent of *Diasenna Nicolai* was senna.

**Diehl,** C. Lewis (1840–1917), German-born American pharmacist active in almost all branches of pharmacy: as owner of a pharmacy in Louisville; as professor of pharmacy at the Louisville College of Pharmacy; in pharmaceutical industry; and as a contributor to pharmaceutical literature. His reports on the progress of pharmacy in the *Proceedings* of the American Pharmaceutical Association offered an all-around survey of great value. See England: *First Century Philadelphia College of Pharmacy,* p. 217, Philadelphia, 1922; *J.A.Ph.A. 6*:423, 1917.

**Digby** (Digbi), Sir Kenelm (1603–1665), secretary of the navy under the English Kings Charles I and II, who left comprehensive collections of secret drug formulas, which were published after his death. See A. C. Wootton: *Chronicles of Pharmacy,* London, 1910. *I,* p. 193; *Dictionary* (English) *National Biography, XV,* p. 60.

**Dioscorides,** Greek physician and botanist (first century A.D.), author of *"Perihylé,"* Latinized materia medica, which for 1500 years was one of the standard works on medicine, pharmacy and botany. See *Dictionary Scient. Biog.*; also J. Berendes: *Des Pedanios Dioskurides aus Anazarbos Arzneimittellehre,* Stuttgart, 1902; Robert T. Gunther: *The Greek Herbal of Dioscorides;* New York, 1959 (English translation of the Materia Medica).

**Dispensary.** The room or place where articles are dispensed; in pharmaceutical practice the dispensary of a hospital, of a physician, of a factory, etc. Contrast with **Medicine chest**.

***Dispensatorium.*** From *dispensare,* "to dispense." As a title for a book of formulas, etc. (directions for the making of preparations) it was employed before the designation "pharmacopeia" came into use, and pre-20th century books thus titled may or may not contain drug standards in a form legally compulsory. Thus we refer to the *Dispensatory of Valerius Cordus, q.v.,* or the *Nürnberg Pharmacopoeia.* The English dispensatories of the seventeenth century and later were for the most part commentaries or English translations from the Latin of the London and other pharmacopeias, and expanded into more or less comprehensive reference books. Such commentaries, partly including texts of the respective pharmacopeias, became common in the United States. See, e.g., *Coxe's Dispensatory,* the *United States Dispensatory,* the *American Dispensatory,* the *National Dispensatory.* Cf. **Pharmacopeia.**

**Dispensatory.** See ***Dispensatorium.***

**Dispenser.** See **Personnel,** and, for terms designating, see **Dealers.**

**Distillation apparatus.** See Gildemeister-Hoffmann-Kremers: *The Volatile Oils,* pp. 51–82, Milwaukee, 1900; H. Schelenz: *zur Geschichte der pharmazeutisch chemischen Destilliergeräte,* Miltitz, 1911; R. J. Forbes: *Short History of the Art of Distillation,* Leiden, 1948.

**Döbereiner,** Johann Wolfgang (1780–1849), German pharmacist and professor of chemistry at Jena. He discovered the catalytic effect of platinum, and used it in converting alcohol into acetic acid (1821) and into acetaldehyde (1832). Finally, by the same means, he converted $H_2SO_3$ into $H_2SO_4$. He produced formic acid by treating manganese with acetic acid and prepared synthetically methyl alcohol. By his "theory of triads" (1829), based on his discovery that there are groups of three elements in which the atomic weight of the one is the mean of those of the other two, Döbereiner created one of the forerunners of the periodic system.

**Dohme,** A. R. L. (b. 1867), a son of Charles Dohme, succeeded his uncle, Louis, as president of Sharp and Dohme until this firm and Mulford and Co. merged (1911–1929). Author. See *Who Was Who in America, 21,* p. 784; *American Men of Science,* ed. 8.

**Dohme,** Charles E. (1843–1911), German-born American pharmacist and pharmaceutical manufacturer. See *Pharm. Era 45*:40, 1912; *J.A.Ph.A. 1*:82, 1912.

**Doliber,** Thomas (1836–1912), pharmacist in Boston and president of the Mellin's Food Company. See *J.A.Ph.A. I*:777, 1912.

**Dorvault,** François Laurent Marie (1815–1879), French pharmacist and writer on pharmaceutical subjects. He not only organized the *Pharmacie centrale de France,* but edited *L'officine, répertoire général de pharmacie practique,* which has been published in many editions as a standard French work on practical pharmacy.

**Dow,** Cora M. (b. 1871), Cincinnati pharmacist and entrepreneur who built one of the first chains of pharmacies. See *Pharm. Era 43*:489, 1910.

***Drogist,*** German for druggist, a merchant specializing in drugs not legally restricted to pharmacies and in spices, cosmetics, technical chemicals, paints, varnishes, etc. As a group separate from pharmacy they established themselves in Germany in the second half of the 19th century.

***Droguiste,*** French for druggist, a sort of third-class pharmaceutical practitioner discontinued in the 20th century.

**Druce,** George Claridge (1851–1932), considered the greatest British field botanist of his time. From a practicing pharmacist in Oxford, where he was mayor (1900), he developed into an influential member of Oxford University. His contributions to botanical literature were extensive. See *Chem. & Drugg. 116*:255, 1932.

**Drug.** French *drogue,* German *Droge.* In its restricted sense, the word has been used to designate so-called "crude" drugs of mineral, vegetable or animal origin, in contrast with galenic preparations or chemicals. In its wider sense, as defined in state and national laws, the term includes all preventive and therapeutic agents. Its derivation is in doubt. Formerly it was regarded as being derived from the Dutch verb *droog,* "to dry," i.e., a product of either vegetable or animal origin preserved by drying (German *Pflanzendrogen, Medizinaldrogen,* as contrasted with vegetables dried for culinary purposes). C. F. Seybold (*Zeitschr. für deutsche Wortforschung 10*:218, 1908) traces it back to the Arabic *dowa*, a remedy.

**Druggist.** (Derived from "drug," *q.v.*), "dealer in drugs." In its original usage in the Anglo-Saxon world the term referred to a wholesaler in drugs. In North America it gradually became the designation for the common type of pharmacist. As "chemist and druggist," the word became part (1868) of the official designation of the English pharmaceutical practitioners, when an act of Parliament required all future "chemists and druggists" to pass examination and be registered.

**Drugs, designations of dealers in.** See: **Dealers in drugs.**

**Dumas,** Jean Baptiste (1800–1884), French chemist who started his career as a pharmaceutical apprentice and received the highest honors in science, as well as in the political life of his country. His determinations of the vapor densities of iodine, sulfur, phosphorus, mercury, etc., were important for theoretic chemistry. He determined the chemical formula for methyl alcohol, chloroform and iodoform, and laid the ground for modern structural formulas. He is considered one of the founders of physical chemistry and "one of those great chemical researchers . . . who served as landmarks" (A. W. v. Hofmann). He held the positions of Secretary of Agriculture and of Commerce in the French government (1849 to 1851) and was subsequently a senator. See *Am. J. Pharm. 56*:351, 1884; Dictionary Scien. Biog.

**Du Mez,** Andrew G. (1885–1948) was active in a series of official and teaching positions and, after 1926, dean of the School of Pharmacy, University of Maryland. Of his numerous publications, the *Year Book* of the American Pharmaceutical Association, edited by him from 1921 to 1935, and after 1935 the *Pharmaceutical Abstracts,* made him especially well known. See *J.A.Ph.A. 28*:p. 67, 1939.

**Duncan,** Andrew (1744–1828), physician and professor at Edinburgh University. Besides his *New Dispensatory,* Duncan wrote several other books on medicine. See *Dictionary of* (English) *National Biography, XVI,* p. 161.

**Dunning,** Henry A. B. (1877–1962), an industrial pharmacist and philanthropist, particularly active in the American Pharmaceutical Association, including chairmanship of two committees culminating in construction of present headquarters building, Washington, D.C. (dedicated 1934). Leader of the firm, Hynson, Westcott and Dunning. See *J.A.Ph.A. 13*:593, 1924 and *18*:3, 1929; *Who Was Who in America.*

**Durand,** Elias (1794–1873), French-born Philadelphia pharmacist. See England, *First Century of the Philadelphia College of Pharmacy,* p. 357, Philadelphia, 1922; *Am. J. Pharm. 45*:432, 509, 1873.

**Dusseau,** Michael, also called du Seau, a French pharmacist (16th century), whose early textbook for pharmaceutical apprentices was used in various editions for more than a century.

**Dyott,** T. W. (about 1775–1850), English-born pharmacist of Philadelphia. See *Bul. Pharm. 18*:237, 1904.

**Ebers,** Georg (1837–1898), German Egyptologist and novelist. He discovered and described the medicinally important papyrus named after him. See ***Papyrus Ebers.***

**Ebert,** Albert Ethelbert (1840–1906), German-born pharmacist in Chicago; professor of pharmacy at the Chicago College of Pharmacy. He invented the sulfurous process for the manufacture of starch and glucose. His name is commemorated by A.Ph.A.'s Ebert Prize for Scientific Research. See M. M. Weinstein and R. G. Mrtek: *J.A.Ph.A.* ns *11*:664–669, 1971, and *Pharm. Hist. 13*:77–88, 1971. *Proc. A.Ph.A. 55*:iii, 1907; Drug. Circ. *51*:84, 1907.

**Eger,** George (1836–1900), German-born and educated American pharmacist. See *Proc. A.Ph.A. 49*:40, 1901.

**Ehrlich,** Paul (1854–1915), German physician and leader of the Institute for Experimental Therapy at Frankfurt-on-the-Main, founded as a means for his research. He was a pioneer in merging descriptive cellular pathology with experimental intracellular chemistry, and in testing and using the microchemical reaction of the tissues to dyestuffs. His best known research was the production of Salvarsan (arsphenamine) which he carried out in collaboration with Hata. See Sigerist: *The Great Doctors,* p. 384, New York, 1933; H. Loewe: Paul Ehrlich, Stuttgart, 1950.

**Electuary.** Latin *electuarium* and *electarium,* from *ecligma* (Greek *ek,* "out," and *leichein,* "to lick.") In classical Latin, "a medicine that melts in the mouth." A soft preparation made by mixing powders and other ingredients with a sweet juice, honey, or a solution of sugar. Cf. ***Confectiones.*** For details see "*Latwerge,*" in Trommsdorff's *Handwörterbuch.*

***Elève.*** See **Personnel.**

**Ellis,** Charles (1800–1874), original member

of the Philadelphia College of Pharmacy as well as of the American Pharmaceutical Association, pharmacist in Philadelphia. See *Drug. Circ. 51*:84, 1907; J. W. England, *First Century of the Philadelphia College of Pharmacy*, p. 355, Philadelphia, 1922; *Proc. A.Ph.A. 55*:583, 1907.

***Enchiridion.*** See **Pharmacopeia.**

**Enema.** Greek *enjénai,* to send in. See **Clyster.**

***Farmocopen.*** See: **Pharmacopeia.**

***Farmacopin.*** See: **Pharmacopeia.**

***Farmocopoea.*** See: **Pharmacopeia.**

***Farmakopo.*** See: **Pharmacopeia.**

**Farr,** John (1791–1847), English-born chemist and founder of the manufacturing firm later known as Powers and Weightman. See England: *First Century of the Philadelphia College of Pharmacy*, p. 33, Philadelphia, 1922.

**Fée,** Antoine Laurent Apollinaire (1789–1874), French pharmacist. He became professor of botany at the University of Strasburg (1833). Fée published his *Cours d'histoire naturelle pharmaceutique* in 1828; and his famous *Commentaires sur la botanique et la matière medicale de Pline* in 1853. See *Dictionary Scient. Biog.*

**Fehling,** Hermann von (1812–1885), German pharmacist and physiologic chemist. He developed the method for the determination of sugar and starch by means of an alkaline copper sulfate solution in the presence of alkali tartrates, which has been named after him. His discovery of paraldehyde is also noteworthy. See *Pharm. J. 45*:83, 153, 1885; *Am. J. Pharm. 57*:463, 1885.

**Ferrand,** Claude-Henry (1740–?), French *pharmacien-en-chef* with the French auxiliary corps in the American Revolutionary War. See A. Balland: *Les pharmaciens militaires Français,* p. 89, Paris, 1913.

**Firmin,** Giles, Jr. (1614 or 1615–1697), born in England, came to Boston first for a brief visit in 1632 and returned 1637, after having studied medicine in England. He is said to have delivered the first anatomic lectures to students in this country. Later on, he returned to England, where he entered the ministry.

**Fischelis,** Robert P. (1891–     ), pharmaceutical administrator, teacher, editor, writer, former executive secretary of the New Jersey Board of Pharmacy (1926-44); pharmacy dean at Rutgers and Ohio Northern universities; director, Division of Chemicals, Drugs and Health Supplies, Office of Civilian Requirements, War Production Board (1941–1945); Secretary and General Manager, American Pharmaceutical Association (1945–1959); consultant to various governmental agencies, advisor to the American delegation to the International Health Conference of 1946, and member of executive committee, National Health Assembly 1948–49. A list of the many honors bestowed on him, and of the various capacities in which he has served American pharmacy, can be found in *American Men of Science,* ed. 8, p. 780, 1949; *Who Was Who in America;* and *J.A.Ph.A.* (Pract. Ed.) *6*:11–12, 1945.

**Flückiger,** Friedrich August (1828–1894). Swiss pharmacist and professor of pharmacy at the University of Strasburg. He was the first of modern pharmacognosists and wrote fundamental books on this subject. He also contributed important articles on the history of pharmacy. See Häfliger, *Fr. A. Flückiger,* Gesellschaft für Geschichte der Pharmazie, Mittenwald, 1928; *Pharm. Rund. 10*:107,1892; F. Hoffmann: *Am. J. Pharm. 67*:65, 1895; *Pharm. J. 54*:538, 1894.

**Foesius,** Anutius (1528–1595), French physician living in Metz (Lorraine). His unlatinized name was Foès. His *Pharmacopoeia Mediomatrica* (Pharmacopeia of Metz) was widely used.

**Foster,** Thomas A. (1896–1973), American pharmacist in community practice (Birmingham, Ala., 1919–1932), then entered U. S. Public Health Service (1932–1960). Distinguished service in Office of the Surgeon General (U.S.P.H.S.), Office of Defense Mobilization, and other posts; helped to advance the role of pharmacy in Federal government service. Retired in rank of Pharmacist Director. *A.Ph.A. Newsletter* 20 Jan. 1973, p. 2.

***Formularium.*** See: **Pharmacopeia.**

**Fourcroy,** Antoine François, Count of (1755–1809), French physician and chemist. He was a teacher of Vauquelin, *q.v.*; with him he worked intimately. He analyzed many medicinal chemicals.

**Fourneau,** Ernest F. A. (1872–1949), French pharmacist who became one of the foremost representatives of chemotherapeutic research. Fourneau, who had been the owner of a pharmacy in Paris for years, was director of the pharmaceutical concern of Poulenc Frères (1901 to 1910) and (1911 to 1945) director of the chemotherapeutic laboratory of the Pasteur Institute for more than 30 years. See George Urdang: *Pharmacy's Part in Society*, pp. 70, 71, Madison, Wis., 1946.

**Fowler,** Thomas (1736–1801), English apothecary and physician. See Wootton: *Chronicles of Pharmacy, II,* pp. 133, London, 1910.

**Fownes,** George (1815–1849), English professor and chemist. His *Manual of Elementary Chemistry* (1845) was widely used in America as well as England. See Ferchl: *Chemisch-Pharmazeutisches Bio-und Bibliographicon*, p. 162, Mittenwald, 1937.

**Francke,** Don E. (1910–    ), American pharmacist of exceptional creativity and influence. Principal founder of *International Pharmaceutical Abstracts, American Hospital Formulary Service,* and *Drug Intelligence and Clinical Pharmacy.* Editor of *American Journal of Hospital Pharmacy* (1944–1966). First American to become (1958) Vice President of International Pharmaceutical Federation. Director of the Audit of Pharmaceutical Service in Hospitals (1956–59) and Director of Scientific Services of American Society of Hospital Pharmacists (1963–1966). Chief hospital pharmacist and professor at Universities of Michigan and Cincinnati. President of Drug Intelligence Publications since 1971. Commemorated by Don E. Francke Medal. See *Who's Who in America*.

**Frank,** Adolf (1834–1916), German pharmacist and one of the most versatile inventors and organizers in industrial chemistry and technology.

**Frederick II,** a Hohenstaufen, German Emperor and King of Southern Italy and Sicily (1194–1250). See **Law for the separation of medicine and pharmacy,** of Frederick II. (*Note* that Frederick II, "The Great," of the House of Hohenzollern, King of Prussia, did not rule until 1712–1786.)

**Fuchs,** Leonhart (1501–1566), physician and botanist. He was the most learned of the contemporary authors of herbals, and, besides his *Neu Kreuterbuch* (1543), wrote many other treatises. His edition of the *Antidotarium* of the Byzantine physician Nicolaus Myrepsus, *q.v.*, with notes, is of special pharmaceutical interest. See *Annual Report of the Smithsonian Institution*, 1917; Eberhard Stübler: *Leonhart Fuchs, Leben und Werk*, Munich, 1928.

**Fuller,** Thomas (1654–1734), English physician and author of several books and pamphlets on medical subjects, including his *Pharmacopeia Extemporanea.* See *Dictionary of National* (English) *Biography, 20,* p. 320.

**Gale,** Edwin Oscar (1832–1913), Chicago pharmacist, historian and poet. See *J.A.Ph.A.* 2:283, 1913.

**Galen** (129/130–199/200), physician from Pergamon, who practiced in Rome. Galen's genius was enormously productive in his time and influential in later times (until ca. 18th century). He spoke for a scientific approach to medicine, even though his codification of humoral pathology and therapeutics inhibited his successors in medical sciences for centuries, through over-respect. In pharmacy Galen's name has been best remembered for centuries through universal use of the term "Galenicals'' as a class designation for medicinal agents prepared without the aid of chemical reactions or changes, and usually with the aid of mixing or solvent-extraction—such as tinctures and decoctions. (The pre-modern term ''galenical'' does not include such modern drug-groups as antibiotics or biologicals.)

**Galenicals,** a broad category for medicinal preparations whose simple ingredients presumably remain unchanged chemically. It includes far more than the drugs advocated or known by Galen, *q.v.*

**Gardiner,** Silvester (1708–1786), American-born physician who studied medicine in London and Paris. He and Wm. Douglass were the first physicians to be adequately educated in England and then to practice in America, and both exerted a marked influence on American medicine. See Henry R. Viets: Some features of the history of medicine in Massachusetts, *Isis 23*:389, 1935; *Dictionary of American Biography, VII,* p. 139.

**Gehlen,** Adolf Ferdinand (1775–1815), German pharmacist and chemicopharmaceutical journalist. Having published chemical journals since 1803 and edited the *Neues Berliner Jahrbuch der Pharmacie,* 1805–1808, he founded in 1815 the *Repertorium für die Pharmacie,* which J. A. Buchner, *q.v.,* continued.

**Geiger,** Philipp Lorenz (1785–1836), German pharmacist and professor of pharmacy at the University of Heidelberg. In 1835 Geiger discovered coniine and, in cooperation with Hesse, isolated atropine, hyoscyamine, aconitine and daturine. From 1824 to 1836, he edited the *Magazin der Pharmazie.* Among his books the *Pharmacopoeia universalis* (started by him in 1835 and continued by Friedrich Mohr) was of greatest importance. See G. Urdang: Philipp Lorenz Geiger, *Pharmazeutische Zeitung 74*:1154, 1929.

**Geoffroy,** Etienne François (1672–1731), French pharmacist and member of a family which gave to the world a number of important scientists. His *Tractatus de materia medica seu de medicamentorum simplicium historia, virtute, et usu delectu* is considered the first book presenting pharmacognosy in a systematic way. With his chemical relationship tables (published first in 1718 in the *Memoirs of the Parisian Academy of Science),* Geoffroy laid the foundation of the theory of relationship between the chemical elements. See: *Dictionary Scient. Biog.*

**Gerard** (Gerarde), John (1545–1612), English surgeon and botanist. Gerard's *Catalogus arborum, fructicum ac plantarum* (1596) and *The herball or general histoire of plantes* (1597) were highly regarded. The latter was issued in an enlarged edition (1633) by the English apothecary Thomas Johnson, *q.v.* See: *Dictionary* (English) *Nat. Biog., XXI,* p. 221.

**Gessner,** Conrad (pseudonym Evonymus Philiatrus) (1516–1565), Swiss physician and botanist. His main work, *Historia plantarum,* was not published until 1751–1771, about 200 years after his death. See Dobler: *Conrad Gessner als Pharmazeut,*Zürich, 1955.

**Ghina (or Ghini),** Luca (1500–1556), Italian physician and botanist. He is assumed to be the inventor of the herbarium, for collecting plants, and for the preservation of the dried pressed mounts.

**Glauber,** Johann Rudolf (1604–1670), German chemist of amazing productivity and versatility. He taught the production of nitric acid by treating saltpetre with sulfuric acid; and of hydrochloric acid by treating sodium chloride with sulfuric acid. He produced sodium sulfate (Glauber's salt), ammonium sulfate, zinc chloride, potassium chloride, etc., and developed numerous methods and technics.

**Glentworth,** George (end of the eighteenth to middle of the 19th century). See England: *First Century of the Philadelphia College of Pharmacy,* pp. 56, 107, Philadelphia, 1922.

**Glyn-Jones,** Sir William (1869–1927), important English chemist and pharmacist, manufacturer, lawyer and legislator. See

*Chem. & Drug. 107*:365, 1927; *J.A.Ph.A. 13*:503, 1924; *16*:894, 1927.

**Gmelin,** Johann Friedrich (1784–1804), German chemist. In addition to many chemical treatises, pharmaceutical and chemical textbooks, etc., he wrote a history of chemistry. He was a member of the Gmelin family, which, descending from a pharmacist at Tübingen, through the generations gave men of importance to pharmacy as well as to the natural sciences in general. See O. Raubenheimer: *J.A.Ph.A. 19*:259, 1930.

**Godfrey.** See **Hanckwitz.**

**Goethe,** Johann Wolfgang von (1749–1832), German poet of highest rank, whose ardent interest in science brought him into close contact with several pharmacists, who became his teachers in chemistry, botany, mineralogy and meteorology. For the relations of Goethe to pharmacists, see G. Urdang: Goethe and pharmacy, Madison, Wis., 1949.

**Goettling,** Johann Friedrich August (1755–1809), German pharmacist and professor of chemistry and pharmacy at the University of Jena. He was one of the first chemists in Germany to repeat and confirm the investigations of Lavoisier, *q.v.*, and, therefore, to abandon the phlogiston theory. In 1780 he started an annual, *Almanach oder Taschenbuch für Scheidekuenstler und Apotheker, q.v.*, the first periodical devoted primarily to the interests of pharmacy.

**Grahame,** Israel J. (1819–1899) was a pharmacist, first in Baltimore and later in Philadelphia. He was professor of pharmacy at the Maryland College of Pharmacy and, in Philadelphia, the principal of several educational institutions for women. His chief merit lies in his research work on percolation. See England: *First Century of the Philadelphia College of Pharmacy*, p. 115, Philadelphia, 1922; *Drug. Circ. 51*:85, 1907.

**Grazzini,** Antonio Francesco, called il Lasca (1503–1584), Italian pharmacist and poet, dramatist and novelist. Several of his books were still republished in the second half of the 19th century.

**Gren,** Friedrich Albert Carl (1760–1798), German pharmacist, physician and chemist. He isolated cholesterin from gallstones and wrote in his short life an amazing number of books and pamphlets.

**Grew,** Nehemiah (1628–1711), English physician. In 1695 he isolated sulfate of magnesium (epsom salt) from the water of Epsom Spring. Grew wrote botanic as well as chemical treatises.

**Griffenhagen,** George B. (1924– ), American pharmacist. Curator of Division of Medical Sciences, Smithsonian Institution (1952–1959); Director of Communications, American Pharmaceutical Association, since 1959, including Managing Editorship of *Journal*, then (since 1962) Editorship. Griffenhagen has been a leader in the American Institute of the History of Pharmacy, prolific historical writer, contributor to drug-abuse control nationally, prominent in international endeavors of organized pharmacy, including historical pharmacy, and a noted topical (pharmaceutical) philatelist.

**Griffith,** Ivor (1891–1961), American pharmacist, born in Wales, professor at the Philadelphia College of Pharmacy, and later President of the College (1912–1961); author of a number of books and articles of a literary as well as a professional nature; editor, *American Journal of Pharmacy* 1921–41. See *Drug Topics*, June 5, 1961, p. 16, and England: *First Century of the Philadelphia College of Pharmacy*, p. 443, Philadelphia, 1922.

**Griffith,** R. Eglesfield (1797–1850), Philadelphia physician, writer on medical and pharmaceutical subjects, (between 1831 and 1836) editor of the *Am. J. Pharm.* See *Am. J. Pharm. 22*:400, 1850.

**Griffits,** Samuel Powell (1759–1826), physician in Philadelphia, professor of materia medica at the University of Pennsylvania. See Kelly and Burrage: *American Medical Biographies*, p. 468, New York, 1920.

**Guignard,** Jean-Louis-Léon (1852–1928), qualified as a French pharmacist, then became a brilliant botanist. Professor of botany (1887–1927) and Director (1900–1910) of the Paris School of Pharmacy; President of the Academy of Sciences (1919). See *Dictionary Scient. Biog.*

**Guthrie,** Samuel (1782–1848), American physician who discovered chloroform at the same time (1831) as the French pharmacist Soubeiran, *q.v.*, and the German chemist Liebig, *q.v.* See *J.A.Ph.A. 20*:482, 1931.

**Häfliger,** Josef Anton (1873–1954), Swiss pharmacist, professor of pharmacy, including the history of pharmacy, at the University of Basle, creator of the pharmaceutico-historical museum which forms an annex to the Pharmaceutical Institute of the University of Basle, and author of numerous pharmaceutical-historical publications. See *Deutsche Apoth. Ztg. 94*:1180–81, 1954.

**Hagen,** Karl Gottfried (1749–1829), German pharmacist and professor of chemistry and physics at the University of Königsberg. He was one of the most eminent and progressive teachers of the sciences of pharmacy in his time. His textbooks dominated the field for many decades. See Gottfried Wallrabe: *Zum Gedächtnis an Karl Gottfried Hagen. Pharm. Zeit. 74*:285, 1929.

**Hager,** Hans Hermann Julius (1816–1897), German pharmacist who wrote commentaries on the German pharmacopeias appearing during his lifetime and, among other treatises, the two which became the most used reference books in the practice of pharmacy: his *Manuale pharmaceuticum* and his *Handbuch der pharmaceutischen Praxis.* The *Pharmazeutische Zentralhalle (Centralhalle)* founded by Hager (1859) was for a long time one of the leading scientific pharmaceutical journals in Germany.

**Hahnemann,** Samuel Christian Friedrich (1755–1843), physician and chemist, creator of homeopathy. Of pharmaceutical interest is the fact that he wrote, besides books concerning his special medical theories, an excellent reference book (lexicon) on the art of the pharmacist, and also several chemical treatises. See Th. L. Bradford: *The Life and the Letters of Dr. Samuel Hahnemann,* Philadelphia, 1895, and Eveline Steinbichler: *Geschichte der homöopathischen Arzneibereitungslehre in Deutschland bis 1872* (Internationale Gesellschaft . . . Bd. 11) Eutin, 1957.

**Hallberg,** Carl Svante N. (1856–1910), Swedish-born American pharmacist, manufacturer, journalist, and professor of pharmacy in the Chicago College of Pharmacy. See England: *First Century of the Philadelphia College of Pharmacy,* p. 195, Philadelphia, 1922.

**Hanbury,** Daniel (1825–1875), English pharmacist and one of the most eminent modern pharmacognosists. His best-known work is the *Pharmacographia,* which he wrote in conjunction with Flückiger, *q.v.* See *Am. J. Pharm. 47*:238, 1875; E. C. Cripps, *Plough Court,* p. 67, London, 1927.

**Hanckwitz,** Ambrosius Gottfried (17th and early 18th centuries). German chemist who, in England, took the name Godfrey (anglicized second given name), instead of Hanckwitz. See R. E. W. Maddison, . . . Hanckwitz family in England, Annals Sci. *11*:64–73, 1955.

**Hancock,** John F. (1834–1909), Baltimore pharmacist. See *Drug. Circ. 51*:107, 183, 1907.

**Hänle,** Georg Friedrich (1763–1824). German pharmacist. In 1823 he founded the *Magazin der Pharmazie.*

**Harrison,** John (second half of the 18th and first half of the 19th century), Philadelphia pharmacist and manufacturer of chemicals. See England: *First Century of the Philadelphia College of Pharmacy,* p. 35, Philadelphia, 1922; S. P. Sadtler: *Am. J. Pharm. 93*:201, 1921.

**Hartshorne,** Joseph (1779–1850). Resident apprentice and apothecary in the Pennsylvania Hospital, later a physician in Philadelphia. See Kelly and Burrage: *American Medical Biographies,* p. 500, New York, 1920.

**Hatcher,** Robert A. (1868–1944), physician and pharmacist, professor of pharmacology and materia medica (1906, to 1935), at Cornell University Medical College; writer on materia medica. See *Who Was Who in America; 20*: p. 1152.

**Heberden,** William (1710–1801), English physician whom Doctor Johnson called: "ultimus Romanorum; the last of our great physicians." His importance to pharmacy lies in his fight against the drugs of old, the use of which was based on out-moded beliefs, rather than on observed effects and/or scientific knowledge. His "Essay on Mithridatum and Theriaca" (1745) exploded a myth, almost 2,000 years old, about these panaceas. See F. H. Garrison: *History of Medicine,* pp. 358, 894, Philadelphia, 1929.

**Hébert,** Louis (about 1580–1627), French pharmacist and pioneer settler in Canada. See A. C. Després: Louis Hébert, premier colon Canadien et sa famille, 2nd ed. Montreal, 1918; also G. Urdang: *Pharmacy's Part in Society;* pp. 50, 52, Madison, Wis., 1946.

**Hebrew** medicine and pharmacy: See, e.g., Otto E. Ruhmer and Arthur G. Zupko: *Some Contributions by Jews to Pharmacy–a Historical Survey,* Madison, Wis., 1960; Harry Friedenwald, *The Jews and Medicine; Essays,* 2 vols., Baltimore, 1944; Solomon Kagan, *Jewish Medicine,* Boston, 1952; L. Glesinger; "Les Juifs et la pharmacie," *Revue Hist. Pharm. 8*:17, 1955; and Oswei Temkin: *Beiträge zur archaischen Medizin,* Kyklos, 1930, *3*:pp. 90-135.

**Hegeman,** William (1817–1875), a New York pharmacist, as early as 1857 operated 4 New York drugstores; hence was one of the earliest forerunners of the chain-store system. See *Drug. Circ. 51*:85, 1907.

**Heller,** William M. (born 1926), American pharmacist. Chief pharmacist, teaching and research, University of Arkansas (1954–1966); first director, *American Hospital Formulary Service* (1955–1963); Director, Scientific Services of American Society of Hospital Pharmacists (1966–1968); Executive Director, U. S. Pharmacopeia (1968–).

**Helmont,** Jean Baptist van (1577–1644), Flemish physician and academic teacher in Leyden. He was a follower of Paracelsus, and some historians consider him (not the later De le Boe Sylvius) as the founder of the Iatrochemical School. However, his theories, like those of his master Paracelsus, were mystifying; while Sylvius, *q.v.*, formulated his physiologicochemical ideas clearly and understandably. Van Helmont made the first attempt at a real analysis of urine. See Garrison: *History of Medicine,* p. 261, Philadelphia, 1929; Sigerist: *The Great Doctors,* p. 157, New York, 1933.

**Herbal.** Title of books of herbs which often also contained special sections on animals, on parts of animals and on minerals used medicinally. Thus they presented the simple drugs not only of the vegetable but also of the animal and the mineral kingdoms. The best introduction to this genre of literature in English is by Agnes Arber: *Herbals; Their Origin and Evolution,* ed. 2, Cambridge 1953.

**Herbalist,** anglicized from of *herbarius q.v.*, a dealer specializing in "herbs," having a world-wide tradition since antiquity, but now dying out in highly developed countries.

**Herbarium.**See ***Herbarius.*** A collection of dried plants; also the title of books on "herbs."

***Herbarius,*** pl. **-*i*,** from Latin *Herba* ("herb"), and *-arius* ("pertaining to"), i.e., a dealer in herbs. Compare French *herbaliste* and *herboriste*, and English "herborist," also "herbarium."

**Herborist,** anglicized form of *herbarius, q.v.* A collector of "herbs."

**Hermbstaedt,** Sigismund (1760–1833), German pharmacist and professor of chemistry at the University of Berlin. Hermbstaedt made an attempt to give phytochemistry a systematic basis in his *Kurze Anleitung zur chemischen Zergliederung von Vegetabilien nach physikalisch-chemischen Grundsätzen* ("Short directions for the chemical analysis of vegetables according to physiochemical principles").

He investigated many technologic problems and was one of the most important chemical engineers of his time.

**Hernandez,** Francisco (1571–1677), wrote on the animals, plants and minerals of Mexico. See Tschirch; *Handbuch der Pharmakognosie,* ed. 2, *I,* Part 3, p. 1546, Leipzig, 1933.

**Hewson,** Thomas Tickell (1773–1848), English born American physician. See: *J.A.Ph.A. 20*:680, 1931.

***Hiera picra.*** Under this name, bitter-tasting powders or *species* were in use from antiquity until about 1800. All contained aloes, except the formula of Scribonius Largus, *q.v.,* which contained colocynth in its place. These powders or species were taken with honey in the form of electuaries. See Wootton: *Chronicles of Pharmacy, II,* p. 138, London, 1910.

**Hildegard of Bingen** (1098–1170), abbess of a cloister at Bingen in Germany, author of a materia medica, called *"physica,"* which according to Tschirch may be considered the first treatise on natural science in Germany. See Tschirch: *Handbuch der Pharmakognosie, I,* Part 2, p. 667, Leipzig, 1910; Gertrude M. Engbring: Saint Hildegard, twelfth century physician, *Bull. Hist. Med. 8*:770, 1940.

**Hippocrates.** (fl. 400 B.C.), a Greek physician, known as the "father of medicine." To him has been attributed the first concept of humoral pathology, *q.v.,* which later on was systematized by Galen, *q.v.,* and, above all, the concept of the sick person as an entity, to be treated as such, instead of merely as the bearer of a particular sickness that had to be treated. This concept, and that of simplicity of medication in connection with adequate diet, has made his name a symbol for movements in medicine, now and again, extolling these principles. See W. S. Jones: *Hippocrates,* with an English translation, London, 1923-1931.

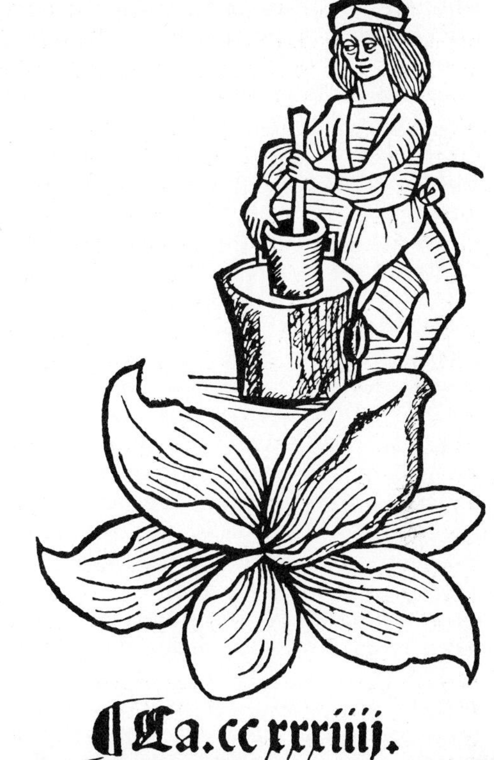

Ca. ccxxxiiij.
Indicus: Sera.li.aggre.cap̄. Ml lech.auct:dyas: Est de ipso dome sticus & silvestris. Et domesticus ē ille q̄ tinctores vtunt: Cuius foliū est simi le folio plantaginis. nisi quia est magis

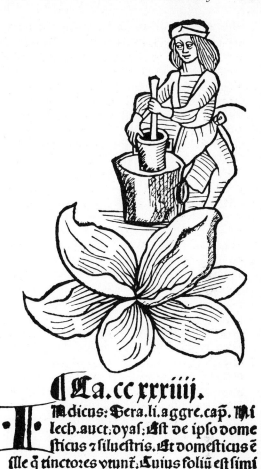

Typical woodcut and excerpt from an herbal *(Hortus sanitatis,* 1491, concerning Indicus (indigo), which was then used as a drug as well as a pharmaceutical coloring agent.

**Hoffmann,** Frederick (1832–1904), German pharmacist, who in more than 30 years of pharmaceutical activity in the United States as a pharmacist, editor, and as analytic chemist, was of the greatest influence in American pharmacy. See *Pharm. Rev. 14*:1, 1896; *23*:1, 1905; *Am. J. Pharm. 78*:144, 1905.

**Hoffmann,** Friedrich (1660–1742), German physician and academic teacher in Halle, who was considered one of the greatest iatromechanists. In pharmacy his name survived in connection with "Hoffmann's drops," which he introduced into therapy. See Garrison: *History of Medicine,* p. 314, Philadelphia, 1929.

**Horus.** The Egyptian god of day, resembling the Greek god Apollo, and one of the gods to whom healing power was attributed. Represented as hawk-headed, he was considered the son of Isis and Osiris.

**Høst-Madsen,** Erik (1883–1974), Danish pharmacist who served as President of the International Pharmaceutical Federation (1935–1953). Co-owner of a Copenhagen pharmacy (1912–1948). Dr. Høst-Madsen's diverse contributions are commemorated by the Høst-Madsen Medal, awarded biennially for scientific achievement in a pharmaceutical field by the International Pharmaceutical Federation.

**Humoral pathology,** the theory that all diseases result from a disordered or abnormal condition of the fluids or humors of the body. As stated in the text, Galen divided the remedies to be used in order to counteract such conditions into three classes. The first class comprised those remedies developing only one of the elementary qualities—warmth, cold, moisture or dryness—drugs with "simple" effect. To the second class belonged those drugs which have, besides one main effect, a secondary effect. Thus their effect is "compound." The third class consisted of drugs with a specific effect, i.e., drugs efficient as "entities." These drugs were supposed to be efficient not because of one or the other "quality," but through their entire substance—hence "entities." They acted as purgatives, emetics, poisons, or antidotes.

Each medicine, and this applied to the drugs of all classes, could exercise its effect in four degrees. Typical of modes of administration is the direction given by Galen for the use of opium: Like all other narcotics, "opium" is, according to its temper, cold. It produces, therefore, in the body a considerable (in the highest degrees, an invincible) cold. Hence in order to soften its effects we have to combine it with heating remedies, the most recommendable of these being Castoreum. See Häuser: *Lehrbuch der Geschichte der Medizin, I,* p. 374, Jena., 1875; Ludwig Israelson: *Die Materia Medica des Kaludios Galenos,* p. 12, 1894.

**Hygeia.** The Greek goddess of health, considered a daughter of Asklepios and often worshipped together with him. Her attributes, a bowl and sacred serpent, have become, in modern times, an international symbol of pharmacy.

**Hynson,** Henry P. (1855–1921), American pharmacist, one of the founders of the firm of Hynson, Westcott and Dunning, Baltimore, and professor in the Department of Pharmacy, University of Maryland.

**Iatrochemistry.** From the Greek *iatros* ("physician"). The doctrine based on a chemical concept of normal and pathologic conditions of the human body. Abnormal chemical conditions naturally were combated by chemical remedies. See **Sylvius.**

***Iatron.*** From Greek *iatros* ("physician"), the room of the physician.

**I-em-hetep.** See: **Imhotep.**

**Imhotep,** originally written I-em-hetep, i.e., "He who cometh in peace," is also known as Imouthes and Imhotpou. He was an architect as well as a physician (about 3000 B.C.), and was deified as a god of medicine and healing about 2500 years after his death. According to Breasted, the Greeks recognized in him their own Asklepios, *q.v.* See Breasted: *A History of Egypt,* p. 113, London, 1921; K. Sethe: *Imhotep, der Asklepios der Aegypter,* Berlin, 1902; J. B. Hurry: *Imhotep, The Vizier and Physician of King Zoser,* Oxford, 1926.

**Imhotpou.** See: **Imhotep.**

**Imouthes.** See: **Imhotep.**

**India.** The name is derived from the river Indus. For ancient Indian medicine and drugs, see G. P. Srivastava: *History of Indian Pharmacy,* Vol. I, ed. 2, Calcutta, 1954; the chapters on "India" or "Indians" in H.

Schelenz: *Geschichte der Pharmazie,* Berlin, 1904; T. Berendes: *Die Pharmazie bei den alten Kulturvolkern,* Halle, 1891; A. Tschirch: *Handbuch per Pharmakognosie, I,* part 2, Leipzig, 1910 and 1933; Henry R. Zimmer: *Hindu Medicine,* Baltimore, 1948. Furthermore, see F. R. Hoernle; *Studies in the Medicine of Ancient India,* Oxford, 1907; G. Piso: *De Indiae utriusque et medica libri XVI* (1658); Jacob Bontius: *De medica Indorum libri IV* (1718). On modern Indian pharmacy, see G. Cecil: Pharmacy in the Indian Native States, *Pharm. J. 117*:674, 1926; and The qualified chemist in India, *Chem. & Drug. 105*:693, 1926.

**Isidorus Hispalensis** (570–636), Bishop of Seville, the best known encyclopedist of the middle Ages. See George Sarton: *Introduction to the History of Science, I*:471–472, Baltimore, 1927.

**Isis.** Egyptian goddess of fecundity and one of the divinities to whom healing power was attributed. She was considered sister and wife of Osiris and mother of Horus and Anubis (Anepu). Isis is sometimes represented as cowheaded. "Isis" has been the title of the journal of the History of Science Society, and was the title of the famous encyclopedic journal edited by the German naturalist, Lorenz Oken, from 1817 to 1848.

**Ives,** Eli (1779–1861), physician. See W. O. Richtmann: *J.A.Ph.A. 20*:681, 1931.

**Jackson,** James (1777–1867), Boston physician, professor at Boston Medical School. See Kelly and Burrage: *American Medical Biographies,* p. 599, New York, 1920.

**Jackson,** Samuel (1787–1872), physician, for some years a pharmacist; first professor of materia medica and pharmacy in Philadelphia College of Pharmacy; from 1827-1863; instructor, then (1835) full professor, at University of Pennsylvania. See J. W. England: *First Century of the Philadelphia College of Pharmacy,* p. 396, Philadelphia, 1922; *Am. J. Pharm. 44*:329, 1872.

**Jacobs,** Joseph (1859–1929), owner of several drugstores in Atlanta, Ga., writer on pharmaceutical subjects and founder of the American Burns Club, an organization of the lovers of the Scottish poet Burns. See J. W. England: *First Century of the Philadelphia College of Pharmacy,* p. 242, Philadelphia, 1922; *Pharm. Era 66*:257, 1929; *J.A.Ph.A. 18*:1095, 1929.

**Japan.** The culture of ancient Japan was derived from China; hence, the known ancient Japanese medicine was Chinese. For details, see the chapters: "Japan" or "Japanese" in H. Schelenz, *Geschichte der Pharmazie;* T. Berendes, *Die Pharmazie bei den alten Kulturvölkern,* Halle, 1891; Tschirch, *Handbuch der Pharmacognosie, I*: Part 2, 1910. Furthermore, see Y. Fujikawa: *Japanese Medicine,* New York, 1934; Charles Rice: Japanese medicine and pharmacy, *New Rem. 6*:20, 1877; K. L. Kaufman, A chronology of some events of pharmaceutical interest in China and Japan, *J.A.Ph.A. 28*:544, 1939. An especially noteworthy book (in Japanese) is by the pharmacist-historian Tootaroo Simizu [or Shimizu], *History of Japanese Pharmacy,* Yokohama, 1960. Medicine and pharmacy in Japan are now Europeanized. The first pharmacopeia following occidental models appeared in 1887.

**Jenner,** Edward (1749–1823). English physician. With his inoculation he "transformed a local country tradition into a reliable prophylactic principle." See Garrison: *History of Medicine,* p. 374, Philadelphia, 1920; Sigerist: *The Great Doctors,* p. 258, New York, 1933.

**Jephcott,** Sir Harry (1891– ). Starting as a practicing pharmacist, Jephcott became one of the leading British pharmaceutical manufacturers, as chairman and managing director of The Glaxo Laboratories. See *Pharm. J. 156*:395, 1946.

**Johnson,** Joseph (1776–1862), physician, wholesale druggist and author. Among his historical publications, *Traditions* and *Reminiscences chiefly of the American Revolution in the South* gained popularity. See *Dictionary of American Biography, X*:p. 108.

**Johnson,** Thomas (d. 1644), English apothecary, botanist and active royal partisan in the struggle between the English crown and Cromwell. See *Dictionary of* (English) *National Biography, XXX:* p. 44.

**Josselyn,** John (d. 1675), traveler and amateur scientist. See *Dictionary of* (English) *National Biography,* XXX: p. 208; *Dictionary of American Biography, X*: p. 219.

**Journalism.** The first pharmaceutical periodical to be classed with the journals (i.e., periodicals issued at more than annual intervals) was Trommsdorff's *Journal der Pharmacie* (1793). The first journal published in the French language appeared (1797) as the *Journal de le sociètè des pharmaciens de Paris.* The first pharmaceutical journal in the English language did not appear in England but in the United States, the *Journal of the Philadelphia College of Pharmacy* (1825). The first Italian journal was the *Giornale di farmacia, chimica e scienze affini* (1824); the first Spanish journal, *El Restaurador Farmaceutica* (1844); the first Portuguese journal, the *Journal da Societada Pharmaceutica de Lisboa* (1840).

Many of the pharmaceutical journals have been published in these languages. English has been employed in British colonies, as well as in the mother country. German-language journals have appeared in Austria and Switzerland (also, for a time, in the United States and Russia). Spanish has been used in former Spanish colonies, and Portuguese in Brazil.

These journals have been devoted to pharmacy as a whole, or to special fields thereof. To a certain extent, the subject matter has been reflected in the titles: *journal* (English, French, German), *bulletin* (English, French; *bolletino,* Italian), *Annals* (German, *Annalen;* French, *Annales*), *Archives* (German and Danish; Italian *Archivio*). Other titles are *Berichte, Magazin, Nachrichten, Zeitung,* etc.

A general bibliography was attempted (1913) by Eugène Guitard in his *Deux siècles de presse au service de pharmacie et cinquante ans de l'Union Pharmaceutique;* a concise bibliography of pharmaceutical journals up to 1894, using the German language (in the United States as well as in other countries) was prepared by F. Hoffmann, editor of the *Pharmazeutische Rundschau* (*12*:7–28). A more complete account will be found in Adlung and Urdang: *Grundriss der Geschichte der deutschen Pharmazie,* pp. 259–271. For American journals, see Minnie Meyer: "Pharmaceutical Journals of the United States," Master's Thesis, University of Wisconsin, 1933. A historical list of journals by states was published in the *J.A.Ph.A. 22*:424, 1933. The best key to currently published journals is the "World List of Pharmacy Periodicals," Theodora Andrews and J. Oslet, eds., *Am. J. Hosp. Pharm. 32*:85–124, 1975 (1st ed., ibid. 1963), republished separately; see also, Henry C. Bolton: *A Catalogue of Scientific and Technical Periodicals, 1665–1895,* ed. 2, Washington, D.C. 1897. See also Appendix 6.

***Kalefactor.*** See: **Personnel.**

**Kebler,** Lyman Fr. (1863–1955), chemist of most versatile activity, worked in governmental service, and in educational and industrial positions; and made contributions on chemical, food and medical subjects, and also on pharmaceutical history; with U.S.D.A. Bureau of Chemistry 1903–29 (chief, Drug division, 1907–23). See *Who's Who in America,* 1938, p. 1386; *American Men of Science,* ed. 8, p. 1317, 1949.

**Kelly,** Evander F. (1879–1944) was professor at the Maryland College of Pharmacy, active in manufacturing pharmacy, pharmaceutical author, and Secretary of the American Pharmaceutical Association from 1926 to 1944. See *J.A.Ph.A. 11*:3, 1922; *Ibid., Pract. Ed. 5*:322–326, 1944.

**Kierstedt,** Hans Taylor (1793–1882), pharmacist in New York. See *Proc. A.Ph.A. 30:*615, 661, 1882.

**King,** John (1813–1893), pioneer eclectic physician and pharmacologist. See H. A. Kelly and W. L. Burrage: *American Medical*

*Biographies,* New York, 1920, p. 661; *Lloyd Libr., Bull.* No. 19, 4, 1912, p. 3.

**Klaproth,** Martin Heinrich (1743–1817), German pharmacist and one of the great chemists of his period. Most of his discoveries he made in the small laboratory of his own pharmacy. He is considered the father of modern analytic chemistry; he was the first to recognize with certainty the elementary character of uranium, titanium and zirconium in 1789; strontium and cerium in 1803. He found fluorine in bones and potassium in feldspar, and was the first to separate barium and strontium. One of his biographers especially stressed that Klaproth never published anything other than his own investigations, and some new facts, and never repeated himself. When the University of Berlin was founded in 1809, he was made its first professor of chemistry. The first Prussian pharmacopeia (1799) bears, in its resolute adoption of the principles of modern chemistry, the impress of this great pharmacist. See Georg Edmund Dann: *Martin Heinrich Klaproth* (1743–1817), Berlin, 1958; George Urdang: M. H. Klaproth, *J.A.Ph.A.* Pract. Ed. *4*:358–31, 1943; and *Dictionary Scient. Biog.*

**Kraemer,** Henry (1868–1924), pharmaceutical teacher and author, was especially known for his botanic and pharmacognostic research work. See J. W. England: *First Century of the Philadelphia College of Pharmacy,* p. 415, Philadelphia, 1922; *J.A.Ph.A. 13*:980, 1924.

**Kremers,** Edward (1865–1941), professor and director of the Course in Pharmacy, University of Wisconsin (1892 to 1935) editor, author, pharmaceutical historian. His example led the way to the modern reform of American pharmaceutical education. See *American Men of Science,* 1938, p. 803; *Who's Who in America,* 1938, p 1457; George Urdang: Edward Kremers in *Am. J. Pharm. Ed.11*:631–658, 1947.

***Laborant.*** See: **Personnel.**

***Laboranten.*** The German term has two meanings: (1) From the 17th to the 19th century, it designated the manufacturers and itinerant sellers—frequently the same persons—of the so-called *Olitäten, q.v.* (2) In more recent times, the term *Laboranten* has referred to people doing laboratory work requiring little or no scientific education.

***Lagerist.*** See: **Personnel.**

**Lasca, Il.** See: **Grazzini.**

**Lascoff,** J. Leon (1867–1943), Russian-born American pharmacist, by example and teaching, made promotion of American professional pharmacy his life task. Starting in 1944 a Lascoff honor award is conferred upon a meritorious pharmacist each year recommended by the evaluation committee of the American College of Apothecaries, which Lascoff helped to found. See *J.A.Ph.A. 26*:199, 1937.

***Laufbursche.*** See: **Personnel.**

**Lavoisier,** Antoine Laurent (1743–1794), French chemist and victim of the French revolutionary tribunal. His fame rests on the recognition of oxygen (discovered almost simultaneously by Priestly, *q.v.,* and Scheele, *q.v.*) as the principle of combustion and on the experimental proof of the part played by oxygen in all chemical and biological changes (oxidation and reduction), thus disproving the phlogiston theory, *q.v.* See Douglas McKie: *Antoine Lavoisier,* Philadelphia, 1935; and Denis Duveen and Herbert Klickstein: A Bibliography of the Works of A. L. Lavoisier, 1743–1794, London, 1954; *Dictionary Scient. Biog.*

**Law for the separation of medicine and pharmacy.** The medical edicts of Frederick II, issued in all probability between 1231 and 1241, had a far-reaching influence on pharmacy, as discussed in the text. A critical edition of Latin texts,* from collating

---

*According to Sudhoff, the law was published in Latin and, simultaneously, in Greek (*Mitt. zur Gesch. der Med.* 13 (1914), p. 180-182). This is important, not only because it allows a comparison of the two texts, but also because it is interesting proof of the fact that at that time Latin and Greek were spoken in the Kingdom of the Two Sicilies.

various manuscripts, has been prepared and given its proper historical setting and interpretation by the pharmacist-historians Wolfgang-Hagen Hein and Kurt Sappert, *Die Medizinalordnung Friedrich II; Eine pharmaziehistorische Studie* (Internationale Gesellschaft, Bd. 12), Eutin, 1957, pp. 48–57 for Latin text and German translation. To convey the general content of the two edicts holding most pharmaceutical interest, we quote a somewhat condensed English version (*Journal of the American Medical Association*, January, 1908; quoted according to J. T. Wash: *The Popes and Science*, p. 419–423).

"Title 46: Every physician given a license to practice must take an oath that he shall fulfill all the requirements of the law, and in addition, whenever it comes to his knowledge that any apothecary has for sale drugs that are of less than normal strength, he shall report him to the court. . . . He (the physician) must not enter into any business relations with the apothecary, nor must he take any of them under his protection nor incur any money obligations in their regard. Nor must any licensed physician keep an apothecary's shop himself. Apothecaries must conduct their business with a certificate from a physician,[1] according to the regulations and upon their own credit and responsibility, and they shall not be permitted to sell their products without having taken an oath that all their drugs have been prepared in the prescribed form, without any fraud. The apothecary may derive the following profits from his sales: Such extracts[2] and simples as he need not keep in stock for more than a year before they may be employed may be charged for at the rate of three tarrenes[3] an ounce. Other medicines, however, which in consequence of the special condition required for their preparation[4] or for any other reason the apothecary has to have in stock for more than a year, he may charge for at the rate of six tarrenes an ounce. Stations for the preparation of medicines may not be located anywhere, but only in certain communities in the Kingdom, as we prescribe below.

"Title 47: In every province of our Kingdom which is under our legal authority, we decree that two prudent and trustworthy men, whose names must be sent to our court, shall be appointed and bound by a formal oath, under whose inspection electuaries and syrups and other medicines be prepared according to law and only be sold after such inspection. In Salerno in particular, we decree that this inspectorship shall be limited to those who have taken their degree as Masters In Physics. . . . We decree also that the growers of plants meant for medicinal purposes[5] shall be bound by a solemn oath that they shall prepare medicines conscientiously, according to the rules of their art, and as far as it is humanly possible that they shall prepare them in the presence of the inspectors. Violations of this law shall be punished by the confiscation of their

[1]A better translation, fitting better the sense of the Latin text, would be: "with the approval of the physicians."

[2]The Latin word *confectiones* cannot be translated by the word "extracts." It means *all* compounded preparations, in contrast to simple drugs.

[3]One *tarrene* equals about 30 cents.

[4]Ex natura means "because of their special nature." There is no reason for an interpretation like that given in the above translation.

[5]The translation is very dubious. The Latin word *conficientes* means, simply, "preparers." Alfred Bäumer translates it as "apothecary" (*Die Aerztegesetzbebung Kaiser Friedrichs II und ihre geschichtliche Grundlage*, Leipzig 1911). That seems to be dubious too, because the duties of the apothecaries, the *confectionarii,* are regulated above, without, however, mentioning the penalties. There is a third and probable possibility of interpretation. The *confectionarius* is the learned apothecary, without respect to the question whether he himself prepares medicines or not. *Conficiens* is anybody who actually prepares something, and *conficientes medicinas* are, therefore, all people who prepare medicines. Thus this term may be used to bring all kinds or preparers of medicines into the frame of the law, whether apothecaries or not.

movable goods. If the inspectors, however, to whose fidelity to duty the keeping of these regulations is committed shall allow any fraud in the matters that are entrusted to them, they shall be condemned to punishment by death."

**LaWall,** Charles H. (1871–1937). LaWall was active in almost all branches of pharmacy: in community practice and in pharmaceutical industry, as an analytic chemist and as a teacher, and in official governmental positions. In addition, he was a prolific writer on pharmaceutical subjects. His *Four Thousand Years of Pharmacy* represents the first attempt at a history of pharmacy written by an American and published in book form in America. See *J.A.Ph.A. 26*:1223, 1937; J. W. England: *First Century of the Philadelphia College of Pharmacy,* p. 420, Philadelphia, 1922.

**LeFebvre,** Nicaise (Nicolas), also called Lefèvre (1610–1674). French pharmacist and chemical author. His *Traité de chymie théorique et pratique,* the fifth edition of which was published under the title *Cours de chymie,* was considered the best chemical textbook of that period and was translated into several languages including English.

***Lefèvre.*** See: **LeFebvre.**

**Lehman,** William (1779–1829), Philadelphia physician and practicing pharmacist, importantly active in scientific and political life. See J. W. England, *First Century of the Philadelphia College of Pharmacy,* p. 352, Philadelphia, 1922.

***Lehr-Bube.*** See: **Personnel.**

***Lehrbursche.*** See: **Personnel.**

***Lehr-Junge.*** See: **Personnel.**

***Lehrling.*** See: **Personnel.**

**Lémery,** Nicolas (1645–1715), French pharmacist who is considered the founder of modern phytochemistry. He taught the analysis of vegetable drugs by the extraction method. In accordance with the traditional classification of all natural objects into three kingdoms, he arranged the materia chemica into mineral, vegetable and animal categories. He was one of the most-translated authors of his time, and his principal books went through many editions. His *Cours de chymie* superseded the book of LeFebvre, *q.v.,* and was for about a century the world's most-used chemistry text. Lémery's *Pharmacopée universelle* appeared in 1697. See C. Guedon: *Isis 65*:212–228, 1974.

**Lespleigney,** Thibault (1496–1567), French pharmacist and writer on pharmaceutical subjects. His *Promptuaire des medecines simples en rythme joyeuse* was reprinted (1898) by Paul Dorveaux.

**Lewis,** William (1714–1781), English physician and chemist. His *New Dispensatory,* containing the theory and the practice of pharmacy, and some of his books on technical chemistry, were translated into German. On the other hand, he translated the pharmaceutical treatise of the German pharmacist Caspar Neumann, *q.v.,* into English. See Edward Kremers: William Lewis, *J.A.Ph.A. 20*:1204, 1931.

**Libavius** (Latinized form of Libau), Andreas (1540–1616), physician and one of the most eminent early chemists. See F. Ferchl: *Chemisch-Pharmazeutisches Bio- und Bibliographikon,* p. 313, Mittenwald, 1937.

**Liebig,** Justus von (1803–1873), German chemist, known especially because of his pioneer work in agricultural and in physiologic chemistry. He was connected with pharmacy by 10 months of pharmaceutical apprenticeship, by a later short activity as inspector of the pharmacies in the Grand Duchy of Hessen, and by collaboration with pharmaceutical chemists throughout his life. In the first laboratory at the University of Giessen, he introduced a type of experimental chemical instruction that became the model for modern chemical instruction the world over. See *Am. J. Pharm. 45*:240, 1873; J. Liebig, an autobiographic sketch, trans. by J. Campbell, *Annual Report* for 1891 of the Smithsonian Institution, p. 257; A. Hofmann, The lifework of Liebig (Faraday lecture, 1875).

**Liggett,** Louis Kroh (1875–1946), American organizer of one of the largest drugstore chains in the world. See Samuel Merwin: *Rise and Fight Againe,* New York, 1935.

**Lilly,** Eli (1838–1898), pharmacist and founder of Eli Lilly and Company, in Indianapolis. See *Proc. A.Ph.A. 46*:48, 1898; *Tile and Till 12*:No. 2, 1926.

**Lilly,** Josiah K. (1861–1948), pharmacist and, in sequence, president and chairman of the board of Eli Lilly and Company. A graduate of the Philadelphia College of Pharmacy (1882), Josiah K. Lilly not only developed his plant into one of the world's greatest pharmaceutical concerns based on scientific research, but made it his task to foster, in fact as well as in idea, the concept of pharmacy as a unit comprised of research, manufacture, wholesaling, dispensing and teaching. For this reason he was given (1942) the highest honor American professional pharmacy grants, the Remington Medal. See McCormick, G. E.: *Pharm. Hist. 12*:57–67, 1970; also, *J.A.Ph.A. 9*:165, 1948.

**Linstead,** Hugh N. (1901– ), distinguished British pharmacist and barrister; son of a pharmacist in Brighton, Secretary of the Pharmaceutical Society of Great Britain, 1926–1964 (previously Asst. Sec.), President of the International Pharmaceutical Federation, 1954–1966. Member of Parliament (1942) and appointed to various governmental bodies. Knighted by the Queen (1953), and decorated and honored by various governments and societies. See: *Who's Who* [British]

**Lloyd,** John Uri (1849–1936). One of the greatest and most versatile pharmacists that America has had. Lloyd was a scientific chemist, a pharmaceutical manufacturer, a teacher and an author of scientific literature as well as of novels; he excelled in all these fields. He was early connected with the Eclectic School of Medicine and played an important part in the development of plant chemistry and drug extraction. The Lloyd Library, initiated by him in Cincinnati, is one of the most comprehensive of its kind and contains not only modern books but also valuable publications out of the pharmaceutical past. See *Dictionary Scient. Biog.*; C. M. Simons: John Uri Lloyd—His Life and Works, 1849–1936, with a History of the Lloyd Library, (private) Cincinnati, Ohio, 1972; also, *J.A.Ph.A. 25*:885, 1936.

***Lohoch,*** from the Arabian *la aka,* "to lick." It was a thick liquid, being of a consistency between a syrup and an electuary.

**Lonicerus,** Adam (1528–1586), municipal physician in Frankfort-on-the-Main. His herbal (1557) continued through more than two centuries, the last (the 20th) edition being issued in 1783.

**Loochs.** See: ***Lohoch.***

***Lumen.*** See: **Pharmacopeia.**

***Luminare.*** See: **Pharmacopeia.**

***Lyekopis.*** See: **Pharmacopeia.**

**Lyman,** Rufus A. (1875–1957), a physician who became one of the most influential pharmaceutical educators of the 20th century in the United States. Founding editor (1937–1955) of the *American Journal of Pharmaceutical Education*; pharmacy dean at the universities of Nebraska and Arizona, and a central figure in the American Association of Colleges of Pharmacy. See J. Tom: *Pharm. Hist. 14*:90–94 & 111, 1972, and M. R. Gibson: *Am. J. Pharm. Edu. 39*:3–9, 1975; personal papers in AIHP Ms. Collection, Madison, Wisc.

**Lyons,** Albert B. (1841–1926), M.D., pharmacist, and professor of chemistry at Detroit College of Medicine, then editor of the *Pharmaceutical Era,* later government chemist and professor in Hawaii and, finally, manufacturing chemist. See *J.A.Ph.A. 15*:411, 1926; J. W. England: *First Century of the Philadelphia College of Pharmacy,* p. 218, Philadelphia, 1922.

**Maben,** Thomas (1855–1937), English pharmaceutical chemist and member of the English staff of the American pharmaceutical firm of Parke, Davis and Company. See *Chem. & Drug. 126*:675, 1927.

**McDonnell,** John N. (1910–1972), American

pharmacist. Practitioner, educator, industrial executive and consultant; government service included Director, Officer of Civilian Penicillin Distribution, War Production Board (1944–45); Editor of *American Professional Pharmacist*—and in other publishing enterprises during 1930's and 40's teamed with the pharmacist-editor Madeline Oxford Holland, his spouse. *J.A.Ph.A.* ns *12*:346, 1972.

**Macfarlan,** John Fletcher (1790–1861), Scottish chemist, pharmacist and physician. A founding member of the Pharmaceutical Society of Great Britain, he also played an important part in medical association work. See *Pharm. J. 20*:488, 1861.

**McIntyre,** Ewen (1825–1913), New York pharmacist. See *J.A.Ph.A. 2*:282, 417, 552, 1913.

**Maimonides** or Abu 'Imran Mûsa ibn Maimon (1135–1204). A Jewish-Spanish physician, who wrote in Arabic. See I. Muenz and H. T. Schnittkind: Maimonides, Boston, 1935; E. H. Rodin: Maimonides, *Calif. and West. Med. 44*:192, 1936; J. J. Wash: *Old-Time Makers of Medicine,* p. 90, New York, 1911; George Sarton: *Introduction to the History of Science, II,* part I, pp. 369–380, Baltimore, 1931. As for the so-called "Prayer of Maimonides," see David Reisman: *The Story of Medicine in the Middle Ages,* p. 64, New York, 1935.

**Maisch,** Henry C. (1865–1901), pharmacist, manufacturing chemist, oldest son of John M. Maisch. See. *Am. J. Pharm. 74*:458, 1902.

**Maisch,** John M. (1831–1893). Maisch entered pharmacy after his arrival in the United States as a German political refugee. He soon became prominent as a teacher, an author and above all as an editor of the *American Journal of Pharmacy*, and the first Permanent Secretary of the American Pharmaceutical Association (1865–1893). See J. P. Remington: J. M. Maisch, *Am. J. Pharm. 66*:1, 1894; J. W. England: *First Century of the Philadelphia College of Pharmacy,* p. 405, Philadelphia, 1922; M. I. Wilbert: John Michael Maisch, an ideal pharmacist, *Am. J. Pharm. 75*:351, 1903. G. Urdang: The fiftieth anniversary of the death of John Michael Maisch, *Am. J. Pharm. 116*:1–11, 1944.

**Mallinckrodt,** Edward (1845–1928), one of the founders and the chief organizer and leader of the firm of G. Mallinckrodt & Co., St. Louis. See *J.A.Ph.A. 17*:208, 1928.

**Manlius de Bosco,** Jacobus (15th century), Italian pharmacist and probably the first pharmaceutical author of a treatise in Italy; compiler of a book on materia medica.

**Marggraf,** Andreas Sigismund (1709–1782), German pharmacist and one of the greatest chemists of his time, Marggraf differentiated between potassium and sodium compounds, identified magnesium, produced compounds of mercury and of silver with organic acids, was the first to prepare potassium cyanide, introduced numerous reagents and discovered sugar in various plants, particularly in the sugar beet. He reported this most important discovery in 1747. In his investigation he used the microscope, the employment of which in chemistry became customary.

**Markoe,** George F. H. (1840–1896), Boston pharmacist, pharmaceutical manufacturer and professor at the Massachusetts College of Pharmacy. See W. L. Scoville: *Am. J. Pharm. 68*:593, 1896.

**Marshall,** Charles (1744–1824), pharmacist in Philadelphia. He was the first president of the Philadelphia College of Pharmacy. See J. W. England: *First Century of the Philadelphia College of Pharmacy,* p. 348, Philadelphia, 1922; E. T. Ellis, *Am. J. Pharm. 75*:57, 1903.

**Marshall,** Christopher, Jr., pharmacist in Philadelphia (eighteenth century). He was the oldest son of Christopher Marshall, Sr., *q.v.*, and for a time, together with his brother, Charles, *q.v.*, owner of the Marshall pharmacy in Philadelphia. See E. T. Ellis: *Am. J. Pharm. 75*:57, 1903.

**Marshall,** Christopher Sr. (1709–1797),

Irish-born pharmacist in Philadelphia. See E. T. Ellis: The story of a very old Philadelphia drug store, *Am J. Pharm. 75*:57, 1903.

**Martius,** Ernst Wilhelm (1756–1849), German pharmacist and professor of pharmacy at the University of Erlangen. He wrote one of the best-known German autobiographies, containing many interesting descriptions of pharmaceutical life.

**Mathioli,** Pietro Andrea (1501–1577), Italian physician and botanist in the service of the German Emperor Maximilian II. His revised and annotated edition of Dioscorides' *De materia medica* meant a revival of the work of the great Greek author. It went through many editions.

**Mayerne,** Theodore Turquet de (1573–1655), French-Swiss physician. Mayerne was forbidden to practice medicine in Paris because he was a Paracelsist and employed antimony in his practice. He went to England, where he became physician-in-ordinary to James I. He published several formulas for chemical remedies. See *Dictionary of National* (English) *Biography, 37*:150; George Urdang: *Pharmacopoeia Londinensis of 1618,* pp. 12, 18–21, 28, 55, 61–64, 72–73, Madison, Wis., 1944.

**Mayo,** Caswell A. (1862–1928), one of the best known American pharmaceutical journalists. See *J.A.Ph.A. 17*:209, 1928.

**Meakim,** John (1812–1863), pharmacist in New York and one of the original members of the American Pharmaceutical Association. See *Am. J. Pharm. 35*:574, 1863; *Proc. A.Ph.A. 12*:23, 1864.

**Mease,** James (1771–1846), physician, editor, author, one of the founders of the Philadelphia Athenaeum. See: *Dictionary of American Biography 12*:486.

***Medicamentarius,*** pl. ***-i.*** from *medicamentum* (cf. the Greek *pharmakon*), "a remedy," and *-arius,* "pertaining to," i.e., a maker of remedies or medicaments.

**Medicine chest.** The chest used by an Egyptian princess (preserved in Berlin) is supposed to have been a medicine chest (possibly also a cosmetic chest). The *apotheca* unearthed in Herculaneum was another such chest. The German language differentiates between *Hausapotheke,* "medicine chest" or "cupboard" for the home; *Reiseapotheke,* a medicine chest convenient while traveling; *Feldapotheke,* or "army chest," used by soldiers in the field. Such regimental chests were prepared at a central station during the American Revolutionary War, for regiments while in the field. (See George B. Griffenhagen: Drug Supplies in the American Revolution, Bulletin 225 [also as Paper 16 in Contributions from the Museum of History and Technology], Smithsonian Institution, Washington, D.C., 1961. Although pioneer physicians carried medical supplies in their saddle bags while on the road, in their surgeries they had small medicine chests.

**Mercer,** Hugh (1725–1777). Scottish-born American physician, who fought in the Revolutionary Army first as a colonel and then as a general, and died from wounds received on the battlefield. The building where he operated a pharmacy and medical office (from 1764) survives in Fredericksburg, Va. (the oldest original structure of its purpose?). See *Dictionary Am. Biog., XII,* p. 541; *J.A.Ph.A. 15*:425, 1926; and J. M. Waterman, *With Sword and Lancet,* Richmond, Va., 1941.

**Merck** in Darmstadt, a German pharmaceutical firm, founded in the twenties of the 19th century, grew out of the "Engel-Apotheke" in Darmstadt, owned by the Merck family since 1668. See: [C. Löw], *Die chemische Fabrik E. Merck-Darmstadt, Darmstadt,* 1952, 78 pp.

**Mesuë,** Johann, Jr. A pseudonym for writings of the 13th century. The books attributed to Mesuë Junior were: (1) The *Grabadin,* from the Arabic *al aqrâbâdhîn* ("compounded remedy"); (2) *Practica medicinarum particularium* or *liber de appropriatis,* often designated a second part of the *Grabadin;* (3) *De medicinis laxativis (solutivis, purgatoriis)* or *De simplicibus* or

*De consolatione simplicium* or *De medicamentorum purgantium simplicium delectu et castigatione*. See A. Tschirch: *Handbuch der Pharmakognosie,* Leipzig, 1910, *I,* part 2, p. 599; G. Sarton: *Introduction to the History of Science, II,* part II, p. 854, Baltimore, 1931 (in section on Samuel Ben Jacob of Capua).

**Mesuë,** Johann, Sr. (777–857), a Christian physician who wrote in Arabic. See A. Tschirch: *Handbuch der Pharmakognosie,* Leipzig, 1910, *I,* part 2, p. 597; G. Sarton: *Introduction to the History of Science, I,* p. 374, Baltimore, 1927.

**Meune,** Odo of (12th century), called also Odo Maydunensis, author of *Macer floridus,* a Latin poem about herbs. The name Macer goes back to the Roman poet Aemilius Macer whom the author wished to honor.

***Migmatopolos***, pl. ***-oi***, seller of mixtures, from the Greek migma (mixture), and polein (to sell).

**Milhau,** John (1795–1874), American pharmacist of French descent and of French pharmaceutical education. Milhau was one of the early leaders of the New York College of Pharmacy. "The passage of the U. S. drug law of 1848 is mainly due to his persistent and conscientious efforts." See G. Sonnedecker in *Veröff. Internatl. Gesell. Gesch. Pharm.*, ns Bd. *42*, p. 141, 1975; also *Am. J. Pharm. 47*:94, 1875; *Drug. Circ. 51*:89, 1907.

**Minderer,** Raymond (1570–1621), physician-in-ordinary to the German Emperor Mathias (1612–1619) and municipal physician in Augsburg. He edited the four earliest 17th-century editions of the *Pharmacopoeia Augustana* and tried to bridge the break between the Galenists, who wanted to restrict therapy to the old drugs known to Galen and his followers, and the Paracelsists, who recommended the employment of chemicals more or less exclusively. His *Medicina militaris,* 1619, represents one of the earliest military pharmacopeias. See Theodor Husemann: introductory essays, in facsimile of the first edition of the *Pharmacopoeia Augustana,* Wisconsin State Historical Society, Madison, Wis., 1927.

**Mitchill,** Samuel L. (1764–1831), physician, chemist, author, editor and senator. See Lyman F. Kebler: S. L. Mitchill, *J.A.Ph.A. 26*:908; 1937.

**Mohr,** Carl Friedrich (1806–1879). German pharmacist and inventor of pharmaceutical and chemical apparatus and technic. Many pieces of auxiliary apparatus used in volumetric analysis were invented by him. His balance for determining specific gravity became a universally used instrument. Among his many books, *Lehrbuch der pharmazeutischen Technik* is especially noteworthy. Upon it were based Redwood's book on *Practical Pharmacy,* in England, and an enlarged edition published by Procter, *q.v.*, in the United States.

**Mohr,** Charles (1824–1901), German-born American pharmaceutical manufacturer and botanist. He was one of the first, if not the first, forester agent of the U. S. Government. See: *Am. J. Pharm. 74*:459, 1902.

**Moissan,** Henri (1852–1907), French pharmacist, discoverer of fluorine and the first to prepare artificial diamonds, recipient of the Nobel prize in chemistry (1906). Before starting teaching at the *École supérieure de pharmacie* in Paris, Moissan had been a pharmaceutical apprentice and a clerk, and had received his diploma as a *pharmacien de première classe.*

**Molière,** pen name of Jean Baptiste Poquelin (1622–1673), a French dramatist famous for his comedies. He often ridicules medical chicanery; *le Médecin malgré lui, le Malade imaginaire* and *l'Amor médecin* contain delightful caricatures of physicians and pharmacists.

**Moore,** J. B. (1832–1909), Philadelphia pharmacist and writer on pharmaceutical subjects. See England, *First Century of the Philadelphia College of Pharmacy,* p. 241, Philadelphia, 1922.

**Moore,** J. Faris (1826–1888), pharmacist in Baltimore and professor at the Maryland

College of Pharmacy. See *Drug. Circ. 51*:88, 1907; *Proc. A.Ph.A. 36*:34, 1888.

**Morgan,** John (1735–1789), American physician, founder of the first American school of medicine and the first influential advocate of the separation of American medicine from pharmacy. See W. J. Bell, Jr., *John Morgan Continental Doctor,* Philadelphia, 1965; M. I Wilbert: John Morgan, *Am. J. Pharm. 76*:1, 1904.

***Morsuli.*** Plural diminutive of *morsus,* a bite (German *Bissen*), from *mordeo,* to bite. *Morselen* or lozenges are hard confections prepared from drugs and sugar. Certain *morsuli* are prepared as much for their taste as for their effect; others are prepared with medicaments, e.g., *China morsellen, Antimonialmorsellen. Wurmmorsellen,* (cf.: ***Rotulae*** and ***Tabulae.***)

**Motter,** Murray Galt (1866–1926), physician, professor of physiology at Georgetown University, director of library service for the Public Health Service; active in U. S. Pharmacopeial work. See *J.A.Ph.A. 15*:125, 1926.

**Moudry,** Frank W. (d. 1971), American pharmacist. Community practitioner in St. Paul, civic leader, authority on pharmacy law enforcement. Secretary of the Minnesota Board of Pharmacy (16 years), and a leader in the National Association of Boards of Pharmacy and in the National Association of Retail Druggists. See *Proc. N.A.B.P.* 1972, p. xxiv; *J.A.Ph.A. 11*:579, 1971.

**Mühlenberg,** Gotthilf Heinrich Ernst (1753–1815), American clergyman and botanist of German descent. Mühlenberg first identified about 100 species and varieties of American plants. See *Am. J. Pharm. 80*:420, 1908; *Pharm. Rund.* 4:119, 1886; *Dictionary Amer. Biog., XIII,* p. 308.

**Mynsicht,** Adrian van (real name Seumenicht) (1603–1683), was a German physician. In his book *Thesaurus et armamentarium medico-chymicum* he for the first time described the preparation of Tartarus emeticus.

***Myrepsos,*** pl. ***-oi,*** maker of ointments, from the Greek myron ("ointment"). See also: ***Myropoeos.***

***Myropoeos,*** pl. ***-oi,*** makers of ointments, from the Greek *myron* ("ointment"). See also: ***Myrepsos.***

**Nees,** von Esenbeck, Theodor Friedrich Ludwig (1787–1837), German pharmacist and professor of pharmacy and botany, first in Leyden and then in Bonn. He was the first to recommend flores koso as a remedy for tapeworm. Among his botanical books his *Plantae Officinales* received much attention.

**Neumann,** Caspar (1683–1737), German pharmacist who was one of the earliest scientific phytochemists. He objected to the pyrochemical method, which yields ashes as therapeutic products. He discovered thyme camphor (thymol) in 1719. An English translation of his lectures by William Lewis appeared (1760) under the title *The Chymical works of Gaspard Neumann Abridged and Methodized with Large Additions.* See P. Stechl, *Pharm. Hist. 12*:51–56, 1970, which includes bibliography of writings.

**Newcomb,** Edwin Leigh (1882–1950), pharmacist, teacher, editor, administrator, one of the most influential leaders of American pharmacy of his period. While teaching at the College of Pharmacy of the University of Minnesota, he established one of the first North American medicinal plant gardens connected with a school of pharmacy. Contributions to the United States Pharmacopoeia and the founding of the Plant Science Seminar (1923). Secretary (from 1927; later executive vice-president) of the National Wholesale Druggists' Association. The founding (1942) and early success of the American Foundation for Pharmaceutical Education was mainly due to

Newcomb's influence. See *J.A.Ph.A.* (Prac. Ed.) *11*:304–305, 1950.

**Newton,** Vandeveer L. (1809–1880), physician and, later on, editor of the *Druggists Circular.* See: *Drug. Circ. 51*:5, 1907.

**Nicolaus Myrepsus** or Alexandrinus (14th century), a physician living in Byzantium, author of a well-known antidotarium. The cognomen Alexandrinus means "the Alexandrian"; the cognomen *Myrepsus,* "ointment cook."

**Nicolaus Praepositus** (about 1500), a French physician who lived in Tours, wrote a well-known antidotarium. The cognomen *praepositus* indicates his position as presiding official, in this case dean.

**Nicolaus Salernitanus.** The presumed author of the oldest antidotarium or formulary associated with the name Nicolaus, an author-name of tangled and obscure literary tradition (note above). Probably formularies associated with the cognomen Nicolaus Salernitanus were based on the anonymous *Antidotarius magnus* (about 1087–1100), whose principal source, in turn, was the Salernitan work of Constantine the African, *q.v.* The name Nicolaus appears nowhere in the *Antidotarius magnus,* and did not become associated with this formulary tradition until after the 12th century. (See Lutz, Alfons: . . . Antidotarius magnus . . . , *Acta Pharmac ae Historica,* No. 1, 1959)

**Occo**, Adolf (or Adolph Occo III, to differentiate him from the two earlier Adolph Occos before him who also were physicians of Augsburg, Germany) (1524–1606). Occo III not only published treatises on medical subjects but also on philosophy, philology and numismatics. See introductory essays by Theodor Husemann, facsimile of the *Pharmacopoeia Augustana, 1565,* Madison, Wis., 1927.

**Oerstedt,** Hans Christian (1777–1851), eminent physicist, son of a Danish pharmacist, in whose pharmacy he passed through an apprenticeship. He even managed for a short time a pharmacy in Copenhagen. H. C. Oerstedt established the principles of electromagnetism and discovered piperine (1820). See Philippe and Ludwig: *Geschichte der Apotheken,* p. 707, Jena, 1855.

**Officina.** See: ***Officine*** and ***Pharmacopeia.***

***Officine.*** From Latin *opus,* "work" (still in common usage in music and literature) e.g., *magnum opus,* and *facere,* "to make" (cf. "factor" and "factory"). The room in which the pharmacist did his work. Later, when a separate laboratory and also a separate storeroom (German *Materialkammer*) were differentiated, the term *officine* was restricted to the dispensing (sales) room in which the pharmacist compounded his prescriptions. The Latin *officina* was Gallicized to *officine,* a designation introduced into English pharmaceuticul literature by the Paris correspondent of the *Chemist and Druggist* of London. The German spelling is *Offizin.* Just as the Dutch *apothek* has been used as a title for a pharmaceutical treatise (e.g., pharmacopeia) so the French word has been used by Dorvault for his handbook *L'officin.*

This designation has been applied not only to the workshop of the pharmacist but also to printing offices, such as the world-famous printing establishment of Plantin and Morehus in Antwerp. On the titlepage of pharmacopeias there is frequently found the reference *ex officina,* followed by the name of the printer.

**Oldberg**, Oscar (1846–1913), Swedish-born American pharmacist. Oldberg was active and instrumental in various fields of pharmacy, as teacher, editor and author of several books. See *Am. J. Pharm. 85*:272, 1913; *J.A.Ph.A. 2*:550, 1913.

**Olitäten** is a German term that designates popular proprietaries of secret composition, prepared since the 17th century, especially in small hamlets in the Silesian mountains and the mountainous parts of Saxony. The term *Olitäten* has been said to derive from the oily consistency of the first and the most popular of these medicines. The peddlers selling these preparations were called *Olitätenhändler*. See A. Adlung and G. Urdang: *Grundriss der Geschichte der deutschen Pharmazie*, pp. 122, 129, 174, Berlin, 1935.

**Oreibasius Pergamenus (Oribasius)** (325–403), physician-in-ordinary to the Roman Emperor Julian the Apostate. Surviving remnants of his work have been edited and translated by Bussemaker and Daremberg in *Oeuvres d'Oribase* (1851–1876). See A. Tschirch: *Handbuch der Pharmakognosie, I*, Part 2, p. 588, Leipzig, 1910.

**Osiris.** The Egyptian god of the underworld and judge of the dead; one of the gods to whom healing power was attributed. He was considered the brother and the husband of Isis, and the father of Horus and Anubis.

**Painter,** Emlen (1844–1890), pharmacist in San Francisco, and pharmaceutical manufacturer, later on, in New York; one of the founders of the California College of Pharmacy and a professor there. See *Pharm. Era* 4:21, 1890; *Druggist's Bull.* 4:36, 1800.

**Papyrus.** (1) The name of a tall sedge, *Cyperus papyrus*, which grows along the banks of the Nile. (2) The name applied to a paper-like material on which the ancient Egyptians painted their hieroglyphics. (3) The name applied to the manuscripts (pl. "papyri") thus prepared. See J. E. Mitchell: The Egyptian papyrus, past and present. *Scient. Am.* 1904, p. 484.

**Papyrus, Ebers,** one of the earliest and most extensive pharmaceutical and therapeutic documents that survives. See B. Ebbel: *The Papyrus Ebers*, translated from W. Wreszinski's hieroglyphic transcript into English, Oxford, 1937; also George Ebers: *Das hermetische Buch über die Arzeimittel der alten Aegypter in hieratischer Schrift*, Leipzig, 1875; H. Joachim: *Papyros Ebers*, translation into German, Berlin, 1890; Walter Wreszinski: *Der Papyrus Ebers, Um Schrift Übersetzung und Kommentar*, Leipzig., 1913.

**Paracelsus,** Aureolus Philippus (or with his original name, Theophrastus Bombastus of Hohenheim) (1493–1541). A Swiss-German physician whom William Osler (*The Evolution of Modern Medicine*, p. 135, New Haven, 1923) calls "the Luther of Medicine, the very incarnation of the spirit of revolt." His importance to pharmacy lies in his studies of drugs and of their effects which led to the systematic introduction of metals into internal therapy and the dawn of pharmaceutical chemistry. See J. M. Stillman: *Paracelsus*, Chicago, 1920; Henry M. Pachter, *Paracelsus*, New York, 1951 (paperback, 1963); and especially Walter Pagel, *Paracelsus; An Introduction to Philosophical Medicine in the Era of the Renaissance*, Basel, 1958.

**Parke,** H. C. (d. 1899), one of the founders of Parke, Davis and Company, Detroit. See *Am. J. Pharm.* 71:208, 1899.

**Parke,** Thomas (1749–1835), well-known Philadelphia medical practitioner. See J. A. Spalding: *Life of Dr. Lyman Spalding*, p. 354, Boston, 1916; and Joseph Parrish in ms. F909 of the Library of the College of Physicians of Philadelphia.

**Parkinson,** John (1567–1650), English apothecary and botanist, author of several treatises on botany. Parkinson was appointed apothecary to King James I, who honored the learned man with the title, "*Botanicus regius primarius.*" See *Dictionary* (English) *National Biography, XLIII*, p. 315.

**Parmentier,** Jean Antoine Augustin (1737–1813), French pharmacist who published a number of fundamental treatises on food chemistry (e.g., his investigations of milk). His distinguished work was recognized by his election to the French academy of Sciences. For a bibliography of his writings, see A. Balland, *La Chimie alimentaire dans l'oeuvre de Parmentier* (Paris, 1902). Most of his career was spent as a military pharmacist, rising to the high post of Inspector General of the *Service de santé des Armées*. See *Dictionary Scient. Biog.* and in *Figures Pharmaceutiques Françaises* . . . pp. 29–34, Paris, 1953.

**Parrish,** Edward (1822–1872), Philadelphia pharmacist and professor at the Philadelphia College of Pharmacy. See England: *First Century of the Philadelphia College of Pharmacy*, p. 404, Philadelphia, 1922; *Am. J. Pharm.* *45*:225, 1873; G. Urdang: Edward Parrish, a Forgotten pharmaceutical reformer, *Am. J. Pharm. Ed.* *14*:223–232, 1950.

**Pasteur,** Louis (1822–1897), French chemist and finally director of the Paris Pasteur Institute, founded to carry on his researches. His purely bacteriologic work was his most important contribution to science and to public welfare. His first investigation, his conversion of dextrotartaric acid into the inactive forms, and his discovery of the splitting of racemic acid into dextro- and levotartaric acid, laid the foundation for modern stereochemistry. See *Dictionary Scient. Biog.*; Sigerist: *The Great Doctors*, p. 360, New York, 1933.

**Patin,** Guy (1601–1672), French physician and head of the anti-Paracelsist group of the French medical world of that time. See F. R Packard: *Guy Patin and the Medical Profession in Paris in the Seventeenth Century*, New York, 1925.

**Patrons of pharmacy.** See: **Deities** and **Saints, Christian.**

**Paullini,** Christian Franz (1643–1712), German physician. Besides his famous *Dreckapotheke*, Paullini wrote numerous books on a multitude of subjects, containing "approximately 18,000 printed pages." See Leo Kauner: Christian Franz Paullini, *Med. Life* *41*:231, 1934.

**Pelletier,** Pierre Joseph (1788–1842), French pharmacist and the first and most successful investigator in the field of alkaloids after Sertürner, *q.v.* He discovered, together with Caventou, *q.v.*, strychnine (1818), brucine (1819), quinine and cinchonine (1820; after Gomes), caffeine (simultaneously with Robiquet and Runge, in 1821). With Dumas, *q.v.*, he discovered narceine, thebaine and pseudomorphine. See *Dictionary Scient. Biog.*

**Pemberton,** Henry (1694–1771), English physician, pupil of Boerhaave, author of several books on medicine, physics and chemistry; pharmacopeial work in England. See *Dictionary of National* (English) *Biography, XLIV*, p. 280.

**Pereira,** Jonathan (1804–1853), English apothecary, physician and finally professor of materia medica, at the School of Pharmacy of the Pharmaceutical Society of Great Britain. See *Am. J. Pharm.* *25*:287, 1853.

**Perkin,** Sir William Henry (1838–1907). In 1856, he discovered aniline mauve in the course of attempts to prepare quinine artificially. The aniline dyestuff, although preceded by the emeraldine of F. Runge, *q.v.*, opened the way for the dyestuff industry, with all its sidelines. See H. Goodman: William Henry Perkin, *Med. Life* *42*:151–162, 1935.

**Persia.** Ancient Persia had its period of highest development between 600 and 330 B.C. (Kyros to Darius III) and included the land southeast of the Caspian Sea, Mesopotamia, Asia Minor and Egypt. In regard to medicine and pharmacy in ancient Persia, see H. E. Sigerist: A History of Medicine, Volume 2: Early Greek, Hindu and Persian Medicine, New York, 1961; also Tschirch's *Handbuch der Pharmakognosie*, Leipzig, 1910, *I*: part 2; T. Berendes: *Die Pharmazie bei den alten Kulturvölkern*,

Halle, 1891; C. Elgood: *Medicine in Persia,* New York, 1934. Concerning modern pharmaceutical practice in Persia, see George Cecil: How pharmacy is practiced in Persia (Iran), *Pharm. Era 57*:43, 1923.

**Personnel.**

Comparable terms in English and German for staff in community pharmacies of the 19th and early 20th centuries:

| English | German |
|---|---|
| Apprentice (French; elève) | Lehrling<br>Lehrbursche<br>Lehr-Junge<br>Lehr Bube<br>Tyro[1] |
| Assistant (French: Compagnon-apothicaire) | Assistent<br>Geselle<br>Subject[1]<br>Adjunkt[1]<br>Defectar[2]<br>Defectuar[2] (Latin: Defectuarius) |
| Dispenser, or prescription clerk | Receptar |
| Manager | |
| | Stoesser[3]<br>Laborant[4]<br>Kalefactor[5] |
| Relief pharmacist | Vertreter |
| Stock-clerk or -boy | Lagerist[6] |
| Porter | Hausknecht |
| Errand boy | Laufbursche |

[1]Designation common in Austria rather than in Germany.

[2]The person who attends to work in the laboratory, as opposed to the *Receptar.*

[3]One who comminutes drugs.

[4]A worker doing manual work in a laboratory.

[5]A person somewhat between the *Stoesser* and the *Laborant.*

[6]Person in charge of the stock.

**Peters,** Hermann (1847–1920), German pharmacist and historian of pharmacy. Of his many publications, the books *Der Arzt und die Heilkunde in der deutschen Vergangenheit* and *Aus pharmaceutischer Vorzeit* especially gained wide acknowledgement. The greatest part of Volume I of *Aus pharmaceutischer Vorzeit* has been translated into English (with some changes) and published by William Netter as *Pictorial History of Ancient Pharmacy.* See introduction to Peters: *Aus der Geschichte der Pflanzenwelt in Wort und Bild,* Gesellschaft für Geschichte der Pharmazie, Mittenwald, 1929.

**Pettenkofer,** Max Joseph von (1818–1901), German pharmacist and professor of medicinal chemistry and hygiene at the University of Munich. He is considered the father of modern hygiene.

***Pharmaceut.*** German for pharmacist, *q.v.,* also spelled **Pharmazeut;** English (obsolete), pharmaceutist.

**Pharmaceutical chemist.** English title introduced by the Pharmacy Act of 1852. Former American degree introduced by the Pharmacy School of the University of Michigan in 1869.

***Pharmacien.*** French for pharmacist, *q.v.,* which succeeded the term *apothicaire.* For some time there were two groups of *"pharmaciens,"* the *Pharmacien de première classe,* entitled to open a pharmacy without restriction, and the *Pharmacien de seconde classe,* allowed to operate a pharmacy only in the district in which he had passed his examination.

**Pharmacist,** from Greek *Pharmakon* ("remedy") and *-ist* ("pertaining to"), a maker of or dealer in remedies. Cf. ***Pharmacopoeus*** and ***Pharmacopolus.*** See also French ***Pharmacien*** and German ***Pharmaceut*** or ***Pharmazeut.*** Cf. also **Pharmaceutical chemist.**

***Pharmacopée.*** See: **Pharmacopeia.**

**Pharmacopeia.** From the Greek word *pharmakon* ("remedy") and *poiein* ("to make"). As the title for a formulary, it was first used by Jacques du Bois (Sylvius) in his *Phar-*

*macopoeae, libri tres,* printed in Lyon in 1548, and by Bretschneider (called Placotomus) in his *Pharmacopoea in compendium redacta,* printed in Antwerp in 1560. In a modern sense, a pharmacopeia is a compilation intended to secure uniformity in medicinal agents as to kind, quality, composition and therapeutic strength, whose specifications are legally obligatory within a defined political area. Since the 18th century the term has been applied largely to treatises in the foregoing or similar sense (e.g., cf. Wittop-Koning, D. A.: *Veröff. Internatl. Gesell. Gesch. Pharm.*, ns Bd. *22*:p. 181, 1963). The spelling varies in different countries: "pharmacopoeia, pharmacopoea, pharmacopea, pharmacopée, pharmaecopee, farmacopoea, farmacopen, farmacopee, farmacopoea, farmakop." Earlier treatises on the preparation of medicaments were known under designations such as: "antidotarium, apotteck, codex, codigo, concordantia, concordia, dispensatorium, enchiridion, formularium, gyógyserkönyi, ljekopis, lumen, luminare, methodus, officina, ratio, receptarium, recettario." Some of the treatises thus titled were legally obligatory in a pharmacopeial sense.

***Pharmacopoeus***, pl. ***-i***, Latinized form of the Greek *pharmakopoeos, q.v.*, maker of remedies. Cf.: ***medicamentarius.***

***Pharmacopola.*** Latinized form of *pharmakopolos.* See also: ***pharmacopolus.***

***Pharmacopolae circumforaneae***, itinerant venders of remedies, the Latinized form of the Greek *pharmakopoloi*; furthermore *circumforaneus* ("of or around the forum or market"). They traveled from market to market. Contrast *sellularii.* See also ***sellularius*** and ***seplasiarius.***

***Pharmacopolus***, pl. ***-i.*** Latinized form of the Greek *pharmakopolos, q.v.* See also: ***pharmacopola.***

***Pharmacotribae, Pharmacotritae***, drug grinders. They are said to have been employed by the ***seplasiarii***, *q.v.* Cf.: ***Rhizotomoi.***

***Pharmacy.*** From Greek ***pharmakon***, *q.v.* ("remedy"). (1) The art and science of the pharmacist; (2) his establishment (synonymous with apothecary shop). Cf. French *pharmacie,* German *Pharmazie* and *Pharmacie,* Italian *farmacia,* etc. Apparently an Egyptian prototype of the term is not to be seen in *ph-ar-maki,* as Schelenz and others supposed, but the etymology perhaps may stem from *phr(t)nhk3w* ("remedy of the sorcerer"). See Frans Jonckheere, *Le 'préparateur de remèdes'. . . .* , Deutsche Akademie der Wissenschaften zu Berlin, Institut für Orientforschung, Veröffentlichung Nr. 29 (*Aegyptologische Studien),* 1955, p. 157 and f.n. 7.

***Pharmakon.*** The Greek word from which many modern terms pertaining to pharmacy, *q.v.*, have been derived. The meaning of the Greek word developed from that of a charm or magic agency, exerted by means of plants with healing but also with poisoning effect (Homer), to that of a remedy without any collateral significance. Often the designation was restricted to purgatives in a real as well as figurative sense. *Pharmacoi* was the name applied to two human scapegoats who, in early Athens, were driven out at the Thargelia feast (the feast of the first bread made of fresh grain), as a symbol of purifying the city from all evil. These men were considered as personified *pharmakon,* in the meaning of "a purifying purgative," hence the name. In addition the word pharmakon could mean "dyestuff." See Walter Artelt: *Studien zur Geschichte der Begriffe 'Heilmittel' und 'Gift'* in *Studien zur Geschichte der Medizin,* Leipzig, 1937.

***Pharmakopoeos***, pl. ***-oi***, "maker of remedies," from the Greek *Pharmakon* ("remedy") and *poiein* ("to make"). Cf. also **pharmacopeia,** "a book that treats of the making of remedies," also, ***Pharmacopolos.*** See the French ***pharmacien,*** English **pharmacist** and **pharmaceutist,** German ***Pharmaceut*** or ***Pharmazeut.***

***Pharmakopolos,*** seller of remedies, "from the Greek *pharmakon* ("remedy") and *polein* ("to sell").

***Pharmazeut.*** German for ***pharmacist,*** *q.v.* Also spelled **Pharmaceut.**

**Philiatrus,** Evonymus. See: **Gessner.**

***Pigmentarius.*** pl. ***-i,*** from *pigmentum* ("paint," also used to designate ointment or pigmented paste and a plant juice); and *-arius,* meaning "pertaining to," i.e., makers of colored cosmetics. Gradually the Roman *pigmentarii* became rather high-class preparers of drugs and dealers in them.

**Pill.** Latin *pila* ("ball").

**Platearius,** Matthaeus (12th century), descendant of a well known Salernitan family of physicians and a renowned physician himself, who wrote the *Circa instans* and the annotated Salernitan *Antidotarius magnus.*

**Pliny.** (23–79 A.D.) Author of the most comprehensive known natural history in antiquity. See *Dictionary Scient. Biog.*; Pliny: *Natural History,* with an English translation by H. Rackham, London, 1938; John Bostock and T. H. Riley: *The Natural History of Pliny* (Bohn's Classical Library), London, 1855–1857; M. E. Littré: *Histoire naturelle de Pline, avec la traduction en français,* Paris, 1877; K. C. Bailey, *The Elder Pliny's Chapters on Chemical Subjects,* London, 1929–1932.

**Potts,** Jonathan (1745–1781). American physician, serving in the Revolutionary War as Deputy Director General and later on as head of the purchasing department for all medical supplies. See L. C. Duncan: *Medical Men in the American Revolution,* p. 184, Carlisle, 1931; *Dictionary Am. Biog., XV,* p. 137.

**Power,** Frederick B. (1853–1927). The organizer and the first director of the school of pharmacy at the University of Wisconsin, scientific director of the Fritzsche Brothers laboratories in New Jersey (1892–1896), director of the Wellcome Research laboratories in London (1896–1914), and head of the phytochemical laboratory of the United States Department of Agriculture (1916–1919). Power became one of the world's best-known research workers in the field of phytochemistry. Power was one of the American pharmacists who completed their professional education by studying at German universities. See *Dictionary of Scient. Biog.*; J. W. England: *First Century of the Philadelphia College of Pharmacy,* p. 410, 1922; *Badger Pharmac.* 1936, No. 16; *J.A.Ph.A. 16*:380, 1927; *Am. J. Pharm. 96*:601, 1924 (containing a chronological record of Power's scientific contributions).

**Powers,** Justin L. (1895– ), an eminent pharmacist, author, and authority on drug standards. From 1940 to 1947, director developmental drug standards laboratory, American Pharmaceutical Association; chairman of the National Formulary Committee for five revisions (1940–1960); active in work on international drug standardization since 1952; editor of the Scientific Edition of the *Journal of the American Phrmaceutical Association* and *Drug Standards* for two decades; educator during most of period 1919–40. See *Who's Who in America* and *American Men of Science.*

**Powers,** Thomas H. (1812–1878), Philadelphia retail and wholesale pharmacist, became (1838) partner of John Farr in the important chemical manufacturing firm later known as Powers and Weightman. See J. W. England: *First Century of the Philadelphia College of Pharmacy,* p. 33, Philadelphia, 1922.

**Prescott,** Albert Benjamin (1832–1905). Without any drugstore practice, the physician Prescott became closely connected with American pharmacy and, as head of the University of Michigan School of pharmacy, one of its most progressive teachers. He was the author of several textbooks, and a member of the United States Pharmacopoeial Convention from 1880 to the time of his death. See: H. R. Manasse, Jr.: *Pharm. Hist. 15*:22–28, 1973; O. Oldberg, *Am. J. Pharm. 77*:251, 1905.

**Procter,** William, Jr. (1817–1874), one of the

most eminent of American pharmacists. Procter was the ninth child of an English-born Quaker and entered pharmacy when the early death of his father forced him to devote himself to a calling. At the age of 20 he was graduated from the Philadelphia College of Pharmacy. Only 4 years later, he acted as secretary to the Committee on Revision of the U.S.P. In 1844 he opened a pharmacy, which he conducted for many years besides carrying on his comprehensive and successful work as experimenter, teacher and author. In 1846 he became a professor of pharmacy at the Philadelphia College of Pharmacy. From 1850 to 1871, he was the sole editor of the *American Journal of Pharmacy*. He published the first textbook on pharmacy by an American pharmacist for American students of pharmacy, which he adapted from a German-British text. No less than 550 original articles in the *American Journal of Pharmacy* bear witness to Procter's indefatigable industry. It was William Procter, Jr., who carried the idea of a national American pharmaceutical association to the Convention of Pharmaceutists and Druggists, held in New York on October 15 and 16, 1851. Thus the first step was taken toward its founding, which took place a year later in Philadelphia. See J. W. England: *First Century of the Philadelphia College of Pharmacy*, p. 402, Philadelphia, 1922.

**Proust,** Joseph Louis (1754–1826), French pharmacist who discovered mannitol (1806) and leucin (1819), and found the element nickel in meteoric iron (1799). He furthermore stated the law of definite and constant proportions in chemical reactions.

**Puckner, W. A.** (1864–1932). Pharmacist, later professor at the Chicago College of Pharmacy, and consulting chemist. In 1907, he became director of the American Medical Association Chemical Laboratory. See *J.A.Ph.A. 21*:1115, 1932; *Indust. & Eng. Chem. News Ed. 10*:255, 1932.

***Pulvis,*** pl. ***pulveres.*** In classical Latin, powder, dust distinguished from coarsely comminuted drugs or *species*. The finely comminuted drugs were designated *pulveres*. Powdering drugs facilitated their administration. Even today, mortar and pestle are the symbol of the art of the pharmacist. The early pharmacopeias designated a special class of preparations as powders. With the advance of iatrochemistry, the term was also applied to mineral preparations in powder form (e.g., allgaroth powder). So far as vegetable preparations are concerned, it was applied to mixtures as well (*e.g., pulvis opii compositus*) and other mixtures containing inorganic chemicals *(Pulvis infantum = Pulvis Rhei compositus)*, or organic chemicals (Tully's Powder = *pulvis morphinae compositus)*.

**Quercetanus.** See: **Quesne,** Joseph du.

**Quesne,** Joseph du, Latinized Quercetanus (1544–1609), French physician and medical author. As a follower of Paracelsus, *q.v.*, he recommended chemicals as remedies, especially preparation of antimony and mercury, without, however, neglecting galenics, He is supposed to have been the first to employ calomel and sulfurated antimony.

**Quincy,** John (d. 1722). English apothecary, later a physician, and a very successful author on medical and pharmaceutical subjects. See: *Dictionary* (English) *National Biography, XLVI*, p. 112.

**Quintessence.** This term was used by Paracelsus for pharmaceutical preparations he considered to represent the most perfect extract of the essential contents of the raw material. His term derives from the fifth essence (Latin *quinta,* "five"), which the Pythagoreans added to the four elements of the ancient Greeks, thought to be a most subtle "ether," a kind of immaterial radiation of the material world.

**Rafinesque,** Constantine Smaltz (1783–1840), botanist of French descent residing in Philadelphia. He wrote several books on history, botany and science, and medical botany. See Alex Berman: C. S. Rafinesque (1783–1840): a challenge to the historian of pharmacy, *Am. J. Pharm. Ed. 16*:409–418, 1952; Alexander Wilder, *History of Medicine*, pp. 421–432, 438, 439, New Sharon, Maine, 1901.

**Ratio.** See: **Pharmacopeia.**

**Raubenheimer,** Otto (1867–1946), German-born Brooklyn pharmacist; a founding member of the *Gesellschaft für Geschichte der Pharmazie;* pharmaceutical historian, author, editor and teacher. See *New York Apoth. Ztg. 47*:159, 1927.

***Receptar.*** See: **Personnel.**

**Redwood,** Theophilus (1806–1892). English pharmacist, editor of the *Pharmaceutical Journal,* and professor of chemistry and pharmacy to the Pharmaceutical Society of Great Britain. He edited, enlarged and translated Friedrich Mohr, *q.v., Lehrbuch der pharmaceutischen Technik.* See: *Am. J. Pharm. 64*:223, 1892.

**Remington,** Joseph P. (1847–1918), one of the most versatile and influential American pharmacists of his time. A graduate of the Philadelphia College of Pharmacy, he first engaged in manufacturing, and then in community pharmacy. He re-entered his alma mater, this time in a teaching position (1871), becoming its dean (1893). Remington was instrumental in the development of the American Pharmaceutical Association and of the *United States Pharmacopoeia* and was for years regarded by many as the outstanding representative of the American profession of pharmacy. In 1919, the New York branch of the American Pharmaceutical Association established the Remington Honor Medal, which is given annually for distinguished service to pharmacy in the United States. The recipients are chosen by majority vote of the living ex-presidents of the Association. See J. W. England: *First Century of the Philadelphia College of Pharmacy,* pp. 407, 408, Philadelphia, 1922.

***Rhizotomos,*** pl. ***-oi,*** literally "root cutters," from the Greek *rhiza* ("root") and *temnein* ("to cut"). The name was also applied to collectors of indigenous drugs.

**Rice,** Charles, German-born American pharmacist (1841–1901), who was pharmacist at the Bellevue Hospital in New York, an excellent chemist, and a man of broadest cultural and scientific background. His phenomenal knowledge of languages gave him an opportunity to keep informed of progress in pharmacy all over the world and facilitated the reform of the *United States Pharmacopoeia,* effected under his chairmanship. See *Proc. A.Ph.A. 49*:45, 1901; J. U. Lloyd: *J.A.Ph.A. 25*:1143, 1936; H. G. Wolfe: *Am. J. Pharm. Ed. 14*:285–305, 1950.

***Ricettario.*** See: **Pharmacopeia.**

**Robiquet,** Pierre Jean (1780–1840), French pharmacist who was one of the most successful phytochemists, he found asparagine simultaneously with Vauquelin (1805); caffeine in collaboration with Pelletier (simultaneously with Runge, 1821); alizarin in collaboration with Colin, 1826; amygdalin (1830); codeine (1832).

**Rondelet,** Guillaume, French physician and academic teacher at the University of Montpellier as well as practicing pharmacist (1507–1566). Besides his *Methodus de materia medicinali et compositione medicamentorum,* he wrote several books, of which *Liber de ponderibus* ("Book of Weights") lived to see several editions.

**Rother,** Reinhold (1843–1889), German born American pharmacist, and writer on pharmaceutical subjects. See: *Am. J. Pharm. 61*:639, 1889.

***Rotulae*** (Latin, rotula, a little wheel). Wheel-shaped lozenges. See: ***Morsuli.***

**Rouelle,** Guillaume François (1703–1770), French pharmacist and chemist. He was the teacher of Lavoisier and one of the most eminent and most diligent chemical authors of his time. He originated the chemical definition of the concept of "salt."

**Rouelle,** Hilaire Marin (1718–1779), French

pharmacist who was the younger brother of Guillaume Francois Rouelle, *q.v.*, and a chemist of high merit. He discovered urea (1773) and hippuric acid (1776); recognized the iron content of the blood; and found natural sulfide of hydrogen.

**Rousseau,** George Louis Claude (1724–1794), German pharmacist of French descent and professor of chemistry at the University of Ingolstadt. Lecturing in the laboratory connected with his pharmacy, he was one of the first teachers of chemistry before Liebig who accompanied his lectures with experiments and gave his students an opportunity for individual experimental work.

**Ruddiman,** Edsel A. (1864–1954), pharmaceutical teacher; from 1901 to 1914, United States food and drug inspector; research chemist; author. See: *Who's Who in America, 50*:2157, 1938; *American Men of Science*, ed. 8, p. 2131, 1949.

**Ruelle,** Jean de, Latinized Ruellius (1474–1537), French physician, canon and writer on botanic and medical subjects. His translation of Dioscorides' *Materia medica,* from the Greek original into Latin, appeared in 1540 with annotations by Euricius and Valerius Cordus (father and son). Among his further translations from Greek into Latin, that of Johannes Actuarius' book, *De compositione medicamentorum,* became especially noted.

**Ruellius.** See **Ruelle.**

**Runge,** Friedlieb Ferdinand (1794–1867), German pharmacist who discovered aniline, which he called "kyanol," in coal tar (1834). Simultaneously, he discovered carbolic acid, rosolic acid and other chemicals in the same substance. This was the beginning of coal-tar chemistry. Likewise, it was he who showed the way to produce dyestuffs with aniline as base. He discovered caffeine (1821). It is of interest to note that aniline had previously been prepared from indigo, first by means of dry distillation by Unverdorben, who called it "krystallin" (1826) and then by Fritzsche, who treated indigo with potassium hydroxide (1841). The designation "aniline" was coined by Fritzsche from the Spanish word *anil-indigo.* Synthetic aniline was prepared by Zinin, by reduction of nitrobenzene with ammonium sulfate (1841). Zinin called his product "benzidam." In 1843 A. W. Hofmann recognized that all these products were identical.

**Rusby,** Henry H. (1855–1940), M.D., botanist and pharmacognosist; professor at the New York College of Pharmacy, 1888–1920; first to identify many South American species; see his book, *Jungle Memories.* See J. W. England: *First Century of the Philadelphia College of Pharmacy*, p. 219.

**Ruth,** Robert J. (1891–1931), pharmacist, teacher, organizer and leader in industrial pharmaceutical service, "father of American Pharmacy Week." See *J.A.Ph.A. 20*:725, 1931; G. Sonnedecker, *Tile and Till 34*:38–41, 1948.

**Sadtler,** Samuel P. (1847–1924), professor of chemistry at Pennsylvania College, then at the University of Pennsylvania, and the Philadelphia College of Pharmacy. See *Am. J. Pharm. 96*:134, 1934.

**Saints, Christian, as patrons of pharmacy.** In the early Middle Ages, the pagan deities associated with medicine and pharmacy, etc., were gradually replaced in the Christian countries by Christian saints, chosen as patrons by the local guilds of physicians and, in the 13th century, of apothecaries, spicers, etc. Most frequently, we meet Cosmas, *q.v.*, and Damian, *q.v.*, as patron saints of the healing arts. Then follow in frequency the Holy Virgin and Mary Magdalene, the latter because she oiled the feet of the Saviour with fragrant oil (a pharmaceutical preparation!). The custom of revering patron saints remained after the time of the Reformation primarily in the Catholic countries. M. Bouvet gives a comprehensive list of such patrons chosen by the apothecaries in the various parts of France. He names S.S. Nicolas, Luke,

Michael, Marcus and Rochus, in addition to Cosmas, Damian, the Holy Virgin, and Mary Magdalene. (M. Bouvet, *Histoire de la pharmacie en France,* p. 259–261, Paris, 1937.

**Salmon,** William (1644–1713), English empiric, who wrote several books and pamphlets on medical and pharmaceutical subjects. See *Dictionary of National* (English) *Biography, 50,* p. 209; W. Kirkby: *Pharm. J. 84*:255–262, 1910.

**Santorio,** Santorio, called Sanctorius (1561–1636), Italian physician and academic teacher at Padua. See Garrison: *History of Medicine,* p. 260, Philadelphia, 1929; Sigerist: *The Great Doctors,* p. 150, New York, 1933.

**Savory,** John (1800–1871), English apothecary. See *Pharm. J. 31*:319, 1871.

**Sayre,** Lucius E. (1848–1925), pharmacist in Philadelphia, later professor at the School of Pharmacy of Kansas State University. See *J.A.Ph.A. 8*:3, 1919; J. W. England: *First Century of the Philadelphia College of Pharmacy,* p. 260, Philadelphia, 1922.

**Scammon,** Frederick (1810–1864), physician and pharmacist, professor of botany of the University of Chicago. See *Alumni Record of the University of Illinois,* p. 431, 1921; *Am. J. Pharm. 36*:277, 1864.

**Scheele,** Carl Wilhelm (1742–1786), one of the greatest chemists of all time, who never left the pharmaceutical profession and made all his discoveries in the laboratories of the pharmacies in which he worked; in the last 11 years of his life, first as manager and then as owner of the pharmacy in the small town of Koeping (Sweden). Among inorganic acids, Scheele discovered arsenic (1771–1772), hydrofluoric (1771), molybdic (1778), and tungstic (1778); among organic acids, citric (1784), gallic (1770), lactic (1780), malic (1784), mucic (1780), oxalic (1770), pyrogallic (1770), tartaric (before 1768) and uric (1776). He identified baryta (1771–1774), chlorine (1774), glycerin (1783), manganese (1773), and milk-sugar (1780); he discovered oxygen (prior to 1773), hydrochloric acid gas (1770), ammonia (1770) and arsenetted hydrogen (1775); and he ascertained the chemical nature of sulfuretted hydrogen (1768). Among the new processes which he invented, those of special interest are for preparing phosphorus (1770), calomel (1774) and benzoic acid (1775). See *Dictionary Scient. Biog.*; O. Zekert: *Carl Wilhelm Scheele. . . ,* Gesell. Gesch. Pharm., 2 vols., 1931–33; and G. Urdang; *The Apothecary Chemist, Carl Wilhelm Scheele,* Madison, Wis., 1942.

**Schelenz,** Hermann (1848–1922), passed the *Staatsexamen* ("state board examination") as *Apotheker* (1873), then operated a pharmacy in Rendsburg, Schleswig (1875 to 1893). Frequent contributor to pharmaceutical journals, more particularly on historical subjects. Author of the following books: *Geschichte der Pharmazie* (1904); *Zur Geschichte der pharmazeutisch-chemischen Destilliergeräte* (1913); *Shakespeare und sein Wissen auf dem Gebiete der Arznei-und Volkskunde* (1914).

He was awarded an honorary M.D. by the University of Freiburg (1920), and he was made an honorary member of the American Pharmaceutical Association (1912). For a more detailed account of his life work, see *Pharm. Ztg. 67*:841, 1922; and, especially, Zimmermann, Walter: H. Schelenz' Lebenswerk, *Pharm. Monatshefte 4*:137, 1923. The last essay by Schelenz published before his death was "American apothecaries in literature," *Pharm. Zeit. 67*:371, 1922.

**Schieffelin,** Henry H., head of the New York wholesale drug firm W. H. Schieffelin and Company from 1814 to 1849 (at that time called H. H. Schieffelin and Company). See *One Hundred Years of Business Life,* 1794–1894. W. H. Schieffelin and Company, New York.

**Schlotterbeck,** Julius Otto (1865–1917), one of the American pharmaceutical teachers who studied at German or Swiss universities. He taught pharmacognosy at the University of Michigan, wrote a number of scientific papers, and later took up industrial work. See *Am. J. Pharm. 89*:336, 1917.

**Schmidt,** Ernst Albert (1845–1921), German pharmacist and professor of pharmacy at the University of Marburg. Schmidt specialized in alkaloid chemistry. His *Ausführliches Lehrbuch der pharmazeutischen Chemi,* highly regarded, has been edited again and again since Schmidt's death. He has, furthermore, the isolation of scopolamine to his credit.

**Schoepf,** Johann David (1752–1800), German physician and botanist. See H. Peters: *Pharm. Rund. 13*:151, 1895.

**Schulze,** F., German military pharmacist (1914 to 1918). See Devin: *Die deutschen Militaerapotheker im Weltkriege,* Berlin, 1920.

**Scoville,** Wilbur L. (1865–1941), pharmaceutical teacher; from 1907–1934 research pharmacist with Parke, Davis and Company; after 1924, head of the analytic department of the firm; author and editor. See *American Men of Science,* p. 1263, 1938; *Who's Who in America, 20*: p. 2221.

**Scribonius Largus** (first century after Christ), Roman physician. The cognomen "Largus" is presumably derived from Latin *largiri,* meaning "the liberal giver." The formulary he wrote was printed in several editions between the 16th and the 18th centuries, under different and sometimes quite arbitrary titles.

**Seaman,** Valentine (1770–1817), New York physician and promoter of vaccination; co-author of the "pharmacopoeia" of the New York Hospital (see p. 258). Kelly and Burrage: *American Medical Biographies,* p. 842, New York, 1920.

***Sellularius,*** pl. ***-i,*** from Lat. *sellula,* "a little seat," and *-arius,* "pertaining to"; hence, people who had sedentary occupations or trades; stationary venders of remedies, as contrasted with ***pharmacopolae circumforaneae,*** *q.v.* They were also called ***seplasiarii,*** *q.v.*

***Seplasiarius,*** from *seplasia,* a street in Capua where unguents (possibly also frankincense and other oriental drugs) were sold, and *-arius,* "pertaining to." Cf. ***sellularius.***

**Sertürner,** Friedrich Wilhelm Adam (1783–1841) German pharmacist who became famous by his discovery of morphine as the *principium somniferum* ("somniferous principle") in opium. His first publications about "meconic acid, which also contained his discovery of the first alkaloid to be prepared in a pure state, appeared in 1805 and 1806 in Trommsdorff's *Journal der Pharmazie, q.v.* It is likely that morphine in a more or less pure state had been obtained before Sertürner by the French pharmacists Derosne and, especially, Seguin. However, the fact that Sertürner discovered the basic nature of the substance called by him morphium, made him the pioneer of alkaloidal chemistry. See F. Kroemecke: *Fr. W. Sertürner,* Jena, 1925.

**Sérullas,** Georges Simon (1774–1832), French Pharmacist who discovered iodoform (1822) and produced several new compounds of bromide.

**Seumenicht.** See: **Mynsicht**.

**Sharp,** Alpheus Pireas (1824–1909), one of the founders of the firm of Sharp and Dohme, Baltimore. "Mr. Sharp read the first scientific paper before the American Pharmaceutical Association," and as an anniversary event "the identical paper was read again at the annual meeting held fifty years later." See *Am. Drug. and Pharm. Rec. 54*:352, 1909.

**Sheppard,** S. A. D. (1842–1915), Boston pharmacist and for 22 years treasurer of the American Pharmaceutical Association. He collected the "Sheppard Library" of about 2,500 volumes, among them about 300 pharmacopeias of different countries and periods, which he bequeathed to the Massachusetts College of Pharmacy. See *Bull. Pharm. 22*:323, 1906; *J.A.Ph.A. 4*:1515, 1915.

**Shoemaker,** Robert (1817–1897), Philadelphia wholesale and retail pharmacist and pharmaceutical manufacturer. Shoemaker is believed to have been the first to manufacture glycerin in the United States (1848). See England: *First Century of the Philadelphia College of Pharmacy,* p. 106.

**Show globes.** There has been much conjecture about the origin of the peculiarly shaped bottles filled with colored liquids which have been used for a long time as a sign of pharmacy, especially in Anglo-Saxon countries. Attempts have been made to trace them back to antiquity. However, there is no mention of such use anywhere before the 17th century. C. J. S. Thompson thinks there is probably a connection between these display bottles and the carboys, use of which for transport and preservation of liquids became general at about the same time. (*The Mystery and Art of the Apothecary,* p. 251, Philadelphia, 1929). It seems highly probable that the bottles filled with colored liquids originated in the early English chemists' shops whose owners wanted to utilize the public attraction of the unusual bottle (apparatus) as well as of the mysterious products (represented by the colored liquids) obtained from the new art of chemistry. Later on, the druggists seized upon these signs, as well as the production or at least the sale of medical chemicals, until both groups merged into the united profession of chemist-and-druggist. See George Urdang: New light on the origin of show globes, *J. Am. Pharm.* (Pract. Ed.) *10*:604–6, 640; see also, George Griffenhagen, The Show Globe, *J.A.Ph.A.* (Pract Ed.) *19*:233–5, 1958 (and *Am. Drugg. 134*:9–11, No. 10, 1956); W. Schneider, in *Pharm. Industrie 17*:29, 1955.

**Simon,** Johann Franz (1807–1847), German pharmacist and physiologic chemist, supposed to have been the first to publish a modern, comprehensive collection of data pertaining exclusively to the "Chemistry of Man." See George Urdang: *Pharmacy's Part in Society,* p. 49, Madison, Wis., 1946.

**Simon,** William (1844–1916), German-born and pharmaceutically educated pharmacist, professor of chemistry at the Maryland College of Pharmacy (1872–1902) at the College of Physicians and Surgeons of Baltimore (1880–1916) and at the Baltimore College of Dental Surgery(1888 to 1916); author of a well-known textbook. See: *J.A.Ph.A. 5*:886, 1916.

**Simmons,** Willard B. (1906–     ) has been Executive Secretary of the National Association of Retail Druggists since 1961, after serving on the Executive Committee, 1953–1961. Practiced pharmacy at Texarkana, Texas (beginning at Bloomburg, 1925). He was prominent in organized civic and business endeavors of East Texas. (*N.A.R.D. Jour.,* pp. 16 and 74, Nov. 6, 1961.)

***Simplicia,*** from the Latin *simplex* ("simple"), generic term for all those drugs not classified as ***composita,*** *q.v.* Lists of such simples were compiled very early. In the 11th century Constantinus Africanus wrote his treatise *De gradibus simplicium* and, in the 12th century, Matthaeus Platearius wrote his famous *Liber de simplici medicina dictus circa instans.* Later on such lists appeared in the pharmacopeias (after the 18th century chiefly under the title of materia medica). In general, only such drugs were listed as *simplicia* as had not passed a process of preparation beyond that of comminution or purification. However, this principle was not strictly followed. Thus the first U.S.P. (1820) mentions, on the one hand, prepared carbonate of lime (a purified simple drug), among the preparations, while on the other hand its materia medica presents "a catalogue of simple medicines together with some prepared medicines which are kept in the shop of the apothecary but not necessarily prepared by him."

**Skoda,** Josef (1805–1881), Bohemian physician and academic teacher in Vienna. He was the leading clinician of the so-called New Vienna School of medicine and the exponent of its therapeutic nihilism. See Garrison: *History of Medicine,* p. 431,

Philadelphia, 1929; Sigerist: *The Great Doctors,* p. 297, New York, 1933.

**Smith,** Daniel B. (1792–1883), Philadelphia pharmacist, who was one of the founders of and leaders in the Philadelphia College of Pharmacy, and a man of high scientific and literary attainments. See England, *First Century of the Philadelphia College of Pharmacy,* p. 353, Philadelphia, 1922.

**Smith,** Peter (1753–1816), American preacher, farmer and medical practitioner, the so-called "Indian Doctor." See *Bull. Lloyd Libr.,* No. 2.

**Soubeiran,** Eugene (1797–1858), French pharmacist. Simultaneously with the American Samuel Guthrie, *q.v.,* and the German Justus v. Liebig, *q.v.,* he discovered chloroform (1831). The trichlormethane found by them was called "chloric ether" by Guthrie, "bichloric ether" by Soubeiran, and "trichloride of carbon" by Liebig. Dumas (1834) gave it the name of chloroform, from formyl (CH) and (tri) chloride.

***Spagiric,*** from the Greek *span* (to separate) and *ageirein* (to combine). The term "spagiric art" used by Paracelsus as a synonym for "chemistry" means, therefore, the art of separating and combining, or of analysis and synthesis.

**Spalding,** Lyman (1775–1821), physician, the principal "father of the U.S.P." See *J.A.Ph.A.* 6:675, 1917; J. A. Spalding: *The Life of Dr. Lyman Spalding,* Boston, 1916.

***Speciarius.*** See: **Species.**

***Species.*** From the latin verb *specio,* to look, to behold, changed in its meaning from the abstract sight to the thing seen. In late Latin, it was specialized to mean goods (wares generally, e.g., wine), but more particularly spices and drugs. Hence *speciarius* (pertaining to *species*), Italian *speziali,* English *spicer,* French *épicier, speciaria* a female spice-dealer. In more modern pharmaceutical practice, the designation species was applied to mixtures of coarsely comminuted (cut or bruised) mixtures of parts of vegetable drugs, such as roots, barks, woods, leaves, flowers, stems, mosses and lichens, seeds and fruits. Occasionally, gums or gum resins were added (Trommsdorff, *Wörterbuch*) e.g., *species pectorales* or German *Brustthee,* and *species laxantes* or "laxative tea." The designation "tea," however, is also applied to unmixed vegetable drugs, e.g., senna tea (leaves), fennel tea (fruit), etc. In this sense, it is also applied to the tea par excellence, Chinese tea, the leaves (or tips of leaves) of *Thea chinensis;* also to its substitutes, e.g., New Jersey tea (leaves of *Ceanothus americanus).* (The word "species" is used in botany to designate a kind, as opposed to "genus.")

**Speck,** William Alfred (1864–1928), American-born pharmacist of German descent, until 1913 owner of a New York pharmacy inherited from his father. From then until his death, he was curator of the unique Goethe Collection created by him at Yale University. See Carl F. Schreiber: William Speck, in memoriam, *Yale University Library Gazette 3*:55, Jan., 1929.

***Spiritus aromatici.*** Like the ***aquae aromaticae,*** *q.v.,* aromatic spirits were made by distillation of aromatic drugs with wine, spirits or even stronger alcohol. Such a preparation was the *eau des Cannes,* which was later introduced into the pharmacopeias as *spiritus melissae compositus.* The terms *spiritus* and *aqua* were used interchangeably. *Spiritus vini* was commonly known as *aqua vitae.* Today they are commonly prepared by the solution of volatile oils in alcohol.

**Squibb,** Edward R. (1819–1900). He was physician, manufacturer, chemist and, in his early days, apprentice and then clerk in a pharmacy from 1837 to 1842. Squibb belongs to the pioneers who became equally important to pharmacy and to medicine. See J. P. Remington: E. R. Squibb, *Am. J. Pharm. 73*:419, 1901.

**Squire,** Peter (1798–1884), English pharmacist. He was appointed chemist-in-ordinary in the court pharmacy of Queen

Victoria and was one of the founders of the Pharmaceutical Society of Great Britain. See *Am. J. Pharm. 56*:400, 1884.

**Stahl,** Georg Ernst (1660–1734), Professor at the University of Halle, later physician-in-ordinary to the King of Prussia and formulator of the phlogiston theory. He developed the ideas of Becher, *q.v.*, to a complete system and coined the name "phlogiston" (from Greek *phlogizein,* "set on fire") for the substantive principle of combustion assumed by Becher. See Garrison: *History of Medicine,* p. 312, Philadelphia, 1929; Sigerist: *The Great Doctors,* p. 183, New York, 1933.

**Starkey** (Stirk), George (about 1620–1665), an American physician who was the only American alchemist of note. He wrote under his own name and under the pen name Eirenaeus Philoponus Philalethes. See *Dictionary Scient. Biog.;* R. S. Wilkinson: Ambix *11*:121–152, 1963.

***Stationarius,*** pl. ***-i,*** from Latin *statio* and *-arius,* "of or belonging to a post or station." Compare the older ***sellularius.*** The term, referring to pharmacist who owns one of the recognized pharmacies at a given locality, appears in the edicts of Frederick II of 1231–1241.

**Stearns,** Frederick (1832–1907), pharmacist, first in Buffalo and then in Detroit; later on, founder of the pharmaceutical manufacturing house of Frederick Stearns and Company of Detroit. See *Drug Circ. 51*:244, 1907. Roland T. Lakey: Frederick Stearns, pharmacist, *J.A.Ph.A.* (Pract. Ed.) *9*:487–489.

**Stillé,** Alfred (1813–1900), Philadelphia physician and professor of medicine at the University of Pennsylvania. His *Elements of General Pathology* (1848), was the first American book on the subject; also co-author of dispensatory. See: *Dictionary Am. Biog., XVIII,* p. 23.

**Stirk,** George. See: **Starkey,** George.

**Stock,** Fred J. (1908–     ). Starting as a practicing pharmacist (1928–1941), Stock became Chief of the U. S. War Production Board, Drugs and Cosmetics Branch during World War II. In this capacity, he headed the War Production Board's drug program, including the overseeing of manufacture and distribution of penicillin, the sulfonamides, and antimalarials. Since the war Stock has been a Vice President of Chas. Pfizer & Co., Inc. (1945–1951) and, since 1952, a Vice-President of Mathieson Chemical Corp. and then of its E. R. Squibb and Sons division. See *Who's Who in America.*

***Stoesser.*** See: **Personnel.**

***Subject.*** See: **Personnel.**

**Swain,** Robert L. (1887–1963), American pharmacist and lawyer, influential on American pharmacy as editor of *Drug Topics* (1939–1960), and through vigorous participation in the affairs of the American Pharmaceutical Association (e.g., Council, 1933–1951 and 1953–1959; President, 1933–1934) and other organizations. Earlier in Maryland he served as editor of *The Maryland Pharmacist* (1925–1940), law enforcement official and professor. See *J.A.Ph.A.* n.s. *3*:1963, 153.

**Sylvius.** See: (1) **Boe, François de le;** (2) **Bois, Jacques du.**

**Sylvius,** Franciscus, or Francois de le Boë Sylvius (1614–1672). A Dutch follower of Paracelsus. He prepared the scientific foundation for the application of chemicals in therapy, preached by Paracelsus, and hence may be regarded as the real founder of the iatrochemical school.He introduced the word and the concept of fermentation; and by means of it he explained the chemical changes that take place within the human body. Not only was the food converted into blood under the influence of the saliva and of glandular secretion, but also the blood itself was transferred by certain "ferments," into a so-called "ether," a hypothetical substance which, according to this theory, is responsible for the life processes. The ultimate products of these changes were acids and alkalies, the proper relation of which in the body guaranteed health. Disturbances produced the so-called *acrimoniae,* which were either acid or alkaline, and were to be corrected by the administration of drugs of alkaline or acid character.

**Symon,** or Simon Januensis (d. 1303), an Italian medical author. The cognomen Januensis means from Genoa.

**Tabernaemontanus.** See **Theodor, Johann.** The word *tabernaemontanus* means "from Bergzabern," his birthplace.

***Tabulae.*** Latin for "board or plank"; also "tablet," diminutive for "table." Comparable to our troches and lozenges.

**Talbor,** Robert, also called Tabor (1642–1681). Talbor started his career as an apprentice to the apothecary Dent in Cambridge, became a (self-styled) physician and, after having cured the English King Charles II with a decoction of cinchona bark, was appointed physician-in-ordinary to His Majesty. See C. J. S. Thompson: *The Mystery and Art of the Apothecary,* p. 232, Philadelphia, 1929; Wootton: *Chronicles of Pharmacy, II,* p. 97, London, 1910.

**Taylor,** Alfred B. (1824–1898), Philadelphia pharmacist. Taylor was the first treasurer of the American Pharmaceutical Association and active in the work of pharmacopeial revision. He was one of the early American pharmacists who combined practical pharmacy with scientific work. See *Proc. A.Ph.A. 46*:51, 1898; J. W. England: *First Century of the Philadelphia College of Pharmacy,* p. 207, Philadelphia, 1922.

***Terra sigillata.*** Clay originating from certain districts of Europe, which was made up into round pastils weighing about ½ ounce. These were stamped with designs alluding to the places of their origin. Such earth tablets were given in dysenteries, internal ulcers and hemorrhages; also in gonorrhea and in pestilential fevers. Externally they were applied to festering wounds. Their use through the ages rested mainly on their recommendation by Galen (*q.v.*). See Wootton: *Chronicles of Pharmacy, II,* p. 53, London, 1910.

**Thacher,** James (1754–1844), American physician. Besides his *American New Dispensatory,* he wrote some other books, among them an *American Medical Biography.* During his service in the Revolutionary Army, he kept a rather full journal, which is one of the most complete diaries of the war. See L. C. Duncan: *Medical Men in the American Revolution,* p. 262, Carlisle, 1931; *Dictionary Am. Biog., XVIII,* p. 387.

**Theodor,** Johann (Jacob), called Tabernaemontanus (1510–1590), German pharmacist, physician, and botanist. The first part of his *New Vollkommentlich Kreuterbuch* ("New Perfect Herbal") was published in 1588 and the second part in 1613 after his death, by Caspar Bauhin, *q.v.*

**Theophrastus Bombastus** of Hohenheim. See **Paracelsus.**

**Theophrastus,** Eresios (371–286 B.C.), pupil of the Greek philosopher Aristotle and one of the oldest botanists whose writings have come down to us. He has been called "the father of botany." See Tschirch: *Handbuch der Pharmakognosie, I,* Part 2, p. 545, Leipzig, 1910; G. Sarton: *Introduction to the History of Science, 1,* pp. 143, 144, Baltimore, 1927.

**Theriac,** also treacle. (Greek *theriake,* Latin theriaca, French *thériaque.*) The Greek term *theriake* was derived from *theriakós* (of wild or venomous beasts); hence, *theriaca* or *theriace* was an antidote, first primarily against the bite of serpents, then against poisons in general. Later it was regarded as a general panacea, although it retained its special reputation as an antidote. Nicander of Colophon, who lived during the second century B.C., is said to have been the first to recommend it. Its highest reputation was gained when prepared according to the supposed formula of Mithridates, King of Pontus in Asia Minor (132–63 B.C.) or according to the modified formulae of Democrates or Andromachus, physicians who lived in Rome during the first century. It was Andromachus who added the "flesh of serpents" to the ingredients of the panacea, and it was the formula of Andromachus which, through Galen, *q.v.*, gained recognition up to the eighteenth century, when the myth of the therapeutic value of theriaca was exploded by William Herberden, *q.v.* During certain periods and in certain countries the composition of theriaca was regarded as being of sufficient importance to have it made by the pharmacist under the supervision of representatives of the medical faculty. See Berman, A.: *Pharm. Hist.*, *11*:5–10, 1969; J. Berendes, *Die Pharmacie bei den alten Kulturvoelkern*, p. 281, Halle, 1891; Peters and Netter, *Pictorial History of Ancient Pharmacy* p. 115, Chicago, 1899; C. J. S. Thompson, *The Mystery and Art of the Apothecary*, p. 58, Philadelphia, 1929; G. Watson: *Theriac and Mithridatium, A Study in Therapeutics*, London, 1966. 165 pp.

**Thompson,** William S. (1822–1894), pharmacist in Baltimore and editor of the *Journal* of the Maryland College of Pharmacy. See: *Proc. Am. Pharm. A. 43*:47, 1895.

**Thoms,** Hermann (1859–1931), German pharmacist and professor of pharmaceutical chemistry at the University of Berlin. The exemplary Institute of Pharmacy at the University of Berlin was the fruit of his endeavor. See *Pharm. Rev. 26*:1, 1908. Thoms was the founder of *Deutsche pharmazeutische Gesellschaft.* Of his discoveries the synthetic substitute for sugar ("Dulcin") found widest recognition. See *Pharm. Ztg. 76*:1349, 1931,

**Thomson,** Samuel (1769–1843). Thomson founded the American botanic school of medical thought, which later on was merged into the eclectic school of medicine. See: *Lloyd Libr. Reprod. Ser.* No. 7; *Dictionary Am. Biog., XVIII,* p. 488; and Alex Berman: *The Impact of the 19th Century Botanico-medical Movement on American Pharmacy and Medicine,* University of Wisconsin, Ph.D. dissertation, 1954.

**Thoth.** Egyptian god of wisdom, magic, and one of the gods to whom healing was attributed. He was represented with the head of Osiris or as dog-headed, and identified with ph-ar-maki.

**Tinctures.** The introduction of tinctures into pharmacy had been credited to a mysterious alchemist, Raymundus Lullus (1235–1315), but most writings ascribed to him may not be his work. However, there is no doubt of the mentioning of such preparations in the *Lullian Corpus,* i.e., pre-Paracelsian writings under the name of Lullus. On the other hand, it was the emphasis put on these liquid extracts of drugs by Paracelsus which was responsible for their introduction into the pharmacopeias and their common use.

The early tinctures, as they are found under this designation in the pharmacopeias of the 16th and even the 17th centuries, differ essentially from the products called tinctures in later times. Minerals, corals, rust (prepared by roasting of vitriol) together with orange peel, red rose petals, aloes, myrrh, crocus, etc., were digested with alcohol and the product called *tinctura corallirum* or *martis e vitriolo* or *proprietatis.* A reddish alcoholic solution of roasted potassium carbonate was called *tinctura tartari.* Preparations like the usual tinctures of later times, i.e., alcoholic or hydroalcoholic solutions of the contents of vegetables or animal drugs produced by maceration are, in the seventeenth century, sometimes enumerated as *aquae cum spiritu vini.* In the language of alchemy, tincture, like elixir, was a term for the mysterious means of transmutation of base metals to gold or silver.

**Trimble,** Henry (1853–1898). He started his career as a pharmacist in Philadelphia and was (from 1883) professor of analytic chemistry at the Philadelphia College of

Pharmacy, and editor (after 1894) of the *American Journal of Pharmacy.* See England: *First Century of the Philadelphia College of Pharmacy,* p. 412, Philadelphia, 1922.

**Trommsdorff,** Johannes Bartholomaeus (1770–1837), German pharmacist. Trommsdorff was a great teacher, devoting his life to the education of pharmacists and to the elevation of pharmacy. He founded a private school of pharmacy in Erfurt, which gained international fame and was the first of its kind, giving laboratory work, in the world. He wrote several textbooks on pharmacy and on chemistry, among them his *Handbuch der Apothekerkunst* (1790), the *Apothekerschule* (1804), the *Allgemeines pharmaceutisch-chemisches Wörterbuch oder die Apothekerkunst in ihrem ganzen Umfange,* in five volumes (1605–1813) and two supplements (1821 and 1822), and the *Handbuch der gesamten Chemie,* in eight volumes (1800–1804). Furthermore, he was the first real pharmaceutical journalist, founding not only the first periodical devoted especially to scientific pharmacy and issued at more than annual intervals, *Trommdorff's Journal der Pharmacie, q.v.,* but trying to write in an interesting way. His research was devoted primarily to pharmaceutical preparations. See Otto Rosenhainer and Trommsdorff: *Trommsdorff's Lebensbild,* Jena, 1913; Curt T. Wimmer, *J.A.Ph.A.* *27*:56, 1938.

***Trommsdorff's Journal der Pharmacie*** (1793–1834). In 1817 the name was changed to *Neues Journal der Pharmacie für Ärzte, Apotheker und Chemiker.* Under this name, the journal was continued until its merger with the *Annalen der Pharmazie* in 1834, the latter journal a substantial contribution by pharmacy to chemistry, which later became *Liebig's Annalen.* See Abe, H. R., et al.: Johann Bartholomäus Trommsdorff (1770–1837) und die Begründung der modernen Pharmazie. Heft 16, Beiträge zur Geschichte der Universität Erfurt, Leipzig, ca. 1972. 295 pp.

**Troth,** Henry (1794–1842), Philadelphia wholesale druggist and one of the most active founders of the Philadelphia College of Pharmacy. See England: *First Century of the Philadelphia College of Pharmacy,* p. 354, Philadelphia, 1922; *Am. J. Pharm. 14*:174, 1842.

**Tschirch,** Alexander (1856–1939). His chief work was the monumental *Handbuch der Pharmakognosie,* which not only supplies detailed accounts of the history of each drug but also contains a comprehensive *Pharmacohistoria.* For further details about his life-work see *Pharm. Zeit. 83*:1293, 1295, 1926. A bibliography, enumerating the publications of Tschirch to January 1, 1923, appeared in *Schweiz. Apoth. Zeit. 60*:730–742, 1922.

**Turner,** William (1515–1568), English physician and pioneer herbalist, and clergyman. He had a private botanic garden at Kew and is considered the father of English botany.

***Unguentarius,*** pl. ***-i,*** from the Latin *unguentum* "ointment," and *-arius,* "pertaining to," i.e., "maker of ointments." Cf.: ***myropoeos*** and ***myrepsos.***

**Urdang,** George (1882–1960), pharmacist, historian, journalist and teacher. Urdang arrived at Madison as a refugee from Hitlerian Germany (1939), to write the Kremers and Urdang *History of Pharmacy,* based on *Kremers' (q.v.)* materials. Urdang was the first Director of the American Institute of the History of Pharmacy (1941–1957) and later became Professor at the University of Wisconsin (history of pharmacy, 1947–1952). In Germany he had been an editor of the *Pharmazeutische Zeitung,* helped to found the German Society for the History of Pharmacy (1926), and earlier in his career had practiced pharmacy in

Rosenberg, Prussia (1910–1919). See: *Pharmacy in History, 5*: Nos. 2 & 3, 1960 (especially H. George Wolfe's article); G. Sonnedecker in *Isis 51*:562–564, 1960 and *Am. J. Pharm. Ed. 24*:536–539, 1960; and *Acta Pharmaciae Historica,* No. 2, 1961.

**Vauquelin,** Louis Nicolas (1763–1829), French pharmacist. He discovered chromium (1797) and asparagine simultaneously with Robiquet (1805); also, nicotine (1811), lecithin (1811) and cyanic acid (1818).

***Vertreter.*** See **Personnel.**

**Virey,** Julien Joseph (1755–1846), French pharmacist, physician, professor of natural history, Virey was one of the co-editors of the *Journal de Pharmacie, q.v.,* and a prolific writer. His *Traité de pharmacie* (1811) was an important work of its kind.

**Wackenroder,** Heinrich Wilhelm Ferdinand (1798–1854), German pharmacist and professor of pharmaceutical chemistry at the University of Jena. He discovered corydaline and carotine and worked intensively in the field of phytochemistry.

**Wall,** Otto A. (1847–1922), professor at the St. Louis College of Pharmacy and author of several books, including *The Prescription* (rev. ed., 1917) See *J.A.Ph.A. 11*:226, 1922.

**Warner,** William R. (1836–1901), American pharmacist and manufacturer. See *Am. J. Pharm. 73*:414, 1901.

**Warren,** John C. (1788–1856), physician, founder of the Massachusetts General Hospital and responsible for the introduction of ether anesthesia. See Kelly and Burrage: *American Medical Biographies,* p. 1196, New York, 1920.

**Wasicky,** Richard (ca. 1885–1971), Austrian physician and pharmacist, who became an internationally renowned pharmacognosist. From the University of Vienna in 1933, he emigrated to Sao Paulo, Brazil, where he became, in 1959, professor at the University of Santa Maria and Director of the Institute of Biomedical Research. See A. Adlung, and G. Urdang: *Grundriss . . .,* p. 310; *J.A.Ph.A.* ns *11*:411, 1971.

**Wayne,** Edward S. (1818–1885), pharmacist in Cincinnati and professor at the Cincinnati College of Pharmacy. See *Drug. Circ. 51*:93, 1907; *Am. J. Pharm. 58*:54, 1886.

**Wedel,** George Wolfgang (1645–1729), German physician and chemist, who wrote many essays on the constituents and the use of vegetable drugs.

**Weightman,** William (1813–1904), English born chemist. In 1878, he became executive head of the American firm of Powers and Weightman, early and important manufacturer of medicinal chemicals. See J. W. England: *First Century of the Philadelphia College of Pharmacy,* p. 33, Philadelphia, 1922.

**Weights and measures.** In general the old systems are built up on the division of a certain unit by 12, the so-called duodecimal system, while the modern system, the decimal system, provides a division by ten. See the general survey by B. Kisch, *Scales and Weights, A Historical Outline* (New Haven and London, ca. 1965).

The Babylonians, Assyrians, Egyptians, Hebrews, Greeks and Romans had their own weights and measures. A comparative survey of the weights used for pharmaceutical purposes from the Babylonian period to the present time is given by Ludwig Winkler, *"Das Apothekergewicht," Pharm. Monatshefte,* 1924, No. 6. An article, "Weights and Measures in History," *Chem. & Drug. 110*:817, 1929, contains 84 photographs of weights and balances which have been used from ancient times to the present, with an explanatory text referring especially to medicine and pharmacy. Further details may be found in such books and articles as W. Ridgeway: *The Origin of Metallic Currency and Weight Standards,* Cambridge, 1892; Ch. Rice: On the origin of our pharmaceutical signs for weights and measures, *New Remedies 6*:212, 1877; H. Sigerist: Masse und

Gewichte in den medizinischen Texten des frühen Mittelalters, *Kyklos* (Leipzig) *3*:439, 1930; G. Sarton: The first explanation of decimal fractions and measures by S. Stevin, *Isis 23*:153, 1935; Oscar Oldberg: Metrology, Parts 4, 5, 6, *Pharm. Era 13*:198, 1895 and The development of our systems of weights and measures, *Pharm. Era 14*:713, 1895; G. Snyder: *Wägen und Waagen*, Ingelheim am Rhein, n.d. [1957]; B. Kisch: *Gewichte-und-Waagemacher im Alten Köln (16.-19. Jahrh.)*, Köln, ca. 1962; H. J. Albert: *Mass und Gewicht; Geschichtliche und tabellarische Darstellungen von d. Anfängen bis zur Gegenwart*, Berlin, 1957; A. M. Merck: *Antigua Metrologia Farmacéutica*, Valencia, 1960; P. Walden: *Mass, Zahl und Gewicht in der Chemie der Vergangenheit. Ein Kapitel aus der Vorgeschichte des sogenannten quantitativen Zeitalters der Chemie*, Stuttgart, 1931; K. M. C. Zevenboom and D. A. Wittop Koning: *Nederlandse Gewichten Stelsels, Ijkwezen, Vormen, Makers en Merken*, Leiden, 1953; and M. Geoffroy: *Dicitionaire des Poids et Mesures*, Baugé, 1907.

**Wellcome,** Sir Henry Solomon (1853–1936), American pharmacist and founder of the English firm of Burroughs Wellcome and Company. Sir Henry Wellcome was a scientific pharmacist as well as an anthropologist, an archaeologist, a writer, a philanthropist, and a collector of all items of historical pharmaceutical and medical interest. See *J.A.Ph.A. 23*:285, 1934; *25*:734, 888, 1936.

**Westrumb,** Johann Friedrich (1751–1819), German pharmacist. He published many papers, especially on technical chemistry, and analyzed many mineral waters.

**Whelpley,** Henry Milton (1861–1926), pharmacist, anthropologist and archaeologist. Professor and dean of the St. Louis College of Pharmacy from 1904, active in a number of offices of the American Pharmaceutical Association. See *J.A.Ph.A. 15*:523, 1926.

**Wiegand,** Thomas S. (1825–1909), Philadelphia pharmacist and pharmaceutical author, for many years registrar at the Philadelphia College of Pharmacy. See *Am. J. Pharm. 81*:502, 1909.

**Wiegleb,** Johann Christian (1732–1800), German pharmacist. An opponent of alchemy, he was at the same time one of the last and most zealous defenders of the phlogiston theory. Among his numerous publications was a precursor of the famous *Chemical Letters*, published half a century later by Liebig.

**Wilbert,** Martin I. (1865–1916). Brilliant and versatile pioneer of American hospital pharmacy; for 17 years a pharmacist at the German Hospital in Philadelphia and, later on (1908–1916) Assistant in the Division of Pharmacology of the Hygienic Laboratory, United States Public Health Service. Wilbert was a voluminous writer on pharmaceutico-historical subjects. For a number of years he edited *Comments and Criticisms on the U.S.P.* See D. F. Burkholder's essay and bibliography of Wilbert's publications, *Am. J. Hosp. Pharm. 25*:330–343, 1968, and J. K. Thum: *Am. J. Pharm. 89*:49, 1917.

**Wilder,** Hans M. (1831–1901), Iceland-born American pharmacist and pharmaceutical author. See *Am. J. Pharm. 73*:411, 1901.

**Willdenow,** Carl Ludwig (1765–1812), German pharmacist, director (after 1801) of the Botanic Garden and (after 1810) professor of botany at the University of Berlin. He was one of the best-known botanists of his time.

**Williamson,** Peter (1795–1886), wholesale druggist and one of the founders of the Philadelphia College of Pharmacy. See England: *First Century of the Philadelphia College of Pharmacy*, p. 351, Philadelphia, 1922.

**Winthrop,** John (1588–1649), governor of Massachusetts Colony. He became important to pharmacy by the list of drugs sent to him from England and used by him in his attempts at caring for the sick in his colony. See *Dictionary of American Biography, XX*, p. 408; W. J. Bell, Jr.: *Early American*

*Science; Needs and Opportunities for Study,* p. 78, Williamsburg, Va., 1955.

**Winthrop,** John, Jr. (1606–1676), governor of Connecticut Colony, one of the earliest preparers of chemicals on North American soil. See R. C. Black: *The Younger John Winthrop,* Irvington, N.Y., 1966; also *Ambix 11*:33–51, 1963 & *12*:24–43, 1964; and *Dictionary of American Biography, XX,* p. 411.

**Wöhler,** Friedrich (1800–1882), German chemist. His artificial preparation of urea in 1828 broke down the supposedly impassable barrier between inorganic and organic chemistry. He first isolated several elements or improved the process of isolation of them, such as potassium, beryllium, aluminum, titanium, boron. Without being a pharmacist himself, as a teacher of students of pharmacy and, for some time, as inspector of the pharmacies of Hannover, he kept in contact with pharmacy. See *Am. J. Pharm. 54*:591, 1882.

**Wood,** George B. (1797–1879), physician, professor at the Philadelphia College of Pharmacy and later at the Medical Department of the University of Pennsylvania. Wood was for several decades the decisive factor in the revisions of the U.S.P. and, in collaboration with Franklin Bache, editor of the *U. S. Dispensatory.* See England: *First Century of the Philadelphia College of Pharmacy,* p. 397, Philadelphia, 1922.

**Wood,** Horatio C (1841–1920), physician, pioneer American pharmacologist, author and professor at the University of Pennsylvania. See *Dictionary Scient. Biog.; Am. J. Pharm. 92*:136, 1920; *Dictionary of Amer. Biog. XX, p. 459.*

**Wood,** Horatio Charles, Jr. (1874–1958), physician, professor at the University of Pennsylvania and, from 1921, at the Philadelphia College of Pharmacy. See *First Century of the Philadelphia College of Pharmacy.* First Supplement, p. 102, Philadelphia, 1934.

**Wulling,** Frederick J. (1866–1947). Professor and dean of the College of Pharmacy, University of Minnesota, 1892–1936, author, zealous advocate of the betterment of American pharmaceutical education. See *J.A.Ph.A. 23*:177, 1934; *Pharmacy Forward,* selections from F. J. Wulling's diary, autobiography, speeches and reports, edited and published by his son, E. G. Wulling, La Crosse, Wis., 1948.

**Ximenez,** Francisco (late 16th to early 17th century), Dominican monk and botanist. See Tschirch, *Handbuch der Pharmakognosie,* ed. 2, *I,* Part 3, p. 1346, Leipzig, 1933.

**Yaple,** Florence (1865–1912), one of the outstanding American woman pharmacists. Miss Yaple was closely connected with the Philadelphia College of Pharmacy and participated, for many years, in the work of editing and managing the American Journal of Pharmacy. See *Am. J. Pharm. 84*:481, 1912.

**Yearbooks.** The annual report is a special type of pharmaceutical serial, popular in the 19th and to some extent still in the 20th century, in various countries and languages. The first pharmaceutical periodical, the *Almanach, oder Taschenbuch für Scheidekünstler und Apotheker.* (1780) was an annual of this sort.

**Youngken,** Heber W. (1885–1963), American botanist and pharmacognosist, professor at the Massachusetts College of Pharmacy, and author. His son, Heber, Jr., in turn, became one of the important pharmacognosists of his generation and then dean of the College of Pharmacy and Vice-Provost at the University of Rhode Island. See England: *First Century of the Philadelphia College of Pharmacy,* p. 418, Philadelphia, 1922.

**Zwelfer,** Johann (1618–1668), at first a pharmacist in Palatine (Germany), later physician in Vienna. His *Animadversiones in Pharmacopoeam Augustanam* (1652) are probably the first known commentary on a pharmacopeia (if we disregard N. Culpeper).

# Notes and References

# Notes and References

## 1. ANCIENT PRELUDE


1. Artelt, W.: Studien zur Geschichte der Begriffe "Heilmittel" und "Gift," Studien zur Geschichte der Medizin *23*:7, 1937; Meyer-Steineg, Th., and Sudhoff, K.: Geschichte der Medizin im Ueberblick, p. 9, Jena, 1921.
2. Srivastava, G. P.: History of Indian Pharmacy, 2nd ed., vol. 1, Calcutta, 1954, (when published, volume 2 will cover the period since 1600). See also the review by Berman, A.: Bull. Hist. Med., *29*:578, 1955. For a summary of some principal facets of classic therapeutics in China and India, see the second edition of Kremers and Urdang: History of Pharmacy, Philadelphia, Lippincott, 1951, pp. 3 to 6 (hereafter referred to as Kremers and Urdang, 2nd ed.). For more information see, for example, from a medical viewpoint: Zimmer, H. R.: Hindu Medicine, 3rd Ser., no. 6, Inst. Hist. Med., Johns Hopkins Univ., Baltimore, 1948; and Müller, R. F. G.: Grundsätze altindischer Medizin, vol. 8, Acta Historica Scientiarum Naturalium et Medicinalium, Kopenhagen, 1951. The latter includes commentary on Charaka's Samhita, whose classic text has been published at least twice in English. On medical services in ancient China: Hume, E. H.: The Chinese Way in Medicine, Baltimore, 1940; Wong, K. C. and Wu, L.-T.: History of Chinese Medicine, Tientsin, 1932; Huard, P. and Wong, M.: La Médecine chinoise, au cours des siècles, Paris, 1959; Evolution de la matière médicale chinoise, Janus *47*:3, 1958, and such German works as those by Franz Huebotter and Gottfried Schramm. There is a comprehensive history of Japanese pharmacy (in Japanese) by Simizu (or Shimizu), Tootaroo: Nihon Yakugakushi, Tokyo, 1949.
3. Jastrow, M.: The medicine of the Babylonians and Assyrians, Proc. Roy. Soc. Med. *7*:109, 1913.
4. Temkin, O.: Beiträge zur archäischen Medizin, Kyklos *3*:90, 1930.
5. Artelt, W.: *op. cit.*, p. 33; Temkin, O.: *op. cit.*, p. 133.
6. Thompson, R. C.: The Assyrian Herbal, London, 1924; On the Chemistry of the Ancient Assyrians, London, 1925; Urdang, G.: Pharmacy in ancient Babylon-Assyria, Palestine and Egypt, Am. J. Pharm. Ed. *7*:50, 1943; Goltz, D.: Mitteilungen über ein assyrisches Apothekeninventar, Arch. int. hist. sci. (Paris) *42*:450 f., 1968.
7. Castiglioni, A.: A History of Medicine, p. 39, New York, 1941.
8. Levey, M.: Chemistry and Chemical Technology in Ancient Mesopotamia, p. 149, Amsterdam, 1959. (Transliterated words have been omitted from the quotation.) An excellent source of information based on the original documents. [See also, Levey, M.: A Sumerian medical text from Nippur of the 3rd millennium B.C., Actes du VIII Congres International d'Histoire des Sciences Collection de Travaux de l'Academie . . . No. *9*:843, 1956; and Kramer, S. N.: First pharmacopeia in man's recorded history, Am. J. Pharm. *126*:76, 1954.]
9. *ibid.*, p. 151.
10. Sigerist, H.: A History of Medicine, vol. 1, Primitive and Archaic Medicine, p. 484, New York, 1955. Probably the best account in English of Babylonian and Egyptian medicine.

11. Meissner, B.: Babylonien und Assyrien, p. 359, Heidelberg, 1925. Von Oefele refers to the "pasisu" in a letter to Hermann Schelenz.
12. Castiglioni, A.: *op. cit.*, p. 38.
13. Dawson, W. R.: Magician and Leech, p. 128, London, 1929.
14. Temkin, O.: Recent publications on Egyptian and Babylonian Medicine, Bull. Inst. Hist. Med., Johns Hopkins Univ., *4*:247, 341, 1936. The names and the estimated dates of the main medical papyri as listed by Temkin are: Kahun, gynecology (also veterinary fragment), ca. 1900 B.C.; Edwin Smith, surgery, ca. 1550; George Ebers, medicine and pharmacy, ca. 1500 B.C.; Hearst, formulary, ca. 1500 B.C.; and between 1350 and 1100 B.C., London 10059, drug therapy and incantations; Berlin 3038 (Brugsch major), therapeutics and fertility tests; Berlin 3027 (Brugsch minor; edited by Erman), diseases, therapy and incantations for childbirth and infants. In addition the short Chester Beatty (BM 10686) papyrus, ca. 1200 B.C., is a formulary for anal diseases. See also, Sigerist: History, 298–318 et passim; Leake, C. D.: The Old Egyptian Medical Papyri, Lawrence, 1952.
15. Grapow, H.: Untersuchungen über die altägyptischen Papyri, I. Teil. Mitt. vorderasiatisch–ägyptische Gesells. *40*: (1), 1935, *et seq.*
16. Ebbell, B.: The Papyrus Ebers, Copenhagen, 1937.
17. Temkin, O.: Isis *28*:126, 1938.
18. Leake, C. D.: Ancient Egyptian therapy, Ciba Symposia, *1*:311, 1940, referring to both the Ebers and the Hearst papyri.
19. Ebbell: *op. cit.*, p. 38.
20. Quantitative measurement in the medical papyri, and drug measurement in particular, is discussed by Leake, C.: Medical Papyri, pp. 18–33.
21. Ebbell: Papyrus, p. 19; cf. p. 29.
22. Sigerist: History, p. 303. For the Smith papyrus, see Oriental Institute Publications, Volumes 3 and 4: "The Edwin Smith Surgical Papyrus," James H. Breasted, translator and editor, Univ. Chicago Press, 1930.
23. Besides present-day flora and ecology, numerous historical asides may be found in Fahmy, I. R.: The medicinal plants of the Middle East, Lebanese Pharm. J. *4*:12, 1956.
24. Dawson, W. R.: Studies in ancient materia medica, Am. Drug. *73*:22, 1925.
25. Breasted, J. H.: A History of Egypt from the Earliest Times to the Persian Conquest, p. 113, London, 1921.
26. Thompson, C. J. S.: The Mystery and Art of the Apothecary, pp. 11, 12, London, 1929.
27. Jonckheere, Frans: Le Preparateur de remèdes dans l'organisation de la pharmacie égyptienne, Publication No. 29, Institut für Orientforschung, Deutsche Akad. Wiss. Berlin, pp. 160–161, et passim, Berlin, 1955. In examining past views in the light of evidence, the author specifically argues against attributing pharmaceutical connotations to "Urma" and to "ph-ar-maki." With regard to the formulas for unguents and perfumed preparations that have been found inscribed on the walls of Ptolemaic temples, the author concludes that these are archival type-formulas for cult ceremonies and festival rituals, without therapeutic purposes. Likewise, the "laboratory" rooms excavated within the walls of the sanctuary, but outside the sacred chambers proper, must have required "pharmaceutical" or "chemical" types of knowledge for their operation, but Jonckheere asks for evidence showing that their products were put to therapeutic use. (See, *ibid.*, pp. 151–157.)
28. Sigerist, History, 343.
29. Grapow, H.: Die ägyptischen medizinischen Papyri, Munich Med. Wochenschr. *82*:135, 958, 1002, 1935.
30. Thompson, C. S. J.: *op. cit.*, p. 24.
31. Especially rich and reliable sources of information about Greek temple medicine are, Kerenyi, Ch.: Le Medecin divin: promenades mythologiques aux sanctuaires d'Asclepios, Basle, 1948, and Edelstein, E. J., and Edelstein, L.: Asclepius. A Collection and Interpretation of the Testimonies, 2 vols., Baltimore, 1945.
32. Osler, William: The Evolution of Modern Medicine, p. 69, New Haven, 1923.
33. Oliver, J. R.: Greek medicine and its relation to Greek civilization, Bull. Inst. Hist. Med., Johns Hopkins Univ. *3*:623, 1935.
34. Edelstein, L.: Peri Deron, und die Sammlung der Hippokratischen Schriften, Berlin, 1931.
35. Jones, W. H. S.: Hippocrates, vol. 1, p. 21, London, 1923. See also Sigerist, H. E.: A History of Medicine, Vol. 2, pp. 320–323, New York, 1961, who interprets the humors already in Hippocratic time as "not mere principles, but are very real."
36. In English, the writings of Jerry Stannard are

of unusual interest concerning Greek pharmacy and drug therapy, such as his Hippocratic pharmacology, Bull. Hist. Med. *35*:497–518, 1961, and Materia medica and philosophic theory in Aretaeus, Sudhoffs Archiv *48*:27–53, 1964. Of earlier work, note especially Dierbach, J. H.: Die Arzneimittel des Hippokrates. . . Heidelberg, 1824; republished Hildesheim, 1969, and the Historische Studien zur Pharmakologie der Griechen, Romer und Araber, in the series, Historische Studien . . . Dorpat (especially R. von Grot in V. I, 1889, pp. 58–133; republished Leipzig, 1968).

37. Jones, W. H. S.: The Doctor's Oath, Cambridge, England, 1924.
38. Tschirch, A.: Handbuch der Pharmakognosie, Leipzig, 1910, 1. (Abt. 3): 1271–1290.
39. Crateuas' drawings are contained in part of the famous Vienna Codex of Dioscorides' writings on crude drugs. It was once possessed by Juliana Anicia, daughter of an emperor of the Western Roman Empire (Anicius Olybirius, 512 A.D.). A beautiful and complete facsimile edition of this manuscript was issued by Graz in Vienna, 1967.
40. The Greek Herbal of Dioscorides: John Goodyer, trans., 1655; Gunther, R. T.: ed., Oxford, 1934 (reprinted Hafner, New York, 1959); see also Cohen, M. R., and Drabkin, I. E.: A Source Book in Greek Science, New York, 1948. On the later influence see, e.g., Stannard, J.: Dioscorides and Renaissance materia medica, *in* Analecta Medico-Historica: Materia Medica in the XVI Century, Oxford-New York, 1966; also note the multivolume Spanish work by Dubler, C. E.: and E. Teres: La 'Materia Médica de Dioscorides. Transmisión medieval y renacentista. . ., Tetuan and Barcelona, 1952–57.
41. Albutt, T. C.: Greek Medicine in Rome, p. 380, London, 1921.
42. Brock, A. J.: Galen on the Natural Faculties, p. ix, London, 1916.
43. Temkin, O.: Galenism, Rise and Decline of a Medical Philosophy, p.112, Ithaca and London, 1973, based on Galen's Ars medica 28 (Kühn edition *1*:383 f.)
44. *Ibid.*, p. 112 f.
45. Pliny, Natural History, bk. 34, ch. 25 (Bostock-Riley edition, vol. 6, p. 195; and footnotes 1, 21, p. 143; and 15, vol. 3, p. 357).
46. For a discussion of some of the evidence and difficulties of interpretation, see Dann, G. E. *in*: Zur Geschichte der Pharmazie No. 1, 1954, pp. 5 and 6 (Beilage der Deutschen Apotheker-Zeitung), based on: Tergolina in Raccolta di scritti in onore di Giulio Conci a cura di A. E. Vitolo (Pisa, 1953). Some comments in Pliny's Natural History on the *seplasiarii*, as cited by Ernst Stieb, may be found at 34.25 (6:195 of the Bostock-Riley edition) and 33.58 (6:143); see also in the Bostick-Riley edition, note 1 at 6:195, note 21 at 6:143, and note 15 at 3:357. One of the most comprehensive sources of information is Schmidt, A.: Drogen und Drogenhandel in Altertum, Leipzig, 1924; (some passages of special pharmaceutical interest have been translated into English by Urdang, G.: Pharmacy in ancient Greece and Rome, Am. J. Pharm. Ed. *7*:160, 1943), and Berendes, J.: Die Pharmacie bei den alten Culturvölkern. Historisch-kritische Studien. 2 vols., Halle, 1891 (republished Hildesheim, 1965).
47. Spencer, W. G.: Celsus De Medicina, vol. 2, pp. xv–lxvii, Cambridge, (Mass) 1938; Castiglioni, A.: Aulus Cornelius Celsus as a historian of medicine, Bull. Hist. Med. *8*:857, 1940; Meinecke, B.: Aulus Cornelius Celsus—plagiarist or artifex medicinae? Bull. Hist. Med. *10*:288, 1941; and Temkin, O.: Celsus' "On Medicine" and the ancient medical sects, Bull. Hist. Med. *3*:249–264, 1935.
48. Schelenz, H.: Geschichte der Pharmazie, p. 165, Berlin, 1904; Schonack, W.: Die Rezeptsammlung des Scribonius Largus, Jena, 1913; Rinne, F.: Scribonii Largi "Compositiones." Dorpat, 1892.
49. Chem. and Drug. *106*:804, 1927.
50. Singer, C.: From Magic to Science, 178, 179.
51. For lists of the plants mentioned by Pliny see Wittstein: Die Naturgeschichte der Caius Plinius Secundus, Leipzig, 1881, and Fée: Commentaires sur la botanique et la matière médicale de Pline, Paris, 1883. For Pliny's chemical knowledge, see Bailey, K. C.: The Elder Pliny's Chapters on Chemical Subjects, 2 vols., London, 1929 and 1932. For a historic paper of great pharmaceutical interest, see Stieb, E. W.: Drug adulteration and its detection, in the writings of Theophrastus, Dioscorides and Pliny, Journal Mondial de Pharmacie *2*:117, 1958.
52. A masterly English translation and commentary may be found in: Adams, F.: The Medical Works of Paulus Aegineta, London, 1844–1847; see also Berendes, J.: Paulos von

Aegina, des besten Arztes sieben Bücher, Leiden, 1914.

## 2. THE ARABS AND THE EUROPEAN MIDDLE AGES

1. Hitti, P. K.: History of the Arabs, p. 174, London, 1937.
2. Baas, J. H.: Outlines of the History of Medicine and the Medical Profession, Handerson, H. E., trans., p. 220, New York, 1889.
3. Campbell, D.: Arabian Medicine and its Influence on the Middle Ages, vol. 1, p. xi, London, 1926.
4. On Theodoq, S. K. Hamarneh cites 'Ali Abu al-Hasan al-Quifti: Ikhbar al 'Ulama bi Akhbar al-Hukama, pp. 74 and 248, Cairo, 1908. Levey, M.: Ibn Māsawaih and his treatise on simple aromatic substances, J. Hist. Med. *4*:394–408, 1961. See also other works by Levey, such as The Medical Formulary or Aqrābādhīn of al-Kindī. . ., Madison, 1966, and The Medical Formulary of Al-Samarquandī. . ., Philadephia, ca. 1967.
5. Said, H. M. (ed. & trans.): Al-Biruni's Book on Pharmacy and Materia Medica. . ., Karachi, 1973. A commentary on al-Biruni's text by S. K. Hamarneh has been issued as Pt. 2 (1973).
6. Sarton, G.: Introduction to the History of Science, 2, p. 663, Baltimore, 1931. For detailed information, see: Von Sentheimer, J.: Grosse Zusammenstellung über die Kräfte der bekannten einfachen Heil- und Nahrungsmittel von Abu Mohammed Abdallah ben Ahmed aus Malaga bekannt unter dem Namen Ebn Baithar, 2 vols., Stuttgart, 1840 and 1842, or Leclerc, L., trans.: Traité des Simples, par Ibn el-Beither, 3 vols., Paris, 1877–1883.
7. The section on Arabic literature has been derived from Hamarneh, S. K.: Origins of Pharmacy and Therapy in the Near East, pp. 54–136, Tokyo, 1973.
8. Ranking, G. S. A.: The life and works of Rhazes, 17th Internat. Congr. Med. *23*:237, 1914; Campbell, D.: *op. cit.*, pp. 60–102; Chem. and Drug. *106*:808, 1927; Ruska, J.: Die Alchemie Al-Razi's, Der Islam *22*:319, 1935; Das Buch der Alaune, p. 12, Berlin, 1935.
9. Sarton, G.: Introduction to the History of Science, I, p. 709, Baltimore, 1927; Meyer-Steineg, Th., and Sudhoff, K.: Geschichte der Medizin in Ueberblick,p. 160, Jena, 1921; Urdang, G.: Zur Geschichte der Metalle in den Amtlichen Deutschen Arzneibüchern, pp. 14, 15, Mittenwald, 1933.
10. Hamarneh, S. K., and Sonnedecker, G.: A Pharmaceutical View of al-Zahrawi (Abulcasis) in Arabic Spain, Leiden, 1963, 176 pp.
11. Meyer-Steineg, Th., and Sudhoff, K.: *op.cit.*, pp. 156, 225, 255; Ruska, J.,and Kraus, P.: Der Zusammenbruch der Jabir Legende, Beilage zum dritten Jahresbericht des Forschungsinstituts f. Geschichte der Naturwiss. in Berlin, 1930; Ruska, J.: Arabische Giftbücher, Fortschritte der Med. *50*:524, 1932.
12. Hamarneh, S. K.: *op. cit.*, but for a general guide to the secondary literature, see his "Bibliography on Medicine and Pharmacy in Medieval Islam," ns Vol. *25*, Veröffentlichungen der Internalionalen Gesellschaft für Geschichte der Pharmazie, Stuttgart, 1964, 204 pp.; also Ebied, R. Y.: Bibliography of Medieval Arabic and Jewish Medicine and Allied Sciences, London, 1971, 150 pp. For a general evaluation of Arabic writings on drugs, see 4 essays by Max Meyerhof, Ciba Symposia *6*:1847–1876, 1944.
13. Hamarneh, S. K., citing Aḥmad 'Isā: Tarikh al-Bimāristānāt fi al-Islām, p. 203, Damascus, 1939.
14. Hamarneh, S. K.: "The Rise of Professional Pharmacy in Islam," Med. Hist. *6*:63, 1962; also his Origins. . ., pp. 49 f.
15. Campbell, D.: *op. cit.*, p. xii.
16. The martyred twins have fascinated a number of artists and writers; e.g., consult Wittmann, A.: Kosmas und Damian; Kultausbreitung und Volksdevotion, Berlin, ca. 1967, 344 pp., and David-Danel, M.-L.: Iconographie des Saints médecins Côme et Damien, Lille, 1958, 257 pp.
17. Fort, G. F.: Medical Economy During the Middle Ages, p. 137, New York, 1883.
18. Meyer-Steineg, Th. and Sudhoff, K.; *op. cit.*, p. 172, and Buck, A. H.: The Growth of Medicine from the Earliest Times to about 1800, p. 238, New Haven, 1917; the quotation is by Sigerist, H. E.: The medical literature of the early middle ages, Bull. Hist. Med. *2*:32, 1934.

19. Castiglioni, A.: (Krumbhaar, E. B., trans.) Italian Medicine, pp. 10, and 3, New York, 1932.
20. Buck, A. H.: *op. cit.*, p. 187.
21. Sigerist, H. E.: *op. cit.*, p. 33. *Ibid.*, p. 40; see also Singer, C.: From Magic to Science, p. 185, New York, 1928.
22. Here are a few examples of early medieval literature of this kind: Extracts from Pliny were compiled for practical use in the so-called *Plinius Valerianus* and a *breviarium*, known as *Medicina Plinii* or *Plini Secundi Junioris de medicina libra*, plagiarized Scribonius. The Pseudo-Apuleius and other contemporary or earlier compilations are the sources of the book *De medicamentis physicis, empiricis ac rationalibus*, written by a high Roman official of Celtic origin, Marcellus of Bordeaux (fl. A.D. 410), who describes drugs of ancient classic literature as well as many medicaments in popular use by his people, the Celts. (See Stannard, J.: Marcellus of Bordeaux and the beginnings of medieval materia medica, Pharm. Hist. *15*:47–53, 1973) About 200 years later a learned Bishop, Isidore of Seville (570–636), wrote his famous encyclopedia, a part of which was devoted to medicine. In this treatise "especially Caelius has been plundered." (Meyer-Steineg, Th., and Sudhoff, K.: *op. cit.*, pp. 171 and 174.)
23. Campbell, D.: *op. cit.*, p. 106. The monasteries of Luxeuil (France), Fulda and Reichenau (Germany), St. Galls (Switzerland) and Bobbio (Northern Italy) were some of their stages. At Reichenau in 825 a German abbot, Walahfried, wrote his *Hortulus*, a Latin poem on plants growing in that district. It became famous not only as poetry but as an excellent description of the appearance and the medicinal virtues of the plants. The intense devotion to medical and pharmaceutical treatment of patients in St. Galls is attested by the plan for a new monastic building, dating from 820. (The building itself was never erected.) It provided not only an infirmary or hospital for the sick, but also a large *armarium pigmentariorum*, i.e., a special room for the preparation and storage of medicines; and a *herbularius*, i.e., a garden for the cultivation of medicinal plants, the names of which are mentioned in the plan.

    About 25 years earlier (794 or 795) the so-called *Capitulare de villis* was promulgated by Louis the Pious (not by the Emperor Charlemagne, as was assumed before the researches of Dopsch). This edict orders and regulates the raising of plants, useful medicinally and otherwise, in all the gardens appurtenant to the royal domain in Aquitania (Southern France). It is important for pharmacy because it represents the first official acknowledgment of the importance of the cultivation of medicinal plants in Western Europe north of the Alps. (Meyer-Steineg, Th., and Sudhoff, K.: *op. cit.*, pp. 175 and 176.)
24. Singer, C.: *op. cit.*, p. 188; Meyer-Steineg, Th., and Sudhoff, K.: *op. cit.*, p. 177.
25. Garrison, F.: An introduction to the History of Medicine, p. 147, Philadelphia, 1929.
26. Sigerist, H. E.: *op. cit.*, p. 28.
27. Castiglioni, A.: *op. cit.*, p. 14.
28. Campbell, D.: *op. cit.*, p. 123. According to Paul Dorveaux (Le livre des simples médecines, Paris, Société française de l'histoire de la médecine, 1913, p. xvi), the *Circa Instans* is only a revised, corrected and considerably augmented edition of Constantine's treatise *(De Gradibus Simplicium)*.
29. Lutz, Alfons: Der verschollene frühsalernitanische Antidotarius magnus in einer Basler Handschrift aus dem 12, Jahrhundert und das Antidotarium Nicholai, Acta Pharmaciae Historica, 1959, No. 1 (an important paper based on Ms. D/III/14 in Basler Universitäts-Bibliothek); on the Antidotarium Nicolai, cf. Van den Berg, W. S.: Eene Middelnederlandsche vertaling van het Antidotarium Nicolai Leiden, 1917.

    The three *Antidotaria Nicolai*, most historians now would agree, may be distinguished as follows:

    (a) Antidotarium Nicolai Salernitani: oldest of the three (written about 1250?).

    (b) Antidotarium Nicolai Myrepsi: the most comprehensive of the three formularies; written in the 14th century by Nicolaus Myrepsus (also called Alexandrinus), a native of Alexandria living at Byzantium.

    (c) Dispensatorium ad aromatarios: presumably written by Nicolaus Praepositus at Lyon about 1500, not a second treatise of the so-called Nicolaus Salernitanus, as previously thought. (Wickersheimer, E.: Nicolaus Praepositus, ein französischer Arzt ums Jahr 1500, Arch. f. Geschichte d. Med. *5*:302, 1912.)

A version written in the 14th and 15th centuries appeared incompletely in French translations, which have been edited and commented on (Dorveaux, P.: L'antidotaire Nicolas, Paris, 1896).

30. Chevalier, A. G.: The 'Regimen Sanitatis Salernitanum, Ciba Symposium, *5*:1732–1737, 1944; Meyer-Steineg, Th., and Sudhoff, K.: *op. cit.*, p. 205. A Latin inscription on the title page indicated that the *Regimen Sanitatis* was prepared by the entire school of Salerno for an English king; but Singer considers this too typical of royal ascriptions often designed solely to achieve greater sale of copies, to be considered alone as convincing evidence. (Singer, C.: *op. cit.*, p. 247.) The work used old medical poetry from Salerno, from other Italian places and France. Additional prose commentary often was printed with the verses.
31. Stillman, J. M.: Paracelsus, p. 45, Chicago, 1920.
32. A scholarly and extensive discussion of this legal milestone in the history of the pharmacist—based on collation and translation of early documents—has been published by W.-H. Hein and K. Sappert: Die Medizinalordnung Friedrichs II (Bd. NS 12, Veröffentlichungen Internat. Gesellsch. Geschichte der Pharmacie), Eutin, 1957. The authors conclude that the main pharmaceutical provisions of the edict were promulgated sometime between 1231 and 1240. (pp. 17–18 and 98) Cf. Adlung, A., and Urdang, G.: Grundriss der Geschichte der deutschen Pharmazie, p. 7, Berlin, 1935. The date of the edict concerning the separation of pharmacy from medicine in the Two Sicilies is given variously in earlier literature (1224, 1231, 1240 and 1241). It has to be kept in mind that the edict was not an isolated legislative act but part of comprehensive legislation to regulate the hygienic conditions of the Southern Italian kingdom, and was started already under the Norman King of Sicily, Roger II, the grandfather of Frederick II. The opinion that the edict concerning the separation of pharmacy from medicine marks the end of this serial legislation, and was promulgated in 1240, was expressed by Huillard-Bréholles in his *Historia diplomatica Friderici Secundi* (Paris, 1854, vol. 4).
33. Häfliger, J. A.: Das Apothekenwesen Basels, p. 31, Mittenwald, 1938; Adlung, A., and Urdang, G., *op. cit.*, p. 52.
34. Neuburger, M.: History of Medicine, (English ed.) vol. 2, pt. I, p. 2, Oxford, 1925.

## 3. CHANGING MEDICAMENTS AND THE MODERN PHARMACIST

1. In the medical field th Greek originals did not replace the medieval Greco-Arabic treatises immediately or extensively. Meyer-Steineg, Th., and Sudhoff, K.: Geschichte der Medizin in Überblick, pp. 247–271, Jena, 1821.
2. The best biography of Paracelsus is by Pagel, W.: Paracelsus: An Introduction to Philosophical Medicine in the Era of the Renaissance, Basel, 1958.
3. Meyer-Steineg, Th., and Sudhoff, K.: *op. cit.*, p. 275.
4. Stillman, J. M.: Paracelsus, p. 106, Chicago, 1920.
5. Multhauf, R.: Medical Chemistry and "The Paracelsians," Bull. Hist. Med. *28*:101, 1954; Debus, A.: The English Paracelsians, New York, 1965.
6. Urdang, G.: How Chemicals Entered the Official Pharmacopeias, Arch. Int. d'hist. Sci. *7*:303–314, 1954.
7. The effect of drugs was explained (in this case mercury bichloride and mercurous chloride) by adherents of the iatrochemical or the iatrophysical theory in the way described by George Urdang: The early chemical and pharmaceutical history of calomel, *in* Chymia, pp. 99–101, Philadelphia, 1948.
8. Ackerknecht, E.: Therapeutics from the Primitives to the 20th Century, p. 60, New York, 1973.
9. Garrison, F. H.: An Introduction to the History of Medicine, p. 314, Philadelphia, 1929.
10. *Ibid.*, p. 438.
11. On homeopathy in the United States, see Kaufman, M.: Homeopathy in America: The Rise and Fall of a Medical Heresy, Baltimore, 1971.
12. Sigerist, H. E.: Man and Medicine, p. 252,

New York, 1932; Adlung, A., and Urdang, G.: Grundriss der Geschichte der deutschen Pharmazie, pp. 361–380, Berlin, 1935.

13. One of the best sources of information on homeopathic pharmacy is: Steinbichler, E.: Geschichte der homöopathischen Arznei Bereitungslehre in Deutschland bis 1872 (Bd. NS 11, Internat. Gesellsch. Geschichte der Pharmazie), Eutin, 1957. A useful work in English is Boericke, F. E.: Three Lectures on Homeopathic Pharmaceutics, Philadelphia, ca. 1878 (by an American homeopathic pharmacist).
14. Ackerknecht, E. H.: A Short History of Medicine, p. 132, New York, 1955.
15. Sigerist, Henry E.: The Great Doctors, p. 293, New York, 1933.
16. ———: Man and Medicine, p. 248. For more substantial historical assessment, see Buess, H.: Zur Frage des therapeutischen Nihilismus im 19. Jahrhundert, Schweiz. Med. Wschr. *87*:304–312, 1957 and Lesky, E.: Von den Ursprüngen des therapeutischen Nihilismus, Sudhoffs Arch. Gesch. Med. *44*:1–20, 1960.
17. ———: The Great Doctors, p. 343.
18. Ackerknecht, E.: Cellular Theory and Therapeutics, Clio Medica *5*:1–5, 1970.
19. For further information, see Parish, H. J.: A History of Immunization, Edinburgh, 1965.
20. On Ehrlich, see Marquardt, M.: Paul Ehrlich, New York, 1951; Loewe, H.: Paul Ehrlich: Schöpfer der Chemotherapie, Stuttgart, 1950; Cowen, D. L.: Ehrlich the Man, the Scientist, Am. J. Pharm. Ed. *26*: 4–11, 1962; and Earles, M. P.: Salvarsan and the Concept of Chemotherapy, Pharm. J. *203*:400–402, 1970. On his receptor theory, see Parascandola, J. and Jasensky, R.: Origins of the Receptor Theory of Drug Action, Bull. Hist. Med. *48*:199–220, 1974.
21. Fleming, Alexander: Chemotherapy, Yesterday, To-day and To-morrow, p. 6, Cambridge, England, 1946.
22. Domagk, G.: Entwicklung der Chemotherapie in den letzten 25 Jahren und Ausblick in die Zukunft, Münch. medizin. Wschr. *100*:2, (reprint) 1958.
23. Osborne, G.: Chemical compounds in the official compendia, Am. J. Pharm. Ed. *26*:22, 1962. For an indication of the character and rate of specific pharmaceutical innovations since the 1930's see, for example: . . . 30 most important drugs of the past 30 years, Amer. Drugg. p. 14, July 6, 1964 (AMA-based); Pharmaceuticals, Gaps in Technology, Paris: OECD, 1969, Annex III (for list of 138 major pharmaceutical innovations since 1950); and FDC Reports for summary of annual reports by Paul De Haen of New York on new USA drug products (e.g., see *32*: pp. 3–5, No. 3, 1970, for a retrospect on developments 1948–1969).
24. Tishler, M.: Impact of Research on Medicinal Chemistry (Division of Medicinal Chemistry, Am. Chem. Soc.), p. 14, (mimeograph) 1959. On the early history of structure-activity relationships, see Parascandola, J.: Structure-Activity Relationships: The Early Mirage, Pharm. Hist. *13*:3–10, 1971 and The Controversy over Structure-Activity Relationships in the Early Twentieth Century, Pharm. Hist. *16*:54–63, 1974.
25. On the history of penicillin, see Florey, H. W., *et. al.*: Antibiotics, London, 1949, vol. I. pp. 1–73, vol. II, pp. 631–671; Hare, R.: The Birth of Penicillin and the Disarming of Microbes, London, 1970; and Elder, A., ed.: The History of Penicillin Production, New York, 1970. The best biography of Fleming is by Maurois, A.: The Life of Alexander Fleming, Discoverer of Penicillin, translated by G. Hopkins, London, 1952.
26. On the early history of antibiotics, see the special issue, J. Hist. Med. *6*: No. 3, 1951. On precursors of Fleming, see the article by J. Brunel, p. 295.
27. Welch, H.: Pharmacology of antibiotics, J. Hist. Med. *6*:348, 1951.
28. For a discussion of this point, see Ihde, A. and Becker, S.: Conflict of Concepts in Early Vitamin Studies, J. Hist. Biol. *4*:1–33, 1971.
29. For further information on the history of vitamins, see McCollum, E. V.: A History of Nutrition, Boston, 1957.
30. On Banting, see Stevenson, L.: Sir Frederick Banting, Toronto, 1946.
31. On the history of oral contraceptives, see Bennett, J.: Chemical Contraception, New York, 1974.
32. Caldwell, A. E.: Origins of Psychopharmacology: From CPZ to LSD, Springfield, Ill., 1970, and Swazey, J. P.: Chlorpromazine in psychiatry, a study of therapeutic innovation, Cambridge, Mass., 1974.

33. See, for example, Lennard, H., *et. al.*: Mystification and Drug Misuse: Hazards in using Psychoactive Drugs, San Francisco, 1971.
34. Meyer-Steineg, Th., and Sudhoff, K.: *op. cit.*, p. 321.
35. Sigerist, H. E.: Man and Medicine, p. 247.
36. Facsimile of the first edition of the Pharmacopeia Augustana, with Introductory Essays by Theodor Husemann, E. Kremers, ed., Madison, Wis., 1927.
37. *Ibid.*, p. xxix.
38. Urdang, G.: The Pharmacopoeia Londinensis of 1618, p. 81, Madison, Wis., 1944.
39. ———: The Great Doctors, pp. 175–184.
40. *Ibid.*, pp. 185–190.
41. Meyer-Steineg, Th., and Sudhoff, K.: *op. cit.*, p. 416.
42. In the 15th century the English physician Howel, in his formulary, recommended "cod oil" in the preparation of a "cere cloth," a kind of cerate to be used on wounds. About 1730, Norwegian fishermen and farmers found that cod-liver oil cured rickets (Brauer, P.: Die Geschichte des Lebertrans. Neue homöopathische Zeitung *9*:437, 1934). In 1770, the English physician Thomas Percival recommended the oil against rheumatism. However, there was no theoretic explanation of the effect of the oil, and the scientific world hesitated to acknowledge it. In 1837 the pharmacist Hopfer de l'Orme in Hanau found iodine in cod-liver oil (Schelenz, H.: Geschichte der Pharmazie, p. 811, Berlin, 1904); and an explanation of its beneficial effect was based on this discovery. The oil entered the pharmacopeias, but as time went on it again fell into disrepute. There was an abundance of other iodine preparations, and according to contemporary theories there was nothing in the iodine content of the oil to explain the peculiar effect attributed to it. Hence it was regarded as of no greater value than other fats and distinguished from them merely by the special disadvantage of bad taste (Kofler, L.: Das Vertrauen zur Arznei im Wandel der Zeiten. Die Vorträge der Hauptversammlung, Basel; Gesellsch. für Geschichte der Pharmazie, P. 138, Mittenwald, 1934). On the history of cod liver oil, see Ihde, A.: Studies on the History of Rickets. II. The roles of cod liver oil and light, Pharm. Hist. *17*:13–20, 1975.

## 4. THE DEVELOPMENT IN ITALY

1. Conci, G.: Pagine di Storia della Farmacia, p. 245, Milan, 1934.
2. Schelenz, H.: Geschichte der Pharmazie, p. 313, Berlin, 1904.
3. *Ibid.*, p. 155. These associations bore the designations *ars collegium, schola,* or even *universitas,* plus a designation of the occupation represented by each guild. These names, adopted in part by the later medieval guilds, do not imply a mainly educational function.
4. Thompson, J. W.: Economic and Social History of Europe in the Later Middle Ages, vol. 1, p. 26, New York, 1931.
5. *Ibid.*, vol. 2, p. 5.
6. Ciasca, R.: L'Arte dei Medici e Speziali, Florence, 1922 and 1927; Staley, E.: The Guilds of Florence, London, 1906; Davidsohn, R.: Geschichte von Florenz, Berlin, 1896–1927.
7. Thompson, J. W.: *op. cit.*, p. 227.
8. Heyd: Geschichte des Levantehandels im Mittelalter, Stuttgart, 1879.
9. Staley, E.: *op. cit.*, pp. 256, 257, 265.
10. *Ibid.*, p. 273.
11. In Verona a guild of the pharmacists *(la magnifica arte degli speziali)* is mentioned in 1221 (Conci, G.: *op. cit.*, p. 241). In Milan the *Paratico apothecariorum spetiariorum et aromatariorum* was founded about 1300. In Piacenza the *speziali* constituted a guild in the 13th century. In Venice (*ibid.*, p. 279) we again find physicians and pharmacists joined in the *capitolare medicorum et spetiatiorum,* founded in 1258. In 1565, the pharmacists parted company with the physicians and formed the *Collegio degli speziali.* Conci (*ibid.*, p. 297) mentions additional pharmaceutical guilds in Monza, Como, Cremona, Siena, Mantua, Volterra, Lucca, Pistoia, Pisa, Perugia, Bologna and Padua.
12. Poce, M.: Pagine storiche sul nobile collegio chimico-farmaceutico, Roma, 1931. This honored institution was founded as the *Universitas aromatariorum,* then after renewal of the charter by the Pope (1429) it was called, *Nobile collegio degli aromatari.*
13. Davidsohn: *op. cit.*, 2, 215.
14. Rosenthaler, L.: Die Drogenliste der Pergolotti, Schweiz, Apoth. Ztg. *60*:89, 1922. In regard to the drugs involved in this trade, see

*La practica della mercatora,* written in the 14th century by the Florentine, Pergolotti, an employee of the Baldi, the great Florentine merchants.

15. Heyd: *op. cit.*
16. Conci: *op. cit.*, p. 291.
17. Schelenz: *op. cit.*, p. 364.
18. Staley, E.: *op. cit.*, p. 241.
19. Pedrazzini, C.: La Farmacia Storica et Artistica Italiana, Milan, 1934. Häfliger, J.: Pharmazeutische Altertumskunde, pp. 27–39, Zürich, 1931.
20. For a comprehensive list see Appendix 5 and George Griffenhagen: Pharmacy Museums, Madison, Wis., 1956. "The most important German private collection" was bought in 1932 by E. R. Squibb & Sons, and about a decade later was presented to the American Pharmaceutical Association. It is now in the United States National Museum (Smithsonian Institution), in Washington, D.C. The contents are described by George Urdang in *The Squibb Ancient Pharmacy,* New York, 1940.
21. Rosenthaler, L.: Die Drogen des Pasi, Pharm. Ztg. *75*:1439, 1930.
22. Castiglioni, A.: Italian Medicine, p. 55, New York, 1932.
23. Ullersperger, J. B.: Geschichtsumriss der Pharmacie im Königreiche Italien, Neues Repertorium für Pharmacie (Buchner, L. A., ed.) *21*:1872, 291. The Austrian regulations were titled *Piano de regolamento per le farmacie della Lombardia austriaca.*
24. Conci: *op. cit.*, p. 301.
25. *Ibid.*, p. 283. Forrester, G. P.: Revolutionary changes in Italian pharmacy, Am. Drugg. & Pharm. Record *61*:27(July), 1913.
26. Personal communication from Prof. Dott. R. Ventura of the University of Pisa (and Mr. Nixon), Prof. Dott. C. Rubiola of Torino 2 Feb. 1975. Gallo, U.: Pharmacy in Italy, J. Mond. Pharm. 1968, No. 1, pp. 23 f.
27. Fleming, D.: A profile of Italian pharmacy, Tile and Till [Lilly], 1961, Sept.–Oct., pp. 68.
28. Urban, E.: Apothekengesetzgebung im Ausland. Thom's Handbuch der praktischen und wissenschaftlichen Pharmazie. vol. 1, p. 203, Berlin, 1924.
29. Ventura, R.: personal communication, 2 Febr. 1975. Pratesi, P., as reported Deutsche Apoth.-Ztg. *43*:1722, 1974.
30. For example, other chairs for medical botany in the 16th century followed at Bologna (1534), Mondovi (1561), and Turin (1566). Hoch, J. H.: A chapter in the history of pharmacognosy, sixteenth century Italy, Am. J. Pharm. *130*:68–73, 1958.
31. The author was Pietro Andrea Mathioli of Siena (1501–1577), physician-in-ordinary to the German Emperor Maximilian II. Some editions of his influential work appeared under the names of editors rather than that of the original author.
32. Thompson, C. J. S.: The Mystery and Art of the Apothecary, p. 129, London, 1929; Zimmerman, L.: Saladini de Asculo Serenitatis Principis Tarenti Physici Principalis Compendium Aromatariorum, Leipzig, 1919.
33. Schelenz, H.: Geschichte der Pharmazie, pp. 334 and 337, Berlin, 1904. Another reflection of the state of pharmacy in the Renaissance, and an important text of its time, was by the physician Quiricus de Augustus of Dertona, The Light of the Pharmacists (*Lumen apothecariorum,* 1495).
34. Schumacher, B.: Das Luminare Majus von Joannes Jacobus Manlius de Bosco 1536, Mittenwald, 1936; Schelenz, *op. cit.*, p. 407.
35. Conci: *op. cit.*, p. 138. One of Sgobbi's predecessors, the German-born Georg Melich, wrote a "practice" of pharmacy, his *Dispensatorium medicum.* The first edition in Italian was published in Venice, 1574; the last in Latin translation in Germany, 1657.
36. Levey, M.: The Italian pharmacopeia and the influence of medieval Arabic pharmacy, Pharm. Hist. *12*:13 f., 1970.
37. Urdang, G.: Pharmacopoeias as witnesses of world history, J. Hist. Med. *1*:47, 1946. For a general discussion of the history of pharmacopeias, including a chronologic international list (but by no means limited to "official pharmacopeias"), see Volckringer, J.: Evolution et unification des formulaires et des pharmacopées, Paris, 1953.

## 5. THE DEVELOPMENT IN FRANCE

1. Hein, W. H., and Sappert, K.: Die Medizinalordnung Friedrichs II (Bd. NS 12, Internat. Gesellsch. für Geschichte der Pharmazie), pp. 76–78, Eutin, 1957, referring to F.

Prevet and quoting a parchment manuscript, the "petit Thalamus," found in the municipal archive in Montpellier.

2. Bouvet, M.: Histoire de la pharmacie en France, Paris, 1937, p. 226.
3. *Ibid.*, p. 252.
4. *Ibid.*, p. 227.
5. Hein, W., and Sappert, K.: *op. cit.*, p. 76.
6. Bouvet, M.: *op. cit.*, p. 60.
7. *Ibid.*, p. 61.
8. *Ibid.*, p. 236.
9. *Ibid.*, p. 71.
10. *Ibid.*, p. 74.
11. *Ibid.*, p. 253.
12. Dr. Louis Irrissou reported (personal communication) that the main importance of the edict of Villers-Cotterets rests on the fact that it made the French language (as spoken in and near Paris) compulsory for official documents, thus reducing the other languages spoken in France at this time, especially Provençal, to dialects and discouraging the use of Spanish, English and German by the population of border areas.
13. Dorveaux, P.: Le livre des simples médecines, p. xx, Paris, 1913.
14. Bouvet, M.: *op. cit.*, p. 64.
15. *Ibid.*, pp. 280–284. It was later ruled that pharmacists who wanted to practice the trade of a spicer could qualify by preparing a special spicer's "masterpiece" (1581), a kind of practical examination. The rights of the competing groups were further adjusted in parliamentary ordinances of 1629, 1689, 1734 and 1742.
16. Personal communication from Dr. Louis Irrissou.
17. In 1957 there remained about one herboristerie to every thirteen pharmacies. (Laurent, J.: La Pharmacie en France: Etude de Géographie Economique, p. 208, Paris, 1959.) The legal bases of French pharmacy had been the royal declaration of 1777 and the law of 1803, which were replaced by the law of September 11, 1941, as amended May 23, 1945.
18. Bouvet, M.: *op. cit.*, pp. 218–224. An example from Molière is the introductory scene to *Le malade imaginaire*.
19. *Ibid.*, p. 42. Philippe's *Histoire des apothicaires* well demonstrates the intensity of recurrent friction between the two professions in France.
20. *Ibid.*, p. 213.
21. *Ibid.*, p. 265, 266. Champier's initial libel was called *Myrouel des apothicaires et pharmacopoles* (1532). It was followed by the *Déclaration des abus et tromperies que font les apothicaires* (1553) by the physician Sébastian Collin (pseudonym: Lisset Benancio), and a lampoon by the physician Jean Surrelh, *L'apologie des médecins contre les calomnies et grands abus de certain apothicaires* (1558). A pharmacist at Lyon (Bernard Palissy?), writing under the pseudonym Pierre Brailler, published a *Déclaration des abus et ignorance des médecins* (1557), then fired the other barrel, *Articulations sur l'apologie de Jean Surrelh* (1558).
22. *Ibid.*, pp. 301–307.
23. Philippe, A.: Histoire des apothicaires, pp. 221–234, Paris, 1853; Bouvet, M.: Histoire de la Pharmacie, pp. 355–357.
24. White, F. A.: French pharmaceutical societies, Amer. Drugg. *71* (No. 9):11, 1923.
25. The Royal Declaration of 1777 and the Law of Germinal 1803—after having formed the legal basis of French pharmacy for about 140 years—were replaced by a law of September 11, 1941, as amended May 23, 1945.
26. Humbert, G.: L'ordre des pharmaciens français, Bull. Féd. Int. Pharm. *21*:155, 1947.
27. Authorized by Article 571 of the Code de la Santé Publique (communication from M. Bouvet and H. Bonnemain, February 23, 1962). The area of Paris and the Seine, with a ratio of about 2,800 to 1, does not yet conform entirely to the general regulation.
28. Bouvet, M.: *op. cit.*, pp. 149, 150.
29. *Ibid.*, p. 138.
30. Deno, R. A.: Pharmacy in France, J.A.Ph.A., Prac. Pharm. Ed. *12*:164, 1951.
31. Lesur, J.: Pharmacists and Biological Analysis, (mimeograph) 1961, 11 pp.
32. Bouvet, M.: *op. cit.*, pp. 66, 310–317.
33. Pegurier, G.: The supervision of pharmacy in France, Chem. and Drugg. *79*:483, 1911.
34. Green, D. S., American Assistant Trade Commissioner at Paris, as quoted in Am. Drugg. *74*:17, 1926.
35. Revue d'histoire de la pharmacie *3*:204, 1932.
36. Berman, A.: The problem of science in 19th century French pharmaceutical historiography, Actes du dixième Congress international d'histoire des sciences, Vol. II, p. 893, Paris, 1964—an informed, perceptive analysis. On the cooperative, see Heger, H.: Apothekerbilder, 2, pp. 88–92, Vienna, 1919;

Sellier, Ch.: La Pharmacie Centrale de France, Paris, 1903. This remarkable "coop" was inititated and steered through its infancy by the pharmacist F. L. M. Dorvault (1815–1879).

37. Bouvet, M.: *op. cit.*, p. 108.
38. *Ibid.*, pp. 78–79.
39. Dulieu, L.: La Pharmacie à Montpellier de ses origines à nos jours, pp. 44 and 247, n.p., 1973. Bouvet, *op. cit.*, pp. 95, 96.
40. Centenaire de l'Ecole supérieure de pharmacie de l'Université de Paris, pp. 9, 10, Paris, 1904.
41. Universities of pharmaceutical studies have been located (under the 1968 law) at Amiens, Angers, Besançon, Bordeaux, Caen, Clermont-Ferrand, Dijon, Grenoble, Lille, Limoges, Lyon, Marseille, Montpellier, Nancy, Nantes, Paris (2), Poitiers, Reims, Rennes, Rouen, Strasbourg and Tours. For the types and locations of pharmaceutical faculties under pre-1968 arrangements, see ed. 3, p. 337, f.n. 43.
42. The "U. E. R." designation in French literature refers to the whole system of "Unités d'enseignement et de recherches" in higher education established by the "loi d'orientation de l'enseignement supérieur du 12 Novembre 1968." Some of these U.E.R. units still keep the old title of "Faculté," but mostly they are grouped into universities.
43. Fabre, R. and Dillemann, G., Histoire de la pharmacie, pp. 62–74, Paris, 1971—a useful, concise synthesis. Personal communications from M. Pierre Julien and M. Georges Viala of Paris, 30 January 1975. The chart is adapted from the German version, Deutsche Apotheker-Zeitung *114*:793, 1974. See also Dillemann, G.: Des ecoles de pharmacie aux "unités d'enseignement et de recherches pharmaceutiques," Rev. Hist. Pharm., *21*:493–504, 1973.
44. Berman, A.: The problem of science in 19th century French pharmaceutical historiography, Actes due dixième Congrès international d'histoire des sciences, Paris, Vol. II, p. 892, 1964.
45. ———: The Cadet circle, Bull. Hist. Med. *40*:108, 1966, quoting Élémens de chymie, ed. 3, Paris, 1796, Vol. I, pp. lxxxi f.
46. ———: The problem, *loc. cit.*, 891. See also Berman's The pharmaceutical component of 19th-century French public health and hygiene, Pharm. Hist., *11*:5–10, 1969, and his especially illuminating paper, Conflict and anomaly in the scientific orientation of French pharmacy 1800–1873, Bull. Hist. Med. *37*:440–462, 1963.
47. André-Pontier, L.: Histoire de la pharmacie, pp. 21–53, Paris, 1900; Bouvet, M.: *op. cit.*, pp. 368–416.
48. Bouvet, *op. cit.*, p. 411.
49. Berman, A.: The scientific tradition in French hospital pharmacy, Am. J. Hosp. Pharm. *18*:110, 1961.
50. *Ibid.*, p. 113.
51. Balland, A.: Les pharmaciens militaires français, p. 2, Paris, 1913.
52. *Ibid.*, p. 5
53. Berman, A.: The scientific tradition, *loc. cit.*, p. 117.
54. ———:The Cadet . . ., Bull. Hist. Med. *40*:111, 1966.

## 6. THE DEVELOPMENT IN GERMANY

1. Häfliger, J. A.: Das Apothekenwesen Basels, pp. 77, 113–115, 125, 126; Mittenwald, 1938; and Schelenz, H.: Geschichte der Pharmazie, p. 531, Berlin, 1904.
2. Schmitz, R.: Das Apothekenwesen von Stadt- und Kurtrier, Frankfurt/Main, 1960. On interpretive problems concerning the emergence of early German pharmacies, see also Schmitz, R.: Mörser, Kolben und Phiolen . . ., pp. 91–95, Stuttgart, 1966.
3. Adlung, A., and Urdang, G.: Grundriss der Geschichte der deutschen Pharmazie, pp. 38–42, Berlin, 1935. The archives in Zerbst preserve a *privilegium,* dated as early as 1303, showing that the Margrave Otto IV of Brandenburg-Landsberg granted Pharmacist Walther, Jr., a salable, hereditary and exclusive right to practice in Prenzlau.
4. *Ibid.*, pp. 42–45.
5. *Ibid.*, pp. 45–47, 497.
6. *Ibid.*,pp. 9, 40; Schelenz, H.: *op. cit.*, p. 465. In the 15th century, for example, such pharmacies were maintained by Lüneburg and Braunschweig and in the 16th century in other north-German cities, such as Güstrow, Hamburg, Hannover, and Hildesheim. Arends, D., and Schneider, W.: Braunschweiger Apotheken-register 1506–1673, p. 18, Braunschweig, 1960.
7. Adlung, A., and Urdang, G.: *op. cit.*, pp. 47, 48.

8. Apotheker-Jahrbuch, Stuttgart, 1951 and 1962, and R. Menge: Die betriebswirtschaftliche Entwicklung der Apotheken, Deutsche Apoth-Ztg., *113*:644, 1973. On cited warnings concerning overcrowding, see Ehrenstein, E.: Pharmacy in West Germany, Amer. Prof. Pharm. *26*:729, 1960 and Klie, W.: 700 Years of Pharmaceutic-System in Germany (mimeograph, n.p., n.d. [Hamburg, c. 1960], p. 3.

8a. Blumhofer, H.: Gesetz über den pharmazeutisch-technischen Assistenten, Dtsche. Apoth.-Ztg. *108*:1691–1694, 1968.

9. Adlung, A., and Urdang, G.: *op. cit.*, p. 3.

10. *Ibid.*, p. 101.

11. See, for example, *ibid.*, pp. 532–542. At least 500 such price lists ("Taxen") for drugs are known, historically, the earliest printed list dating from Dresden, 1553.

12. Flückiger, Fr. A.: Die Frankfurter Liste, Arch. d. Pharmazie, *201*:433–464, 508–521, 1872; Das Nördlinger Register, Arch. d. Pharmazie, *211*:96–115, 1887.

13. Adlung, A., and Urdang, G.: *op. cit.*, pp. 346–361.

14. *Ibid.*, pp. 117–129.

15. For references and comment concerning changes in the regulations and attendant debates, I am grateful for personal communications from Prof. Dr. Wolfgang Schneider of Braunschweig, May 16, 1962, and from Prof. Dr. Erika Hickel of Braunschweig, March 15, 1975. For the issues, probably to be resolved by further legislation, see, e.g.: On initiatives and reasons for the proposed change in 1961 drug law, Walter P.: Aspekte. . ., Pharmazeut. Ztg. *118*:1863–1867; 1973, on the original draft of the proposed law, Entwurf. . ., ibid., *119*:48–66, 1974; and an overview of 1973 debate, ibid., pp. 5–7; and an overview of 1974 debate, Walter, P.: Die Neuordnung. . ., ibid., pp. 1201–1240. The issues included responsibility for side effects; questions of drug safety and effectiveness in permits to market; a pooled fund from manufacturers to cover liability judgments arising from drug-induced injuries; rules governing manufacture in pharmacies and calculation of the government-controlled prices.

16. Adlung, A., and Urdang, G.: *op. cit.*, pp. 131–152.

17. Berendes, J.: Das Apothekenwesen, Stuttgart, 1907, p. 169.

18. Adlung, A., and Urdang, G.: *op. cit.*, pp. 134, 135. Pharmacists of exceptional scientific talent made pharmaceutical chemistry at the Berlin *Collegium medicum* noteworthy. The first professor there in that subject was the pharmacist Caspar Neumann, and the last was M. H. Klaproth, who was later the first professor of chemistry at the University of Berlin (see Glossary).

18a. A particularly rich source of information on the historical development of pharmacy's association with German universities is, Schmitz, R.: Die deutschen pharmazeutisch-chemischen Hochschulinstitute; Ihre Entstehung und Entwicklung in Vergangenheit und Gegenwart, Stuttgart, ca. 1969.

19. For the law on pharmaceutical education, see: Approbationsordnung für Apotheker vom 23. August 1971, Pharmazeut. Ztg. *116*:1250–1257, 1971, which also gives the structure of the curriculum (pp. 1254 f.). For advice and references on recent changes in pharmaceutical law and education, warm appreciation is expressed to Prof. Dr. Erika Hickel of Braunschweig (personal communication, March 15, 1975). For an American assessment of West German pharmaceutical education in the 1950's see, Sonnedecker, G.: Studying Pharmacy in West Germany, Am. J. Pharm. Ed. *22*:169, 1958. and Burckhalter, J. H.: Doctoral and Postdoctoral Study in Germany, Am. J. Pharm. Ed. *22*:18, 1958.

20. Adlung, A., and Urdang, G.: *op. cit.*, pp. 411–421.

21. *Ibid.*, p. 418; Urdang, G.: Goethe and Pharmacy, Madison, Wis., 1949.

22. Adlung, A., and Urdang, G.: *op. cit.*, p. 405.

23. Ferchl, Fritz: Illustrierter Apothekerkalender, Mittenwald, Stuttgart, Berlin, 1925–1939, and the post-war continuation edited by Wolfgang-Hagen Hein; Zur Geschichte der deutschen Apotheke, Berlin, 1933–1942; and Die Apotheke von der Gotik bis zum Biedermeier, Mittenwald, 1920. Beautiful pictorial evidence further supporting this statement may be seen in: Hein, W. H.: Die Deutsche Apotheke; Bilder aus ihrer Geschichte, p. 58, et passim, Stuttgart, 1960.

24. An incident illustrating their resourcefulness occurred during the prolonged German opertions in East Africa during World War I. A military pharmacist, Schulze, succeeded in manufacturing sufficient amounts of quinine from cinchona trees in the Usambara district to ward off malaria; otherwise the prolonged resistance of the troops would not have been possible. (Adlung, A., and Urdang, G.: *op. cit.*, p. 279.)
25. The three were founded within a space of 14 years: the Berliner Apotheker Konferenz in 1794; the Magdeburger Apotheker Konferenz in 1798; and the Erfurter Kraenzchen in 1808. On Nuremberg, see Brunner, L.: Dreihundertjahrfeier des Collegium Pharmaceuticum Norimbergense, Stuttgart, 1932.
26. After the Nazis gained power in 1933 the Deutscher Apothekerverein became first the Standesgemeinschaft Deutscher Apotheker, and in 1935 the Deutsche Apothekerschaft. Its leader had jurisdiction also over the Pharmazeutische Gesellschaft from 1934 to 1945. The Gesellschaft began a reorganization in 1947.
27. On the history of German pharmaceutical associations in general, see Adlung, A. and Urdang, G.: *op. cit.*, pp. 259–271.
28. The *Gremien* in Austria—the first of which was the Wiener Apotheker Gremium (1723)—were unofficial associations but had official approval. In Saxony compulsory bodies similar to those in Bavaria and entrusted with the same tasks were founded in 1865, under the name Pharmazeutische Kreisvereine.
29. Such *Kammern* have existed in Brunswick since 1865, in Prussia since 1901, in Baden since 1906, in Hessia since 1923, in Wuertemberg since 1925, in Thuringia since 1926 and in Bavaria since 1927. In the later totalitarian organizing of the whole life of the German people into groups that guaranteed the desired political character and indoctrination, the Reichapothekerkammer, based upon the Reichapothekerordnung, came into existence (1937). Thus an official and compulsory pharmaceutical body for the "ethical" affairs of all German pharmacists was created. All pharmacists had to belong to the Kammer and were submitted to a rigid control. The leader of the Deutsche Apothekerschaft was also president of the Reichapothekerkammer, exerting a far-reaching power over the professional and, in part, even the private activities of German pharmacists.
30. Hügel, H.: Pharmazeutische Gesetzeskunde, 9th ed., Stuttgart, 1962.

## 7. THE DEVELOPMENT IN BRITAIN

1. Adlung, A., and Urdang, G.: Grundriss der Geschichte der deutschen Pharmazie, pp. 190–192, Berlin, 1935.
2. Cowen, D. L.: Liberty, laissez-faire, and licensure in nineteenth-century Britain, Bull. Hist. Med. *43*:30–40, 1969.
3. Whittet, T. D.: mimeographed essay in Kremers Reference Files, Pharmaceutical Library, University of Wisconsin (at B14a).
4. Trease, G. E.: The "Spicer-Apothecary" of the Middle Ages, The Future Pharmacist, No. 26 (Summer):54, 1957, clarifies the evolution and the function of the different groups; see also his: The Spices and Apothecaries of the Royal Household in the Reigns of Henry III, Edward I and Edward II *in* Nottingham Mediaeval Studies 3 and 19, 1959; and Trease, G. E.: Pharmacy in History, pp. 31–67 passim, London, 1964. The early spicer (or speciarius) dealt in a variety of commodities that Trease found to include spices and crude drugs, prepared medicines and sweetmeats, sugar, rice, dried and candied fruits, perfumes, dyestuffs, alum and a limited number of other chemicals, as well as cotton thread, silk and paper.
5. For a good general account of this period, see Matthews, L. G.: History of Pharmacy in Britain, pp. 35–41, London, 1962; Trease, G. E.: Pharmacy in History, pp. 68–109, London, 1964; and Whittet, T. D.: "Part 6. England and Wales" from his series on the evolution of pharmacy in Britain (in mimeograph form as of 1961).
6. Thompson, C. J. S.: The Mystery and Art of the Apothecary, pp. 86–100, London, 1929; Chem. & Drugg. *108*:855, 1928; Gilmour, J. P.: The origin of British Pharmacy, Quart. J. Pharm. & Pharmacol. *5*:425, 1932; Kirkby, W.: The Supply of Physic, Chem. & Drugg.

*117*:234, 1932. Some prominent 14th century apothecaries mentioned by Thompson (some of them having come from France) were Henry (also Richard) Montpellier, Roger de Frowicke, Pierre de Montpellers, Coursus de Gangeland, and J. Falcand de Luca.

7. Barrett, C. R. B.: Society of Apothecaries of London, p. xv, London, 1905.
8. Pharm. J. *116*:437, 1926.
9. Thompson: *op. cit.,* p. 180. More recent and important histories of the Society are by Underwood, E. A.: A History of the Worshipful Society of Apothecaries of London, London, 1963, and Copeman, W. S. C.: The Worshipful Society of Apothecaries of London—A History, 1617–1967, London, 1967.
10. Barrett: *op. cit.,* pp. 42–49, 79–83, 267–293.
11. At this time it established a special naval stock. In 1811 and for 10 years previously drugs supplied to the navy averaged annually about $100,800. The supply of drugs to the East India Company averaged about $90,350 annually. (Barrett, *op. cit.,* 102, 119, 176.) Considering the change in the purchasing power of English as well as American currency, these figures must be multiplied to compare with present-day values.
12. Whittet, T. D.: The Apothecary in the Great Plague of London of 1665; The Sydenham Lecture for 1965. Worshipful Society of Apothecaries of London, London, n.d. Roberts, R. S.: The Apothecary in the 17th century, Pharm. J. *189*:505, 1962.
13. Kett, J. F.: Provincial medical practice in England 1730–1815, J. Hist. Med. & Allied Sci., *19*:18–20, 1964.
14. Thompson: *op. cit.,* p. 278.
15. Wootton, A.: Chronicles of Pharmacy, I, pp. 152–154, London, 1910; Bayles, H.: The Rose Case, Chem. & Drugg. *133*:9, 1940, (who cites the Journal of the House of Lords for March 15, 1703/04). See, furthermore, Leake, C.: Percival's Medical Ethics, pp. 112–119, Baltimore, 1927.
16. Kett, *op. cit.,* p. 17.
17. Kett, *op. cit.,* p. 20.
18. Matthews, *op. cit.,* p. 67, also 115; "The title of chemist and druggist," Chem. & Drugg. *105*:90, 1926.
19. Kett, *op. cit.,* p. 22, also 19.
20. Bell and Redwood: *op. cit.,* p. 64, and personal communication from T. Douglas Whittet (January 1962). The Apothecary Society's control of medical education in England and Wales continued until the General Medical Council was formed in 1859.
21. Ferguson, T.: The apothecary in Scotland, Chem. & Drugg. *116*:695, 1932; Wilbert, M. I.: John Morgan, Am. J. Pharm. *76*:6, 1904; Pharm. J. *161*:23, 1948.
22. Whittet, T. D.: From Apothecary to Pharmacist, Ireland; and, From Apothecary to Pharmacist, Scotland (mimeograph version), London, 1961.
23. Barrett: *op. cit.,* p. 224.
24. Bell and Redwood: *op. cit.,* pp. 98; 116–119.
25. *Ibid,* pp. 216–218; Pharm. J., *116*:458, 1926, and Earles, M. P.: Pharmacy and its relation to scientific education in nineteenth-century Britain, Pharm. Hist. *11*:48 f., 1969.
26. Pharm. J., *130*:549, 1933.
27. The interpretation of influences upon pharmacy after the 1950's has been based substantially on Matthews, *op. cit.,* pp. 390–393; and Bush, P. J. and Wertheimer, A. I.: Pharmacy and the HMO: The British Experience (Acad. Pharm. Sci. Sec. on Econ., 1973; in Kremers Reference Files, Pharmaceutical Library, University of Wisconsin).
28. Gamble, F. W.: The Conference, Chem. & Drugg. *99*:129, 1923.
29. National Pharmaceutical Union 1921–1946, London, 1946 (20 pp.) contains historical notes and a summary of functions. Matthews, *op. cit.,* pp. 139 f.; see also, The National Pharmaceutical Union; Fifty Years' Service to Independent Pharmacy, London, 1971, 36 pp. The official organ of the Union since 1969 has been the *NPU Times*.
30. Chem. & Drugg. *108*:855, 1928.
31. Barrett: *op. cit.,* p. xxxiv.
32. Bell and Redwood: *op. cit.,* p. 21; Barrett: *op. cit.,* p. 132; Chem. & Drugg. *105*:198, 1926.
33. Ferguson: *op. cit.,* Chem. & Drugg. *116*:696, 1932.
34. The principal acts regulating the practice of pharmacy in Northern Ireland were the Pharmacy and Poisons Act (Northern Ireland, 1925) and the Medicines, Pharmacy and Poisons Act (Northern Ireland, 1945). The corresponding acts in Eire were the Pharmacy Act (Ireland, 1875) and the Pharmacy Amendment Act (Ireland, 1890).
35. Adams, F. W.: The medicines act made plain, Pharm. J. *202*:151 f., 1969; . . . An NPU view of the medicines act, *ibid.,* 289 f.; Howells, A.:

The effect of recent legislation on pharmaceutical practice, *ibid.*, *201*:281–292, 1968.

36. Pharm. J. *116*:566, 1926. In an amendment to the Dental Practitioners Bill of 1878, initiated by the Pharmaceutical Society, the British government provided that druggists should be registrable who had practiced dentistry in conjunction with pharmacy. A large group of druggists in this way became dentists.
37. For background on the case brought by Dickson, an executive of Boots, Ltd., see, e.g., Special reports: Pharmaceutical Society of Great Britain: special general meeting, Pharm. J., *195*:117–128, 1965; Special reports: high court of justice: Dickson v. Pharmaceutical Society: powers of Society questioned, *ibid. 196*:660–681, 1966; House of Lords appellate committee: Society v. Dickson: Pharmaceutical Society Loses, *ibid. 200*:651–660, 1968; Lewis, D. F.: The effect of the Dickson judgment on the profession of pharmacy, *ibid. 201*:252–258, 1968. For other reportage and editorializing on this influential event in 20th-century British pharmacy, see elsewhere in *Pharm. J.* from *195*:59–61, 1965 to the final decision in 1968.
38. Harbingers of the movement toward planned distribution of pharmacies had arisen in the Society already in 1941 and 1961 but the sustained effort came between 1966 and 1974. The sources presently lie mostly in the journalistic accounts of that period. The following references (courtesy of Prof. Ernst W. Steib of the University of Toronto), in abbreviated form, give guidance to the principal journal for those who wish to follow the arguments: Pharm. J. *196*:133 f., 427, 433; 551–544; 1966; *198*:462, 471 f., 1967; *201*:399–402, 1968; *203*:313 f., 329–344, 583 f., 729, 1969; *204*:628 f., 382, 1970; 382; *210*:330 f., 538, 1973; *212*:214, 387, 393, 1974.
39. Quote from Matthews, L. G.: History of Pharmacy in Britain, p. 138, Edinburgh and London, 1962. Interim reforms occurred following the influential W. H. Beveridge report in 1942 *(Social Insurance and Allied Services)*, culminating in 1946 with two complementary enactments, the National Health Services Act and the National Insurance Act. With this legislation the English Ministry of Health (and counterparts in Wales and Scotland) thus "became fully responsible for the general practitioner and pharmaceutical services, hospitals, local authority services, mental health and hygiene (water supplies, sewerage, etc.)," as pointed out by Trease, G. E.: Pharmacy in History, p. 240, London, 1964. The British experience with health insurance generated a large literature (in addition to government publications) of which only a few general examples may be mentioned: Lindsey, A.: Socialized Medicine in England and Wales: The National Health Service, 1958–1961, Chapel Hill,1962; Eckstein, H.: The English Health Service; Its Origins, Structure and Achievements, Cambridge, Mass.,1958. On more specifically pharmaceutical aspects see, e.g., Martin, J. P.: Social Aspects of Prescribing, London, 1957; The British National Health Service—A Short Survey with particular reference to the pharmaceutical services, London: The Pharmaceutical Press, 1961, 21 pp.; on the 1974 reorganization see: Pharm. J. *212*:258 and 352, 1974.
40. Thompson: *op. cit.*, pp. 162, 166, 167.
41. *Ibid.*: p. 263. In Scotland, more of the pharmacies retained a dignified apearance, T. D. Whittet believes (personal communication, 1962).
42. Wootton: *op. cit.*, I. p. 365 and 141; Thompson: *op. cit.*, pp. 266–268.
43. Pharm. J. *116*:437, 1926.
44. Ferguson: *op. cit.*, Chem. & Drugg. *116*:697, 1932.
45. Barrett: *op. cit.*, p. xxxii, gives the full text.
46. *Ibid.*, pp. 5, 103, 197.
47. Bell and Redwood: *op. cit.*, pp. 104, 167, 175. See also, Wallis, T. E.: History of the School of Pharmacy, University of London, London, 1964; and Earles, M. P.: The pharmacy schools of the nineteenth century, *in*: Evolution of Pharmacy in Britain, pp. 79–95, London, 1965. Also on the earlier period, see Sage, C. E.: School of Pharmacy of the Pharmaceutical Society of Great Britain, Pharm. Era, Dec. 31, 1896 pp. 869–871.
48. Fairbairn, J. W.: Pharmaceutical education in Great Britain—a comparative study, Am. J. Pharm. Ed. *22*:1, 1958.
49. The degree of Bachelor of Pharmacy may be taken at the universities of Leeds, London, Nottingham, Wales, Bath and Edinburgh; and the Bachelor of Science in Pharmacy at the universities of Glasgow and of Manchester. There are some optional 4-year programs, and

Manchester makes it the minimum for a degree. Technical colleges that gave courses of instruction qualifying for the examinations of the Pharmaceutical Society, and now offer qualifying degrees in their own right are in Aberdeen, Birmingham, Brighton, Bristol, Cardiff, Liverpool, Plymouth, Portsmouth, Sunderland. Bradford, Strathclyde and Aston—which include pharmacy departments—were upgraded to university status and expanded. On the Bradford "sandwich" plan, see Pharm. J. *205*:50 f., 1970. Examples of a feature of the British system of higher education that permits the awarding of degrees outside the university framework, if under the control and approval of a Council for National Academic Awards (i.e., CNAA institutions), are Brighton, Leicester, Liverpool, Portsmouth Colleges of Technology, Robert Gordon's Institute of Technology, and Sunderland Polytechnic. (Pharm. J. *202*:340, 1969), which are pharmacy faculties unaffiliated with a university. The pharmaceutical Society ended the last phase of its long involvement in pharmaceutical education when it examined its last pharmacy student in 1970.

For a good summary 1939–1966 see, Maplethorpe, C. W.: Pharmaceutical Education in 1966, Pharm. J. *197*:491–493, 503, 1966. For the various undergraduate and graduate programs, see, e.g., The schools of pharmacy, Pharm. J. *209*:20–22, 1972.

When the two registers of pharmacists, representing the two different levels of qualification, were amalgamated, a mark of deference to the Pharmaceutical Chemists was preserved when the Society designated them as PSGB "Fellows." Thereafter, a pharmacist might earn Fellowship status in the Society by accomplishing postgraduate research, but in recent years the distinction is conferred only as an honorary recognition of outstanding services to British pharmacy.

50. Other reciprocal arrangements made by Great Britain incude Australia, New Zealand and South Africa.
51. In a significant document concerning the character and outlook of British pharmacy since mid-century, an expanded use of "pharmaceutical assistants" was foreseen (Report of the Committee on the General Practice of Pharmacy, Pharm. J., Sept. 30, 1961). There have been variants on the theme and training program—for "shop assistants," for "dispensary assistants," and the giant chain store, Boots Ltd., operated its own training program. In Scotland there has been a training program for hospital-pharmacy technicians operating under the aegis of the Scottish Association for National Certificates and Diplomas. (Training of . . ., Pharm. J. *198*:559 f., 1967; *199*:68–70, 1967). On the revised "PATB" syllabus, see: Step forward in training technicians, Pharm. J. *202*:180, 1969.
52. In incorporating the more recent history of British pharmacy in this chapter, I am greatly indebted and appreciative to the historians of pharmacy, Dr. Ernst W. Stieb of the University of Toronto and Dr. Melvin P. Earles of the Chelsea College of Science for information and many references cited.
53. Urdang, G. Pharmacopoeia Londinensis of 1618, Madison, Wis., 1944.
54. Cowen, D. L.: The Spread and Influence of British Pharmacopoeial and Related Literature, n.s. Bd. 41, Veröffentlichungen d. Internat. Gesel. f. Gesch. d. Pharm., Stuttgart, 1974.
55. Bell and Redwood: *op. cit.*, p. 163.
56. The investigations of T. Douglas Whittet of London permit a more adequate documentation of British pharmaceutical contributions to science than heretofore. See also, e.g., Schofield, M.: A pharmacist turned chemist, Pharm. J. *160*:22, 1948.
57. Cripps, E. C.: Plough Court, pp. 25–51, London, 1927.
58. Chem. & Drugg. *114*:749, 1931; *116*:711, 1932; *118*:667, 1933; *120*:732, 1934; *124*:737, 1936. See also, Established 100 years, Pharm. J. *146*:153, 1941, and anniversary publications by Howard, G. E.: Howards 1797–1947, Ilford, 1947, and Barker, H. J.: The History of Duncan, Flockhart & Co., Edinburgh, 1947.

## 8. SOME INTERNATIONAL TRENDS

1. Schelenz, H.: Geschichte der Pharmacie, Berlin, 1904, p.432.
2. Thompson, C. J. S.: The Mystery and Art of the Apothecary, London, 1929, p. 233.

3. Personal communication from Howard Bayles of England.
4. Schelenz: *op. cit.*, p. 579.
5. Wootton, A.: Chronicles of Pharmacy, 1, pp. 319–322, London, 1910.
6. Encyclopaedia Britannica, 11th ed., vol. 20, p. 903, 1901.
7. Langenhan, H. A.: Liquor potassii arsenalis. Bull. Univ. Wis., Ser. No. 1153, Gen. Ser. No. 936. The English patent law of 1852, which required preliminary disclosure, began an era of real invention, as is shown by patents granted in the years 1854–1856: use of glycerin in cosmetics (1854, No 85, John Henry Johnson); capsules (1855, No. 824, Jules Denoual); first aniline dye (1856, No. 1984, William Henry Perkin); use of "paraffine" in hair oils and ointments (1856, No. 2945, Charles Humphrey). (Chem. & Drugg. *124*:758, 1936)
8. Inlow, E. B.: The Patent Grant (Johns Hopkins U. Studies in Historical and Political Science. Series 68, No. 2), pp. 36–38, 43 and 48, Baltimore, 1950.
9. Markham, J. W.: The Patent System and the Ethical Drug Industry, p. 36 (mimeographed, PMA, revised draft), n. p., 1961.
10. Fischelis, R. P.: What is a patent or proprietary medicine? Am. J. Pharm. Ed. *2*:163 f., 1938.
11. Schechter, F. I.: The Historical Foundations of the Law Relating to Trade-Marks, pp. x and 19–21, New York, 1925.
12. The History of Pharmacy in Pictures, commissioned by Parke, Davis & Company, recreates in painting No. 7 a general impression of the scene as Lemnian earth was being made into one of the very earliest "trademarked" drugs. (This and other paintings in the series created by the artist Robert Thom in collaboration with George Bender may be consulted in Great Moments in Pharmacy, Detroit, 1966 and other printed forms.
13. XI. Congrés international de la pharmacie: Compte rendue, La Haye (The Hague), 1913, pp. 143–153; Chem. & Drugg., Year Book, p. 382, London, 1945.
14. Schechter: *op.cit.*, pp. 139–141 et passim. The various national laws have been revised repeatedly. The first American law had to be re-enacted in 1876 to make it constitutional and was subsequently revised in 1881, 1905, 1920, and 1946. For a readable handbook on the purposes, provisions, and legislative history of the Lanham Act, see Toulmin, H. A., Jr.: The Trade-Mark Act of 1946, Cincinnati, Ohio, 1946. 224 pp. and 1947 Supplement.
15. Wilbert, M. I.: On the problem of proprietary and trade names, Proc. A.Ph.A. *51*:529, 1903.
16. Editorial. On the promotion of drugs, N. Eng. J. Med., *263*:44, 1960.
17. National Pharmaceutical Council, Statements of Generic Equivalency, New York, p. 1–2 (loose-leaf service).
18. Drug Bioequivalence; A Report of the Office of Technology Assessment, Drug Bioequivalence Study Panel, pp. 58 f. et passim, Washington, D. C. [1974], an important and controversial document. Daddario, E. Q.: OTA and the drug bioequivalence study, J.A.Ph.A. ns *14*: 554 f., 1974 and ibid., 403–416. Cf., e.g., PMA Newsletter, p. 2, Jan. 13, 1975.
19. Representative reports bracketing the decade, which stress the limitations of prescription-drug "equivalency" are: Levy, G. and Nelson, E.: Pharmaceutical formulation and therapeutic efficacy, J.A.M.A. *177*: 689, 1961 and, Academy of Pharmaceutical Sciences (A.Ph.A.), Drug product quality, J.A.Ph.A., ns *10*:107–116, 1970. See also for various viewpoints of 1960–61, J. Mondial de Pharmacie *3*:331, 1960; J.A.Ph.A. n.s. *1*:92 ff, 1961; Am. J. Hosp. Pharm. *18*:443, 1961; N. Eng. J. Med. *263*:21, 1960.
20. Prohibiting prescription drug brand names, J.A.Ph.A., ns *14*:492, 1974.
21. U. S. Department of Health, Education and Welfare Office of the Secretary, Task Force on Prescription Drugs, Final Report, Washington, D.C. 1969.
22. A useful summary, if not balanced account, of many relevant questions and references that cannot be given here, is in Silverman, M. and Lee, P. R.: Pills, Profits and Politics, pp. 143-170, Berkeley, 1974. The authors adduced from their information that perhaps a half dozen to a dozen drugs involve proved instances in which two products meeting accepted standards performed significantly different in patients (p. 149). They acknowledge the reality of the problem but do not see trademarking as the long-term solution.

23. Adlung, A., and Urdang, G.: Grundriss der Geschichte der deutschen Pharmazie, p. 200, Berlin, 1935.
24. Urdang, G.: Pharmacy's position under regulated community medicine, J.A.Ph.A. *27*:702, 1938; Urdang, G., and Murphy, J.: Position of Pharmacy in Sickness Insurance, pp. 14-20, Madison, Wis., 1942.
25. Adlung and Urdang: op. cit., pp. 211–218. In 1888 Austria established a health plan similar to that of Germany.
26. Sulzbach, W.: German Experience with Social Insurance, p. 7, New York, 1947.
27. A brief discussion of possible influences is included in Sonnedecker, G.: Government health insurance—in historical perspective, J.A.Ph.A., ns *2*:654, 1962.
28. Farman, C. H., and Hale, V. M.: Social Security Legislation Throughout the World, Social Security Administration, Bureau Report No. 16, Washington, D.C., 1949, 176 pp. Pharmaceutical coverage is not identified separately in Farman's 1954 report: Old-Age, Survivors, and Invalidity Programs Throughout the World, Social Security Administration, Bureau Report No. 19; Follmann, J. F., Jr.: Trends in the future of voluntary health insurance, Proceedings, 1961, Ann. Conf. County Med. Soc. Officers (reprint), p. 6; and Hall, R.: World drug [insurance] programs, J.A.Ph.A., ns *9*: 604–610; 634, 1969.
29. Eckstein, H.: The English Health Service; Its Origins, Structure and Achievements, p. x, Cambridge, Mass., 1958. For a good concise survey with special reference to pharmacy, see The British National Health Service, London (Pharmaceutical Press), 1961, 22 pp.
30. Linstead, H. N.: Pharmacists and machines, J.A.Ph.A. *2*:346, 1962.
31. On the initiative of a pharmacist, Sir William Glyn-Jones, who was a member of Parliament, the enactment of 1911 contained a clause prohibiting "arrangements for the dispensing of medicines being made with persons other than persons, firms, or bodies corporate entitled to carry on the business of a chemist and druggist under the provision of the Pharmacy Act." (Pharm. J. *131*:60, 1933.)
32. Bull. Fed. Internat. Pharm. 7:57, 1926.
33. Hauser, V.: The Impact of Sickness Societies on Retail Pharmacy (mimeographed), p. 4, Internat. Pharm. Fed. London, 1955.
34. Follman, J. F., Jr.: Trends . . ., op, cit., pp. 3 f., and The Cost of Medical Care, p. 153, Geneva, 1959.
35. See Field, M. G.: Doctor and Patient in Soviet Russia, Cambridge, Mass., 1957.
36. House of Delegates 1920, J. A. M. A. *74*:1319, 1920.
37. "Statement of the position of the American Pharmaceutical Association with respect to compulsory national health insurance, J.A.Ph.A. (Pr. Ph. Ed.) *10*:294f., 1949, and "Resolutions . . .," ibid., 471.
38. For the period up to World War II, a particularly good source of information is Anderson, O. W.: The Health Insurance Movement in the United States; A Case Study of the Role of Conflict in the Development and Solution of a Social Problem (unpublished Ph.D. thesis, Univ. of Michigan, Ann Arbor, 1948); see also his Family Medical Costs and Voluntary Health Insurance, a Nationwide Survey, New York, 1956. Also publications of the Health Information Foundation.
39. Health Insurance Institute as cited in Pharmaceutical Payment Programs—an Overview . . . , p. 8, P.M.A., Washington, D.C., 1973.
40. *Ibid.*, 9 f., and Kramer, J. R.: Medical care: as costs soar, support grows for major reform, Science *166*:1128, 1969.
41. De Salvo, R. J. and McEvilla, J. D.: Prescription drug programs available to labor union members, J.A.Ph.A. ns *10*: 509, 1970; Pharmaceutical Payment . . . , *op. cit.*, 17.
42. Street, J. P.: An overview of third party payment programs, Wis. Phar., *15*:137–141, 1972; and on impending prospects: The great national health insurance debate, J.A.Ph.A., ns *14*:558–562, 1974. Note also Braverman, J.: Group practice prepayment plans . . . J.A.Ph.A., ns *11*:563, 1969, and his National compulsory health insurance . . . , J.A.Ph.A., ns *10*:266–275, 1970.
43. On the slow emergence of a concept and understanding of addiction, see Sonnedecker, G.: Emergence of the concept of opiate addiction, J. Mondial Phar., No. 3, 1962, pp. 275–290 and No. 1, 1963, pp. 27–34.
44. Eddy, N. B., et al.: Drug dependence: its significance and characteristics, Bull. Wld. Hlth. Org. *32*:721–733, 1965, and World Health Organization, Technical Report No. 273, 1964.
45. Terry, C. E., and Pellens, M.: The Opium Problem, New York, 1928, is rich in historical

information. See Renborg, B. A.: International Drug Control, Washington, D.C., 1947 (276 pp.) for an excellent historical account and the situation current in the 1940's. Convention [1961] narcotic drugs, J. mondial de pharm. No. 3, 1962, p. 291.

46. Twelve Congresses were held as follows: Braunschweig, 1865; Paris, 1867: Vienna, 1869; St. Petersbourg, 1874; London, 1881; Brussels, 1885; Chicago, 1893; Brussels, 1897; Paris, 1900; Brussels, 1910; The Hague, 1913; Brussels, 1935. After 1935, the International Congress, in its old sense, was supplanted by the "General Assemblies" of the International Pharmaceutical Federation. To clarify this organizational question a special Commission of the Council recommended in 1956 that international meetings sponsored by the Federation be considered "congresses" whether devoted to professional or scientific pharmacy. The general or professional part includes the General Assembly, a body organized to act for the constituent national societies (Ordinary Members); the part programmed by the Scientific Sections has been presented (since 1958) as an International Congress of Pharmaceutical Sciences (annually, the 35th at Dublin in 1975). The scientific congresses have been held, variably, either in conjunction with the General Assemblies and/or separately (on alternate years).

    The General Assemblies convened since the founding of the Federation (biennially when international conditions permit) have been held as follows. They are designated by a numbering separate from the pre-1912 Congresses.

    1. The Hague 1912
    2. Ghent 1913
    3. Brussels 1922
    4. London 1923
    5. Lausanne 1925
    6. The Hague 1927
    7. Paris 1928
    8. Stockholm 1930
    9. Brussels 1935
    10. Copenhagen 1937
    11. Berlin 1939 (not held)
    12. Zurich 1947
    13. Amsterdam 1949
    14. Rome 1951
    15. Paris 1953
    16. London 1955
    17. Brussels 1958
    18. Copenhagen 1960
    19. Vienna 1962
    20. Amsterdam 1964
    21. Madrid 1966
    22. Hamburg 1968
    23. Geneva 1970
    24. Lisbon 1972
    25. Rome 1974

    An excellent critical commentary on the early Congresses is Hoffmann, Fr.: The international pharmaceutical congresses, Am. J. Pharm. *73*:315, 373, and 431, 1901; see also Oldberg, O.: The international pharmaceutical congresses, Western Drugg. *15*:24, 1893, and especially Griffenhagen, G.: Participation of U. S. Pharmacists in International Congresses, Am. J. Hosp. Pharm. *20*:121–131, 1963.

47. The *Bulletin* of the Federation, established in 1912, became the *Journal Mondial de Pharmacie*, 1957–1972. The *Bulletin d' Informations* has been published since 1967. The Federation's *Acta Pharmaceutica Internationalis*, 1948–1952, published or re-published selected scientific articles, but did not offer a sufficiently distinctive service in relation to existing scientific literature to survive.

48. Reinstein, J. A.: The history and objectives of the International Pharmaceutical Students' Federation, J. Am. Pharm. Assoc., Prac. Phar. Ed. *19*:88 f., 1958. For operational details of the pharmacy student exchange program, see Samuels, J. D.: International Pharmaceutical Students' Federation, J.A.Ph.A. ns *2*:355 f., 1962. The A.Ph.A. authorized full membership of its Student Section in 1957; the earlier associate membership of the Association's University of Wisconsin Branch apparently was the first American participation by an organization.

49. Exemplifying American views is the report, International relations, J.A.Ph.A. ns *8*:374–378, 1968; and on some differences of view, see "Statement on A.Ph.A.-F.I.P. Relationships, submitted to the A.Ph.A. Council 26 March 1966, by Don E. Francke (mimeograph, 9 pp.) in Kremers Reference Files, F. B. Power Pharmaceutical Library, University of Wisconsin. For historical data, see especially Wittop Koning, D. A.: Federation Internationale pharmaceutique 1912–1962, J. Mondial de Pharm., No. 2(May–Aug.) 1962, pp. 181–219.

"History of the Federation," *in* Official Handbook, 16th General Assembly, Féd. Internat. Pharm., London, 1955, pp. E17–19. See also Sonnedecker, G.: One world for pharmacy? Modern Pharmacy *41* (No. 3): 12, 1956; also J.A.Ph.A. *12*:1070, 1932, and Bull. Féd. Internat. Pharm. *21:22*, 1931.

50. International meetings, J.A.Ph.A. ns *12*:610, 1972; Bull. d' Inform. (F.I.P.), No. 3, 1974, pp. 10, 16–18, and no. 4, 1974, p.4.
51. Hampshire, C. H.: The International Pharmacopoeia of the World Health Organization, Bull. Féd. Internat. Pharm. *24*:123, 1950–51.
52. Power, Fr. B.: Unification of potent medicaments, Am. J. Pharm. *75*:1, 1903. Second International Conference . . . Final Protocol and Draft of the International Agreement, ms. in Kremers Reference Files, University of Wisconsin.
53. Hamphshire, C. H.: Interim report of the Technical Commission of Pharmacopoeial Experts, League of Nations, Bull. Health Org. *12*:112, 1945–46.
54. Miller, L. C.: An International Pharmacopoeia, Food Drug Cosmetic Law J. *8*:299 f., 1953. The quotation is from the Pharmacopoea Internationalis, Supplement, p. xx, Geneva, 1959. Cook, E. F.: The international pharmacopoeia . . . Bull. Amer. Soc. Hosp. Pharm. *12*:120–124, 1955; see also the series of articles in.: Bull. Féd. Internat. Pharm. *24*:123, 1950–51.; and Rasmussen, H. B.: fifty years' endeavor to create an international pharmacopoeia, Bull. Féd Internat. Pharm. *24*:20, 1950–51. See also P. Blanc (W.H.O.) to G. Sonnedecker (U. Wis.), 13 December 1963 concerning volunteer workers and centers for reference standards: in Kremers Reference Files, Pharmacy Library, U. Wis.
55. For good discussions from different viewpoints, see Miller, L. C.: International nonproprietary names, The Trade-Mark Reporter *43*:133, 1953; and Levy, M. W.: Who authorized it?, The Trade-Mark Reporter, 229.
56. Stainier, C.: Les sphères d'influence des pharmacopées nationales, de la pharmacopée Européenne et de la pharmacopée internationale, J. mondial de pharm., No. 1: 1969, 43; also J.A.Ph.A. ns *15*:705, 1975.
57. These triennial Pan-American Congresses have been held as follows:
    (1) Havana, Cuba, 1948
    (2) Lima, Peru, 1951
    (3) Sao Paulo, Brazil, 1954
    (4) Washington, D.C., 1957
    (5) Santiago, Chile, 1960
    (6) Mexico City, Mexico, 1963
    (7) Buenos Aires, Argentina, 1966
    (8) Caracas, Venezuela, 1969
    (9) Panama City, Panama, 1972
    (10) Punta del Este, Uruguay, 1975
58. Orfila, A.: Manuscript address in the Edward Kremers Reference Files, Univ. of Wisconsin (filed C36 [h] III), p.1.
59. Haddad, A. F.: The first Middle East Pharmaceutical Conference, Lebanese Pharm. J. *4*:221, 1956: See also Winters, J. H. M.: F.I.P. and international pharmacy, supplement to Bull. d'inform. (F.I.P.), No. 2, 1967. On Asian federation, see J. mondial de pharm. No. 2, 1963, 138 f. and J. Philip. Assoc. No. 4, 1963, 126–132.
60. Linstead, H.: Pharmacists and machines, J.A.Ph.A., ns *2*:376, 1962.

## 9. THE NORTH AMERICAN COLONIES

1. See for example, Bartels, K. H.: Drogenhandel und Apothekenrechtliche Beziehungen zwischen Venedig und Nürnberg, Frankfurt/M., 1966.
2. Hein, W-H.: Die Preisverzeichnisse des Grazer Codex 311. 1. Mitteilung: Eine Drogenpreisliste von der Nördlinger Messe im Jahre 1447, Pharm. Zeit. *118*:1148, 1973.
3. Cowen, D. L.: The British North American Colonies as a Source of Drugs, Veröff. d. Intl. Gesell. f. Gesch. d. Pharm. *28*:47, 1966.
4. Morgan, J.: The Birth of the American People, pp. 32, 33, New York, 1930.
5. *Ibid*.: p. 166. "Pennsylvania remained culturally more German than English until the revolutionary era." According to Franklin about one-third of the inhabitants of Pennsylvania, at the time of the revolution, were Germans.
6. Haggis, W. A.: Fundamental errors in the early history of Cinchona, Bull. Hist. Med. *10*:417, 568, 1941.
7. Kremers, E.: Drugs of North American Indians, Pharm. Rev. *23*:130, 1905, Youngken, H. W.: The Drugs of the North American Indians, Am. J. Pharm. *96:*485, 1924, *97:*158, 257, 1925, Corlett, T. W.: The Medicine Man of the American Indian, p. 318, New York, 1935.

8. Roys, R. L.: Ethno-botany of the Maya, Pub. No. 2, Mid. Am. Res. Ser., Tulane University, New Orleans, 1931.
9. Gruz, M. de la: The Badianus Manuscript; an Aztec Herbal of 1552, Introduction, translation and annotations by Emily Walcott Emmart, Baltimore, 1940. See also, Standley, P. C.: The flora of Yucatan, Pub. No. 279, Field Mus. of Nat. Hist., Chicago, 1930. See also Weinland, J. L.: Some U.S.P. drugs used by early Central American Indians, Purdue Pharm., 11, No. 2, pp. 6-8; No. 3, p.3.
10. For an extensive bibliography on the drugs of the North American Indian, see Note 8 on pp. 348–349 of the Third Edition. In addition, in a long appendix on "Contributions to Pharmacology," Vogel, V. J.: American Indian Medicine, pp. 267–414, Norman 1970 lists, in alphabetical order, drugs used by the Indians and provides interesting historical monographs on each. Vogel also provides (pp. 519–539) a valuable index of botanic names.
11. Vogel: *op. cit.*, p. 267.
12. Ettinger, A. A.: James Edmund Ogelthorpe, p. 120, Oxford, 1936; Church, L. F.: Oglethorpe, pp. 95–96, London, 1932; Wilson, R. C.: Pharmacy in the Life of Georgia, pp. 6–15, Atlanta, 1959; Krafka, J., Jr.: An account of the Attempt of the Society of Apothecaries to Establish the Drug Trade in Colonial Georgia. J.A.Ph.A., *28:*616–619, 1939.
13. Richtmann, W. O.: A history of the cultivation of medicinal plants in the U.S., J.A.Ph.A. *9*:816, 1920; Cowen, *op. cit.*, pp. 51, 53.
14. The title of the complete work was Historia Medicinal de las Cosas que se traen de Nuestras Indias Occidentales, que Sirven en Medicina. On Monardes and the various editions, translations and influences of his work, see Guerra, F.: Nicolas Bautista Monardes; Su vida y su obra, Mexico, D.F. 1961, 226 pp.
15. Stuenzer, K.: Die Schrift des Monardes über die Arzneimittel Amerikas, Halle, 1895.
16. Among them was Francisco Hernandez's Quatro libros de la naturaleza y virtudes de la plantas y animales que estan recevidos en el uso de medicina en la Nueva Espana . . . (Mexico, 1615); Guielmo Piso's De medicina Brasilensi libri 4 (Amsterdam, 1648), Wm. Hughes' The American Physician . . . (London, 1672); and Pouppé Desportes' Traité ou Abrégé des Plantes Usuelles des Domingue (Paris, 1770). See also in Cowen, D.: America's Pre-Pharmacopoeial Literature, p. 28, Madison, Wis., 1961.
17. Hartwich, C.: Die Bedeutung der Entdeckung von Amerika für die Drogenkunde. Berlin, 1892.
18. Lib. I, Chaps. 25 to 75: Historia de las Indias, by Las Casas, printed for the first time in 1875–1876 *in* the Coleccion de documentos ineditos para la historia de España.
19. Major, R. H.: Select letters of Christopher Columbus, Hakluyt Society, No. 2, 1847.
20. Cowen, D. L.: Colonial laws pertaining to pharmacy, J.A.Ph.A. *23:*1242, 1934.
21. Birkett, H. S.: The History of Medicine in the Province of Quebec, 1535–1838, New York, 1908.
22. Thwaites, R. G.: Jesuit Relations, p. 155, 1897. Thwaites' index volume includes 9 other references to pharmacist Hébert.
23. Bradley, Th. J.: The first pharmacist in North America, J.A.Ph.A. *25:*628, 1936.
24. Giovanni, Sister M.: The Role of Religious in Pharmacy Under Canada's 'Ancien Regime,' p. 59, Toronto, 1962.; See also Kremers, E.: History of American pharmacy, Am. Drugg., *68*:10, 1920.
25. Liot, A.: Les apothicaires dieppois du 16 au 19 siècle, Chap. 4, Rouen, 1912.
26. Parkman, F.: History of La Salle, Boston, 1892; Sayre, D. E.: Orvietan or Theriac, Amer. Drugg. & Pharm. *44:*71, 1904.
27. Lafitau, J. F.: Mémoire, La plante du Ginseng de Tartaire en Canade, Paris, 1718.
28. Duffy, J., ed.: The Rudolph Matas History of Medicine in Louisiana, pp. 87–89; 117, Baton Rouge, 1958.
29. Morgan: *op. cit.*, p. 119.
30. Ward, Chr.: New Sweden on the Delaware, p. 134, Philadelphia, 1938.
31. Johnson, A.: The Instruction for John Printz, Governor of New Sweden, p. 30, Philadelphia, 1930.
32. New Netherland Register: *1*:89, 1911.
33. Shrady, J.: Med. Reg. of New York *25*:233, 1887, and New Netherland Register *1*:26, 1911.
34. Many of Kierstedt's descendants have been identified in the medical profession. His great-great-grandson, the late general Henry T. Kierstedt, of Harlem, at his well known drugstore on Broadway, dispensed the "Kierstedt ointment," made from a recipe left by Dr. Hans. This Henry T. Kierstedt was

president of the American Pharmaceutical Association (1860–1862), one of two presidents who have held the office for 2 years. Shrady: *op. cit.*, pp. 232, 233: Raubenheimer, H.: Early American pharmacy, Med. Life *33*:57, 1926.

35. Morgan: *op. cit.* p. 38.
36. Cowen: British North American Colonies, p. 49.
37. *Ibid.*, pp. 49–50.
38. *Ibid.*, pp. 50–54.
39. Blanton, W. B.: Medicine in Virginia in the Seventeenth Century, pp. 8,9, Richmond, 1930.
40. *Ibid.:* pp. 30, 31.
41. *Ibid.:* p. 116.
42. Viets, H. R.: Some features of the medicine in Massachusetts during the Colonial period, 1620–1770, Isis *23*:390, 1935.
43. Cowen, D. L.: The Boston Editions of Nicholas Culpeper. J. Hist. Med. & Allied Sciences, *11*: 156–158, 165, 1956.
44. Judd, S.: History of Hadley, pp. 438–444. Springfield, Mass., 1905.
45. Bradley, W. T.: Medical practices of the New England aborigines, J.A.Ph.A. *25*:146, 1936. The kinds of native drugs employed in the first decades of the settlement can be learned particularly from William Wood's *New England's Prospect* and John Josselyn's *New England Rarities.*
46. Reprint with comments, Badger Pharmacist No. 15, 1937; Kremers, E.: American Pharmaceutical Documents, 1643 to 1780, Madison, Wis., 1944.
47. Viets: *op. cit.*, p. 392.
48. Browne, C. A.: Some relations of early chemistry in America to medicine, J. Chem. Ed. *3:*268, No. 3.
49. *Ibid.:* pp. 270, 271, 273.
50. Drug list of King Philip's War: Badger Pharm., No. 25, 1939.
51. Bradley, W. T.: Giles Firmin, Sr., J.A.Ph.A. *26*:250, 1937.
52. Holmes, Oliver Wendell: Works, Medical Essays. vol. 9, pp. 312-369, Boston, 1895. Massachusetts was not unique in this respect. Similar variations in title were to be found in 17th century New Jersey, for example. Cowen, D. L.: Medicine and Health in New Jersey: A History. p. 5, Princeton, 1964.
53. Wilbert, M. I.: The beginnings of pharmacy in America, Am. J. Pharm. *79*:400, 1907.
54. Bull. Mass. Coll. Pharm. 3, No. 4:39, 1914.
55. Griffenhagen, G.: Bartholomew Browne, Pharmaceutical Chemist of Salem, Massachusetts, 1698–1704, Essex Institute [Mass.] Historical Collections, January 1961, pp. 19–30; summarized in Pharmacy in History 7:1, 1962.
56. Viets: *op. cit.*, p. 397.
57. Cowen, D. L: The New Jersey Pharmaceutical Association 1870–1970, p. 117, Trenton, 1970.
58. Waring, J. I.: A History of Medicine in South Carolina 1670–1825, p. 65, Charleston, 1964.
59. Shryock, R. H.: Medicine and Society in America, p. 9, New York, 1960.
60. Norris, G. W.: Early History of Medicine in Philadelphia, p. 603, Philadelphia, 1866.
61. Duncan, L. C.: Medical Men in the American Revolution, p. 187, Carlisle Barracks, Pa., 1931; Eberle, E. G.: Hugh Mercer, J.Am.Pharm.A. *15*:424, 1926; Waterman, J. M.: With Sword and Lancet, Richmond, Va., 1941.
62. Publications of the Colonial Society of Massachusetts, vol. XIV, p. 159, Boston, 1913.
63. Cowen, D. L.: The New Jersey Pharmaceutical Association, p. 115.
64. Schoepf, J. D.: Reise durch einige der mittlern und südlichen Vereinigten Staaten . . . , Erlangen, 1788.
65. Cowen, D. L.; The New Jersey Pharmaceutical Association, p. 118.
66. *Ibid.*
67. Van Doren, C.: Benjamin Franklin, p. 128, New York, 1938; Wilbert, M. I.: Benjamin Franklin, Am.J.Pharm. *78*:219, 1906.
68. [Franklin, B.:] Some Account of the Pennsylvania Hospital, p. 29, Philadelphia, 1754; Van Doren, *op. cit.*, p. 429.
69. Cowen, D. L.: A Store Mixt, Various, Universal, J. Rutgers U. Lib. *25*: *passim,* 1961.
70. E.g., on May 1, 1774 Drs. John Griffith and Moses Scott of New Brunswick, N.J. entered into a joint partnership and "purchased a quantity of Drugs Shop furniture and other necessaries for carrying on the druggists business and Practice of Physick & Surgery." Moses Scott, Physician's ledgers, Rutgers U. Libr.
71. Wilbert, M. I.: Beginnings of American pharmacy, Am. J. Pharm. *79:*400, 1907.
72. Griffenhagen, G.: Drug Supplies in the American Revolution, Smithsonian Bulletin 225, p. 113, Washington, 1961.
73. *Ibid.*, p. 117.

74. Pharm. Era, *33*:200, 1920.
75. Troth, S. A.: A retrospect of pharmacy, Am. J. Pharm. *77*:426, 1905.
76. Hoch, J. H.: The History of Pharmacy in South Carolina, p. 72, Charleston, 1951.
77. Hoch, J. H.: The History of Pharmacy in South Carolina, p. 72, Charleston, S.C., 1951.
78. Smith, D. B.: Christopher Marshall, J. Phil. Coll. Pharm. *2*:255, 1830; Ellis, E. T.: The story of a very old Philadelphia drugstore, Am. J. Pharm. *75*:57, 1903; England, J. W.: First Century of the Philadelphia College of Pharmacy, p. 28, Philadelphia, 1922.
79. Gill, H. B., Jr.: The Apothecary in Eighteenth-Century Williamsburg, p. 10, Williamsburg, 1970.
80. The quotation is taken from David L. Cowen's article, "Colonial laws pertaining to pharmacy," J.A.Ph.A. *23*:1236,1934. The Virginia Act of 1736 was first published as chapter 10 of the acts of 1736. (At a General Assembly . . . continued to the fifth day of August–1736, p. 26, Williamsburg, 1736.) Cowen says furthermore: "Various authorities have erroneously dated this act as 1636. See Wickes, 'History of Medicine in New Jersey' (Newark, 1879), page 54; F. H. Garrison, An Introduction to the History of Medicine (Philadelphia, 1914), pages 233, 682; *Ibid.*, 1929 ed., pages 304, 824; and La Wall (4000 Years of Pharmacy), pages 331, 571 . . . . Wickes cites as his authority the 'Half Yearly Compendium of Medical Science, Jan. 1878 (page 66). This, however, gives the date correctly as 1736." The mistake of Wickes, obviously a mere slip of writing or printing, in this way became perpetuated.

    According to Cowen, the reference to a New Jersey act of 1664 as the "earliest law regulating apothecaries in the new world" (LaWall, C.: 4000 years of Pharmacy, p. 572, Philadelphia, 1927) is baseless. The first assembly ever convened in New Jersey met May 26 to 30, 1668.
81. Cowen, D. L.: Colonial laws pertaining to pharmacy, J.A.Ph.A. *23*:1241, 1934.
82. This early history of the hospital by Franklin once again has become readily available through a reprint edition, with an introduction by I. Bernard Cohen, Baltimore, 1954.
83. Wilbert, M. I.: John Morgan, Am. J. Pharm. *76*:5, 1904.
84. *Ibid.*, p. 6.
85. *Ibid.*: p. 9; see also Kredel, F. E., and Hoch, J. H.: Early relations of pharmacy and medicine in the United States, J.A.Ph.A. *28*:704, 1939, Blanton; W. B.: Medicine in Virginia in the Eighteenth Century, pp. 12, 32, Richmond, 1931.
86. Bell, W. J.: John Morgan, Continental Doctor, p. 241, Philadelphia, 1965.
87. See Austin, R. B.: Early American Medical Imprints: A guide to works printed in the United States 1668–1920, Washington 25, D.C., 1961, for bibliographic information on early American pharmaceutical literature and on libraries where copies may be found. See also, Cowen, D. L.: *America's Pre-Pharmacopoeial Literature*, Madison, 1961.
88. Bell, W. J., Jr.: *op. cit.*, p. 106 ff.

## 10. THE REVOLUTIONARY WAR

1. Duncan L. G.: Medical Men in the American Revolution, p. 18, Carlisle Barracks, Pa., 1931.
2. Robert Bishopp, George Brown, Michael Croker, Arthur Edwards, Richard Huddleston, John Johnston, Benjamin Mace, Daniel Maudeville, William Payne, Richard Proctor, John Watson, Gregory West, and John Rush. The last was a surgeon who was "appointed apothecary to the general hospital." Shrady, J.: Med.Reg. New York, *19*:194, 1881.
3. The names of Becker, Keller, Rudolph and Schirmer have come down. *Ibid.*
4. Balland, A.: Les pharmaciens militaires français, Paris, 1913, pp. 9, 89.
5. Bouvet, Maurice: Histoire de la pharmacie de France, Paris, 1937, p. 331. Other French compatriots who, at one time or other, served as pharmacists in Rochambeau's army were Jean Baunach, Berry, Dessenis, Gourdon, Claude-Charles Humbert, Benjamin Magenc, Maheux and Vancalbeck (or Vancattelech), as given by Bouvet in his unique work: Le service de santé français pendant la Guerre d'Indepéndance des Etats-Unis (1777–1782), Paris, 1934, p. 38.
6. Duncan, L. C.: *op. cit.*, p. 22.
7. ———: *op. cit.*, p. 60.
8. The medical directors who succeeded each other (see Gibson, James E.: Dr. Bodo Otto, and the Medical Background of the American Revolution, Springfield, Ill., p. 185) were Benjamin Church, John Morgan, William Shippen, and John Cochran (Duncan, L. C.: *op.*

*cit.*, pp. 61, 78, 79, and 276; see also Wilbert, M. I.: John Morgan, Am. J. Pharm. *76*:1, 1904).

9. Gibson, J. E.: *op. cit.*, p. 106.
10. Jour.Cont.Cong.: 7:232, 1777. The statement that Congress provided for two "Apothecaries" is not correct; a recommendation to that effect *(Ibid.*, p. 199) was not approved.
11. *Ibid.*, *22*:410, 1782.
12. A list of known or purported apothecaries in the American forces in the Revolution gleaned from a variety of sources follows. Clearly the records and the literature are incomplete and confused:

Andrew Caldwell:
—"Apothecary's Mate," at Philadelphia Medical Store, Nov. 1783
—"Apothecary's mate," Southern Dept., ca. 1782–1784.

John Carn (Carne, Caine, Carns, Crane) of South Carolina:
—"Deputy Apothecary," appointed by Congress, Sept. 20, 1781;
—"Apothecary," 1780–1781.
—"Deputy Apothecary," Hosp. Dept. South. Army, ca. 1782–1784.

Patrick Carne(s) of South Carolina:
—"Surgeon's Mate," 1777;
—"Deputy Apothecary, Southern Department, 29 Feb. [sic]–1781 to end of war,"perhaps in confusion with John Carne.

William Cobb of Virginia:
—"Apothecary."

Andrew Craigie of Massachusetts:
—"Commissary of Stores," later "Apothecary" to Massachusetts troops, 1775;
—"Apothecary" in Continental Army, 1776;
—"Apothecary General" "of the Middle Department," 1778, of the "Continental Army," 1777–1780;
—(Chief) "Apothecary of the Army," appointed by Congress October 7, 1780, to Nov., 1783.

Henry Crow:
—"Assistant Apothecary," Middle Department, June, 1778.

John B. Cutting of Massachusetts (on whose Muster he appears but he is usually listed as from New York):
—"Apothecary's mate" and "assistant apothecary" at hospitals in Cambridge, Roxbury, New York and Newark, 1776;
—"Apothecary," Middle Department, 1777;
—"Apothecary," Eastern Department, July 10, 1777–1779;
—Oaths of allegiance as "Apothecary General of the Middle Department," 29 and 30 May, 1778;
—"Apothecary," Middle Department, 1779–10 June 1780;
—"Apothecary General," at Valley Forge and Yellow Springs, 1777, 1778;
—"Apothecary General to the Army," Paramus, N.J., 1780;
—"Apothecary" to end of war.

Anthony T. Dixon:
—"Apothecary" at the Alexandria, Va. hospital, July 1, 1776 on.

John Douglass:
—"Apothecary's mate," Southern Dept., 1783–1784.

Dr. Henry C. Flagg:
—"Deputy Apothecary," Southern Department, 1781;
—"Apothecary," and "Apothecary General," Southern Department, 1782 to close of war.
—"Deputy Apothecary," Southern Dept., 1783–1784

———Fraley:
—"Assistant Apothecary," at Valley Forge, 1777.

A. Giles:
—"Apothecary" at Cambridge and New York Hospitals, July, Aug., 1776.

Joseph Hay:
—"Mate," "Surgeon," and "Apothecary" at Williamsburg, Va. hospital.

George Ickman:
—"Assistant Apothecary" at Valley Forge, 1777.

William Johonot (Johnonott) of France:
- —"Assistant Apothecary," appointed by Congress, October 7, 1780;
- —"Apothecary" at Fishkill, N.Y., 1781.

Evan Lewis of South Carolina (Georgia?):
- —"Surgeon's Mate," Continental Hospital, Charleston;
- —"Apothecary's Mate," Continental Hospital, Charleston, 1780;
- —"Deputy Apothecary," 1780.

William McKenzie:
- —"Apothecary's mate," Southern Dept., ca. 1782–1784.

Joseph Prescott:
- —"Hospital Mate," "Surgeon's Mate," "Surgeon";
- —"Apothecary of Southern Department," at Hillsborough, N.C. Hospital, 1780.

Thomas Prudden:
- —"Apothecary's mate," Southern Dept., ca. 1782–1784.

Israel Root, of Connecticut:
- —"Apothecary General, Northern Department," 1779–1783. (Perhaps the same man as the following.)

Josiah Root, of Connecticut:
- —"Surgeon's mate, Apr. 1, 1777–July 31, 1780;
- —Warrant as Assistant *to* Apothecary General in Northern Dept., 1 Aug. 1777;
- —"Assistant Apothecary General";
- —"Apothecary General."

Daniel Smith of South Carolina:
- —"Deputy Medical Purveyor":
- —"Apothecary."

Nathaniel Smith:
- —"Apothecary's mate," Southern Dept., ca. 1782–1784.

Francis Wainwright:
- —"Apothecary's mate," South. Dept., ca. 1782–1784;
- —"Surgeon's mate," Southern Dept., 1782–1783.
- —"Apothecary's mate" in charge of medical stores at New Windsor, Nov., 1783.

John Willson:
- —"Apothecary's mate," South. Dept., ca. 1782–1784.

13. Duncan, L. C.: *op. cit.*, p. 329; Jour. Cont. Cong.: *18*:910, 1780.
14. Jour. Cont. Cong.: *21*:981, 1781.
15. Duncan, L. C.: *op. cit.*, pp. 158–159. The man chosen for the post was Dr. William Smith of Pennsylvania.
16. ———: *op. cit.*, p. 41.
17. Kebler, L. F.: Andrew Craigie, J. Am. Pharm. A. *17*:66, 1928. Later, when Morgan succeeded Church as medical director, it seems probable that Craigie was transferred for a short period, rather than being forced "out of office" temporarily, as Kebler inferred.
18. Duncan, L. C.: *op. cit.*, pp. 330–331.
19. Griffenhagen, George: Drug Supplies in the American Revolution, Paper 16 in Contributions from the Museum of History and Technology, United States National Museum, Bulletin 225, Washington 25, D.C., 1961, and also separately; see pp. 130–133.
20. For example, on April 22, 1776, Director-General Morgan advised Washington that he had collected "a noble store of medicines." Bell, W. J.: John Morgan, Continental Doctor, p. 188, Philadelphia, 1965. See also, Bell, W. J.: *op. cit.*, p. 204; Duncan, L. C.: *op. cit.*, p. 125; Griffenhagen, G. B.: *op. cit.*, pp. 115–116.
21. For example, see the efforts of Dr. Potts. Griffenhagen, G. B.: *op. cit.*, pp. 126, 128; Gibson, J. E.: *op. cit.*, p. 154.
22. Griffenhagen, G. B.: *op. cit.*, p. 112.
23. *Ibid.*, p. 123.
24. *Ibid.*, p. 122.
25. *Ibid.*, p. 122.
26. Gibson, J. E.: *op. cit.*, p. 155.
27. Griffenhagen, G. B.: *op. cit.*, pp. 127–128.
28. Gibson, J. E.; *op. cit.*, p. 155.
29. *Ibid.*, p. 153.
30. Griffenhagen, G. B.: *op. cit.*, p. 127.
31. This quotation and most of the information given on drug supply in the Revolution is taken from Griffenhagen, *ibid.*, pp. 129 f., *et passim.* On the pharmaceutical content of the "standardized field boxes," see also Gibson, J. F.: *op. cit.*, p.167; and on a drug inventory

of the general hospital (1775) by Craigie, see Kebler, L. F.: *op. cit.*, p. 73.

32. Griffenhagen, G. B. Medicine Chest. The Antiques Dealer for October, 1974, p. 34; Bell, W. J.; *op. cit.*, p. 189; Gibson, J. E.: *op. cit.*, p. 166.
33. Gibson, J. E.: *op. cit.*, p. 166.
34. *Ibid.*, pp. 166, 177.
35. *Ibid.*, p. 166.
36. Torres-Reyes, R.: Morristown National Historical Park 1779–80 Encampment A Study of Medical Services, p. vi, Washington, 1971.
37. Orderly Book of the New Jersey Brigade, p. 56, Hackensack, N.J., 1922.
38. Jour. Cont. Cong.: *22*:409, 1782.
39. Gibson, J. E.: *op. cit.*, p. 158; Griffenhagen, G. B.: Drug Supplies, p. 126.
40. Packard, F. R.: The History of Medicine in the United States, p. 278, Philadelphia, 1901.
41. Torres-Reyes, R.: *op. cit.*, p. 84.
42. Blanton, W.: Medicine in Virginia in the Eighteenth Century, p. 281, Richmond, 1931,
43. Waring, J. I.: A History of Medicine in South Carolina 1670–1825, p. 341, Charleston, 1864.
44. *Ibid.*, p. 98.
45. Proc. N.J. Hist. Soc., *3*:98, 1848–49.
46. Gahn, B. W., and Kebler, L. F.: Dr. William Brown, J. Am. Pharm. A. *16*:1090, 1927.
47. Berman, Alex: The Beth Holim Formulary of London (1749). Am. J. Hosp. Pharm. *17*:24, 1960.
48. Badger Pharmacist, Nos. 22 to 25, 1938; Kremers, E.: American Pharmaceutical Documents, 1643–1780, Madison, Wis., 1944; Adlung, A., and Urdang, G.: Grundriss der Geschichte der deutschen Pharmazie, Berlin, 1935, pp. 4 and 317; Urdang, G.: Zur Geschichte der Metalle in den amtlichen deutschen Arzneibüchern, Mittenwald, 1933, p. 40.
49. Translation by Sister Mary Francis Xavier, as published by Rho Chi (Eta) in the Badger Pharmacist, Nos. 22 to 25, 1938 (Lititz Pharmacopoeia) and Nos. 27 to 30, 1940 (Coste's compendium); re-published as part of Kremers, Edward (ed.): American Pharmaceutical Documents, 1643–1780, Madison, Wis., 1944. In addition, a facsimile of the original Latin text of the Lititz Pharmacopoeia was published as a separate pamphlet by the American Pharmaceutical Association, Washington, D.C. (no date), 32 pp. (reprinted from England, Joseph: The First Century of the Philadelphia College of Pharmacy, Philadelphia, 1922).
50. Cowen, D. L.: America's Pre-Pharmacopoeial Literature, p. 20, Madison, 1961. For a facsimile, translation and commentary of Coste's work, see The Badger Pharmacist, Nos. 27 to 30, 1940.

## 11. YOUNG REPUBLIC AND PIONEER EXPANSION

1. Wilbert, M. I.: Some early botanical and herb gardens, Am. J. Pharm. *80*:412, 1908; and sections on natural history and botany in Struik, Dirk J.: Yankee Science in the Making, Boston, 1948, and Hindle, Brooke: The Pursuit of Science in Revolutionary America 1735–1789, Chapel Hill, 1956.
2. Maisch, J. M.: G. H. E. Muehlenberg als Botaniker, Pharm. Rund. *4*:123, 1886.
3. *Ibid.*: p. 124.
4. Bull. Lloyd Libr., Repro. Ser. No. 1.
5. *Ibid.*: Repro. Ser. No. 4.
6. Maisch, J. M.: *op. cit.*, p. 123.
7. Wilbert, M. I.: *op. cit.*, p. 424.
8. Flexner, J. T.: The Traitor and the Spy, p. 7, New York, 1953.
9. Wilbert, M. I.: *op. cit.*, pp. 425–426.
10. Bull. Lloyd Libr., Repro. Ser. No. 7, p. 15; details about Thomson remedies, p. 75.
11. Berman, A.: The Impact of the Nineteenth Century Botanico-Medical Movement on American Pharmacy and Medicine (unpublished Ph.D. dissertation, University of Wisconsin), p. 319, Madison, 1954.
12. Cowen, D. L.: America's First Pharmacy Laws, J.A.Ph.A (Pract. Pharm. Ed.) *3*:168, 1942.
13. Berman, Alex: The Impact of the Nineteenth Century Botanico-Medical Movement on American Pharmacy and Medicine (unpublished Ph.D. dissertation), University of Wisconsin, Madison, 1954, *passim*. See also Berman's excellent published papers, such as Bull. Hist. Med. *25*:405–428 and 519–538, 1951 (on original Thomsonians); J. Hist. Med. *11*:133–155, 1956 (on neo-Thomsonians); and Bull. Hist. Med. *30*:1–25, 1956 (on their scientific aspirations).
14. Wilder, A.: History of Medicine, p. 655, New Sharon, Maine, 1901.

15. Bull. Lloyd Libr., Repro. Ser. No. 7, p. 75.
16. Wilder, A.: *op. cit.*, p. 438.
17. *Ibid.*, p. 429.
18. *Ibid.*, p. 431.
19. *Ibid.*, p. 430; Berman, A.: C. S. Rafinesque (1783–1840): a Challenge to the Historian of Pharmacy, Am. J. Pharm. Educ., *16*:411–415, 1952.
20. Berman, A.: Impact of Nineteenth Century Botanico-Medical Movement, p. 321.
21. Wilder, A.: *op. cit.*, pp. 659–660.
22. Kaufman, M.: Homeopathy in America, p. 28, Baltimore, 1971; Kett, J. F.: The Formation of the American Medical Profession, p. 136, New Haven, 1968.
23. Kett, J. F.: *op. cit.*, pp. 136–138.
24. Kaufman, M.: *op. cit.*, p. 29.
25. *Ibid.*, pp. 29, 166.
26. *Ibid.*, pp. 166, 173.
27. The pharmacists were: "Drs." Lewis Sherman, J. Wilkinson Clapp, Henry M. Smith, James F. Gross, William Boeridke, and A. F. Worthington. The Homeopathic Pharmacopoeia of the United States, Seventh Edition, p. 22, Philadelphia, 1964.
28. *Ibid.*, p. 24.
29. See Cowen, D. L.: Liberty, Laissez-Faire and Licensure in Nineteenth Century Britain, Bull. Hist. Med. *63*:30–40, 1969.
30. Shryock, R. H.: Medical Licensing in America, 1650–1965, pp. 28–29, Baltimore, 1967.
31. Shafer, H. B.: *op. cit.*, p. 211; Shryock, R. H.: *op. cit.*, pp. 23, 30.
32. Shafer, H. B.: *op. cit.*, p. 214; Shryock, R. H.: *op. cit.*, p. 31.
33. Brewer, W. A.: Reminiscences of an old pharmacist, Pharm. Rec. *4*:326, 1884. Young, James Harvey: The Toadstool Millionaires: A Social History of Patent Medicines in America before Federal Regulation, Princeton, 1961, appears to be the best book of its scope.
34. Shrady, John: Med. Reg. N.Y. *22*:245, 1884.
35. Shrady, John: Med. Reg. N.Y. *24*:264, 1886. A good insight into the kind and the amount of drugs usually imported by American druggists may be found in two invoices (1785) concerning shipments of drugs from London to druggists in Philadelphia. Reproductions of these invoices with comments are available (Kremers, E.: Two invoices of 1785, J. Am. Pharm. A. *20*:682, 1931). They supplement the Colonial lists of drugs previously mentioned. Together, they make possible a comparative study of the drugs used in the North American settlements.
36. Sadtler, S. P.: Influence of pharmacists on the development and advance of modern chemistry, Am J. Pharm. *93*:197, 1921.
37. Ellis, E. T.: The story of a very old Philadelphia drugstore, Am. J. Pharm. *75*:57, 1903; W. A. Brewer, Sr., *op. cit.*, pp. 210, 232, 255, 282, 304, 326, 348, 410, 424, 442, 460, 475, 494.
38. LaWall, C. H.: The founding of the Philadelphia College of Pharmacy and Science, Am. J. Pharm. *93*:172, 1921; Arny, H. V.: Pharmacy 100 years ago, Am. J. Pharm. *93*:188, 1921.
39. Cowen, D. L.: Louisiana, Pioneer in the regulation of pharmacy, Louisiana Hist. Quart. *26*:5, 1943.
40. *Ibid.*: pp. 7–11.
41. Hoch, J. H.: The first American board of pharmacy, Am. J. Pharm. *104*:750, 1932.
42. Ellis, E. T.: *op. cit.*, p. 59.
43. Shrady, John: Med. Reg. N.Y. *17*:178, 1879. On New York City, see Kellocks' New York Directory, 1786.
44. England, J. W.: The First Century of the Philadelphia College of Pharmacy, Philadelphia, 1922, p. 55.
45. Arny, H. V.: *op. cit.*, p. 184.
46. Shrady, John: Med. Reg. N.Y. *25*:243, 245, 1887; and Kredel, F. E., and Hoch, J. H.: Early relation of pharmacy and medicine in the United States, J. Am. Pharm. A. *28*:796, 1939.
47. Sharpless, Isaac: Two Centuries of Pennsylvania History, Philadelphia, 1900, p. 239.
48. Lindley-Hawes-Schneider-Quaife: The Ordinance of 1787 and the Old Northwest Territory, Marietta, Ohio, 1937, p. 31. In the resolutions of October 6, 1780, concerning reorganization of the medical department of the army it is stated that the several officers of the medical staff also "shall at the end of the war be entitled to a certain provision of land, in the proportion following: the Apothecary the same as a Lieutenant-Colonel. Assistant Apothecary the same as Major." (Kebler, L. F.: Andrew Craigie, J. Am. Pharm. A. *17*:172, 1928.)
49. Lindley-Hawes-Schneider-Quaife: *op. cit.*, p. 30.
50. Sigerist, H. E.: American Medicine, New York, 1934, p. 58.

51. Cf.: An American physician-apothecary of 1793, Pharm. Ern *48*:298, 1915.
52. Sealsfield, George: Lebensbilder aus der westlichen Hemisphaere; more specifically in the chapter: Ein Nachtstück am untern Mississippi; and Thwaites, R. G.: Early Western Travels, vol. 4; Pharm. Rev. *23*:15, 1905.
53. Kremers, E.: The history of American pharmacy, Am. Drugg. *68*(May), 1920; Badger Pharmacist No. 5, 1930.
54. Lindley-Hawes-Schneider-Quaife: *op. cit.*, p. 82.
55. *Ibid.*: p. 65.


## 12. THE GROWTH OF ASSOCIATIONS


1. Davenport, B. F.: History of the Massachusetts College of Pharmacy, p. 7, Cat., Mass. Coll. Pharm. 1882–83.
2. England, J. W.: The First Century of the Philadelphia College of Pharmacy, p. 46, Philadelphia, 1922.
3. *Ibid.*: p. 54.
4. *Ibid.*: p. 356.
5. LaWall, C. H.: The founding of the Philadelphia College of Pharmacy and Science, Am. J. Pharm. *93*:175, 1921.
6. *Ibid.*: p. 63.
7. Kremers, Edward: The teaching of pharmacy during the past 50 years, Drugg. Circ. *51*:61, 1907.
8. England, J. W.: *op. cit.*, p. 352.
9. Am. J. Pharm. *45*:513, 1873; see also England, *op. cit.*, p. 352.
10. *Ibid.*: p. 373; W. Procter, Jr., Necrology, Am. J. Pharm. *18*:315, 1846.
11. England, J. W.: *op. cit.*, p. 57.
12. *Ibid.*: p. 72.
13. *Ibid.*: p. 70.
14. *Ibid.*: p. 71.
15. Marshall, E. C.: Early History of the Massachusetts College of Pharmacy, Quart. Bull. Mass. Coll. Pharm. *3*:9, 1911.
16. Davenport, B. F.: *op. cit.*, p. 8.
17. Marshall, E. C.: *op. cit.*, p. 10.
18. *Ibid.*: p. 15.
19. Robbins, D. C.: Address, Alumni Association Representative, New York College of Pharmacy, 1872.
20. A centennial history was published by Wimmer, C. P.: The College of Pharmacy of the City of New York, New York, 1929, supplemented by Ballard, C. W.: A History of the College of Pharmacy, Columbia University, New York, 1954.
21. Proc. A.Ph.A. *7*:87, 1858.
22. The Graduate, p. 18, Cincinnati College of Pharmacy, 1925.
23. *Ibid.*: p. 381; Am. J. Pharm. *26*:380, 1854.
24. Proc. A.Ph.A. *7*:86, 1858; Am. J. Pharm. *37*:157, 1865.
25. Meyer Brothers' Drugg. *39*:48, 1918; Am. J. Pharm. *37*:158, 1865.
26. Day, W. R.: The School of Pharmacy, Illinois Alumni Record, 1921.
27. Among these were the Richmond Pharmaceutical Society, founded in 1852 (Am. J. Pharm. *24*:385, 1852), which later on adopted the name Richmond College of Pharmacy (Proc. A.Ph.A. *8*:104, 1859) and was revived in 1873 as the Richmond Pharmaceutical Association (Am. J. Pharm. *45*:575, 1873), "a social scientific union in Boston" (Proc. A.Ph.A. *6*:74, 1857) which was reorganized as the Boston Druggist's Association in 1875 (Drugg. Circ. *51*:171, 1907); the Pharmaceutical Association of Washington City (Proc. A.Ph.A. *6*:6, 1857); and the San Francisco Pharmaceutical Association, which was founded in 1858 (Proc. A.Ph.A. *7*:88, 1858) and died out in 1860 (Proc. A.Ph.A. *9*:67, 1860). Such city organizations were founded, disappeared and revived again and again all over the country. In large cities pharmaceutical associations existed at that time and continue to exist, which were organized because of very different motives. In New York City, a multiplicity of such associations strives for cooperation in an organization founded in 1910 under the name of New York Pharmaceutical Conference and reorganized, in 1935, as the New York Pharmaceutical Council. There are no fewer that 14 local pharmaceutical groups affiliated with the Council, among them the New York German Apothecaries' Society and the New York Italian Pharmaceutical Association J.A.Ph.A. *26*:369, 1937). The New York organization of Chinese druggists does not consist of licensed pharmacists.
28. Adlung, A., and Urdang G.: Grundriss der Geschichte der deutschen Pharmazie, p. 417, Berlin, 1935. In the small German principality of Baden, for example, 30 physicians and 20 pharmacists left their native country after the defeat of the uprising.
29. Eberle, E. G.: Old druggists in Texas, Drugg.

Circ. *51*:187, 1907; see also Mayo, C. A.: The Lloyd Library and its makers, Bull. Lloyd Library, No. 28, p. 10, 1928.

30 Am. J. Pharm. *28*:90, 1856. See Article XI, par. 2 of the Society's by-laws of October 1, 1851. In 1852 the *Leseverein* changed its name to *Deutscher Pharmazeutischer Verein* and, in 1875, to *Deutscher Apotheker-Verein von New York.*

31. Schleussner, C. F., and Lehman, R. S.: History of the German Apothecaries Society, p. 24, New York Deutscher Apotheker Verein, New York, 1926. A quite different type of local association originally influenced by the German element is called Veteran Druggists' Association. The first such association was organized in 1898, and after World War I the idea spread to many of the larger American cities, largely as social clubs for aging pharmacists, then in more recent decades declined.

32. Proc. A.Ph.A. *53*:74, 1905; *54*:21, 93, 1906.

33. On the development of professional fraternities in American Pharmacy see, e.g., Brown, L. N.: A brief history of Phi Delta Chi fraternity, J.A.Ph.A. *11*:351–352, 1922; Knox, J. W. T.: Historical sketch of Phi Chi fraternity, Proc. A.Ph.A. *52*:439, 1904; Bliss, A.: A brief history of the Kappa Psi fraternity, J.A.Ph.A. *11*:352, 1922; Bowers, R. A., and Cowen, D. L.: Rho Chi Society; Development of the Honor Society of American Pharmacy, ed. 2, Indianapolis, 1961; Boonshoft, Jerome, and Kirschner, Robert: 40 Years of AZO; A Complete and Factual History of the Events and Activities of Alpha Zeta Omega Pharmaceutical Fraternity, n.p., 1960; Bonow, E. R.: The Pearl of Kappa Epsilon [Madison, Wis.], 1951; Bonow, E. R.: The history of professional pharmaceutical fraternities for women, Am. J. Pharm. Ed. *18*:410–413, 1954.

34. Am. J. Pharm. *40*:88, 1868

35. Am. J. Pharm. *50*:460, 1878; Proc. A.Ph.A. *28*:586, 1880. Proc. A.Ph.A. *29*:536, 1881. Am. J. Pharm. *26*:475, 1890; Proc. A.Ph.A. *40*:1107, 1892.

36. Am. J. Pharm. *52*:382, 1880.

37. Proc. A.Ph.A. *32*:26, 1884.

38. Drugg. Circ. *51*:116, 1907; Proc. A.Ph.A. *50*:40, 1902.

39. Cowen, D. L.: The New Jersey Pharmaceutical Association, New Jersey J. Pharm. *18*:(No. 12) 16, 17, 1945.

40. Am. J. Pharm. *43*:280, 1871.

41. *Ibid.*: p. 329. Another type of medical influence may be seen in the reorganization of the West Virginia association (1881). Among the pharmacists thus active were "a number of physicians who maintained stores in various localities." (Proc. West Virginia State Pharm. Assoc., p. 34, 1931.)

42. The list in Drugg. Circ. *51*:115, 1907, has been corrected and completed from various sources; e.g., see West. Drugg., Extra, *15*:39, 1893; H. M. Whelpley: Pharm. Era *16*:887, 1896; C. W. Holmes: Am. Drugg. & Pharm. Rec. *36*:194, 1900; West. Drugg. *24*:209, 1902.

43. For example, in Michigan (1883), Mississippi (1891), where pharmacy laws were enacted in 1885 and 1892, and in West Virginia (1881) and Maine (1890), where pharmacy laws were amended in 1882 and 1891. Proc. A.Ph.A. *15*:18, 1867. Am. J. Pharm. *45*:329, 422, 1873. Proc. A.Ph.A. *46*:1128, 1898.

44. Elliott, E. C. (ed.): The General Report of the Pharmaceutical Survey, p. 56, Washington, D.C., 1950.

45. Drugg. Circ. *51*:100, 1907.

46. Shafer, H. B.: The American Medical Profession, 1783–1850, p. 230, New York, 1936. As to the medical influence on legislation concerning the adulteration of drugs, see Nitardy, F. W.: Notes on early drug legislation, J.A.Ph.A. *23*:1122, 1934. The quotation is from Drugg. Circ. *51*:100, 1907.

47. Am. J. Pharm. *23*:290, 1851.

48. *Ibid.*: *24*:85, 1852.

49. *Ibid.*: *24*:86, 1852. Ibid., *24*:87, 1852; as quoted by Urdang, G.: The founding . . ., in: Tribute in Bronze to the Founding . . .p. 8, Philadelphia, 1964.

50. For further information about the prominent part played by William Procter, Jr., see Urdang, G.: College of pharmacy associations, Am. J. Pharm. Ed. *17*:334, 1944.

51. Am. J. Pharm. *25*:13, 1853.

52. England, J. W.: *op. cit.*, p. 127.

53. Am. J. Pharm. *26*:290, 1854.

54. Hoffman, F.: A retrospect of the development of American pharmacy and the American Pharmaceutical Association, Proc. A.Ph.A. *50*:122, 1902. LaWall, C. H.: A history of the pharmaceutical codes of ethics, J.A.Ph.A *10*:895–961, 1921. J.A.Ph.A. *11*:728, 1922. The Code has since undergone two major revisions, in 1952 and 1969, and a Judicial Council

for interpreting the principles in terms of practice and for encouraging compliance was authorized by by-law in 1969.

55. Cf. Constitution and By-laws of the American Pharmaceutical Association, Washington, D.C.: [1961], p. 2 (current version available from Association on request). The interpretation of the objectives was discussed by the chairman of the House of Delegates in 1958, Lansdowne, J. W.: Seven objectives, J.A.Ph.A. (Pract. Ed.) *19*:728, 1958.
56. J.A.Ph.A. *1*:928–929, 1079–1084, 1912.
57. APhA Resolutions . . ., J.A.Ph.A. ns *4*:428, 1964; and House of Delegates, ibid., ns *5*:272, 1965.
58. The Proceedings of the American Pharmaceutical Association and, since 1912, the Journals are the most satisfactory sources of the history of the Association. Short surveys are published in anniversary numbers of several pharmaceutical journals, e.g., C. L. Diehl, Pharm. Era *16*:878, 1896; Drugg. Circ. *51*:100, 1907; F. Hoffmann, Retrospect, Proc. A.Ph.A. *50*:100, 1902; J. H. Beal, Address, J.A.Ph.A. *16*:799, 1927.
59. On Remington and the founding of the Sections see Proc. A.Ph.A. *35*:472 f. and 485, 1887. The best single source on the history of the Sections is: The Sections of the American Pharmaceutical Association—A Symposium, Madison, Wis., 1953 (also in Am. J. Pharm. Ed., vol. 17, No. 3, 1953). On the evolving Academy structure, see the annual proceedings issue of the J.A.Ph.A.; on the change from military to federal section, see J.A.Ph.A. ns *13*:479 f., 1973.
60. Drugg. Circ. *51*:73, 1907; Maisch, John M.: Die Conference der Fachschulen der "Colleges of Pharmacy," Pharm. Rundschau *1*:182, 1883; and Sonnedecker, Glenn: The conference of schools of pharmacy—a period of frustration, Am. J. Pharm. Ed. *18*:389–401, 1954.
61. Kraus, E. H.: American Association of Colleges of Pharmacy, J.A.Ph.A. *14*:981, 1925; and Sonnedecker, Glenn: The section on education and legislation, Am. J. Pharm. Ed. *17*:371–375, 1953.
62. *Notes and Journal* of the N.A.R.D., Am. J. Pharm. Ed. *13*:358–375, 1949; The National Association of Retail Druggists, Drugg. Circ. *51*:104, 1907.
63. Boards of pharmacy, Drugg. Circ. *51*:137, 1907; see especially, National Association of Boards of Pharmacy 1904–1954, Madison, Wis., 1955 (also in Proc. N.A.B.P., 1954).
64. J.A.Ph.A. *16*:842, 1927.
65. J.A.Ph.A. *16*:842, 1927; Swain, R. L.: The principles of law enforcement, J.A.Ph.A. *21*:1319, 1932; Dretzka, S. H.: Proc. Natl. Assoc. Bds. Pharm. 1944, pp. 170 f., and 1949, pp. 94 and 110–113.
66. Stieb, E. W. American College Apothecaries; The First Quarter Century 1940–1965, n.p., 1970, 98 pp. The "conference" was preceded by the Association for the Advancement of Professional Pharmacy in New York in 1939; J.A.Ph.A. (Pract. Ed.) *28*:938, 1939 & *2*:334, 1941.
67. Stieb, E. W.: American Institute of the History of Pharmacy—Through Two Decades, Madison, Wis., 1961. Also in 1941 the Friends of Historical Pharmacy Inc. was formed and has since dedicated its effort to maintaining the restored apothecary shop of the colonial physician-pharmacist Hugh Mercer, at Fredericksburg, Va. J.A.Ph.A. (Pract. Ed.) *2*:177, 1941. The General Report of the Pharmaceutical Survey 1946–49, Washington, D.C., 1950, p. 47 f., also gives reliable sketches on other national organizations.
68. Urdang, George: The precedents of the N.A.R.D. and its founding fifty years ago, Am. J. Pharm. Ed. *13*:3tin xoro.
69. Beal, J. H.: Proposed merger of the American Pharmaceutical Association and the National Association of Retail Druggists, pp. 1–2 & 7–9, [1935], ms. in folder 13, box 13, AIHP mss 149, USPC Papers, State Historical Society of Wisconsin, Madison.
70. Kelly, E. F., and Dargavel, John: Report on historic A.Ph.A.–N.A.R.D. Conference, J.A.Ph.A. (Pract. Ed.) *4*:394, 1943; also, Second annual A.Ph.A.–N.A.R.D. Conference, J.A.Ph.A. (Pract. Ed.) *6*:13, 1945.
71. While the A.Ph.A. maintained an aloof silence publicly, the deep split that occurred is suggested by the bitter denunications under such raucous headlines as "Druggists sold down the river. Plotters use A.Ph.A. in betrayal . . .," (N.A.R.D. Journal *73*:730 f., 1951); see also Misguided and weasel opposition, N.A.R.D. Journal *72*:1499, 1950; Destructive confusion confounded, *ibid., 72*:1835, 1950; and Fischelis of the A.Ph.A. aligns himself with manufacturers against N.A.R.D. bill, *ibid, 73*:808 and 826–836, 1951. Hurling such adjectives as "inane" and "befuddled," the

latter article scarcely left doubt that "coordination" and joint conferences were temporarily ended.

72. Agenda, ground Rules . . ., and proposed resolution, for "APhA/ASHP/NARD Conference on Unified Organizational Structure [for] Friday, March 3, 1972"; photocopy-ms., 5 pp., in Kremers Reference Files (at C36(e)I), Pharmaceutical Library, University of Wisconsin-Madison.
73. Benson, G. E.: NARD and APhA—common goals and objectives, J.A.Ph.A. ns *13*:485 f., 1973; also Shinnick, H. J.: A framework established, J.A.Ph.A. ns *14*:505, 1974.
74. Latiolais, C. J.: Service to the public—our permanent interest, J.A.Ph.A., ns *13*:471, 1973; also on integration, Parks, L. M.: Time for decisions; changes, J.A.Ph.A. ns *12*:266 f., 1972.
75. Berman, Alex: The American Society of Hospital Pharmacists—a tribute, Am. J. Hosp. Pharm. *19*:212, 1962; Austin, E. C.: Training hospital pharmacists, Drugg. Circ. *65*:87–88, 1921.
76. The Sections of the APhA; A Symposium, pp. 358 f., Madison, 1953 (reprinted from Am J. Pharm. Edu.).
77. Reports of officers, Am. Jour. Hosp. Pharm. *30*:947 f., 1973. For an economic interpretation of the remarkable growth, see Oddis, J. A.: The evolving program . . ., Drug Intell. & Clin. Pharm. *6*:435–440, 1972.
78. Francke, D. E.: Origin and development of the American Hospital Formulary Service, Drug Intell. & Clin. Pharm. *6*:448–456, 1972.
79. Berman, A.: Historical currents in American hospital pharmacy, Drugg. Intell. & Clin. Pharm. *6*:447, 1972. See also, Ten years of the American Society of Hospital Pharmacists, Bull. Am. Soc. Hosp. Pharm. *9*:No. 4, 1952. Berman, A.: The American Society . . ., a Bicentennial Perspective, n. p., c. 1975. 16 pp.
80. Stieb, E. W.: American College of Apothecaries; The First Quarter Century 1940–1965, pp. 2–6, n.p. 1970. Stieb's study, upon which the A.C.A. section is largely based, shows the diverse origins and key components of such an academy-type organization in pharmacy; see also Selby, C. V.: The American College of Apothecaries as I see it, Bull. Am. Coll. Apoth. 3: No. 5, p. 4, 1943.
81. Ibid., 19. Martin S. Ulan served as Secretary, 1950–51, in the interim between Selby and Abrams.
82. Ibid., p. 23. Representative A.C.A. serials have been the *ACA Bulletin* (f. 1941); the *ACA Secretaries Newsletter* (f. 1946); *The Voice of the Pharmacist* (f. 1957; published through a separate corporation); *Physician's Newsletter* (from 1954 on regular basis) *Facts on the Operation of Prescription Pharmacies* (annually from 1953).
83. *Ibid.*, p. 31.
84. *Ibid.*, p. 33 f.; 37.
85. As one of its activities, the College has conferred periodically, since 1944, the J. Leon Lascoff Award honoring exceptional professional achievement in pharmacy and commemorating a New York pharmacist of distinction who was one of the principal founding members. (ibid., p. 63).
86. General Report of the Pharmaceutical Survey, p. 39.
87. Shannon, M. C.: The first national organization for employee-pharmacists (1910–1934), Pharm. Hist. *17*:58–68, 1975.
88. General Report of the Pharmaceutical Survey, p. 186.
89. Pharm. Era *16*:901, 1896; Harding, H. B.: Proprietary articles, Am. Drugg. & Pharm. Rec. *36*:190, 1900; Drugg. Circ. *51*:112, 1907.
90. For sketches on manufacturing organizations see the General Report of the Pharmaceutical Survey, pp. 42, 46 and 53; on founding the N.A.M.M.P. see Drugg. Circ. *56*:158, 1912; A.P.M.A. see Maltbie, B. L.: A Quarter Century of Progress in Manufacturing Pharmacy, New York, 1937; on P.A.A., see Kemp, E. F.: Some notes on the history of the Proprietary Association, J.A.Ph.A. *15*:973–979, 1926.
91. Pharm. Era *16*:896, 948, 1896; Drugg. Circ. *51*:110, 1907; Proc. Nat. Wholesale Drugg. Assoc., especially 1924, p. 28, and A History of the National Wholesale Druggists Association, from Its Organization to 1924, New York, 1924.
92. The association was formed by buying clubs of retail druggists. See 50th Anniversary, Federal Wholesale Druggists Association Inc., 1915–1965, n.p., 1965, 60 pp.
93. Some national examples not discussed in another context in this book would be the American Society of Pharmacognosy (f. 1959), Plant Science Seminar (f. 1923; see Claus, E. P.: A brief history of the Plant Science Seminar, Am. J. Pharm. Ed. *17*:433–436, 1953), Metropolitan Drug Association Secretaries, Friends of Historical Pharmacy (f. 1941, primarily to maintain the Hugh Mercer

Apothecary Shop; see General Report of the Pharmaceutical Survey, p. 48), National Drug Trade Conference (f. 1913; see, *ibid.*, p. 51). National Conference of State Pharmaceutical Association Secretaries (f. 1927; *ibid.*)., National Pharmaceutical Council (f. 1953; J.A.Ph.A. (Pract. Ed.) *15*:28 and 214, 1953), Association of Food and Drug Officials of the United States (f. 1897; before 1938 titled American Dairy, Food and Drug Officials), National Conference on Pharmaceutical Research (1920–1941; see J.A.Ph.A. *12*:623, 1923).

Associations that thus far remain largely regional in their scope include the American College of Pharmacists (f. 1944), American Congress of Pharmacists (f. 1960) [Drug Topics, May 9, 1960, pp. 12 and 62], Drug, Chemical and Allied Trades Section of the New York Board of Trade (voting membership restricted to firms within 75-mile radius of New York City), Society of Doctors of Pharmacy (mainly California), and Jewish Pharmaceutical Society of America (mainly New York area).

94. Smith, H. A. and Kuhn, N. A.: Study in pharmaceutical polity . . . affiliation on the move, J.A.Ph.A. ns *5*:17, 1965.
95. Francke, D. E.: Editorial: American pharmacy's federation—false hope or bright future, Am. J. Hosp. Pharm. *19*:209, 1962. The far-reaching decision taken by the Association at the 1962 meeting was reported: J.A.Ph.A. ns *2*:270 and 281, 1962.

## 13. THE RISE OF LEGISLATIVE STANDARDS

1. Duffy, John: The Rudolph Matas History of Medicine in Louisiana, Baton Rouge, 1958, vol. 1, pp. 326–327.
2. Cowen, D. L.: America's first pharmacy laws, J.A.Ph.A. *3*:168, 1942. Key legal issue was a provision that the New York College of Pharmacy should bring suits and itself receive the $150 penalty from the convicted.
3. Cowen, D. L.: Louisiana, pioneer in the regulation of pharmacy, Louisiana Hist. Quart. *26*:334, 1943.
4. Charter of the City of Louisville of 1851, and Ordinances of the City, Louisville, 1869, p. 431.
5. Proceedings of the American Pharmaceutical Association, 1868, Philadelphia, 1869, p. 370.
6. Laws of Pennsylvania, 1866, Harrisburg, 1866, p. 679.
7. Am. J. Pharm. *44*:137, 1872; Apothecaries' Union of New York City, Report of the Executive Committee, New York, 1871; Pharm. Rev. *21*:465, 482, 1903; *22*:31, 155, 1904.
8. Proc. A.Ph.A. *20*:150, 1872.
9. Cowen, D. L.: America's first pharmacy laws, J.A.Ph.A. *3*:162–169, 214–221.
10. *Ibid.*: pp. 162–166.
11. *Ibid.*: pp. 166–167.
12. *Ibid.*: pp. 167–168. An interesting sidelight of the legislative history in Georgia was the provision for the licensing of "Botanic or Thomsonian apothecaries" in an 1847 act.
13. *Ibid.*: p. 168.
14. Cowen, D. L.: A roster of the licensed apothecaries of Louisiana, J. New Orleans Coll. Pharm. *8*:3–4, 20–21, 1943.
15. Cowen, D. L.: America's first pharmacy laws, J.A.Ph.A. *3*:214.
16. Hoch, J. H.: History of Pharmacy in South Carolina, pp. 40, 73–76, Charleston, 1951. The surviving license of Abraham A. Solomons "to carry on the Business of Apothecary and Druggist" in South Carolina, dated December 15, 1835, is the oldest known.
17. Cowen, D. L.: America's first pharmacy laws J.A.Ph.A. *3*:169.
18. *Ibid.*: p. 215.
19. Partial lists of early state laws on adulteration and poison are to be found in Cowen: Louisiana, pioneer in the regulation of pharmacy, Louisiana Hist. Quart. *26*:334, 335.
20. Some facts on early poison legislation are given by Wilbert, M. I.: The evolution of laws regulating the sale and use of poisons, J.A.Ph.A. *1*:1259–1261, 1912.
21. Proc. A.Ph.A. *17*:51, 1870.
22. Beal, J. H.: The evolution of pharmacy laws in the United States, Am. Drug. & Pharm. Rec. *36*:179, 1900.
23. Am. J. Pharm. *44*:137, 1872.
24. Kremers, Edward: The history of American pharmacy, Am. Drugg., *68*(No. 5):14, 1920.
25. Am. J. Pharm. *44*:137, 1872.
26. Beal, J. H.: A general form of pharmacy law, Proc. A.Ph.A. *48*:309, 1900; Pharm.Rev. *18*:203, 1900.
27. As to pharmaceutical activities left to general merchants by the state pharmacy acts, see

Robert Fischelis: A survey of state pharmacy laws with reference to the sale of drugs and medicines by several merchants. J.A.Ph.A. *20*:1331, 1931.

28. On the national examination, see, e.g., A Candidate's Guide to the Blue Ribbon Examination . . ., (R. Greising, ed.), Chicago, ca. 1972; on the 1972 resolution of the N.A.B.P. and its model bill directed to the state legislatures, see: The Continuing Education Pamphlet: Uniform Continuing Education Act, Chicago, n.d. [ca. 1972]. See also Sica, A. and Greising, R.: . . . Standard Exam for Licensure, Proc. N.A.B.P. 1971, pp. 127–133.
29. The annual *Proceedings* volume (since 1906) provides communication between the N.A.B.P. and the profession, and among the state boards, supplemented by the *N.A.B.P. Bulletin* (1935–1967), succeeded since 1971 by an *N.A.B.P. Newsletter*, and by the proceedings of the annual joint conferences of the regional Districts.
30. Sonnedecker, Glenn: The birth of the National Association of Boards of Pharmacy fifty years ago, in National Association of Boards of Pharmacy 1904–1954, Madison, Wis., 1955, pp. 23–33; also published in Proceedings of the National Association of Boards of Pharmacy, 1954.
31. Wiley, H. W.: Education of a Hoosier, Indiana Mag. Hist. *24*:94 f., 1928.
32. Editorial, Bull. A.Ph.A. *5*:391, 1910.
33. Editorial, Pharm. Era *14*:512, 1895.
34. For the evidence and judicious accounts of the complex background to the law, see Young, J. H. "Social History of American Drug Legislation" in: Drugs in Our Society (P. Talalay, ed.), pp. 217–226, Baltimore, ca. 1964; and his The Toadstool Millionaires, Princeton, ca. 1961; Anderson, O. E., Jr.: The Health of a Nation; Harvey W. Wiley and the fight for Pure Food, Chicago, 1958; and Wilson, Stephen: Food and Drug Regulation, Washington, 1942.
35. Report of committee on drug reform, Bull. A.Ph.A. *5*:655, 1910.
36. See, e.g. Proc. A.Ph.A. *55*:241, 1907, and Bull. A.Ph.A. *4*:467, 1909.
37. Wallace, J. C.: The chairman's address, J.A.Ph.A. *1*:939, 1912. For an account of one segment of the state endeavors in this field before Federal legislation, see Sonnedecker, Glenn, and Urdang, George: Legalization of drug standards under state laws in the United States of America, Food, Drug, Cosmetic Law J. *8*:741–760, 1953; see also for the legal aspect—Sonnedecker, Glenn: The section on education and legislation of the American Pharmaceutical Association, Am. J. Pharm. Ed. *17*:362–383, 1953.
38. Dunn, C. W.: Our food and drug law, with some observations on its major statute, Food, Drug, Cosmetic Law J. *9*:385, 1954. The only other major statutes controlling interstate commerce earlier than the Federal Food and Drug Act of 1906 were the Interstate Commerce Act (1887) and the Sherman Antitrust Act (1890). This avenue of Federal control took on new significance with the revised Food and Drug Act of 1938, which Dunn calls "of profound legal importance, in itself and as a modern administrative law; and because it . . . makes an extreme use of the congressional power over interstate commerce, to regulate intrastate commerce as well." Administration of the Federal law at first was placed with the U. S. Department of Agriculture's Bureau of Chemistry (from 1927 part of a Food, Drug and Insecticide Administration). After revision of the law, the F.D.A. was transferred, executively, to the Federal Security Agency, (an agency absorbed into the present Department of Health, Education, and Welfare). [*ibid.*, p. 385]
39. Senate Document No. 124, 75th Congress, 2d Session; this report on a case is reprinted in Herrick, A. D., and Smith, A. E.: New Drugs, p. 157, New York, 1946.
40. "Editorial" [E. F. Kelly, Secretary], J.A.Ph.A. *27*:369, 1938; see also Winne, A. L. E.: Proc. Natl. Assoc. Bds. Pharm., p. 58 f., 1938.
41. Veldee, M. V.: Federal regulation. II. U. S. Public Health Service, J.A.Ph.A. *8*:161–163, 1947. The revised act of 1944 was PL 410-78th Congress. On the transfer of function from U.S.P.H.S. to F.D.A., see e.g., Drug Topics, p. 4, June 19, 1972, and P.M.A. Newsletter, p. 2, May 26, 1972.
42. Herzog ,S. A.: Durham-Humphrey—two years after, Food Drug Cosmetic Law J. *10*:119–128, 1955.
43. See, Hearings Before the Subcommittee on Antitrust and Monopoly of the Committee on the Judiciary, United States Senate, Eighty-Sixth Congress, Second Session: Administered Prices in the Drug Industry, Wash-

ington, D.C., 1961, especially parts 14 through 26; see also, "Report" on same to the Eighty Seventh Congress, First Session, Report 448, Senate.

44. For a factual review of events leading to enactment of the Drug Amendments of 1962 (signed October 10), see Stempel, Edward: The impetus of thalidomide on drug legislation and regulation, Am. J. Pharm. *134*:355–364, 1962. For the provisions of the enactment and discussions of possible implications in practice, see J.A.Ph.A. ns *2*:638-646, 1962; and on the thalidomide aspect particularly, FDC Reports *24*:No. 32 (Aug. 6) and No. 33 (Aug. 13), 1962. For the argument that costs may exceed benefits from the 1962 amendments, see, e.g., Peltzman, Sam: Regulation of Pharmaceutical Innovation—The 1962 Amendments, American Enterprise Institute for Public Policy Research, Washington, 1974, or Landau, R. L. ed.: Regulating New Drugs, Chicago, 1973, a symposium addressed primarily to interpreting diverse effects of the 1962 amendments; and Wardell, W. M. and Lasagna, L.: Regulation and Drug Development, Washington, D.C., 1975.
45. On the erratic evolution of our understanding of addiction, see Sonnedecker, Glenn: Emergence of the concept of opiate addiction, J. mondial Pharm., opiate addiction, part 1, J. mondial Pharm. No. 3 (Sept.-Dec.), pp. 275–290; part 2, J. mondial Pharm. No. 1 (Jan.–Mar.), 1963, pp. 27–34.
46. On this Committee's work, see Proc. A.Ph.A. *49*:465, 1901; *50*:567–574, 1902; *51*:471, 1903.
47. Supplemental Federal acts have included the Narcotic Drugs Import and Export Act of 1922 (revising the Act of 1909), the Marihuana Tax Act of 1937 (subsequently placed in the Internal Revenue Code, and later ruled unconstitutional), the Opium Poppy Control Act of 1942, Public Law 729 of 1954 (an amendment important to practicing pharmacists), and the Narcotic Control Act of 1956 (which provided remarkably punitive penalties for unlawful sale or possession of narcotic drugs and marihuana). With few exceptions, state laws substantially followed a model issued in 1932, as a "Uniform State Narcotic Law," with the joint backing of medical, pharmaceutical and government agencies.
48. Drug Topics, p. 2, col. 1, Dec. 17–31, 1962.
49. National alarm over a spreading "drug abuse problem" and frustration in Congress over the limited effectiveness of government agencies of control help account for legal and administrative changes since the mid-1960's. In 1965 the Drug Abuse Control Act was passed (covering stimulants, depressants, hallucinogens, and—for the first time nationally—counterfeit drugs). For administration and enforcement, a Bureau of Drug Abuse Control was set up in the Department of Justice. In 1968 enforcement of this act and the old Harrison Narcotics Act was combined (by Executive Order) through a new Bureau of Narcotic and Dangerous Drugs, also in the Justice Department. This agency continued to handle regulation and enforcement until absorbed (Executive Order, 1973) into a new Drug Enforcement Administration. Provisions notably affecting the practice of pharmacy (effective May 1, 1971) were contained in the Controlled Substances Act of 1970 (PL 91-513).
50. Musto, D. F.: The American Disease; Origins of Narcotic Control, p. 244, New Haven, 1973. Now the most comprehensive single source on the subject, but see also Musto's "American Reactions to International Narcotic Traffic," Pharm. in Hist. *16*:115–122, 1974.

## 14. THE DEVELOPMENT OF EDUCATION

1. Wilbert, M. I.: The beginnings of pharmacy in America, Am. J. Pharm. *79*:406, 1907.
2. LaWall, C. H.: The founding of the Philadelphia College of Pharmacy and Science, Am. J. Pharm. *93*:169, 1921.
3. Hoch, J. H.: Dr. Lewis Mottet's projected Institute of Pharmacy, J.A.Ph.A. *27*:1260–61, 1938.
4. Wolfe, H. G.: James Cutbush—author, teacher, apothecary general, Am. J. Pharm. Ed. *12*:89–125, 1948.
5. LaWall, C. H.: *op. cit.*, p. 170.
6. Kremers, Edward: The Old Northwest Territory and Pharmaceutical Education, p. 7, Purdue University, Lafayette, Indiana, 1934.
7. England, J. W.: The First Century of the Philadelphia College of Pharmacy, p. 463, Philadelphia, 1922.
8. Proc. A.Ph.A. *3*:14, 1854; Am. J. Pharm. *26*:388, 1854.
9. Am. J. Pharm. *18*:148, 1846.
10. England, J. W.: *op. cit.*, p. 143.

11. *Ibid.*: p. 404.
12. Wilbert, M. I.: John M. Maisch, Am. J. Pharm. *75*:356, 1903.
13. Osborne, G. E.: David Stewart, M.D., first American professor of pharmacy (1833–1899), Am. J. Pharm. Ed. *23*:219–230, 1959; see also Meyer Bros. Drugg. *17*:200, 1896.
14. Parrish, Edward: American pharmacy, Am. J. Pharm. *26*:216, 1854.
15. Sonnedecker, Glenn: American Pharmaceutical Education Before 1900, unpublished Ph.D., dissertation, University of Wisconsin, Madison, 1952, Pt. 2, p. 461 ff., and Urdang, George: The part of doctors of medicine in pharmaceutical education, Am. J. Pharm. Ed. *14*:546–556, 1950. See also Kremers, Edward: The teaching of pharmacy during the past fifty years, Drugg. Circ. *51*:68, 1907.
16. Day, W. B.: The school of pharmacy, Alumni Rec., University of Illinois, p. xxvi, 1921.
17. England, J. W.: *op. cit.*, p. 147.
18. *Ibid.*: p. 406.
19. Shafer, H. B.: The American Medical Profession 1783–1850, p. 43, New York, 1936.
20. Am. J. Pharm. *44*:189, 1872.
21. *Ibid.*: p. 233.
22. Am. J. Pharm. *19*:256, 1847.
23. Sonnedecker, Glenn: *op. cit.*, p. 115. About that same time some pharmacy was taught at the neighboring University of South Carolina, but it had a tenuous connection because of exigencies of the reconstruction period; and apparently there were no graduates until 1886. The first place where pharmacy instruction began within a general college program (1865) probably was Baldwin University, a small institution in Berea, Ohio.
24. Proc. A.Ph.A. *19*:425, 1871; and Manasse, Jr., H. R.: Albert B. Prescott's Legacy . . ., Pharm. Hist. *15*:22–28, 1973.
25. Comparative data on practical-experience requirements in 54 countries are given by Dieckmann, Hans: Geschichte und Probleme der Apothekerausbildung, in erster Linie in Frankreich und Deutschland, pp. 187–195, with commentary, 121 ff., Frankfurt a/M, 1954.
26. Proc. A.Ph.A. *19*:96, 1871.
27. *Ibid.*, p. 47.
28. Letter of J. O. Schlotterbeck, written November 12, 1906, in Kremers Reference Files, Pharmaceutical Library, University of Wisconsin-Madison.
29. Pharm. Rev. *21*:362, 1903.
30. Sonnedecker, Glenn: American Pharmaceutical Education Before 1900, pp. 113–120.
31. The comparative comments are based upon Scoville, W. L.: Proc. Am. Conf. Pharm. Facul., p. 17, 1905, and the A.Ph.A. Pharmaceutical Directory, 1975. Colleges not affiliated with a general institution of higher learning were those of Massachusetts, St. Louis, Philadelphia, and the school of the Medical University of South Carolina. States not yet having a school of pharmacy (1975) were Alaska, Delaware, Hawaii, Maine, Nevada, New Hampshire and Vermont.
32. World Directory of Schools of Pharmacy 1963. Geneva: W.H.O., 1966. Sweden and Spain, indeed, reported about three times as much population per school of pharmacy than the U.S.A. average.
33. Cf. Cowen, D. L: Notes on pharmaceutical training in New Jersey before 1900, Am. J. Pharm. Ed. *12*:303, 1948; and Parrish, Edward: The preliminary education of apprentices, Proc. A.Ph.A., *20*:178, 1872.
34. At Purdue a "good common school education" or an equivalent examination and 2-year apprenticeship were required in 1884 (Lee, C. O.: The first courses in pharmacy, Am. J. Pharm. Ed. *4*:60, 1940). At Michigan those with practical experience could defer the examination covering preliminary education and receive other concessions (Annual Announcement . . . Michigan, 1887–88, pp. 8–10; see also Pharm. Rundschau *5*:128, 1887).
35. Bastin, E. S.: Pharmacal education, West. Drugg. *10*:403, 1888.
36. Sonnedecker, G.: American Pharmaceutical Education Before 1900 (unpublished Ph.D. thesis, University of Wisconsin), pp. 264 f.
37. Beal, J. H.: Report on preliminary education requirement, Proc. A.Ph.A. *46*:548, 1898.
38. By-laws of the American Conference of Pharmaceutical Faculties, in: Proc. Am. Conf. Pharm. Fac., pp. 45, 46, 1906.
39. See Blauch, L., and Webster, G.: The Pharmaceutical Curriculum, pp. 14 f. on this point and the development of prerequisites in the present century.
40. Mayo, C. A.: The prerequisite law in New York, Bull. Pharm. *18*:502, 1904.
41. England, J. W.: The First Century of the Philadelphia College of Pharmacy, p. 182; The status of prerequisite laws and pharmaceutical licensure, Am. J. Pharm. *93*:539, 1921.
42. Elliott, E. C., ed.: The General Report . . ., p.

225, Washington, 1950. This section on apprenticeship relies substantially on the historical introduction to the pioneering research by Des Roches, B. P.: A Comparative Study of the Pharmacist as Preceptor in Wisconsin and Ontario (unpublished Ph.D. dissertation, University of Wisconsin), pp. 1–29, Madison, 1970, and Brown, V. J.: The year of apprenticeship; its use and misuse, Am. J. Pharm. Edu. *26*:39–51, 1962.

43. Proc. Natl. Assoc. Bds. Pharm. 1969, pp. 214 and 530, Chicago, n.d. The transition of usage from the trade-based term "apprenticeship" to the profession-based "internship" was signaled in 1953 when the N.A.B.P. recommended that the term "apprenticeship" be discontinued in pharmacy. (Brown, loc. cit., p. 40).
44. On N.A.B.P. developments see, e.g., Proc. Natl. Assoc. Bds. Pharm., 1969, pp. 210–212; *ibid.*, 1971, p. 484 (on new standard) and *ibid.*, 1972, p. 65; *ibid.*, 1973, pp. 159–163; Accreditation Manual, Seventh Edition . . . Effective from July 1, 1974, p. 14, Chicago: A.C.P.E., 1975 (concerning clinical experience). Historical experience in Europe suggests that the exact time-length of supervised experience is not crucial to competency; during the early 1970's the country-to-country variation appeared to be from a few months to 1½ years.
45. On the rise and demise of the Syllabus Committee, and the subsequent development, see: Blauch, L. E., and Webster, G. L.: The Pharmaceutical Curriculum, pp. 18–27. See also the Committee's report, The Pharmaceutical Syllabus, 1910, 146 pp.
46. Am. J. Pharm. *41*:472, 1869.
47. Proc. Am. Assoc. Coll. Pharm., p. 27, 1926.
48. Blauch, L. E., and Webster, G. L.: The Pharmaceutical Curriculum, p. 16, Washington, D.C. A few schools continued 3-year courses optionally until as late as 1939.
49. Elliott, E. C., ed.: The General Report of the Pharmaceutical Survey, pp. 105 and 230 (note f.n. 6); Report . . . Proposal C (A.A.C.P.), Am. J. Pharm. Educ. *14*:655, 1950; and Brodie, D. C.: Is pharmaceutical education prepared to lead its profession?, Rho Chi Report 1973, pp. 6–12.
50. Brady, E. S.: The six-year program, Am. J. Pharm. Ed. *17*:448, 1953, and *26*:62, 1962. A 6-year (Pharm. D.) program was adopted by the University of California in 1956, and by the University of Michigan (particularly in hospital pharmacy) in 1962.
51. Tice, L. F.: Pharmacy education for today and the future, pp. 6–9, mimeographed address, Charleston, S.C. 28 October, 1966; in Kremers Reference Files, Pharmaceutical Library, University of Wisconsin, Madison.
52. Task Force on Prescription Drugs; Final Report, pp. xvii and 20, Washington, D.C. (H.E.W.), 1969.
53. Report on the current status of clinical pharmacy education programs, Am. J. Pharm. Edu. *36*:403, 1972. About half the schools were offering the equivalent of 6 to 7 semester-credits; 21 schools were offering between 300 and 1000 clock-hours of such instruction, the others less. Report of the American Council on Pharmaceutical Education, *ibid.*, p. 395. Among 73 colleges, 40 did not yet have clinical externship or clerkship out in community pharmacies; and among those that did, at least optionally (including California), the average was 19 clock-hours. Only 6 schools had yet responded to the advent of pharmacy technicians by instructing students how to supervise and apply control systems in utilizing technicians (*ibid.*, p. 394).
54. Weaver, L. C.: Address of the Vice President (A.A.C.P.), Am. J. Pharm. Edu. *37*:396, 1973; and Knapp, D. A.: Comments on curriculum length and content, *ibid.*, *37*:287–289, 1973.
55. Hynson, H. P.: Historical notes on degrees in pharmacy, Drugg. Circ. *51*:80, 1907.
56. Scoville, W. L.: American Pharmaceutical Colleges, p. 16, Am. Conf. Pharm. Faculties, 1905. Ten years later (1915) the School of Pharmacy of Northwestern University still offered a 1-year course leading to the degree of Graduate in Pharmacy. The degree of Pharmaceutical Chemist was awarded after a second year of study. Before the American Conference of Pharmaceutical Faculties (1918) A. Koch reported, "The Ph.G. degree is conferred by 39 institutions for a two-years' course, and by one school after 4 years; the degree of Bachelor of Science in Pharmacy by 20 schools for a four-years' course, by one for three years and by one for two years; the Doctor of Pharmacy degree by three schools for three years, by one for four years, by three schools for six years and by one for a seven-years' course. The Master of Pharmacy degree is conferred by one school for three years, and

the Master of Science in Pharmacy by three schools for a five-years' course." (Proc. Am. Conf. Pharm. Fac., p. 44, 1918).

57. Urdang, George: Edward Kremers (1865–1941), reformer of American pharmaceutical education, Am. J. Pharm. Ed. *11*:650, 1947. Parascandola, J. and Sonnedecker, G.: Ground and background for the historical marker . . ., Wis. Pharm., p. 366, Nov. 1974. Oswald Schreiner of Maryland, B.S. in Pharm., 1897, was the first pharmacy graduate to earn a Ph.D. "for work in the pharmaceutical sciences under the direction of Edward Kremers. This degree clearly marks the beginning of doctoral training in the pharmaceutical specialties in America, although technically the degree had to be awarded through the Chemistry Department because the Department of Pharmacy did not yet have the administrative authority to offer the Ph.D. . . ."
58. Green, M. W.: Progress and problems in graduate instruction in pharmacy, Am. J. Pharm. Ed. *19*:467 ff., 1955; *38*:250 ff., 1974; and General Report of the Pharmaceutical Survey, p. 110.
59. Sonnedecker, Glenn: *op. cit.*, pp. 282–287.
60. Pharm. Era *16*:384, 1896.
61. Proc. West Virginia Pharm. Assoc., p. 341, 1931. See also Cook, R. B.: The Annals of Pharmacy in West Virginia, pp., 31 ff., Charleston, 1946.
62. Pharm. Era *17*:499, 1897.
63. Proc. A.Ph.A. *54*:200, 1906.
64. For example, see the account of subsequent diploma peddling by the "dean" of pharmacy at the erstwhile "Lincoln-Jefferson University": "Teacher of Pharmacy." The unsavory story. . . . J.A.Ph.A. (Pract. Ed.) *7*:196–202, 1946.
65. The Apothecary *1*:4, 1891; and Circular of Information for 1892, Northwestern University School of Pharmacy, 37–39, Chicago, n.d. Purchasers of Oldberg's book could obtain guidance through sets of questions sent by the author periodically. Earlier Oldberg had issued for the same home-study purpose an *Outline of a Course in Practical Pharmacy* (1885).
66. Christensen, H. C.: What legal difficulties may we get into when we abolish assistant registration, Am. J. Pharm. Ed. *1*:44 and 47, 1937. A comprehensive survey of the question of the assistant pharmacist and its historical development is given by John Grover Beard in J.A.Ph.A. *15*:119, 1926. A case study by G. Sonnedecker of the "cram school" technic can be found in the article entitled "Teacher of pharmacy . . ." J.A.Ph.A. (Pract. Ed.) *7*:196–202, 1946.
67. Oldberg, Oscar: The principles of university and school extension applies to pharmaceutical studies, The Apothecary *1*:3, 1891.
68. Buerki, R. A.: Historical Development of Continuing Education in American Universities (unpublished Ph.D. dissertation, Ohio State University), pp. 58, 94, 177 f., 185, 380 f., 382–385. The account of the evolution of 20th-century continuing education relies largely upon Dr. Buerki's extensive study. See also, General Report of the Pharmaceutical Survey, pp. 231 f.
69. Sonnedecker, G.: Exploratory Paper for a Proposed National Study of Pharmacy . . . (mimeographed, American Pharmaceutical Association), pp. 87 f., n.p., 1965.
70. The Continuing Education Pamphlet; Uniform Professional Continuing Education Act, p. 5, n.p.: N.A.B.P., ca. 1972.
71. By 1975 more than a fifth of the states had adopted some legal requirement of continuing education for pharmacists. Some of the points at issue in the development of mandatory continuing education are reflected in the final report of the A.Ph.A.-A.A.C.P. Task Force on Continuing Competence in Pharmacy; for its recommendations see A.Ph.A. Newsletter, *13*:No. 29, p. 1, 1974 (Dec. 14). In addition the 1974 report of the A.A.C.P.'s Academic Affairs Committee expressed concern "about the opportunistic and fragmented nature of most continuing education in pharmacy" (mimeograph, p. 6). See also Jobe, B. D.: Mandatory continuing education—an overview and update, Louisiana Pharm. *32*:12–15 (May) 1973.
72. The foregoing discussion is based on the following article and the sources there cited: Sonnedecker, Glenn: The Conference of Schools of Pharmacy—a period of frustration, Am. J. Pharm. Ed. *18*:389, 1954; on Maisch, see Pharm. Rundschau *1*:193, 1870.
73. Proc. A.Ph.A. *38*:243 f., 1890.
74. A copy of Dr. James H. Beal's memoirs was put at the disposal of the author of this book by his son, Dr. George D. Beal.

75. Proc. Am. Conf. Pharm. Fac. pp. 7 and 8, 1902.
76. Weaver, L. C.: Address of the Vice President, Am. J. Pharm. Edu. *37*:395, 1973; see also Schwarting, A.: *ibid.*, *36*:352, 1972; Petersen, R. V., *ibid.*, *37*:390, 1973; and A.A.C.P. circular to members, 7 January 1975, 4 pp.
77. See Mahaffey, F. T.: Annual Report to the Sponsors . . . p. 9, n.p., March 15, 1972; Accreditation Manual, Seventh Edition . . . (Chicago, 1975). See also, Green, M. G.: Pharmacy looks at accreditation, Am. J. Pharm. Educ. *23*:430–438, 1959; and Dickey, F. G.: Accreditation and licensure . . . Proc. Natl. Assoc. Bds. Pharm. 1973, pp. 239–248, Chicago, n.d. General Report of the Pharmaceutical Survey 1946–49, pp. 70 f. and 214 ff. Standards were first published by the Council in 1937. As a temporary measure after World War II the Council used a classification system in rating schools (A, B, C, Y) but has been able to return to a simple designation of "accredited" (or non-accredited). A list of accredited schools may be obtained on request to the Council at 1 East Wacker Drive, Chicago, Ill. 60601.
78. Newcomb, E. L.: Chronological facts relating to the birth . . ., in: National Wholesale Druggists' Association Year Book for 1948, pp. 477–494—an important document for understanding the A.F.P.E. origins.
79. Briggs, W. P.: American Foundation for Pharmaceutical Education—25th Anniversary Year, 1967, n.p., 12 pp.; see also the Foundation's annual reports.
80. Charters, W. W.: Basic Material for a Pharmaceutical Curriculum, p. v, New York, 1927.
81. *Ibid.*, p. xiii.
82. Proc. Am. Assoc. Coll. Pharm., p. 24, 1927.
83. J.A.Ph.A. *16*:351, 1927.
84. J.A.Ph.A. (Sci. Ed.) *32*:368, 1943.
85. Am. J. Pharm. Ed. *7*:574, 1943; *8*:245, 246, 1954.
86. The three Assistant Directors of the Pharmaceutical Survey (Lloyd E. Blauch, J. Solon Mordell, and H. H. Remmers) each had unusual expertise in his field and helped to produce special monographs as offshoots of the Survey as well as the General Report. An active advisory committee of 15, drawn from various segments of the pharmaceutical field and the laity, was chaired by the aging director of the survey of the 1920's, W. W. Charters. The Findings and Recommendations of the Pharmaceutical Survey, 1948 (Washington, D.C.) were preprinted as a booklet separate from the General Report.
87. Francke, D. E., et al.: Mirror to Hospital Pharmacy . . ., Washington, D.C., ca. 1964, 244 pp.
88. "Resolutions-1966," J.A.Ph.A. ns *6*:293, 1966. Sonnedecker: An Exploratory Paper . . . loc. cit.
89. Schwarting, A.: President's Address, Am. J. Pharm. Ed. *36*:353 f., 1972. The report of the Millis commission was published December 1975.
90. Lyman, R. A.: The American Institute of the History of Pharmacy and the Pharmaceutical Press (mimeograph address), p. 5, Madison, Wis., 1942.

## 15. THE ESTABLISHMENT OF A LITERATURE

1. Trans. New York M. Soc., p. 131, 1807–1831.
2. England, J. W.: The First Century of the Philadelphia College of Pharmacy, p. 94, Philadelphia, 1922.
3. Trans. Coll. Phys. Phila.: Ser. 3, *9*:101, 1887.
4. Collections for an Essay towards a Materia Medica of the United States, read before the Philadelphia Medical Society, February 21, 1798, and published in the same year; the second part was published in 1804. See reprint in Bull. Lloyd Libr. vol. I, Part 1, p. 32 and Part 2, p. 6.
5. Proc. Conn. Med. Soc.: reprint; p. 191 and 196.
6. Alden, E.: Historical Sketch of the Origin and Progress of the Massachusetts Medical Society, Mass. Med. Soc. Comm. *6*:56, 1838.
7. Pharmacopoeia, Mass. Med. Soc., Boston, 1808: p. v.
8. The Medical Repository, New York, 5, 1808.
9. Pharmacopoeia, Mass. Med. Soc., p. v.
10. Burrage, W. L.: A History of the Massachusetts Medical Society, 1781–1822, p. 75, Norwood, Mass., 1923.
11. Minutes Med. Soc. South Carolina, 1808.
12. U.S.P., 1820, p. 19.
13. Minutes Med. Soc. South Carolina, 1808.
14. Niles, E. H.; The Massachusetts Pharmacopoeia of 1808, J.A.Ph.A. *25*:542, 1936.
15. Cowen, D. L.: The New York Hospital and its pharmacopoeia, N.Y. St. Jour. Med. *73*:901, 1973.
16. Pharmacopoeia Nosocomii Neo-Ebora-

censis, pp. vi–ix, New York, 1816. On the 1811 edition see, Sonnedecker, G.: Earliest formulary for a civilian hospital, U.S.A., Drug Intell. and Clin. Pharm. *6*:425–434, 1972. For criticism of the 1811 edition see, e.g., Am. Med. & Philos. Reg. *4*:602, 1814. The sources for this earlier edition are so far unknown; the 1816 edition stated that, besides drug formulas from the Hospital's staff, it drew principally on the London, Edinburgh, and Dublin pharmacopeias.

17. Quotations from Berman, A.: Historical currents in American hospital pharmacy, Drug Intell. and Clin. Pharm. *6*:443, 1972.
18. Francke, D. E.; Origin and development of the American hospital formulary service, *ibid.*, pp. 448–454.
19. Kebler, L. F.: S. L. Mitchill, J.A.Ph.A. *26*:908, 1937. Kebler states that the correct spelling of the name is Mitchill and not Mitchell.
20. U.S.P., 1820: p. 5.
21. Trans. New York State M. Soc. p. 112 and 130, 1807–1831.
22. U.S.P., 1820: p. 9. The first two circulars of the Committee were issued on March 4 and November 21, 1818. Kebler: *op. cit.*, p. 912.
23. U.S.P., XI, 1937: p. xix.
24. On the founding and the men who participated see, Sonnedecker, Glenn: The men who participated in the founding convention, pp. 13–15, et passim, and also historical articles by others, in Founding of the United States Pharmacopeia 1820; Dedication of a Painting . . ., New York, 1957.
25. As quoted by Lord, R. A.; Lyman Spalding and the U.S. Pharmacopoeia, Pharm. Hist. *17*:22 f., 1975; Mr. Lord also has published, from an extensive biographical study being completed: Dr. Lyman Spalding. . . , Northern Light [Masonic] June 1974, pp. 8 f. & 13.
26. Trans. Coll. Phys. Phila.: Ser. 3, *9*:135, 1887; U.S.P., 1820; p. 15.
27. Trans. Coll. Phys. Phila.: *loc. cit.*
28. Eberle, E. G.: A Copy of Proof Sheets U.S.P. I, Baltimore, 1932. The copy preserved and reproduced was the one assigned to Dr. DeButts and apparently returned by him with his suggestions to the chairman.
29. U.S.P., 1820: p. 26.
30. *Ibid.*: p. 22.
31. Phil. J. Med. & Phys. Sci. *2*:367, 1821.
32. Spalding, J. A.: The Life of Dr. L. Spalding, p. 363, Boston, 1916.
33. The first edition of the U. S. Pharmacopeia was changed more for the second issuance than had been thought before the study by Laurence D. Lockie, The Second (1828) Edition of the Pharmacopeia of the United States (mimeograph, Section on Historical Pharmacy, American Pharmaceutical Association, 1958; 5 pp.). Lockie reported that type was re-set, the copyright changed, typographical errors corrected, 3 changes made in the materia medica lists, and 7 changes made in procedural directions.
34. Med. Repos.: pp. 363, 364, 1821.
35. For information on the schism and the two second editions, see J. Phila. Coll. Pharm. *3*:64–65 and 68, 1832; U.S.P., 1830: title page and pp. 3–6; U.S.P., 1831: pp. vii, ix, xxix; Trans. Coll. Phys. Phila.: Ser. 3, *9*:135, 1887.
36. On early pharmaceutical cooperation, see England, J. W.: *op. cit.*, p. 96; Trans. Coll. Phys. Phila.: *loc. cit.*; U.S.P., 1831: pp. xiv and xxviii.
37. Am. J. Pharm. *14*:122, 1842; see also England, J. W.: *op. cit.*, p. 120; Thrush, M. C.: U.S.P. and its predecessors, Drugg. Circ. *51*:46, 1907.
38. U.S.P., 1873: pp. xiii and xviii.
39. Proc. A.Ph.A. *24*:631–33 and 646, 1876.
40. Am.J. Pharm. *49*:209, 1877.
41. Trans. Am. Med. Assoc. *28*:109, 1877.
42. Proc. A.Ph.A. *25*:538, 1877.
43. Proc. A.Ph.A. *26*:668, 879, 1878.
44. Am. J. Pharm. *54*:638, 1882. The book appeared in October 1882, but in a reprinting necessary the next year the title page was re-dated 1883.
45. U.S.P., 1893: p. xxvi. On pre-1906 drug standards, see Sonnedecker, G., and Urdang, G.: Legalization of drug standards under state laws in the United States of America, Food Drug Cosmetic Law J. *8*:753, 1953.
46. U.S.P., 1905: p. xxv, and later editions: A facsimile of the Certificate of Incorporation in Pharm. Rev. *18*:546, 1900; first three paragraphs in Urdang, G.: Pharmacy's Part in Society, p. 13, Madison, Wis., 1946.
47. Proc. A.Ph.A. *38*:263, 1890.
48. U.S.P., 1905: p. xxxi.
49. *Ibid.*: p. xxxix.
50. *Ibid.*: p. xxx.
51. U.S.P., 1916: xliii.
52. On the role of the Spanish edition see King, N.: Development of drug standards in Latin America, Pharm. Hist. *13*:11–26, 1971.

53. Succeeding Remington for the unexpired term of office was the pharmacist Charles H. LaWall, professor at the Philadelphia College of Pharmacy.
54. U.S.P., 1936: p. xxxiv.
55. Cook, E. F.: The new Pharmacopoeia, J.A.Ph.A. *14*:864, 1925.
56. Pharmacopoeial Board of Trustees, U.S.P.: J.A.Ph.A. *28*:1011, 1939. The U.S.P. once observed, "No funds are received from either government or private sources, although the conservatively estimated monetary value of the talent and time contributed from these sources exceeds the actual expense of the revision activities." (Preface, U.S.P. XV, 1955, p. xiii.)
57. U.S.P., 1936: p. xiv.
58. *Ibid.*: p. xi; p. xiii; a harbinger of U.S.P. reference standards was the offer in U.S.P. X (1926, p. 4) from the Bureau of Chemistry of the U.S. Department of Agriculture to "supply standard substances conforming to the pharmacopoeial requirements" in biologic assays.
59. U.S.P., 1942: p. xxv (preface).
60. This decision was to "become effective in time for the 1950 Convention." The amendment to the by-laws providing for the full-time director was among the changes inaugurated by the adjourned meeting of the Pharmacopeial Convention held in Cleveland, Ohio, in 1942.
61. Am. Prof. Pharm. *15*:435–439, 470, 1949. As temporary quarters, the Pharmacopeia had purchased a building in Philadelphia and established offices there in 1945.
62. Miller, L. C.: Stewardship of our legacy *in* Founding of the United States Pharmacopeia 1820, p. 30, New York, 1957.
63. For a good discussion of the changing circumstances and Latin usage, see Urdang, G.: The place of Latin in the official standards of pharmacy, Bull. Natl. Form. Comm. *12*:201–220, 1944.
64. U.S.P. XV, 1955: p. xi (preface).
65. U.S.P. XVI, 1960: pp. xvi and xxvii.
66. A spur to the merger of the U.S.P. and N.F. was the appearance of *Drug Bioequivalence: a Report of the Drug Bioequivalence Study Panel,* the Office of Technology Assessment (Washington, D.C. [1974], 78 pp.), which implied that the standard-setting function might be done better by the government. This and some other conclusions have been challenged by representatives of the sciences and professions concerned. Not at issue, however, was the possibility of improvement; and by 1975 the U.S.P.C. had contracted with an outside consultant to "analyze the organization and administration of the USPC for the purpose of recommending specific changes necessary to fulfill the clear and urgent needs identified by the Study Panel." (Wm. M. Heller, U.S.P., to Edward M. Kennedy, U. S. Senate, September 9, 1974; copy in Kremers Reference files, Pharmacy Library, University of Wisconsin-Madison).
67. England, J. W.: The First Century, pp. 72, 73. This tract exposed the formulas of some of the popular "patent medicines" often requested, under the title, *Formulary for the Preparation of Eight Patent Medicines Adopted by the Philadelphia College of Pharmacy* (Philadelphia, 1824).
68. Proc. A.Ph.A. *6*:81, 1857; *7*:230, 1858.
69. Am. Drugg. *15*:199, 1886.
70. U.S.P., 1882: p. xxx.
71. Proc. A.Ph.A. *34*:558, 1885.
72. *Ibid.*
73. Sonnedecker, G., and Urdang, G.: Legalization . . . (note 45), p. 754.
74. As an important participant from 1940 until his retirement, Justin Powers offers much insight into the character of the American standard-setting mechanism in two lectures on "Drug Standards in the United States" in: The Pharmaceutical Sciences; Third Annual Visiting Lecture Series, pp. 231–250, Austin, Texas, 1960.
75. Cook, E. F.: J.A.Ph.A. *30*:469, 1941; and Powers, J. L.: *ibid,* p. 477.
76. Quoted from editorial, J. Pharm. Sci. *63*: p. i, 1974. A convenient source of further historical facts on the evolution of drug standards in the United States is the historical introduction in each edition of both the *U. S. Pharmacopeia* and the *National Formulary*. The numbered editions of the *National Formulary* together with the year in which they became effective ("official") are: 1st, 1888; 2nd, 1896; 3rd, 1906; 4th, 1916; 5th, 1926; 6th, 1936; 7th, 1942; 8th, 1947; 9th, 1950; 10th, 1955; 11th, 1960; 12th, 1965; 13th, 1970; and

14th, 1975. (For the first 3 editions, before there was a date of "officiality," the year of publication is listed.) See also, Powers, J. L.; Trends in official drugs and a preview of the new National Formulary (VIII), Bull. Natl. Form. Comm. *14*:124f., 1946; and Osborne, G. E., and Lee, C. O.: Graphic story of official galenicals, Bull. Natl. Form. Comm. *15*:185–204, 1947.

77. The nine editions are dated 1806, 1810, 1814, 1818, 1822, 1825, 1827, 1830, and 1831. On early dispensatories of America and related works see Cowen, D. L.: America's Prepharmacopoeial Literature, pp. 19 ff., Madison, Wis., 1961.
78. Alden, E.: *op. cit.* (note 6), p. 57. The four editions were 1810, 1813, 1817, and 1821.
79. The eleven editions edited jointly by Wood and Bache appeared in 1833, 1834, 1836, 1839, 1843, 1845, 1847, 1849, 1851, 1854 and 1858.
80. Wood, H. C., Jr.: The history of the U.S. Dispensatory, J.A.Ph.A. *20*:792, 1931.
81. Since the 15th edition, additional editions have appeared in 1888 (16th), 1894 (17th), 1899 (18th), 1907 (19th), 1918 (20th), 1926 (21st), 1937 (22nd), 1943 (23rd), 1947 (24th), 1960 (25th), 1967 (26th) and 1973 (27th).The consistent popularity and distinction of the *Dispensatory* represents a long and successful cooperation between the editors previously mentioned and their publishers. Grigg and Elliot of Philadelphia published the first 8 editions. Then Lippincott—at that time called Lippincott, Grambo and Company—bought out Grigg and Elliot. For more than a century (from 1851, the 9th edition, until the present) the book has been published by Lippincott.
82. A 2nd edition (revised) appeared already the same year and had to be reprinted the following year, in 1880. Further editions appeared in 1884 (3rd), 1889 (4th), and 1894 (5th), the latter reprinted with a supplement in 1896.
83. Am. Drugg. & Pharm. Rec. *24*:195, 1894.
84. Steinbichler, E.: Geschichte der homöopathischen Arzneibereitungslehre in Deutschland bis 1872, Internationale Gesellschaft . . ., n.s. Bd. 11, Eutin, 1957.
85. Homoeopathic Pharmacopoeia of the United States, p. 17, 7th ed., Philadelphia and Chicago, 1964.
86. J.A.Ph.A. *1*:168, 366, 505, 637, 760, 1307, 1912; *4*:1178, 1915; Lascoff, J. S.: The value of the recipe book to the pharmacist, J.A.Ph.A. *16*:714, 1927. See also the Historical Introduction in the respective R. B. editions.
87. New and Non-official Remedies, 1909, pp. 9 and 10.
88. *Ibid.*
89. Silverman, M. and Lee, P. R.: Pills, Profits, and Politics, pp. 109 and 292, Berkeley, c. 1974.
90. New Drugs Evaluated . . . , p. iii, Chicago, 1965, and J. Am. Med. Assoc. *223*:371, 1973. Although refusing to continue the Council on Drugs in November 1972, the A.M.A. House of Delegates resolved to use "all appropriate AMA resources . . . to delineate clearly the independent A.M.A. policy on drugs and drug therapy." One response to this policy was publication of a new volume, *AMA Drug Evaluations* (1st ed., Chicago, 1971).
91. In the title of the book by Redwood and Procter, Mohr has been erroneously given the Christian name Francis.
92. Am. J. Pharm. *21*:120, 1849.
93. *Ibid.,*: p. 213.
94. England, J. W.: The First Century, p. 403.
95. Am. J. Pharm. *28*:10, 1856.
96. Am. J. Pharm. *27*:574, 1855.
97. In 1859, a 2nd edition and in 1864 a 3rd edition appeared. In this latter the title *Introduction to Practical Pharmacy* was changed to the less specific title *A Treatise on Pharmacy*. The reason for dropping the word "practical" is to be found in the enormous increase in theoretical and scientific matter. After the death of Parrish in 1872, Thomas S. Wiegand published a 4th edition in 1874 and a 5th edition in 1884.
98. The editions of 1885, 1889, 1894, 1905, 1907, and 1917 appeared under the editorship of the original author. Among the many collaborators, E. Fullerton Cook and Charles LaWall, assistants to Remington in the Philadelphia College of Pharmacy, were the most active. Thus it was only natural that after the death of Remington (1918), these two men, more particularly Cook, edited the next (7th) edition, which appeared in 1926, and the 8th edition, issued in 1936. After the death of LaWall in 1937, Cook chose Eric W.

Martin as his partner in the task of editing a 9th edition of Remington's *Practice of Pharmacy* (1948). Martin continued as editor-in-chief for the 12th edition, which appeared in 1961.

99. Am. J. Pharm. *60*:270, 1888; Pharm. Rundschau *6*:148, 1888.

100. A 2nd edition appeared in 1901, a 3rd in 1906, a 4th in 1910 and a 5th in 1916. One year later, in 1917, Charles Caspari, Jr., died. The editorial task of revision was taken over by E. F. Kelly, long assistant and associate of Caspari on the faculty of the Maryland College of Pharmacy. Kelly, in addition to continuing the work, returned to the original intent of making a concise book. The 6th revision, published in 1920, with its 954 pages, still retained the volume to which the book had gradually grown. However, the 7th edition (1926) was condensed to 615 pages, and the 8th edition (1939) to 553 pages.

101. The 2nd edition appeared in 1917, the 3rd in 1926, and the 4th, edited by Arny with the collaboration of R. P. Fischelis, in 1937. A noteworthy feature of Arny's *Principles* was its comprehensive bibliography at the end of each chapter, giving direct reference to the literature covered in the text.

102. Glenn, L. Jenkins was senior editor for the 9th edition appearing in 1957. A more concise competitor, which also has not survived, was by J. H. Beal, titled *Prescription Practice and General Dispensing: an elementary treatise for students of pharmacy* (1908). An interesting attempt to meet the needs of "students of medicine and of pharmacy who desire to acquire a complete knowledge of what a prescription was, is, and should be" (preface to the 4th, 1917, edition) was made by Otto A. Wall, Ph.G., M.D., in his book *The Prescription, Therapeutically, Pharmaceutically, Grammatically, and Historically Considered,* 1888. The most popular book devoted exclusively to the problem of incompatibilities was published by Edsel A. Ruddiman in 1897 under the title *Incompatibilities in Prescriptions.* A 2nd edition appeared in 1900, a 3rd in 1908, a 4th in 1917, a 5th in 1925 and a 6th in 1936.

103. Among them L. E. Sayre's *Organic Materia Medica and Pharmacognosy* (1894), and more recently textbooks by Youngken (first edition in 1922) and by Mansfield (first edition in 1926). The *Textbook of Pharmaceutical Botany* by Heber Youngken was issued from 1914 until 1951, in 7 editions. Much used by students of pharmacy were Bastin's *Elements of Botany,* first published in 1887, the name of which was later changed to *College Botany,* and the books of Henry Kraemer, *Applied Economic Botany* and *Scientific and Applied Pharmacognosy*, both first published in 1915. Based on the 3rd edition of Kraemer's book, E. N. Gathercoal and E. H. Wirth published their *Pharmacognosy* (ed. 2, 1947). A modern view is represented by Robertson Pratt and Heber W. Youngken, Jr., in *Pharmacognosy* (ed. 1, 1951), and Emil Ramstad in *Modern Pharmacognosy* (ed. 1, 1959).

104. John Uri Lloyd's *Chemistry of Medicines* had appeared in 1881. In 1884, William Simon published the 1st edition of his *Manual of Chemistry*. In 1887, Oscar Oldberg and John H. Long published a *Laboratory Manual of Chemistry, General and Pharmaceutical.* In 1894, an *Elementary Course in Inorganic Pharmaceutical Chemistry,* written by F. J. Wulling, appeared, and in 1895 S. P. Sadtler and H. Trimble published their *Textbook of Chemistry for the Use of Pharmaceutical and Medical Students.*

Several pharmacists wrote books on analytic chemistry, one of the first being the *Manual of Chemical Analysis, as applied to the examination of medicinal chemicals,* published by Frederick Hoffmann in 1873 (1883, ed. 2). In 1885 Trimble's *Handbook of Analytic Chemistry* appeared. Of books of more recent vintage, the following are exemplary: E. V. Lynn, *Organic Chemistry, with Applications to Pharmacy and Medicine* (1941); G. L. Jenkins and others, *Quantitative Chemistry* (1931; ed. 3, 1949); G..L. Jenkins and W. H. Hartung, *The Chemistry of Organic Medicinal Products* (1941 ed. 3, 1949); L. M. Parks, Paul J. Jannke, Loyd E. Harris, John E. Christian, *Inorganic Chemistry in Pharmacy* (1949).

104a. Bell, J. E.: A comparative evaluation of drug interaction publications, Am. J. Hosp. Pharm. *28*:938–944, 1971. In the vanguard were works in 1970 by N. J. Sawyer, et al., by E. A. Hartshorn, and by M. S. Cohon; and, in 1971, by S. Garb and, notably, by P. D. Hansten.

105. England, J. W.: The First Century, p. 100; see p. 278 for a history of the journal; also Am. J. Pharm. *76*:223, 1904.

106. The *New York Journal of Pharmacy* (1852-1854)

of the New York College of Pharmacy was revived several times and under different titles. The *Journal and Transactions of the Maryland College of Pharmacy* (1858–1862), *The Pharmacist* (1868–1885) of the Chicago College of Pharmacy, and *the Apothecary* (1891–1897) of the Illinois College of Pharmacy all had only a short existence.

107. Sonnedecker, G.: The Journal [of A.Ph.A.] is born, J.A.Ph.A., ns *1*:744–5 and 776-7, 1961.
108. Sonnedecker, G.: Two decades of progress with the American Journal of Hospital Pharmacy, Am. J. Hosp. Pharm. *19*:215-225, 1962.
109. Other state associations which soon journalized their proceedings were Texas (1926), Maryland (1926), New Jersey (1928) and Wisconsin (1933). More rapid was the development of journals of county and city associations (Meyer, M. M.: The pharmaceutical journals in the U.S., unpublished Master of Science thesis, University of Wisconsin, 1934. The geographic list was published in the J.A.Ph.A. *22*:424, 1933). Sometimes the development went another way: In February, 1927, there appeared the first number of *The New York Pharmacist,* "Official Journal of the N.Y. Pharmaceutical Conference, Inc.," which in July, 1932, became the organ of the New York State Pharmaceutical Association as well. The title changed (1935) to the *New York State Pharmacist,* becoming exclusively the official organ and property of the New York State Pharmaceutical Association. Some of these publications disappeared after a time, became merged with independent commercial journals, or continued as such with changed names.
110. J.A.Ph.A. *22*:424, 1933.

## 16. ECONOMIC AND STRUCTURAL DEVELOPMENT

1. England, J. W.: The first Century of the Philadelphia College of Pharmacy, p. 28, Philadelphia, 1922; Ellis, E. T.: The story of a very old Philadelphia drugstore, Am. J. Pharm. *75*:57, 1903.
2. Proc. A.Ph.A. *2*:24–42, 1853; *3*:34, 1854; *50*:124, 125, 1902.
3. Drugg. Circ. *51*:181, 1901.
4. *Ibid.*
5. Leach, J. G.: History of the Bringhurst Family, pp. 39, 41, 52, Philadelphia, 1901.
6. *Ibid.*: p. 52.
7. Parchen, H. M.: Early days of Montana pharmacy, Drugg. Circ. *51*:191, 1907.
8. Bull. Pharm. *16*:100, 1902; see also Mrtek, M. B., et al.: . . . Philo Carpenter (1805–1886), Pharm. Hist. *12*:151–155, 1970.
9. Besides France, Holland and Switzerland especially practiced for many decades this means of restricting the number of pharmacists.
10. Bull. Pharm. *18*:267, 1904.
11. Rorem, C. R., and Fischelis, R. P.: The Costs of Medicine, p. 207, Chicago, 1932. In regard to the drug purchases of medical practitioners, see p. 92.
12. Young, J. H.: Pioneer nostrum promoter: Thomas W. Dyott, J.A.Ph.A. ns *1*:290, 1961.
13. Liggett, L. K.: Pharmacy in the past 25 years, Pharm. Era *47*:52, 1914.
14. Mason, H. B.: A remarkable pharmacy, Bull. Pharm. *18*:144, 1904.
15. *Ibid.*: p. 229.
16. Drugg. Circ. *51*:105, 1907.
17. A decree entered in the United States Circuit Court for the District of Indiana, May 9, 1907, under the Sherman Antitrust Act, declared all the essential and effective measures of the agreement to be illegal.
18. Drugg. Circ. *51*:434, 1907.
19. N.A.R.D. J. *52*:629, 1931.
20. Decision of December 7, 1936 in the Old Dearborn Case. Wilson, Stephen: The background and operation of the Pennsylvania fair trade law in the drug trade, J.A.Ph.A. *28*:541, 1939.
21. Statement of Maurice Mermey . . . at public hearing, Wednesday, May 25, 1955, before the Special Sub-Committee in Connection with the Study of the Anti-Trust Laws of the Committee on the Judiciary of the U. S. House of Representatives, mimeograph, Bureau of Education on Fair Trade, New York, 1955, p. 3; and, Are we heading for a federal price-fixing law?, Consumer Reports, May, 1958.
22. Statement of Lewis A. Engman, Chairman . . . on S. 408 (mimeograph, Federal Trade Commission), Washington, D.C. February 18, 1975. 4 pp.; and, A Revolt Against Fair Trade . . . , Weekly Pharmacy Reports, *24*:3, 1975 (Feb. 24).
23. Parsons, L. C.: Some economic and social implications of fair trade legislation, J.A.Ph.A. *28*:539, 1939. The account of recent

developments in fair trade is based partly upon Helfand, W. H.: The fair trade movement, American Institute of the History of Pharmacy (unpublished paper), 1962.

24. National Prescription Audit, General Information Report, 12th ed., p. 6, Ambler, Pa., 1973.
25. On price-cutting of prescriptions, for examples see Drug News Weekly, pp. 4 and 5, April 11, 1962, and other issues of this tradepaper. On compounding that survives, see: Market Research Report, Abbott Laboratories (mimeographed), North Chicago, p. 1, July 26, 1962, and National Prescription Audit, loc. cit.
26. Weekly Pharmacy Reports, *12* (No. 2):3, January 14, 1963.
27. Rorem and Fischelis, The Costs of Medicine, p. 85.
28. Mason, H. B.: A new economic order in pharmacy, Proc. A.Ph.A. *49*:470, 1901.
29. Stephenson, H.: Drug store, Am. Drugg. *88*:224, 1933.
30. Garcha, B. S.: The merger jigsaw puzzle, Drug Topics, p. C6, April 16, 1973—an article that offers considerable insight in general concerning the scale and fluidity of amalgamation and expansion since the late 1960's.
31. Delgado, F. A.: Chain and independent drug store, J.A.Ph.A. *26*:931, 1937; N.A.R.D. J. *69*:1424, 1947; and, on population, What the Drug Chains Mean to You, p. 6, New York, N.A.C.D.S., c. 1947.
32. Drug Topics' Drug Trade Marketing Guide, New York, 1961, pp. 10, 12, et passim; also Chain Store Age (Drug Store Manager's Edition), June 1950 [Silver Jubilee Issue], pp. J5 and 14 ff.; and Olsen, in Drug Topics, p. 75, April 8, 1963.
33. Walgreen Pepper Pod (50th Anniversary Issue, June 1951, pp. 19 and 28f.; "Walgreen enters discount house field. . . , Drug Topics, p. 12, April 9, 1962. On sales growth, note Am. J. Pharm. Edu. *38*:313, 1974 and Chain Store Age, May 1973, pp. 79f. It is noteworthy that by 1907 Pharmacist George B. Evans of Philadelphia had, in his 5-unit chain, one drugstore of a "supermarket" type that extended over two floors, and in the prescription department had what might be termed a technician typing labels and maintaining the records for 5 "dispensers." (Mason, H. B.: A million dollars a year, Bull. Pharm., pp. 277–271, 1907)
34. Frank, G.: Pharmacists. . . in economic life, J.A.Ph.A. *19*:1049f., 1930.
35. Drugg, Circ. *51*:149, 1907.
36. Amer. Drugg. & Pharm. Rec. *41*:328, 344, 1902.
37. Rorem and Fischelis: *op. cit.*, p. 74; and Rexall Drug and Chemical Co. Annual Report, p. 7, 1961.
38. Rexall Drug and Chemical Co., Annual Report, pp. 1, 4, 17, and 22, 1962.
39. Amer. Drugg. & Pharm. Rec. *47*:115, 275, 1905.
40. Rorem and Fischelis, *op. cit.*, p. 74.
41. *Ibid.*: p. 75.
42. Drugg. Circ. *51*:149, 1907. Among them we find the New York Consolidated Drug Company "doing business as a regular wholesale institution" and turning over "its $60,000 capital stock about ten times a year"; the Brooklyn Consolidated Drug Company, the Calvert Drug Company of Baltimore; the Washington Wholesale Drug Exchange; and the Philadelphia Wholesale Drug Company (Drugg. Circ. *51*:149, 1907). The latter, founded in 1886 as "Apothecaries' Union, Limited," is one of the oldest American retail druggists' buying clubs, "so successful as virtually to monopolize the wholesale drug business in Philadelphia." Its sales to its 800 members and to other retail dealers in 1930 exceeded $12,000,000.
43. Rorem and Fischelis, *op. cit.*, p. 126.
44. There existed at that time buying clubs of larger importance in 13 cities: Philadelphia, Baltimore, Washington, Providence, New York, Rochester, Buffalo, Cincinnati, Indianapolis, St. Louis, Kansas City, Atchison and Minneapolis. In addition, Weld mentions "a company in Cleveland with branches in Chicago, Columbus, and Detroit, which operates in a similar manner to that of the cooperatives, but which is owned and operated largely as a private enterprise." (Weld, L. H. D.: Cooperative buying by retail druggists, Drugg. Circ. *61*:120, 1917.)
45. 50th Anniversary; Federal Wholesale Druggists' Association Inc. 1915–1965, pp. 7–9, n.p., 1965; Rorem and Fischelis, *op. cit.*, p. 126.
46. *Ibid.*: p. 128.
47. *Ibid.*: pp. 127, 128, Founded as Olcott and McKesson in New York (1833), the name changed to McKesson and Robbins, Inc. in 1853.

48. Road to Market; 125 Years of Distribution Service [by McKesson & Robbins], 1833–1958, New York, 1958. The corporation's growth is all the more remarkable in view of the scandal of fraudulent mismanagement discovered in 1938 (see, e.g., McKesson breakdown, Drug & Cosmetic Ind. *43*:683–685, 1938; and *ibid.*, *44*:37, 1939).
49. Chain Store Age (Drugstore Edition), pp. 41, 46, 51, 53, 55, Oct. 1973. It was with this issue that the Drugstore Edition changed its policy so that henceforth "the two groups—chains and co-ops/voluntaries—will be treated editorially as one entity that controls over 70% of the nation's retail drug volume." (p. 3) The proportion of this volume pharmacy-related (in the sense of prescriptions, other medicaments, toiletries and cosmetics) was at this time 74.4 per cent in the affiliated independent drugstores as compared with 58.3 per cent in the drug chains.
50. Liggett vs. Baldridge, 278 U.S. 105 (1928), decided U. S. Supreme Court, November 19, 1928. Pharm. Era *65*:355, 1928.
51. Beal, J. H.; Directing the trend of evolution in pharmacy, Pract. Drugg. *48*:14, Sept. 1930; Rorem and Fischelis, *op. cit.*, p. 181.
52. Powers, W. E.: Address of the president, Proc. Natl. Assoc. Bds. Pharm., pp. 29 f., 1956.
53. Snyder's Drugstores vs. Minnesota State Board of Pharmacy, District Court, Second Judicial District, File No. 324715, 17 Dec. 1962.
54. Greenberg, Emil, and Sharenow, I. L.: The Constitutional Basis of a Pharmacy Ownership law (mimeographed), p. 11, 1962; and Mellon, L. P.; Legislation, can it effectively limit practice of pharmacy to pharmacists?, J.A.Ph.A. ns *2*:647, 1962.
55. State of Florida vs. Leone, 118 S. 2d 781, as quoted by Leonard F. Mellon in J.A.Ph.A. ns *2*:648, 1962.
56. *Ibid.*: p. 649, quoting a proposal drafted by Judge Andrew Salvest, attorney (1960) for the New Jersey board of pharmacy.
57. *Ibid.*: p. 650.
58. In the Supreme Court of the United States, October Term 1973: No. 72-1176. North Dakota State Board v. Snyder's Drug Stores, Inc.; . . . Joint Brief Amicus Curiae of the American Pharmaceutical Association and the National Association of Retail Druggists, pp. 6 and 11 f.; on the background of the case, North Dakota Supreme Court rules. . . , J.A.Ph.A. ns *14*:390 f., 1974.
59. For the text of the decision, see: Supreme Court of the United States No. 72–1176, North Dakota State Board of Pharmacy v. Snyder's Drug Stores, Inc., December 5, 1973, in: J.A.Ph.A. ns *14*:12–15 (see also editorial, *ibid.*, p. 11).
60. J.A.Ph.A. ns *14*:476, 1974, and A.Ph.A. Weekly, p. 3, April 12, 1975.
61. Francke, D. E.: Editorial: The Supreme Court's Reversal of the Liggett Decision, Drug Intell. & Clin. Pharm. *8*:7, 1974.
62. Data extracted from the Era Druggists Directory and the Statistical Abstracts of the United States.
63. Licensure Statistics 1948, Proc. NABP, pp. 46–57, Chicago, 1948, to which national total I added 6000 as a rough compensation for the missing figure for Illinois. For the 1974 estimate I am indebted to Prof. W. Michael Dickson for permitting access to preliminary data from the Pharmacy Manpower Information Project of the American Association of Colleges of Pharmacy, and applying a preliminary average adjustment factor to the data (publication pending). On the prescription volume increase see, e.g., Manpower, J.A.Ph.A., *19*:541, 1958.
64. Appreciation is expressed to Drs. C. A. Rodowskas, Jr. and W. M. Dickson for access to their preliminary project data. (*Ibid.*)
65. Licensure Statistics. . ., Chicago: National Association of Boards of Pharmacy, in annual Proceedings and as a separate; Dickson, W. M. and Rodowskas, C. A., Jr.: Women in pharmacy—projections for the future, J.A.Ph.A. ns *13*:632, 1973. On women in 19th-century pharmacy see Culp, R. W.: The education, career. . . , Trans. Coll. Physicians Phila, 4th ser., *41*:211–227, 1973, and Sonnedecker, G.: Women as pharmacy students. . . , Veröffent. Internatl. Gesel. Gesch. Pharm., ns 40, pp. 135–141, 1972.
66. Appreciative acknowledgment is made to Paul O. Williams while at the University of Wisconsin for comparative analysis of data for 1948 to 1960. The statistics used are mainly from annual surveys reported in the Proceedings of the National Association of Boards of Pharmacy. Griffenhagen is quoted from his Philadelphia address, World-wide census of pharmacy, J.A.Ph.A., ns *3*:370 f.,

1963. Community pharmacy was included in a business census by the U. S. Bureau of the Census 7 times in the 33 years 1929–1962; while these data are useful, they are complicated by the inclusion of nonpharmacies that sell a certain range of packaged drugs, in all but two of the surveys, and by vagaries of definition.
67. World Directory of Schools of Pharmacy 1963, Geneva, 1966, which gives data for 1963 supplied by governments (except for stated exceptions); and Griffenhagen, G.: A "U.N." of Pharmacy (mimeographed address, 1963), pp. 19 and 21; and published J.A.Ph.A. ns *3*:370 f., 1963.
68. Riley, J. J.: A History of the American Soft Drink Industry, pp. 3, 6, 9 f., 52-57, Washington, D.C., 1958. This carefully written volume includes information on the scientific as well as the commercial background, and on the European as well as American developments.
69. Youth of the fountain, Amer. Drugg. *88*:75, 208, Oct. 1933; J. W. England: *op. cit.*., p. 357; on Elias Durand, see Am. J. Pharm. *45*:508–517, 1873, also *ibid.*, p. 432.
70. Amer. Drugg. *88*:214, Oct. 1933.
71. Delgado, F. A.: *op. cit.*, p. 929. Walgreen Pepper Pod (50th Anniversary Issue), pp. 6 and 12, June 1951. In the early 1920's Charles Walgreen, Sr., experimented with serving hot foods from an "annex" room of his second drugstore; "by 1925–26 we began expanding our fountain menu to include hot foods, chop suey, soups, etc."
72. Expectations by physicians and laymen that the pharmacist will provide food service is cited by Delgado, F. A.: The Professional Pharmacy, ed. 2, p. 1, Washington, 1935, and Rorem and Fischelis, *op. cit.*, p. 65.
73. Drug Topics' Drug Trade Marketing Guide, New York, 1961, pp. 57 f., and N.A.R.D.-Saturday Evening Post: The Independent Druggist, Report No. 1, p. 61, Philadelphia, 1945 and U. S. Census Bureau, for 1972 (through American Druggist, personal communication).
74. The application of this term to any business to the exclusion of others is wrong. All business should be conducted on an ethical basis. The commercialization of the drugstore, as distinguished from professionalization, is not necessarily unethical.
75. England, J. W.: *op. cit.*, p. 65.
76. Sonnedecker, G.: A Franco-American Pharmacist: John T.G.F. de Milhau (1795–1874), Veröffent. Internatl. Gesel. Gesch. Pharm., ns 42, pp. 141–152, 1975.
77. Mason, H. B.: The Metcalf pharmacy in Boston, Bull. Pharm. *22*:279, 1908.
78. Drugg. Circ. *51*:167, 1907. For observations of New York pharmacy in 1903 from a British viewpoint (Thomas Maben), see Am. Drugg. & Pharm. Rec. *42*:132&134, 1903.
79. Liggett, L. K.: Pharmacy in the past 25 years, Phar. Era *47*:51, 1914—a revealing, if biased, look at a pivotal period in pharmacy's history.
80. For example, when Walgreen Drug Stores acquired the three units of Globe Discount City, each unit covered "over 100,000 square feet," of which the prescription department measured about 20 by 20 feet; and other "departments common to drugstores" (including toys and tobacco) measured about 3,000 square feet. (Walgreen enters discount house field . . . , Drug Topics, p. 12, 9 April 1962).
81. Jordan, C. B.: Address, J.A.Ph.A. *20*:812, 1931.
82. Delgado, F. A.: The Professional Pharmacy, p. 1.
83. Am. Prof. Pharm. *11*:905, 1945.
84. Olsen, P. C.: What pharmacy graduates should know . . . , Drug Topics, p. 75, 8 April 1963.
85. The concentration of high-volume prescription practice in a much smaller number of pharmacies is cited from surveys by manufacturers' representatives for the journal *American Professional Pharmacist;* see The Clark-O'Neill Indicia, vol. 5, p. 4, Feb. 1963. A striking claim by *American Professional Pharmacist* (although not corroborated by Olsen's data) is that approximately one third of the American community pharmacies were providing about three fourths of all prescriptions dispensed. (e.g., Am. Prof. Pharm., July 1961, p. 34, n.; Business Publications Audit of Circulation; and personal communication from editor I. Rubin, 15 August 1961). For Olsen's vigorous rebuttal, see Drug Trade News, p. 4, April 6, 1959.
86. The "medication profile" as an element of the clinical approach to practice had beginnings as early as 1946–47; e.g., Aaron Silnutzer, J.A.Ph.A. ns *14*:352, 1974; cf. Jack W. Dorsey, *ibid.*, 353.
87. Apple, W. S.: Reformation in pharmaceutical practice, J.A.Ph.A. ns *5*:188f. and 216, 1965; also White, E. V.; *ibid.*, 532–535 and 552–554.

Ryan, M. R. and Huffman, D.C., Jr., Practicing pharmacy the private-office way, Drug Topics, pp. 25–27, Aug. 20, 1973.

88. Drug Topics, p. 2, 25 April 1949, and Drug Topics' Drug Trade Marketing Guide, p. 28; and Delgado, F. A.: Prescription Department Sales Analysis in Selected Drug Stores, p. 1, Department of Commerce, Washington, D. C.

88*a*. Campbell, N. A. and Hammel, R. W.: Development of the third party payment concept for [American] medical and pharmaceutical services, Pharm. Hist. *15*:117–123, 1973; also PMA . . . Fact Book, pp. 24 & 67, Washington, 1973.

89. Charters, W. W., *et al.*: Basic Material for a Pharmaceutical Curriculum, p. 19, New York, 1927; cf. Delgado, F. A., and Kimball, A. A.: Prescription Department Sales Analysis in Selected Drug Stores, p. *22*; Elliott, E. C. (ed.): The General Report of the Pharmaceutical Survey, pp. 226-228, Washington, D.C., 1950; and "1961 prescription survey," Abbott [Laboratories] Market Research Report (mimeographed, 26 July 1962); National Prescription Audit; General Information Report, p. 3, Dedham, Mass., 1962; ibid., p. 6, Ambler, Pa. Data are not entirely comparable because of varying definitions of what constitutes a "compounded" prescription.

90. *Ibid.*, p. 2, 1973 ed.

91. Charters, W. W.: *op. cit.*, pp. 259 f.; Delgado and Kimball: Prescription Department Sales Analysis, pp. 31 and 35; Mordell, J. S.: The Prescription Study of the Pharmaceutical Survey, pp. 11 and 261 f., Washington, 1949; and Abbott Market Research Report. The reason could not be discerned for the marked difference in proportion of proprietary prescriptions between Charters' 10.29 per cent about 1926 and Delgado's 25 per cent in 1931–32 (20% if considering the most-prescribed ingredients alone). Delgado's figure would be still higher if added to the further 25 per cent that were a mixture of official, proprietary and other nonofficial drugs.

92. Ruth, R. J.: The history of National Pharmacy Week, J.A.Ph.A. *20*:696, 1931; and Sonnedecker, G.: National Pharmacy Week—a pharmacist's vision fulfilled, Tile and Till *34*:38–41, 1948.

93. Abramson, Robert: A brief history of National Pharmacy Week, J.A.Ph.A. (Prac. Ed.) *17*:449, 1956. For the Truman letter, see *ibid.*: *9*:153, 1948.

94. American Social Hygiene Association, J.A.Ph.A. (Prac. Ed.) *1*:65–68, 1940; and committee reports in the Proceedings in following years. See also, Clarke, Walter: Pharmacy's role in the social hygiene program, *ibid.*, *5*:16, 1944; also *9*:295 and 348, 1948.

95. On the developing program and sample materials, see Henderson, Jean: Pharmacies become health information centers, J.A.Ph.A. (Pract. Ed.) *9*:348 ff., 1948; and Fischelis, R. P.: *ibid.*, p. 721. See also, Fischelis, R. P.: The role of the pharmacist in the cancer program (mimeographed address), Public Health Cancer Assoc., New York, Oct. 24, 1949.

96. See special issue on theme of the pharmacist as a health educator, J.A.Ph.A. ns *4*: No. 10, 1964; also, *ibid.*, ns *5*:250 and 472, 1965.

97. Jinks, M.: The contribution of clinical pharmaceutical education to professional practice, Am. J. Pharm. Edu. *38*:712–718, 1974, as a typical characterization of the clinical pharmacy role and potential. Apple, W. S.: Reformation in pharmaceutical practice, J.A.Ph.A. ns *5*: 188 f. and 216, 1965.

98. Van Itallie, P. H.: The beginnings of hospital pharmacy, Pulse of Pharmacy *17*:3, No. 2, 1963.

99. Some Account of the Pennsylvania Hospital . . . , p. 29, Philadelphia, 1754; for Thomas Boulton's indenture, see the reproduction in The First Century of the Philadelphia College of Pharmacy 1821–1921, (J. W. England ed.) p. 22, Philadelphia, 1922.

100. England, J. w.: Pharmacy in a great hospital, Bull. Pharm. *15*:188, 1901, quoting the Philadelphia Hospital Report of 1890, as to earlier conditions.

101. Sonnedecker, G.: Earliest formulary . . ., Drug. Intell. & Clin. Pharm. *6*:430, 1972.

101a. Ott, B.: Hospital pharmacy and its opportunities, J.A.Ph.A. *15*:392, 1926.

102. Landefeld, S.: The rise of the modern hospital idea: 1900–1913, Synthesis; Undergrad. J. Hist. Philos. Sci. *1*:19, No. 3, 1973; citing J.A.M.A. *35*:885, 1900.

103. This segment of the account rests mainly on the work of Prof. Alex Berman, especially Historical currents in American hospital pharmacy, Drug Intell. & Clin. Pharm., *6*:441–447, 1972, and Ten years of the American Society of Hospital Pharmacists 1942–1952 (with Gloria Niemeyer and Don E.

Francke), Bull. Am. Soc. Hosp. Pharm., *9*:No. 4, 1952.

104. Francke, D. E., Latiolais, C. J., Francke, G. N., and Ho, N. F. H.: Mirror to Hospital Pharmacy, a Report of the Audit . . ., p. 36, Washington, D.C., c. 1964.
105. *Ibid.*, p. 58.
106. *Ibid.*, p. 60.
107. *Ibid.*, p. 122f.
108. *Ibid.*, p. 131; and Prescription Drug Data Summary 1971, pp. 29f., Washington, D.C., HEW-SS Pub 59–71 (5–71), 1971.
109. National Prescription Audit, General Information Report, 12th ed., p. 48, Ambler, Pa., 1973.
110. The principles were jointly adopted by the American Hospital Association, American Medical Association, American Pharmaceutical Association, and American Society of Hospital Pharmacists (Amer. J. Hosp. Pharm. *21*:40–41, 1964). For an excellent discussion of the formulary system (and, in the present connection, pp. 139f.), see Francke, D.: *op. cit.*
111. Francke, D. E.: The importance of an historical perspective, Drug Intell. & Clin. Pharm. *8*:55, 1974. The great difference in conservatism and in perspective between hospital pharmacy and pharmaceutical education, attributed by Dr. Francke, tends to be illustrated from a different viewpoint by J. A. Oddis, A.S.H.P. Executive Secretary, in his address, "Facing Up to Hospital Pharmacy Manpower Needs" (ASHP mimeograph), Washington, D.C., November 18, 1966, 16 pp. See also Francke, G: Evolvement of 'clinical pharmacy,' Drug Intell. *3*:348, 1969, and Report of task force on the pharmacist's clinical role, J.A.Ph.A. ns *11*:482, 1971.
112. 100 Years of Business Life, p. 32, Schieffelin & Co., New York, 1894.
113. Drugg. Circ. & Chem. Gaz. *10*:236, 1866; see also *12*:350, 1868; Drugg. Circ. *51*:110, 1907.
114. Moxley, G. B.: Address, Proc. Natl. Wholesale Drugg. Asso., p. 29, 1924.
115. Fisher, Albert: Facts, p. 19; How the Magic Pipeline Works (N.W.D.A. pamphlet), ed. 3, p. 12, New York, 1962. (The latter pamphlet has a useful glossary of business terms used in the drug field, particularly wholesaling.) For an analysis still significant, see Rorem and Fischelis: *op. cit.*, p. 133 et passim.
116. FDC Reports, p. T & G9, June 10, 1974; *ibid.*, p. T & G10, Jan. 13, 1975.
117. Statistical Abstracts of the United States, p. 846, Washington, 1961. On earlier figures and comparative margins, see Historical Statistics of the United States, Colonial Times to 1957, pp. 524 and 525, Washington, 1960. On postwar drop in profit, see Fisher, A. B.: Facts on. . . Service Wholesale Druggists, N.W.D.A. Bull. No. 49, p. 16, New York, 1954. On the changing marketing practices mentioned, see, e.g., Waterman, C. G. *in* Pharmaceutical Wholesalers Association Report of the Year 1960–61, p. 4; on the diagnosis concerning proportional distribution costs, see Werble, Wallace, The revolution in pharmaceutical wholesaling, *ibid.*, p. 27.
118. This section is partly a condensation of Sonnedecker, G.: The rise of drug manufacture in America, Emory Univ. Quart., *21*:73–87, 1965, which was part of a special issue on "The American Drug Scene." I thank Emory University Quarterly for the opportunity to use some of the material here. See also Cowen, D. L.: The role of the pharmaceutical industry, pp. 72–82, in: Safeguarding the Public; Historical Aspects of Medicinal Drug Control (J. B. Blake, ed.), Baltimore, 1970.
119. Sadtler, S. P.: Influence of pharmacists on the development and advance of modern chemistry, Am. J. Pharm. *93*:200, 1921; England, J. W.: The First Century, p. 31.
120. Haynes, W.: American Chemical Industry, Vol. I, p. 211, New York, 1954.
121. England J. W.: *op. cit.*, p. 111, quoting Poulson's Advertiser of Aug. 18, 1826.
122. *Ibid.*, p. 112.
123. *Ibid.*, p. 32.
124. *Ibid.*, p. 32.
125. *Ibid.*, p. 33.
126. Chemical industry's contribution to the nation, 1635–1935, Suppl. to Chem. Industries, p. 41, May, 1935.
127. Its original name was George K. Smith and Company. Successively, it became Smith and Shoemaker, Mahlon K. Smith and Company, and the Smith and Kline Company. The firm was incorporated under its present name, the Smith Kline & French Laboratories, in 1891 (Pharm. Era p. 283, March 12, 1903; also, SK&F: More Than a Century of Progress, Philadelphia, 1963). "The nucleus of the present house of Smith, Kline & French was formed in 1863, when Smith & Shoemaker succeeded to the business of George K. Smith & Co.," according to one interpretation of the transition from a small

pharmacy (Pharm. Era p. 955, Dec. 31, 1896); see also, The Klines of SKF . . ., Med. Times *88*:775–780, 1960.

128. In 1876, after John Uri Lloyd had entered into partnership, the H. M. Merrell Company changed its name to Merrell, Thorp and Lloyd; in 1881 to Thorp and Lloyd Brothers; in 1885 to Lloyd Brothers and in 1924 to Lloyd Brothers Pharmacists, Inc. Under John Uri Lloyd the concern assumed a leading position in the field of plant preparations of every kind and, moreover, one of the valuable sources of progress in plant chemistry, colloidal chemistry and new pharmaceutical methods and devices. A list of the earliest "drug houses" still in existence, valuable if the meaning of some of the dates is understood, appears in Drug and Cosmetic Industry *70*:29, Jan., 1952. (This includes additions and corrections to all previous lists published by Drug and Cosmetic Industry.)
129. Lee, C. O.: The Shakers as pioneers in the American herb and drug industry, Am. J. Pharm. *132*:178–193, 1960; Andrews, E. D.: The New York Shakers and their industries, N.Y. State Mus. Circ. *2*:5, 1930; Hoffman, G. N.: Mt. Lebanon medicine makers, the Shakers, Pharm. Era *53*:197, 1920.
130. Pharm. Rec. *23*:141, 1905.
131. New Idea, *27*:(No. 1):3, 1905; and Lakey, R. T.: Frederick Stearns, pharmacist, J.A.Ph.A. (Pract. Ed.) *9*:486–489, 1948.
132. Pharm. Rundschau *10*:276, 1892; England, J. W.: The First Century, p. 216; Remington, J. P.; E. R. Squibb, Am. J. Pharm. *73*:420, 1901. For a full-length biography see Blochman, L. G.: Doctor Squibb; The Life and Times of a Rugged Idealist, New York, 1958, 371 pp.
133. Smith, G. W.: The Squibb laboratory in 1863, J. Hist. Med. *13*:382–394, 1958.
134. Pharm. Rundschau *5*:250, 1887.
135. England, J. W.: The First Century, p. 107.
136. Pharm. Era *16*:941, 1896; Foote, P. A; Tablets, Madison, Wis., Bull. of the Univ. of Wisconsin, Ser. No. 1566, Gen. Ser. No. 1340, Dec. 1928; Griffenhagen, G., and Sonnedecker, G.: A history of sugar-coated pills and tablets, J.A.Ph.A. (Pract. Ed.) *18*:486–488 and 553–555, 1957; Urdang, George: Compressed tablet, What's New (Abbott Labs.), p. 16, Fall 1943.
137. *Ibid.,*: especially Foote, pp. 95 f., and Urdang, p. 16.
138. Facts about Pharmacy and Pharmaceuticals, New York, 1958, pp. 12f., Brown, Francis C.: The Pharmaceutical Industry, pp. 20 f. (republished separately, from Glover and Cornell: The Development of American Industries, New York, 1951).
139. Taylor, F. O.: 45 years of manufacturing pharmacy, J.A.Ph.A. *4*:468, 1915.
140. J. Chem. Ed. *8*:477, 1931.
141. Tile and Till *12*:30, 1927.
142. *Ibid.*, p. 50.
143. Mallinckrodt Chemical Works: Saint Louis Exhibition, 1904, p. 3.
144. Chemical industry's contribution, *op. cit.*, p. 139.
145. The discussion concerning Sterling Drug Incorporated is based on, and partly literally from, The Sterling Story, published by the firm in 1947.
146. Dunn, C. W.: Pharmaceutical industry progress, Drug & Cosm. Ind. *72*:554, 1953.
147. PMA Prescription Drug industry Fact Book, p. 13, Washington, 1973; and Administered Prices: Hearings Before the Subcommittee on Antitrust and Monopoly of the Committee on the Judiciary, U. S. Senate, 86th Congress, 2nd Session, Part 19, Washington, D.C.,1960, p. 10,760.
148. Statistical Abstract of the United States, 1948, p. 840; cf., Statistical Abstract of the United States, 1961, p. 782 (for changing census classification, see also p. 776). Facts about Pharmacy and Pharmaceuticals, pp. 12 f., New York, 1958.

    Unless otherwise specified, 1972 data come from the PMA's Prescription Drug Industry Fact Book, Washington, D.C., 1973. 101 pp. For access to further information on the American drug industry, see especially Southern, W. A.: Sources of drug market data, Drug & Cosm. Ind. *73*:328–9 and 417–21, 1953, and Weindling, N.: Statistical Sources for Pharmacists, J.A.Ph.A. ns *14*:26–30, 1974.
149. Searle, J. G., *et al.*: The pharmaceutical industry, J. mondial Pharmacie, No. 3, p. 211, 1961.
150. Rorem and Fischelis, *op. cit.*, pp. 109–110.
151. *Ibid.*, p. 114.
152. *Ibid.*, p. 102 and 104.
153. Olsen, P. C.: Marketing drug products, Drug Trade News, p. 20, April 6, 1959; and Drug Topics, p. 75, April 8, 1963. Also Drug Topics, pp. 1 and 55, Sept. 27, 1948.
154. Statistical Abstract of the United States 1961, pp. 880 and 882; and FDC Reports, *25*:16, April 22, 1963;. . . Fact Book, p. 59, 1973.

155. Pharmaceutical Manufacturers Association, Ethical Drug Industry Survey of Research and Development Expenditures 1960–61, p. 1, Washington, D.C., June, 1961; Pharmaceutical Manufacturers Association Yearbook 1962–63, pp. 178 and 180, Washington, D.C., n.d. The sample consisted of 86 PMA firms.
156. PMA Prescription Drug Industry Fact Book, p. 47, Washington, D.C., 1973. For somewhat different and more detailed analysis see, de Haen, Paul: Review of Drugs, 1941–1961; Single Chemical Entities Introduced in the United States and Patent Status (multilith, Pharmaceutical Manufacturers Association), Washington, D.C., 1962; see especially the revision sheets. On the early history, Weikel, M. K., and Sonnedecker, G.: Emergence of Research as a Function of American Pharmaceutical Industry (mimeograph, University of Wisconsin), Madison, 1963.
157. FDC Reports, *25*:11, April 22, 1963, based on the studies of Paul de Haen of New York. Lasagna, L. and Wardell W.: Regulation and Drug Development, Washington, 1975.
158. For an informative exposition of some of the issues since the 1950's from a viewpoint not atypical of industry's critics, see Silverman, M. and Lee, P. L.: Pills, Profits, and Politics, Berkeley and Los Angeles, ca. 1974. 403 pp.
159. See also, Francke, D. E., Latiolais, C., Francke, G. and Ho, N.: Mirror to Hospital Pharmacy; A Report of the Audit . . ., pp. 36 (sec. 2.0) & 38 (sec. 2.5), Washington, 1964, for illuminating comment on the relationships between pharmaceutical industry and the professions and the public interest.

## 17. THE AMERICAN PHARMACIST IN PUBLIC SERVICE

1. England, J. W.: The First Century of the Philadelphia College of Pharmacy, pp. 348, 351, 352, Philadelphia, 1922.
2. *Ibid.*: p. 353; Urdang, G. : The influence of the Quakers on Philadelphia institutions, Am. J. Pharm. *118*:81–88, 1946.
3. England, J. W.: *op. cit.*, p. 356.
4. Maisch, J. M.: G. H. E. Mühlenberg als Botaniker, Pharm. Rundschau *4*:119, 1886.
5. Am. Prof. Pharm. *29*:58-64, 1963. For some other examples see Drug Topics, p. 40, Feb. 2, 1959; p. 15, March 16, 1959; p. 46, Aug. 17, 1959; p. 2, Sept. 28, 1959.
6. The types of service by pharmacists that have been needed are described by Shriver, R. S.: The pharmacists and the Peace Corps, J.A.Ph.A. ns *2*:353–354, 1962, and Goldsmith, D. and McTigue, J.: Pharmacists in the Peace Corps, J.A.Ph.A. ns *3*:618 f., 1963.
7. Information concerning pharmacists and their services in humanitarian work, either religious or secular, is invited for the historical record by the American Institute of the History of Pharmacy, whose address is: Pharmacy Building, Madison, Wisconsin 53706. While no central registry has come to light, two of the pharmacist-missionaries–Henry C. Kammerer of Trenton, N.J. (about 1954) and James S. Palmgren of 532 Sheridan Road, Evanston, Ill.—served their colleagues well by compiling information, and they have kindly supplied most of the following names of American pharmacist-missionaries: Albert S. Bauman, Miss Frances Bell, Richard Blakney, Muriel Clemenger, H. S. Cliff, Mr. and Mrs. Ronald G. Coppola, Ronald Esson, Mrs. Max Gray, Lorraine Gribbons, Miss Barbara Hartman, Larkin E. Harvey, Dorothy Ireland, Miss Betty K. Job, Henry Kammerer, Mrs. B. Koschade, Samson Huri Lal, C. O. Lee, Jack Lesshafft, Kennie M. Linn, William Wayne Logan, Donald Lutes, Curtis Matthews, Richard McLean, Harold E. McMillan, Robert A. McRuer, E. N. Meuser, James S. Palmgren, R. T. Roberts, Mr. Ronnesson(?), Neil Solvik, Miss Emmie Stevens, Raymond E. Watson, Norman Whipple and Miss J. S. Williams. Lorraine Gribbens wrote from Borneo in Am.J. Pharm. Ed. *26*:475-480, 1962, and J.A.Ph.A. *3*:610–614, 1963. Stilwell, D.: MAP—international medical help, J.A.Ph.A., ns *12*:631 f., 1972
8. The project was conceived by a physician, and the American Pharmaceutical Association helped to raise funds. On the project, see Health mission to the world, J.A.Ph.A. (Pract. Ed.) *21*:764–765, 1960; on experiences of one of the pharmacists, see Sherwood, M. F.; Letters from S. S. Hope, J.A.Ph.A. ns *2*:708–710, 1962, S. S. Hope headed for scrap pile, Wi. State J., Feb., 13, 1975, sec., 6, p. 1.
9. Griffenhagen, G. B.: American pharmacists in political life, J.A.Ph.A. ns *6*, 376 and 378, 1966.
10. J.A.Ph.A. *16*:592, 1927; N.A.R.D. J. *65*:564,

1945; Costello, P. H.: Survey of pharmacy laws, p. 62, Proc. Natl. Assoc. Bds. Pharm., 1955; personal communication from American Pharmaceutical Association (G. Griffenhagen), June 26, 1961; see also A.Ph.A. Newsletter, p. 3, June 30, 1962, and Costello, *ibid.*, p. 67, 1961. For representative accounts of pharmacists as mayors see, e.g., Drug Topics, 1959: Aug. 17, p. 2; Aug. 31, p. 4; Sept. 14, p. 58; Oct. 26, p. 3; and Nov. 23, p. 4; and 1960: Feb. 15, p. 2, and Aug. 15, p. 2. For a special issue on the pharmacist in political and civic life see J.A.Ph.A. ns 2(No. 7), July, 1962.

11. King, R. O.: The city that druggists run, Am. Drugg. *88*:26, 90, Dec., 1933.
12. Griffenhagen, G. B.: Stepping stones in Golden State pharmacy, Pac. Drug Rev., 1950; a reprint was issued under the title "The Story of California Pharmacy" by the American Institute of the History of Pharmacy, Madison, Wis., 1950.
13. Ewe, George: David Henshaw—From druggist to secretary of the Navy, J.A.Ph.A. *24*:858, 860, 1935; also see Cyclopaedia of American Biography.
14. On Carl Durham (b. 1892) see the feature "Nuclear pharmacist," New York Times, Feb. 20, 1957, and on Hubert Humphrey (b.1911) see Time magazine, Feb. 1, 1960, pp. 13–16. Griffenhagen, G. B.: American pharmacists in political life, J.A.Ph.A. ns *6:* 380 and 382, 1966.
15. Wolfe, H. G.: James Cutbush—author, teacher, Apothecary General, Am. J. Pharm. Ed. *12*:89, 125, 1948.
16. Am. J. Pharm. *34*:93, 1862.
17. Rittenhouse, H. N.: U. S. Army medical storekeepers, Am. J. Pharm. *37*:87 ff., 1865; Stevens, Hennel: The medical purveying department of the United States Army, Am. J. Pharm. *37*:91 ff., 1865.
18. Fell, E. R.: The pharmaceutical department of the U. S. A. Hospital, Am. J. Pharm. *37*:107, 1865. Smith, G. W.: Medicines for the Union Army; the United States Army Laboratories During the Civil War, pp. 9–10, Madison, 1962.
19. Proc. A.Ph.A. *42*:vi, 1894; *43*:75 ff., 1895.
20. Proc. A.Ph.A. *46*:72, 1898; *Ibid., 47*:117 ff., 1899.
21. Proc. A.Ph.A. *50*:201, 1902.
22. Proc. A.Ph.A. *51*:111, 1903; Drugg. Circ. *46*:218, 1903.
23. J.A.Ph.A. *5*:1037, 1408, 1916.
24. J.A.Ph.A. *11*:764, 1922, and *13*:263, 1924.
25. J.A.Ph.A. *26*:1051, 1937.
26. For a good review especially of developments from the 1930's until after World War II, by the Chairman of the Joint Committee on Status of Pharmacists in Government Service, see: Einbeck, A. H.: Pharmacy in the army and navy, Merck Report, pp. 22–26, Jan., 1947.
27. Committee on Pharmacists in Government Service, J. Am. Pharm. Assoc. ns *3*:330, 1963. Donehew, G. R.: The career and training of an Army pharmacy officer, J.A.Ph.A., ns *14*: 679–681, 1974.
28. This professional level was authorized (1946) by Public Law 293, 79th Congress.

    Trygstad, V. O.: Utilization of Pharmacists in Veterans Administration (mimeographed address, Pharmacy Section, Association of Military Surgeons of the United States), Nov. 11, 1953, in Kremers Reference Files, Pharmaceutical Library, University of Wisconsin, Madison; on author Trygstad, then Director of the V.A. Pharmacy Service, see Drug Topics, March 25, 1963, p. 20.
29. Promotions up to the grade corresponding to Captain in the Army were available at this time. See: Parker bill passed by Congress, Bulletin No. 5 (mimeograph, American Pharmaceutical Association), April 18, 1930 (in Kremers Reference Files, Pharmaceutical Library, University of Wisconsin).
30. Archambault, G. F.: Benjamin E. Holsendorf 1874–1944, Am. J. Pharm. Edu. *14*:305–309, 1950.
31. Archambault, G. F.: Your profession in the U. S. Public Health Service, J.A.Ph.A. (Pract. Ed.) *9*:39–41, 1948; Archambault, G. F., Foster, T. A., and Kinsey, R. D. : Pharmacy in the U. S. Public Health Service . . . then and now, J.A.Ph.A. (Pract. Ed.) *9*:345–347, 376–384, 1948.
32. In a personal communication, George F. Archambault stated, "The utilization of pharmacists *per se* in the present U. S. Public Health Service program is due in main to the foresightedness of three individuals, Dr. R. C. Williams, Assistant Surgeon General, Chief of the Bureau of Medical Services; Dr. Otis L. Anderson, Medical Director, Chief of the Division of Hospitals; and Dr. G. Halsey Hunt, Senior Surgeon, Assistant Chief of the Division of Hospitals.
33. Einbeck, A.; Report of the [joint] Committee

on the Status of Pharmacists in Government Service (mimeographed, American Pharmaceutical Association meeting), (in Kremers Reference Files, Pharmaceutical Library, University of Wisconsin). The quotation is from Winship, H. W. III: [U.S.P.H.S.] Pharmacy goes west: cultivating the Navajo Indians, J.A.Ph.A. ns *4*:599, 1964. On Foster, see Am. J. Hosp. Pharm. *17*:377 f., 1960; on Archambault, see Who's Who in America, and Am. J. Hosp. Pharm. *16*:543, 1959.

34. Besides the Kremers Reference Files, Pharmaceutical Library, University of Wisconsin, the following sources of biographical information were consulted: on Power, Am. J. Chem. Ed. *31*:258, 1954; on Giordano, Who's Who in America and Drug Topics, July 30, 1962, pp. 3 and 44; on Bransky, Am. J. Pharm. *132*:352, 1960; on Gasen, J.A.Ph.A. (Pract. Ed.) *6*:183, 1945. On Smithsonian, see Hamarneh, S. K.: History of the Division of Medical Sciences. . . , in Contributions from the Museum of History and Technology, U. S. National Museum Bull. 240, pp. 269–300, Washington, D.C., 1964.
35. HEW's Weikel discusses MAC. . . , A.Ph.A. Newsletter, Jan. 4, 1975, pp. 2–4. In a somewhat related category is pharmacist William Murfin who gave up practice in Ft. Pierce, Fla., to become Associate Commissioner of the Small Business Administration (1969) in the Federal government (Drug Topics, March 31, 1969, p. 10).
36. Hutchins, Harold: Heroic druggists triumph over flood, Am. Drugg. *93*:24, 66, May, 1936.
37. Emergency pharmacy. . . , Drug Topics Oct. 18, 1965, p. 6.
38. See the civil defense issue of J.A.Ph.A. *21*: No. 10, 1960, particularly (Burney) p. 623 and (Dodge) p. 629. For other examples, see J.A.Ph.A. ns *5*:545, 622, & 659, 1965.

## 18. CONTRIBUTIONS BY PHARMACISTS TO SCIENCE AND INDUSTRY

1. Sadtler, S. P.: Influence of pharmacists on the development and advance of modern chemistry, Am. J. Pharm. *93*:198, 1921.
2. Dictionary of National [British] Biography, London *14*:186, 1888.
3. Bouvet, Maurice: Histoire de la pharmacie en France, p. 368 ff., Paris, 1937.
4. André-Pontier, L.: Histoire de la pharmacie, p. 53, Paris, 1900. The note concerning Pasteur in Ferchl: Chemischpharmazeutisches Bio-und Bibliographikon, p. 396, Mittenwald, 1937, as an "apothecary's apprentice in Besançon," is erroneous. André-Pontier states that Pasteur, "who never was a pharmaceutical apprentice, visited with an apothecary of his town during his college time at Besançon, as frequently as possible, in order to become familiar with the chemical reactions."
5. Nordenskiöld, Erik: The History of Biology, p. 377, New York, London, 1928; Urdang, G.: Berzelius and Pharmacy, J.A.Ph.A. *37*:481–485, 1948.
6. Hoefer, Ferdinand: La chimie, p. 3, Paris, 1865.
7. On the role played by pharmacists in chemical education, see Urdang, G.: Pharmacy's Part in Society, pp. 22–31, Madison, Wis., 1946.
8. For a discussion of Scheele's life and work, see Urdang, G.: The Apothecary Chemist Carl Wilhelm Scheele, Madison, Wis., 1942. On the role played by pharmacists in the acceptance of Lavoisier's views, see Urdang, G.: Lavoisier's "Chemical Revolution" and Pharmacy, Am. J. Pharm. Ed. *18*:216–222, 1954. For a good analysis of the complex of circumstances surrounding the discovery of oxygen, and Scheele's claim to priority, see J. R. Partington: The discovery of oxygen, J. Chem. Edu. *39*:123–125, 1962.
9. "The Forgotten Chemist," The Laboratory (Fisher Scientific Co., Pittsburgh), vol. 7, no. 2, p. 19.
10. On Klaproth, see Dann, G. E.: Martin Heinrich Klaproth (1743–1817). Ein deutscher Apotheker und Chemiker, Berlin, 1958; Urdang, G.: M. H. Klaproth, J.A.Ph.A. (Pract. Ed.) *4*:358–361, 1943.
11. Lieben, Fritz: Geschichte der physiologischen Chemie, p. 44, Leipzig, Wien, 1935.
12. On Marggraf, see the article by M. S. Staum in the Dictionary of Scientific Biography, vol. 9, pp. 104–107, New York, 1974. See also Kopp, Hermann: Geschichte der Chemie, vol. 1, pp. 208–211, Braunschweig, 1843.
13. Walden, Paul: Tobias Lowitz, ein vergessener Physiko-Chemiker, Diergart's Beiträge zur Geschichte der Chemie, Gedächtnisband für G. W. A. Kahlbaum, Leipzig, Wien, 1909, p. 533; Bloch, M.: Tobias Lowitz, in Bugge: Buch der grossen Chemiker, *1*, p. 362, Berlin, 1929.
14. Bouvet, M.: *op. cit.*, p. 372.

15. Speter, Max: Liebig oder Soubeiran, Chem. Ztg. *55*:781, 1931.
16. Lieben, F.: *op. cit.*, p. 70.
17. The Laboratory, *loc. cit.*, p. 18.
18. Wallrabe, Gottfried: Zum Gedächtnis an Karl Gottfried Hagen, Pharm. Ztg. *74*:286, 1929.
19. Communications de l'Académie de Médicine de 1829 à 1833, quoted after Bouvet, M.: *op. cit.*, p. 380.
20. Bouvet, M.: *op. cit.*, p. 371.
21. Rappaport, R.: G. F. Rouelle: An Eighteenth-Century Chemist and Teacher, Chymia *6*:82, 1960; Leicester, H. and Klickstein, H.: A Source Book in Chemistry 1400–1900, pp. 75–79, Cambridge, Mass., 1963.
22. Morton, A. A.: Laboratory Technique in Organic Chemistry, p. 202, New York, London, 1938.
23. *Ibid.*: pp. 38, 214.
24. For further information on many of the chemical discoveries, theories and techniques discussed in this section, see Ihde, A. J.: The Development of Modern Chemistry, New York, 1964.
25. Rosenthaler, Ludwig: Die Entwicklung der Pflanzenchemie von Du Clos bis Scheele, Ber. deutsch. pharm. Gesellsch. *14*:295, 1904.
26. A translated excerpt from Sertürner's 1817 paper appears in Holmstedt, B. and Liljestrand, G.: Readings in Pharmacology, pp. 72–76, Oxford, 1963.
27. On the work of these men, see Delépine, M.: Joseph Pelletier and Joseph Caventou, translated by Ralph Oesper, J. Chem. Ed. *28*:454–460, 1951; also see the articles by Alex Berman in the Dictionary of Scientific Biography, vol. 3, pp. 159–160, New York, 1971 (Caventou) and vol. 10, pp. 497–498, New York, 1974 (Pelletier).
28. Zaunick, Rudolph: Albert Niemann, der Entdecker des Kokains, die Pharmazie *4*:475–477, 1949.
29. Mayer, F. F.: Assay of Alkaloids, Am. J. Pharm. *35*:20–29, 1863; Hoffmann, Fr.: Zur Geschichte des Mayerschen Alkaloid Reagenz und Ferdinand F. Mayer's, Pharm. Rund. *12*:125–131, 1894. Mayer's claims were not entirely unchallenged (Am. J. Pharm. *37*:5–16, 1865).
30. Pharm. J. & Pharm., London *117*:726, 1926.
31. Griffith, Ivor: Frederick Belding Power, Am. J. Pharm. *99*:252, 1927. See also the same author: A half century in plant chemistry, Am. J. Pharm. *96*:601, 1924.
32. The comment and the examples concerning the remarkable contribution of French hospital pharmacists are based entirely on Berman, Alex: The scientific tradition in French hospital pharmacy, Am. J. Hosp. Pharm. *18*:116, 1961.
33. Ihde, A. J.: *op. cit.*, p. 162.
34. Lieben, Fr.: *op. cit.*, p. 395.
35. *Ibid.*: p. 340. On Lowitz, see Leicester, H.: Tobias Lowitz—Discoverer of Basic Laboratory Methods, J. Chem. Edu. *22*:149–151, 1945.
36. *Ibid.*: p. 42.
37. *Ibid.*: p. 597.
38. Graduate Enrollment Data, October, 1973 and Graduate Study in Member Colleges, 1974–1975, Am. J. Pharm. Ed. *38*:250–268, 1974.
39. Urdang, G.: Pharmacy's Part in Society, *op. cit.*, pp. 70, 71; see also Delépine, M.: Life and Works of Ernest Fourneau, 1872–1949, Bull. soc. chim., 1950, pp. 953–982; Henry, T. A.: Ernest Fourneau, 1872–1949, J. Chem. Soc., 1952, pp. 261–266.
40. Chen, K. K.: In Pursuit of Science, J. Am. Ph. Assoc. ns *6*:27, 1966.
41. Binz, Arthur: Chemie, Technik und Weltgeschichte, Z. ang. Chemie *40*:450, 1927.
42. Kopp, H.: *op. cit.*, p. 227.
43. Kränzlein, G.: Zum hundertjährigen Gedächtnis der Arbeiten von F. F. Runge, Z. ang. Chemie *48*:1, 1935, p. 1.
44. *Ibid.*: p. 2; Urdang, G.: Der Anilinentdecker F. F. Runge, Pharm. Ztg. *80*:526, 1935.
45. Adlung, A. and Urdang, G.: Grundriss der Geschichte der deutschen Pharmazie, p. 488, Berlin, 1935.
46. The inventor of the caoutchouc synthesis Fritz Hofmann wrote the letter quoted in response to a request of Urdang, then editor of the Pharmazeutische Zeitung. It was published in Pharm. Ztg. *79*:999, 1934, under the title: Der Vater der Kautschuksynthese, Apotheker Fritz Hofmann. For biography, see: Schneider, Wolfgang: Fritz Hofmann, Pharm. Industrie *19*:38–41, 1957, and Zimmermann, Walther: Fritz Hofmann, Deutsch. Apoth. Ztg. *87*:1286–88, 1938.
47. Urdang, G.: Hermann Thoms, Pharm. Ztg. *76*:1351, 1931.
48. Ritsert, E.: Über den Werdegang des Anästhesins, Pharm. Ztg. *70*:1006, 1925.
49. Urdang, G.: Die deutsche Apotheke als Keimzelle der Deutschen pharmazeutischen Industrie, Die Vorträge der Hauptversammlung der Gesellschaft für Geschichte der Pharmazie in

Wien, 1931, p. 93, Mittenwald, 1931; Urdang, G.: Retail pharmacy as the nucleus of the pharmaceutical industry, Bull. Hist. Med., Suppl. No. 3, pp. 325–346, 1944.

50. Dannemann, Friedrich: Vom Werden der naturwissenschaftlichen Probleme, p. 269, Leipzig, 1928.
51. Adlung and Urdang: *op. cit.*, p. 440.
52. Gilbert's Annalen *7*:525, 1801.
53. Ferchl, F. and Süssenguth, A.: Kurzgeschichte der Chemie, p. 169, Mittenwald, 1936. (English edition under the title, A Pictorial History of Chemistry, pp. 182–183, London, 1939.)
54. Adlung and Urdang: *op. cit.*, p. 452.
55. *Ibid.*: p. 470.
56. Green, J. Reynolds: A History of Botany, 1860–1900, Oxford, p. 232.
57. André-Pontier, L.: *op. cit.*, p. 51.
58. Pharm. J. *146*:143, 1941.
59. Personal communication from Mr. Howard Bayles, Norwich, England; Chem. & Drug. *116*:255, 295, 1932.
60. Sigerist, H. E.: The Great Doctors, pp. 374–378, Garden City, N.Y., 1958 (Doubleday Anchor paperback edition).
61. Heimen, H.: Apotheker Pilâtre de Rozier, der erste Luftschiffer, Pharm. Ztg. *69*:1120, 1924.
62. Urdang, G.: Berühmte Berliner Apotheker, Pharm. Ztg. *77*:1239, 1932. See also, Seabra, P.: Oxidase in biology and in flying research, Med. Times, Dec., 1943; and Urdang, G.: Pharmacy and aviation, Bull. Hist. Med. *15*:324–326, 1944.
63. Urdang, G.: Pharmacy's Part in Society, *op. cit.* offers a more detailed and pictorially documented (47 illustrations) study of the subject dealt with in this chapter.

## APPENDIX 5. PHARMACY'S HISTORY—A GROWING AWARENESS

1. Versuch einer Geschichte des Apothekenwesens in der freyen Reichsstadt Nürnberg, Nuremberg, 1722 (facsimile edition, Nuremberg, 1932). Wolf, E.: Ueber die Anfaenge der Pharmaziegeschichtschreibung; von Johannes Ruellius, 1529, bis David Peter Hermann Schmidt, 1835, (inaugural dissertation), Marburg, 1965, 164 pp.
2. For example, those of the pharmacists J. C. Wiegleb, J. Fr. Gmelin, and J. B. Trommsdorff. J. A. Buchner's text (Vollständiger Inbegriff der Pharmacie, 1822–1827) achieved a more elaborate account. (On these authors, see Glossary.) Much attention also was paid to pharmacy in an early history of chemistry (1843–1847) by H. Kopp.
3. For example, see the note "Bibliography" in Appendix 7, as well as the "Notes and References" to each chapter of this volume, and Sonnedecker's bibliographic essay in Remington's Pharmaceutical Sciences (J. E. Hoover, ed.), pp. 16–18, 15th ed., Easton, 1975.
4. Urdang, G.: The pharmaceutico-historical movement, Am. J. Pharm. Ed. *16*:214, 1952. See also his, The idea and the task of the history of pharmacy, J. Am. Ph. Assoc. *27*:909–913, 1938.
5. For information on the Academy and its individual members, see: Académie Internationale d'Histoire de la Pharmacie, Acta Pharmaciae Historica; Edition à l'occasion du XXeme anniversaire de la fondation (G. Folch Jou and H. Tartalja, eds.), Madrid, 1974, 207 pp. The ordinary (full) members from the USA 1952–1975 have been George Urdang, Glenn Sonnedecker, and George Griffenhagen.
6. Stieb, E. W.: American Institute of the History of Pharmacy, Through Two Decades, Madison, Wi, 1961, 25 pp.; see particularly the annual Proceedings Issue of *Pharmacy in History* for subsequent years.
7. Sonnedecker, G.: A survey of the status of history of pharmacy in American pharmaceutical education, Am. J. Pharm. Ed. *16*:21, 1952 and Grosicki, T. S.: History of Pharmacy in the Five-Year Program, Am. J. Pharm. Ed. *27*:237, 1963.
8. Urdang, G.: History of pharmacy as an academic discipline, J. Hist. Med., *3*:5–10, 1948 (his first lecture as full professor at Wisconsin). On the man, see Pharm. in Hist., *5*:1960, Nos. 2 & 3; and on Kremers see, Urdang, G.: Edward Kremers (1865–1941): reformer of American pharmaceutical education, Am. J. Pharm. Ed. *11*:631, 1947.
9. Griffenhagen, G.: Pharmacy Museums, p. 8, Madison, 1956. For information on the evolution of museums both in general and pharmaceutically, see also Hamarneh, S. K.: Temples of the Muses and a History of Pharmacy Museums, Tokyo, Japan, 1972.
10. Ibid., p. 8.
11. Ibid., pp. 9 & 11; Häfliger, J. A.: Pharmazeutische Altertumskunde. . ., p. 9, Zürich, 1931. The latter is a kind of prototypical monograph on pharmaceutical artifacts, as well as on a specific collection. (The Univer-

sity of Basel still remains outstanding internationally for its richness of rarities.)

12. Hamarneh, S. K.: History of the Division of Medical Sciences, U. S. National Museum Bulletin, No. 240, pp. 269–300, Washington, D.C., 1964.
13. Urdang, G.: New light on the history of show globes, J.A.Ph.A. (Pract. Ed.) *10*:604–606 & 640, 1949; Griffenhagen, G.: The show globe—a symbol of pharmacy, in: Readings in Pharmacy (P. A. Doyle, ed.), pp. 111–117, New York, 1962.
14. These four references may be especially helpful to novice collectors for the guidance they offer to further literature. Three are inexpensive paperbacks published by the American Institute of the History of Pharmacy (Pharmacy Building, Madison, WI 53706, U.S.A.): Hamarneh, S. K.: Pharmacy Museums . . . U.S.A. (1972), with a bibliography in 11 topical categories partly relevant to collecting (pp. 41–49). Griffenhagen, G. and Stieb, E. W.: Tools of the Apothecary; A Select Bibliography (1975), a valuable collector-oriented listing of historical publications on specific types of equipment classified under topical headings. The unique Historical Hobbies for the Pharmacist, G. A. Bender and J. Parascandola, eds. (1974), in which five pharmacists tell of their experiences in five fields and the literature that they found useful.

    For a combination of practical value (identification and dating) and sheer pleasure, most collectors of pharmaceutical Americana place high value on the annual catalogs issued by large wholesale druggists, which had become by the 1880's profusely illustrated bound volumes. One of these volumes still can be discovered occasionally at dealers in out-of-print books; and the copies held by libraries around the country have been charted (extensively, though not completely) in, Romaine, L. B.: A Guide to American Trade Catalogs 1744–1900, pp. 127–137 (Chapt. 19: Drugs and Pharmaceuticals), New York: R. R. Bowker, 1960.

## APPENDIX 6. PHARMACEUTICAL LITERATURE

### Italy

1. Thompson, C. J. S.: The Mystery and Art of the Apothecary, p. 129, London, 1929; Zimmerman, L.: Saladini de Asculo Serenitatis Principis Tarenti Physici Principalis Compendium Aromatariorum, Leipzig, 1919.
2. Schelenz, H.: Geschichte der Pharmazie, p. 334, Berlin, 1904 (reprinted, 1965).
3. *Ibid.*, p. 337.
4. Schumacher, B.: Das Luminare majus von Joannes Jacobus Manlius de Bosco 1536, Mittenwald, 1936; note also Schelenz, *op. cit.*, p. 407.
5. Conci. *op. cit.*, p. 138. One of Sgobbis' predecessors, the German-born Georg Melich, wrote a "practice" of pharmacy, the *Dispensatorium medicum,* of which the first edition in Italian was published in Venice in 1574, the last in Latin translation in Germany in 1657.
6. The most definitive paper to date on the question of the "first pharmacopeia," and the *Nuovo receptario* particularly, is by Alfons Lutz: Studien über die pharmazeutische Inkunabel 'Nuovo Receptario' von Florenz, Bd. 13 NS, Internatl. Gesellsch. für Geschichte der Pharmazie, Stuttgart, 1958. The title of the Florentine book was later changed to *Ricettario fiorentino,* under which name it was reissued until 1789. Although the first edition is dated 1498, Lutz shows that by our calendar it would have been printed January 21, 1499.
7. The *Antidotarium Bononiense* (1574) in Bologna, the *Pharmacopoea Bergamensis* (1580) in Bergamo, the *Antidotarium Romanum* (1583) in Rome the *Pharmacopoea Veneta* (1618) in Venice, the *Antidotarium Messanense* (1629) in Messina, the *Antidotarium Neopolitanum* (1649) in Naples, the *Pharmacopoea Ferrariensis* (1725) in Ferrara, the *Pharmacopoea Taurinensis* (1736) in Turin, the *Pharmacopoea Sardoa* (1773) in Sardinia, the *Formulario farmaceutico* (1791) in Genoa, and lastly the *Pharmacopoea Parmiensis* (1823) in Parma.

### France

8. Jean de Ruelle (Latinized, Ruellius) published in 1536 his *De natura stirpium.* The Parisian Jacques du Bois (Latinized, Sylvius) issued in 1541 his *Methodus medicamenta componendi . . .*, and in 1548 his *Pharmacopoeae, libri tres,* which was translated into French by André Caille. In 1556 G. Rondelet of Montpellier published his famous *Materia medica*.
9. Cordonnier, E.: Sur le plus ancien traité de pharmacie rédigé en français, *L'enchirid ou manipul des miropoles,* de Michel Dusseau (1561), Janus *5*:471.
10. For example, the pharmacist Thibaut

Lespleigney wrote a versified description of drugs (1537). Joseph du Chesne (Latinized, Quercetanus), physician-in-ordinary to King Henry IV, may be mentioned here as a zealous partisan for Paracelsian ideas, which are reflected in his *Pharmacopoea dogmaticorum restituta* (1603).

11. Titles and dates of some of the outstanding works of this period are the *Pharmacopée royale* of Moise Charas (1676); *Traité de la chymie* (also as *Cours de chymie)* of N. Lefebvre (1660); *Cours de chymie* (1675), *Traité universel des drogues simples,* and *Pharmacopée universelle* (1697) of Nicholas Lémery; *Elémens de pharmacie* of A. Baumé (1762); *Manuel du pharmacien* of J. F. Demachy (1788); and the *Tractatus de materia medica* of E. F. Geoffroy (1741, posthumously).
12. Next was the *Formulaire de Blois* (1634); then the first *Codex medicamentorum seu pharmacopoeia Parisiensis* (1638); followed by the *Pharmacopoeia Lillensis* (1640) and the *Pharmacopoeia Burdigalensis* (1643) and others, the last local standard appearing in Lyons (1778).
13. On the history of the French journals from 1665 to 1860 see especially Guitard, E.-H.: Deux Siècles de presse au service de la pharmacie, Paris, 1913.

    In 1809 the *Bulletin de pharmacie* was founded. In 1814 its title was changed to *Bulletin de pharmacie et des sciences accessoires* (one year later the word "bulletin" was replaced by "journal"). After 1842 it had been known as the *Journal de pharmacie et de chimie.* In 1942, this time-honored scientific voice of French pharmacy merged with the *Bulletin des sciences pharmacologiques* (established in 1899), to form the *Annales pharmaceutiques françaises,* the organ of the Académie de Pharmacie since its establishment in 1946.

    Among well-known French pharmaceutical journals which have been discontinued is *Le répertoire de pharmacie,* founded in 1844. It was merged in 1926 with *L'union pharmaceutique,* a journal issued since 1869 by the French cooperative, *Pharmacie centrale de France,* as an "organe des intérêts scientifiques, pratiques et moraux de la profession." This journal was a victim of the troubled times of 1940. *La pharmacie française,* until discontinued, had a special place as the journal of French students of pharmacy (1896–1970).

**Germany**

14. Here are some of the best known examples of such books: The *Arzneibuch* of a supposed physician, Ortolff von Bayrlandt, is a compilation of Latin medical books available at the beginning of the 15th century. The *Gart der Gesuntheit,* also called the little *Hortus sanitatis,* probably was written by the physician Joh. Wonnecke of Caub and published in 1485. (Schelenz, *op. cit.,* pp. 326 and 327) These books were followed by the so-called large *Hortus sanitatis* (1491), an anonymous comprehensive work in Latin (Fischer, H.: Mittelalterliche Pflanzenkunde, pp. 95–109, Munich, 1929); an enormously influential distillation book by the surgeon Hieronymus Brunschwig, who lived from about 1450 to before 1512 (*ibid.,* pp. 109-113); the herbals of the so-called "fathers of botany": Otto Brunfels (1488–1534), Hieronymus Bock (1498–1554), and Leonhart Fuchs (1501–1566); and also the herbals of Adam Lonicerus (1528–1586) and Johann Theodor, who was called Tabernaemontanus (1520–1590). (Nissen, C.: Die botanische Buchillustration, Geschichte und Bibliographie, Stuttgart, 1951).
15. It was republished with annotations by Joachim Camerarius in 1588, B. Verzasha in 1678, and Ph. Zwinger in 1696. All three were physicians.
16. By 1647 Wecker's book had appeared in nine Latin and two French editions. The book is curious for its special chapter on excrements used as medicaments, which stemmed from primitive medicine and old superstitious beliefs about the nature of disease. Excrementa came into new vogue—reflecting the lack of critical attitudes and of reliable technics for evaluating materia medica—and reached a climax with the book *Dreckapotheke,* published by the physician Paullini in 1696.
17. Schroeder's book was published in Latin in 1641 and translated not only into German but also into English, under the title The Compleat Chymical Dispensatory.
18. Gugel, K. F.: Johann Rudolph Glauber 1604–1670, Leben und Werk, Würzburg, 1955; and Klutz, M.: Die Rezepte in Oswald Crolls 'Basilica Chymica' (1609) und ihre Beziehungen zu Paracelsus, Bd. 14, Veröff. Pharm. gesch. Seminar. . . , Braunschweig, 1974.

19. In 1740 the *Praelectiones chymicae* of the pharmacist Caspar Neumann were published posthumously. This book, based on his own experiments, represented a much more critical spirit than the book of Schroeder and became very popular. In 1777, J. Ch. Wiegleb (1732–1800) published his *Deutsches Apothekerbuch* (German practice of pharmacy). One year later, in 1778, J. F. A. Goettling (1755–1809) published his *Einleitung in die Pharmazeutische Chemie* (introduction to pharmaceutical chemistry). Between 1778 and 1782, K. G. Hagen in Koenigsberg (1749–1829) published his *Lehrbuch der Apothekerkunst* (textbook on the practice of pharmacy), which until the middle of the 19th century was the most-used book in the scientific education of the apprentices. In 1790, Joh. Bartholomaeus Trommsdorff began his long series of textbooks on pharmacy, among them his *Handbuch der pharmazeutischen Warenkunde,* the first textbook on pharmacognosy written in German, and his *Allgemeines pharmazeutisch-chemisches Wörterbuch oder die Apothekerkunst in ihrem gesamten Umfange* (pharmaceutico-chemical dictionary or the art of pharmacy in its entire extent). In 1792, S. Hermbstaedt (1760–1833) published his *Katechismus der Apothekerkunst* (catechism of the art of the apothecary) and, in 1795, J. F. Westrumb (1751–1819) published his *Handbuch der Apothekerkunst fuer Anfaenger* (textbook on pharmacy for beginners).
20. Vershofen, W.: Die Anfänge der chemisch-pharmazeutischen Industrie, Bd. 1, Berlin-Stuttgart, 1949; Bd. 2, Aulendorf, 1952; Bd. 3, Aulendorf, 1958 (beginnings to 1914).
21. Lutz, A.: Das Nürnberger Dispensatorium des Valerius Cordus vom Jahre 1546, die erste amtliche Pharmakopöe, *in* Festschrift z. 75. Geburtstag von Ernst Urban, pp. 107–125, Stuttgart, 1949. Cf., Urdang, G.: The Development of Pharmacopoeias, p. 9, New York, 1950. See also Winkler, L.: Die älteste deutsche Pharmakopoea von Valerius Cordus, Mittenwald, 1934. We cannot expect agreement on "first" pharmacopeias without a definition held in common. A more meaningful focus is that there were *several* kinds of attempts in several places to give force to drug standards, suggesting a recognized need by the mid-16th century going beyond an isolated, local concern.
22. In the 17th century, the series of Augsburg pharmacopeias was particularly notable (for example, 1613, 1640 [for the first time with a Mantissa hermetica], 1684, etc.). The Cologne pharmacopeia appeared in a new edition in 1627, the Nuremberg in 1612 and 1666. *A Facsimile of the First Edition of the Pharmacopoeia Augustana* was published by the State Historical Society of Wisconsin, Madison, 1927.
23. Seven editions followed under the title *Dispensatorium Borusso-Brandenburgicum,* the title signalizing the fact that the duchy of Prussia had been made a kingdom (1701), and the electorate of Brandenburg had been assigned second place in the union of the two states. When the Holy Roman Empire of the German Nation disappeared (1806), additional state pharmacopeias were published in Württemberg (1741, 1750, 1754, 1760, 1771, 1785, 1798), Braunschweig (1777), the Palatinate (1764, 1802), Hessia (1806), and in the hierarchic principalities of Fulda (1787, 1791), Münster (1739) and Würzburg-Bamberg (1778, 1782, 1796). Dispensatories of municipalities were issued in the same period in Bremen (1792), Hamburg (1716, 1768, 1772) and Regensburg (1727, 1737).
24. It was supplemented by a collection of official formulas published in a *Catalogus medicamentorum compositorum.* Up to 1722 all subsequent editions of the *Augustana* remained in force. In 1729, the first Austrian pharmacopeia printed in Austria appeared under the title *Dispensatorium Pharmaceuticum Austriaco-Viennenense,* which lived through six further editions, until 1770. In 1774, there appeared the *Pharmacopoeia Austriaco-provincialis.* The name signified that Austria was but one of the many provinces of the Empire. The last editions of this treatise were issued in 1794 (Latin) and 1795 (German). It was followed in 1812 by the first *Pharmacopoea Austriaca* (Zekert, Otto: Oesterreichische Pharmakopoeen, Pharm. Monatshefte *12*:2, 22, 55, 75, 1931). This name was a reflection of the fact that Austria was no longer one of the constituents of the Holy Roman Empire of the German Nation. It had become a separate unit, one of a new empire embracing all countries belonging to the Austrian line of the princely house of Habsburg, to the exclusion of most of the German states. The ninth edition of the *Pharmacopoea Austriaca* appeared in 1961.

25. Urdang, G.: Zur Geschichte der Metalle in den amtlichen deutschen Arnzeibüchern, pp. 36–38, Mittenwald, 1933.
26. Adlung, A., and Urdang, G.: *op. cit.*, pp. 308, 309, 331, 332.
27. According to R. Folch y Andreu, the situation in Spain was the reverse. In Spain the galenical pharmacopoeias were prepared by pharmacists who, when chemicals for internal use were introduced into the official books, were replaced by physicians. (Die praehispanischen offizinellen pharmakopoeen, in: Die Vorträge der Hauptversammlung der Gesellschaft für geschichte der Pharmazie in Basel, 1934, pp. 212–223, Mittenwald, 1934.)
28. Adlung, A., and Urdang, G.: *op. cit.*, pp. 333, 334.
29. Schneider, W.: Vorgeschichte der ersten Pharmacopoea Germanica, Pharm. Ztg. *104*:495, 519, 1085, 1959. An excellent book that considers German drug standardization within a broad framework is, Hickel E.: Arzneimittel-Standardisierung im 19. Jahrhundert in den Pharmakopöen Deutschlands, Frankreichs, Grossbritanniens und der Vereinigten Staaten von Amerika, Stuttgart, 1973.
30. In regard to the development of pharmaceutical journalism in Germany, see Adlung, A., and Urdang, G.: *op. cit.*, pp. 259–271.
31. Among them was *Gehlen-Buchner's Repertorium für die Pharmacie* (1815). Subject to frequent changes were the *Annalen der Pharmacie* (which first appeared in 1832), combining Haenle-Geiger's *Magazin für Pharmacie* (founded in 1823) with the *Archiv des Apothekervereins im noerdlichen Teutschland* (founded in 1822; first issued two years previously as *Pharmaceutische Monatshefte).* In 1834 *Trommsdorff's Journal* merged with the *Annalen.* However, the *Archiv* regained its independence under the title *Archiv der Pharmacie* (1835). Woehler, in his capacity as one of the editors, suggested that the original title *Annalen der Pharmacie* be changed to *Annalen für Chemie und Pharmacie.* After the death of Liebig the word pharmacy was dropped. Since 1874 this lost child of pharmacy has borne the title *Justus Liebig's Annalen der Chemie.* (Schneider, W.: Justus von Liebig und das *Archiv der Pharmazie,* Arch. Pharm. *286*:165, 1955.)
32. Schneider, W.: 100 Jahre Pharmazeutische Zentralhalle, Pharm. Zentralhalle *98*:330, 347, 1959.
33. ———: 100 Jahre Deutsche Apotheker-Zeitung. Vom Pharmaceutischen Wochenblatt aus Württemberg über die Süddeutsche Apotheker-Zeitung zur Deutschen Apotheker-Zeitung, D. Apoth. Ztg. *101*:761, 1961.
34. After 1933 the *Apotheker-Zeitung* became known as the *Standeszeitung Deutscher Apotheker* and after 1934 as *Deutsche Apotheker-Zeitung.* Having disappeared at the end of the war (1945), it revived in 1949, to be merged (1950) with the *Süddeutsche Apotheker-Zeitung.* The *Jahresbericht der Pharmazie,* published annually since 1841, has been issued since 1906 by the Apothekerverein.

**Great Britain**

35. Anon.: Side-lights on English pharmacy 1550–1650, Chem. & Drugg. *120*:720, 1934; and Singer, C.: Sketches in the history of English medicine, Chem. & Drugg. *112*:800, 1930.
36. Thompson: *op. cit.,* p. 150.
37. Bell and Redwood: *op. cit.,* p. 14.
38. Kirby, W.: A quack of the seventeenth century, Pharm. J. *84*:255, 1910.
39. Kremers, E.: William Lewis, J.A.Ph.A. *20*:1204, 1931; and, for a history and bibliography of Lewis' dispensatory (et al.), see Cowen, D. L.: The Edinburgh dispensatories, Papers Bibliog. Soc. Amer. *45*:85–96, 1951.
40. Cowen, D. L.: The Spread and Influence of British Pharmacopoeial Literature; an Historical and Bibliographic Study, Bd. 41, Veröff. Internatl. Gesell. Gesch. Pharm., Stuttgart, 1974.
41. Urdang, G.: Pharmacopoeia Londinensis of 1618, Madison, Wis., 1944, pp. 24, 77–81.
42. *Ibid.*: pp. 36, 54; Wootton: *op. cit.,* 2, pp. 2–4, 61–64. Wootton speaks of 1028 simples in the second issue of the London Pharmacopoeia of 1618. He takes this number from Munk (The Rolls of the Royal College of Physicians of London, 1878, 3, p. 376), who counted only the individual paragraphs and not the different drugs sometimes listed in the same paragraph; as a result, his numbers are too low.
43. Urdang, G.: *op. cit.,* pp. 61–63.

44. Wootton: *op. cit.*, 2, pp. 64–69. Editions of the London Pharmacopoeia were published in 1617, 1650, 1677, 1721, 1746, 1788, 1809, 1824, 1836 and 1851.
45. An excellent paper, with definitive bibliographic information, is by Cowen, David L.: The Edinburgh pharmacopoeia, Medical History *1*:123, 340, 1957; see also his guide: Library Holdings of the Edinburgh Pharmacopoeia (mimeographed) Rutgers University, 1957, 14 pp., surveying libraries in twelve countries. Cowen identifies the twelve editions as published in 1699, 1722, 1735, 1744, 1756, 1774, 1783, 1792, 1803, 1817, 1839, 1841.
46. Cowen: Spread and Influence, pp. 15 f. and 18.
47. Bell and Redwood: *op. cit.*, p. 329.
48. A volume of *Additions* was issued in 1874. New versions were published in 1885 (with an *Addendum* in 1890) and in 1898. In 1900 and thereafter, there appeared an *Indian and Colonial Addendum* which was incorporated into the *Pharmacopoeia* of 1914. The *Pharmacopoeia* issued in 1932 showed for the first time the influence of a closer cooperation with the Committee on Revision for the *United States Pharmacopoeia.* Addenda were published in 1936, 1940, 1941 (two), 1942, 1943 and 1945.
49. Cowen, D. L.: The Edinburgh pharmacopoeia, Med. Hist. *1*:130, 1957, and Barrett: *op. cit.*, p. 157, 168.
50. Bell and Redwood: *op. cit.*, p. 208.
51. British Pharmacopoeia, London, 1973, pp. vii, xiii.
52. Bell and Redwood: *op. cit.*, p. 329; see also, Urdang G., and Sonnedecker G.: "Authoritative English language drug compendia supplementing pharmacopoeias," Food Drug Cosmetic Law J. *8*:485, 1953.
53. Among these were *The Chemist* (1804–1858); *The Chemical Gazette* (f. 1842), which merged with *The Chemical News* in 1859; *The Annals of Chemistry and Practical Pharmacy* (1842–1843); *The Pharmaceutical Times* (1846–1849); *Annals of Pharmacy and practical Chemistry* (1852–1854) (Bayles, H.: Six journals for chemists, Chem. & Drugg. *146*:244, 1944). Typical of the erratic evolution that often makes journal bibliography perplexing (and suggestive of changes occurring on a broader historical stage) is the journal founded in 1884 as the *British and Colonial Druggist,* which became the *British and Colonial Pharmacist* (1915), then the *British and Overseas Pharmacist* (1952), next broadening its scope to *British and Overseas Pharmacy and Medicine* (1958), moving further into medicine as the *Chemotherapy Review* (1960), then appearing (since 1961) as the *Medical Observer and Chemotherapy Review.*
54. Chem. & Drugg. *75*:136, 1909. See also the *Chem. & Drugg. Centenary Number, 1859–1959;* and (concerning the PSGB's *Journal)* Brocklehurst, E. A.: The Society's publishing activities, *Pharm. J. 200*:91–95, 1968. Another monthly (which included useful historical features) was the *Pharmacy Digest* (titled *The Alchemist* 1920–1958), which ceased publication in 1966.

**U.S.A.**

55. Meyer, M. M.: The Pharmaceutical Journals in the United states (unpublished M. Sc. thesis, U. Wis.), p. 10, Madison, 1934.
56. Among regional journals the old *Pacific Drug Review* (1888-1964, thereafter (called *Western Pharmacy*, 1961–1964) and the *North Western Druggist* (f. 1892) showed particular strength; also serving the far West were the *Rocky Mountain Druggist* (f. 1888) and *West Coast Druggist* (f. 1928, combining *Stirring Rod,* f. 1906, and the *California Retail Drug Journal*, f. 1915). The Middle West has been similarly served by *Midwestern Druggist* (f. 1925) and the *Central Pharmaceutical Journal* (f. 1947); the South is served by the *Southern Pharmaceutical Journal* (f. 1908) and the *Southeastern Drug Journal* (f. 1926); and in the East *The Apothecary* (founded, 1888, as *The New England Druggist*) and the *Mid-Atlantic Apothecary* (replacing, 1953, the *Mid-Atlantic Pharmacist*, f. 1951).
57. Hoffmann, F.: A century of American pharmaceutical literature, Amer. Drugg. & Pharm. Rec. *36*:164, 165, 1900.
58. Kassner, H. C.: How we learn, Am. Drugg. *88*:280, 1933.
59. It was edited by Hoffmann and Edward Kremers until 1900; and from 1901 to 1909, by Kremers. In 1909 it was consolidated with the *Midland Druggist,* remaining alive under the title *Midland Druggist and Pharmaceutical Review* until 1926. At this time the title was changed to *Interstate Journal*. The *Pharmaceu-*

*tical Review* became the cradle of another monthly, the *Pharmaceutical Archives,* (6 vols., 1898–1903; revived 1936–1945), which possibly can be considered the first American pharmacy periodical mainly devoted to research, under the sponsorship and editorship of Edward Kremers.

60. There existed in 1875 a *Deutsch-Amerikanische pharmaceutische Zeitung,* for pharmacists and druggists as well as for physicians of German origin, published in Belleville, Ill. In New York the *Apotheker-Zeitung* appeared from 1880 to 1933 (beginning 1895, it was the official organ of the New York German Apothecaries Society). From 1885 to 1897 this Society published the *Monatsblatt des New Yorker deutschen Apothekervereins,* which was revived in 1934. Other foreign language publications, though short-lived, were the *Gaceta medico-farmacéutica de Nueva York* (1892–1898); *Monitor medico-farmacéutico* (1883); *Revista americana de farmacia* (1895–1921) (Meyer, M.: *op. cit.,* p. 14). *Pharmacy International* (in English, f. 1947), *El Farmacéutico* (in Spanish, f. 1925) and *La Farmacia Moderna* (in Spanish, f. 1945) were examples of private American journals designed to serve pharmacy abroad and promote international trade, rather than serve a resident ethnic group.
61. *The Philadelphia Druggist and Chemist,* founded in 1878, changed its name a year later to the *Monthly Review of Medicine and Pharmacy* (1879–1882) and was followed in 1895 by a *Monthly Retrospect of Medicine and Pharmacy,* also published in Philadelphia (1895–1902). In New York a journal with the title *Physician and Pharmaceutist* (from 1871 on, *Pharmacist*) was published from 1868—in 1879 changing its name to *Physician and Pharmacist and the Bulletin of the Medical-Legal Society;* a few months later, dropping the word *Pharmacist,* it was continued as the *Physician and Bulletin of the Medico-Legal Society.*
62. Kassner, H.: *op. cit.,* p. 280.
63. These publications served those engaged in making and marketing drugs. The firms, in turn, produced a periodical literature of "house organs" designed to interest practicing pharmacists, hence provide a vehicle for promoting the company concerned. Perhaps the first such house organ of substance was the vigorous *New Idea* published (1879–1924) by Frederick Stearns and Company of Detroit (a firm absorbed by Winthrop). Following Stearns by a year, Meyer Brothers and Company of St. Louis transformed their price list into a house organ (1880), the *St. Louis Drug Market Reporter,* surviving until 1964 as the *Meyer Druggist.* Meanwhile, house organs have appeared in almost every type and format of pharmaceutical periodical known, then tended to die out during the course of the present century under the impact of rising publishing costs and increasing competition among pharmacy journals of free circulation (i.e., supported by advertising rather than paid subscriptions). To discuss them in a text lacking space even to mention some important independent and association journals, would go too far; some additional details may be found in the 2nd edition, pp. 397–399.
64. Cowen, D. L.: The Boston editions of Nicholas Culpeper, J. Hist. Med. *11*:156–165, 1956.
65. For bibliographic clarification, see Cowen, D. L.: America's Pre-pharmacopoeial Literature, pp. 20 f.
66. The editions of King's *American Dispensatory* that represent actual revisions are dated 1864, 1870, 1889 and 1900.

# Index

Numbers in *italics* indicate illustrations; the letter "t" after a number indicates a table. The Glossary (Appendix 7), containing notes on names and terms significant in pharmaceutical history, is not included in the Index.